LHRH and Its Analogs

Contraceptive and Therapeutic Applications

Advances in Reproductive Health Care
Series Editor: **E. S. E. Hafez**

LHRH and Its Analogs: Contraception and Therapeutic Applications
Edited by B. H. Vickery, J. J. Nestor Jr. and E. S. E. Hafez

Spontaneous Abortion
Edited by E. S. E. Hafez

Voluntary Termination of Pregnancy
Edited by E. S. E. Hafez

Biomedical Aspects of IUDs
Edited by H. Hasson, W. A. A. van Os and E. S. E. Hafez

Prostaglandins and Fertility Regulation
Edited by M. Toppozada, M. Bygdeman and E. S. E. Hafez

Male Fertility and Its Regulation
Edited by T. Lobl and E. S. E. Hafez

Advances in Reproductive Health Care

LHRH and Its Analogs

Contraceptive and Therapeutic Applications

Editors

B. H. Vickery
J. J. Nestor Jr.
and E. S. E. Hafez

MTP PRESS LIMITED
a member of the KLUWER ACADEMIC PUBLISHERS GROUP
LANCASTER / BOSTON / THE HAGUE / DORDRECHT

Published in the UK and Europe by
MTP Press Limited
Falcon House
Lancaster, England

British Library Cataloguing in Publication Data

LHRH and its analogs.—(Advances in reproductive health care;)
1. Generative organs—Diseases—Chemotherapy
2. Luteinizing hormone releasing hormone—Therapeutic use
I. Vickery, B. H. II. Nestor, J. J.
III. Hafez, E. S. E. IV. Series
616.6′5061 RC877

ISBN 0–85200–732–9

Series ISBN 0–85200–781–7

Published in the USA by
MTP Press
A division of Kluwer Boston Inc
190 Old Derby Street
Hingham, MA 02043, USA

Library of Congress Cataloging in Publication Data

Main entry under title:

LHRH and its analogs.

(Advances in reproductive health care;)
Bibliography: p.
Includes index.
1. Luteinizing hormone releasing hormone—Agonists —Congresses. 2. Luteinizing hormone releasing hormone—Antagonists—Congresses. 3. Luteinizing hormone releasing hormone—Physiological effect—Congresses. 4. Contraceptive drugs—Congresses. I. Vickery, B. H. (Brian H.), 1941– . II. Nestor, J. J. (John J.), 1945– . III. Hafez, E. S. E., 1922– . IV. Series. V. Title: L.H.R.H. and its analogs.
RG137.6.L78L46 1984 612.6 84–4532

ISBN 0–85200–732–9

Typeset by Macmillan India Ltd, Bangalore.
Printed by Butler and Tanner Ltd, Frome and London

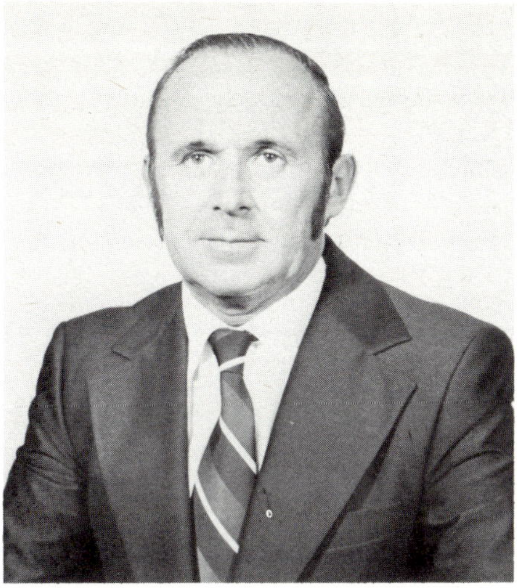

Andrew V. Schally

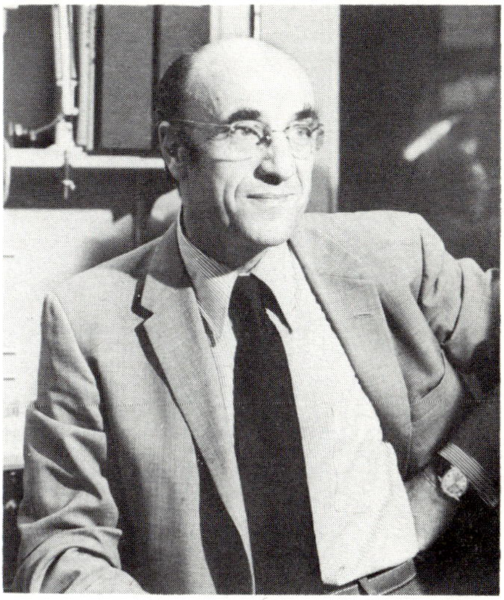

Roger Guillemin

DEDICATION

The present advanced status of our knowledge of the mechanism of interaction of the hypothalamus and adenohypophysis rests on the solid foundation laid down by many workers over the past four decades. Foremost amongst these contributions have been the isolation, structure determination and syntheses of hypothalamic releasing factors in the laboratories of Drs Andrew V. Schally and Roger Guillemin. These contributions were recognized in 1977 by the award of the Nobel Prize in Chemistry to Dr Guillemin and Dr Schally.

'For their discoveries concerning the peptide hormone production of the brain'.

It is with great pleasure that we dedicate this volume to Drs Andrew Schally and Roger Guillemin and their co-workers.

B. H. Vickery
J. J. Nestor Jr.
E. S. E. Hafez

Contents

List of Contributors

Fatima Bint Akhtar
Department of Experimental Endocrinology
University Women's Hospital
Domagkstrasse 11
D-4400 Munster, F. R. Germany

A. Nancye Alexander
Rabin Associate

Shabir Anik
Staff Researcher
Institute of Pharmaceutical Sciences
Syntex Research R1-140
3401 Hillview Avenue
Palo Alto, CA 94304 USA

Ricardo H. Asch
Jane & Roland Blumberg
Professor of Obstetrics & Gynecology
Department of Obstetrics & Gynecology
University of Texas Health Science Center
7703 Floyd Curl Drive
San Antonio, TX 78284 USA

Thomas M. Badger
Assistant Professor
Department of Obstetrics & Gynecology
Vincent Research Laboratories
Massachusetts General Hospital
Boston, MA 02114 USA

J. P. Balmaceda
Assistant Professor
Department of Obstetrics and Gynecology
Univ. Texas Health Science Centre
7703 Floyd Curl Drive
San Antonio, TX 73230 USA

C. Wayne Bardin
Director, Center for Biomedical Research
The Population Council
Rockefeller University
York Avenue & 66th Street
New York, NY 10021 USA

Jeffrey L. Barron
Department of Chemical Pathology
University of Cape Town Medical School
Observatory 7925
Cape Town, South Africa

Alain Bélanger
Molecular Endocrinology Laboratory
Le Centre Hospitalier de l'Universite Laval
2705 Lauvier Boulevard
Quebec G1V 4G2 Canada

Christer Bergquist
Section for Reproductive Endocrinology and Infertility
Department of Obstetrics and Gynaecology
University Hospital
S-751 85 Uppsala
Sweden

Mario Borghi
Postdoctoral Fellow
Department of Obstetrics and Gynecology
Univ. Texas Health Science Centre
7703 Floyd Curl Drive
San Antonio, TX 73230 USA

William J. Bremner
Chief, Endocrine Section
Division of Endocrinology/ Metabolism
University of Washington
Medical Center
Veterans Administration Hospital
4435 Beacon Avenue South
Seattle, WA 98108 USA

Frank A. Carone
Morrison Professor and Deputy Chairman of Pathology
Northwestern University Medical School
303 E. Chicago Avenue
Chicago, IL 60611 USA

Melvin D. Chaplin
Principal Scientist
Institute of Pharmacology & Metabolism
Syntex Research A3-146
3401 Hillview Avenue
Palo Alto, CA 94304 USA

Richard N. Clayton
M.R.C. Senior Clinical Research Fellow & Honorary Consultant Physician
Department of Medicine
University of Birmingham
Edgbaston
Birmingham, B15 2TH UK

Florence Comite
Clinical Center
Developmental Endocrinology Branch
NICHD
NIH Bldg. 10, Room 10B09
Bethesda, MD 20205 USA

Alan Corbin
Associate Director
Biological Research (Endocrinology)
Wyeth Laboratories
P.O. Box 8299
Philadelphia, PA 19101 USA

David H. Coy
Research Professor
Department of Medicine
Tulane University School of Medicine
1430 Tulane Avenue
New Orleans, LA 70112 USA

Laurence W. Crim
Memorial University of Newfoundland
Marine Sciences Research Laboratory
St. John's Newfoundland
Canada A1C 5S7

William F. Crowley
Assistant Professor of Medicine
Endocrinology & Metabolism
Vincent Research Laboratories
Massachusetts General Hospital
Boston, MA 02114 USA

Gordon B. Cutler
Developmental Endocrinology Branch
National Institute of Child Health and Human Development
National Institutes of Health
Building 10, Room 10B09
Bethesda, MD 20205
USA

Laurence M. Demers
Pathology
The Milton S. Hershey Medical Center
P.O. Box 850
Hershey, PA 17033
USA

Zvi Dïckerman
Sackler School of Medicine
Tel Aviv University
Israel

Gregory C. Doelle
Fellow, Department of Medicine
Division of Endocrinology
School of Medicine
Vanderbilt University
Nashville, TN 37232 USA

Maria Dufau
Department of Health and Human Service
National Institutes of Health
Bethesda, MD 20205
USA

Richard A. Edgren
Director, Scientific Affairs
Syntex Labs L-2001
3401 Hillview Avenue
Palo Alto, CA 94304 USA

Robert M. Evans
Doelle associate

Nacia Faure
Research Associate
Laval University
Hospital St. Francors D'Assize
10 Rue de l'Espinay
Quebec G1L 3L5 Canada

Atilla T. A. Fazekas
Medical Department
Hoechst Canada Inc.
4045 Cote Vertu
Montreal, Canada, H4R1R6

George Flouret
Professor
Department of Physiology
Northwestern University Medical School
303 E. Chicago Avenue
Chicago, IL 60611 USA

Hamish M. Fraser
MRC Reproductive Biology Unit
Centre for Reproductive Biology
37 Chalmers Street
Edinburgh EH3 9EW
Scotland

E. C. Griffiths
Physiology Department
University of Manchester
Stopford Building
Manchester M13 9PT UK

E. S. E. Hafez
Reproductive Health Center
Medical University of South Carolina
Department of Physiology
171 Ashley
Charleston, SC 29455 USA

Do Won Hahn
Section Head
Reproductive Research Section
Ortho Pharmaceutical Corporation
Route 202
Raritan, NJ 08869 USA

Joachim Happ
Professor
Department of Radiology
Division of Nuclear Medicine
University of Frankfurt on Main
Theodore Stern-Kai 7
6000 Frankfurt/Main
West Germany

Wolfgang Hardt
Assistant Professor
Department of Obstetrics & Gynecology
Free University of Berlin
Universitats-Frauenklinik
Charlottenburg
Pulstrasse 4-14
1000 Berlin-19, West Germany

Michael J. K. Harper
Professor
Department of Obstetrics & Gynecology and Department of Physiology
University of Texas Health Science Center
770 Floyd Curl Drive
San Antonio, TX 78284 USA

Harold A. Harvey
Associate Professor of Medicine
Division of Oncology
The Milton S. Hershey Medical Center
The Pennsylvania State University
Hershey, PA 17033 USA

David Heber
Associate Director and Assistant Professor of Medicine
G.C.R.C.
Harbor-UCLA Medical Center
1000 W. Carson
Torrance, CA 90509 USA

Milan Henzl
Clinical Medicine
Syntex Research
3401 Hillview Avenue
Palo Alto, CA 94304
USA

Teresa L. Ho
Staff Researcher
Institute of Bio-Organic Chemistry
Syntex Research R6-201
3401 Hillview Avenue
Palo Alto, CA 94304 USA

Andrew R. Hoffman
Department of Medicine
Division of Endocrinology
Stanford University Medical Center
Stanford, CA 94305 USA

Aaron J. Hsueh
Associate Pofessor
Research Center
School of Medicine
Department of Reproductive Medicine M-025
University of California – San Diego
La Jolla, CA 92093 USA

Phillip B. C. Jones
A. Hsueh Associate

Stanley Kushinsky
Senior Scientist
Head, Department of Analytical and Metabolic Chemistry
Institute of Pharmacology & Metabolism
Syntex Research A3-165
3401 Hillview Avenue
Palo Alto, CA 94304 USA

Fernand Labrie
Professor
Department of Molecular Endocrinology and Medicine
Le Centre Hospitalier de l'Universite Laval
2705 Laurier Boulevard
Ste-Foy, Quebec PQ
G1V 4G2 Canada

Zvi Laron
Institute of Pediatric and Adolescent Endocrinology
The Beilinson Medical Center
Petah Tikva
Israel

Andre Lemay
Professor Adjoint
Departement d'obstetrique et gynecologie
Universite Laval
Endocrinologie de la Reproduction
Hopital Saint-Francois d'Assise
10, Rue de l'Espinay
Quebec P.Q.
Canada GIL 3L5

A. Lipton
Harvey Associate

D. Lynn Loriaux
Developmental Endocrinology Branch
National Institute of Child Health and Human Development
National Institutes of Health
Building 10, Room 10B09
Bethesda, MD 20205 USA

Devorah Max
Assistant Director
Clinical Research
Abbott Laboratories
North Chicago, IL 60064 USA

John L. McGuire
Vice President of Basic Sciences
Research and Development
Ortho Pharmaceutical Corportion
Route 202
Raritan, NJ 08869 USA

Georgia I. McRae
Staff Researcher
Department of Physiology
Institute of Biological Sciences
Syntex Research R2-101
3401 Hillview Avenue
Palo Alto, CA 94304 USA

Robert P. Millar
Department of Chemical Pathology
University of Cape Town Medical School
Observatory 7925
Cape Town, South Africa

Mary J. Nekola
Research Associate Professor
Department of Medicine
Tulane University School of Medicine
1430 Tulane Avenue
New Orleans, LA 70112 USA

Clinton Nerenberg
Staff Researcher
Department of Analytical and Metabolic Chemistry
Institute of Pharmacology and Metabolism
Syntex Research A3-165
3401 Hillview Avenue
Palo Alto, CA 94304 USA

John J. Nestor
Head, Department of Peptide Research
Institute of Bio-organic Chemistry
Syntex Research R6-201
3401 Hillview Avenue
Palo Alto, CA 94304 USA

Eberhard Nieschlag
Max Planck Clinical Research Unit for Reproductive Medicine
University Women's Hospital
Steinfurter Strasse 107
D-4400 Munster, F.R. Germany

Sven J. Nillius
University Hospital
Department of Obstetrics & Gynecology
S-75014 Uppsala 14 Sweden

Marilyn H. Perrin
Peptide Biology Laboratory
The Salk Institute
10010 North Torrey Pines Road
La Jolla, CA 92037 USA

Darryl R. Peterson
Associate Professor of Physiology
Department of Basic Sciences
University of Illinois College of Medicine at Peoria
P.O. Box 1649
Peoria, IL 61656 USA

Rachel M. Popkin
H. Fraser Associate

John Porter
Peptide Biology Laboratory
The Salk Institute
10010 North Torrey Pines Road
La Jolla, CA 92037 USA

Ruth Prager-Lewin
Institute of Pediatric and
Adolescent Endocrinology
Beilinson Medical Center
Petah Tikva
Israel

David Rabin
Professor
Division of Endocrinology
Department of Medicine
Vanderbilt University Medical School
Nashville, TN 37232 USA

Catherine Rivier
Peptide Biology Laboratory
The Salk Institute
10010 North Torrey Pines Road
La Jolla, CA 92037 USA

Jean Rivier
Associate Research Professor
The Salk Institute
P.O. Box 85800
San Diego, CA 92138 USA

Lynda M. Sanders
Staff Researcher
Institute of Pharmaceutical Sciences
Syntex Research R1-140
3401 Hillview Avenue
Palo Alto, CA 94304 USA

Richard Santen
Division of Endocrinology
Milton S. Hershey Medical Center
Pennsylvania State University
Hershey, PA 17036 USA

Andrew V. Schally
Professor & Chairman
Department of Medicine
School of Medicine
Tulane University
1430 Tulane Avenue
New Orleans, LA 70112 USA

Bruce D. Schanbacher
U.S. Meat Animal Research Center
SEA-AR
U.S. Department of Agriculture
Clay Center P.O. Box 166
Nebraska 68933 USA

Manfred Schmidt-Gollwitzer
Professor, Department of Obstetrics & Gynecology
Free University of Berlin
Universitats-Frauenklinik
Charlottenburg
Pulstrasse 4-14
1000 Berlin-19, West Germany

Richard M. Sharpe
H. Fraser associate

Joseph A. Smith
Assistant Professor of Surgery
Division of Urology
University of Utah Medical Center
50 N. Medical Drive
Salt Lake City, Utah 84132 USA

Mary Alie Stetler-Stevenson
Research Associate
Department of Physiology
Northwestern University Medical School
303 E. Chicago Avenue
Chicago, IL 60611 USA

Kalyan Sundaram
Scientist
The Population Council
Center for Biomedical Research
1230 York Avenue
New York, N.Y. 10021 USA

Ronald S. Swerdloff
Professor and Chief
Division of Endocrinology
Department of Medicine
Harbor-UCLA Medical Center
UCLA School of Medicine
1000 W. Carson Street
Torrance, CA 90509 USA

Ram M. Tahilramani
Chemist
Institute of Bio-Organic Chemistry
Syntex Research RS-201
3401 Hillview Avenue
Palo Alto, CA 94304 USA

George Tolis
Director, Endocrine Division
Hippokrateion Hospital,
Athens, Greece

G. Tsalacopoulos
Obstetrics and Gynaecology
University of Cape Town Medical School
Observatory, 7925 Cape Town,
South Africa

Wylie Vale
Research Professor
Peptide Biology Laboratory
The Salk Institute
P.O. Box 85800
San Diego, CA 92138 USA

Brian H. Vickery
Senior Scientist
Head, Department of Physiology
Institute of Biological Sciences
Syntex Research R2-101
3401 Hillview Avenue
Palo Alto, CA 94304 USA

Barry Warner
Instructor
Department of Medicine
Milton S. Hershey Medical Center
Penn State University
Hershey, PA 17033 USA

E. Jean Wickings
Department of Experimental Endocrinology
University Women's Hospital
Domagkstrasse 11
D-4400 Munster, F.R. Germany

Preface

A. CORBIN

Investigations on LHRH and its analogs have just completed their first decade. We have witnessed a veritable explosion of chemical, physiologic and pharmacologic data on this hypothalamic peptide and the approximately 1500 agonist and antagonist analogs that have been synthesized. In order to track this expanding field, I was asked to organize an international symposium on basic and clinical aspects of LHRH analogs as part of the Reproductive Health Care: CDS Symposium held in Maui, Hawaii, in October 1982. This meeting brought together a number of the leading investigators in the field. Much new state-of-the-art information was presented which I and my colleagues felt deserved a wider audience. Drs Vickery, Nestor, and Hafez consented to undertake this task.

Upon review of the literature, it was apparent that there was no recent text which fully covered the breadth of developments in the field. Accordingly, the editors decided to use the symposium as a nucleus on which to build a singular, comprehensive state-of-the-art analysis of this rapidly growing discipline, and the application of such knowledge to reproductive medicine. As exemplified by the various areas of expertise provided by the individual contributors, it becomes obvious that the scope of the subject matter, while relating solely to a well-defined chemical class (LHRH analogs) and a circumscribed physiologic and pharmacologic entity (reproduction), has expanded enormously. Thus, the basic animal studies on these molecules, and our perception of their biologic properties, have guided us from the conceptive and contraceptive realm into novel practical and therapeutic clinical and veterinary applications, including the potential management of an array of reproductive pathologies.

Introduction

J. J. NESTOR Jr. and B. H. VICKERY

The suggestion that the anterior pituitary was controlled by the central nervous system through an array of stimulatory and inhibitory signals of a chemical nature (Harris, 1955) received support from the demonstration that hypothalamic extracts (McCann *et al.*, 1960; Igarashi and McCann, 1964) contained a substance that could directly release luteinizing hormone (LH) and follicle stimulating hormone (FSH) from pituitary gonadotropes. The final proof of this concept came with the isolation and chemical synthesis of several of these factors (Schally *et al.*, 1979). It is now clear that these factors are secreted from neural elements of the mediobasal hypothalamus and that these releasing or inhibiting factors travel to the anterior pituitary by means of the hypothalamo-hypophysial portal system (Figure 1).

The secretion of LH and FSH was thought to be under the control of separate releasing factors but the decapeptide LH/FSH-releasing hormone, <Glu-His-Trp-Ser-Tyr-Gly-Leu-Arg-Pro-Gly-NH_2 (LHRH), was shown to stimulate the release of both gonadotropins (Schally *et al.*, 1971). In the anterior pituitary, LHRH binds to specific membrane bound receptors on the gonadotropes which are stimulated to secrete and synthesize LH and FSH (Chapter 4). The determination of the structure of this releasing hormone from porcine (Matsuo *et al.*, 1971*a*) and ovine (Burgus *et al.*, 1972) sources and its chemical synthesis (Matsuo *et al.*, 1971*b*) have permitted the explosion of work on its chemistry, pharmacology and clinical applications which forms the basis of this book. The lengthy scientific struggle which clarified the role of the brain in the control of the anterior pituitary gland was recognized by the award of the Nobel Prize in Medicine in 1977 to Roger Guillemin and Andrew Schally.

LHRH is a decapeptide with blocked N- and C-termini. It is resistant to exopeptidase cleavage but is rapidly cleared *in vivo* (Bennett and McMartin, 1979) by endopeptidases and glomerular filtration ($T_{\frac{1}{2}} \sim 5$ min). Proteolytic cleavage was demonstrated at the < Glu–His, Trp–Ser, Tyr–Gly, and Pro–Gly bonds when various tissue homogenates were used, but the significance of these enzymes during metabolism is unclear. Well over 1000 analogs have been synthesized and include both agonists (Chapters 1 and 3) and antagonists (Chapters 2, 3, 10) with high potency and prolonged duration of action (see Chapters 1 and 10 for reviews). The most potent

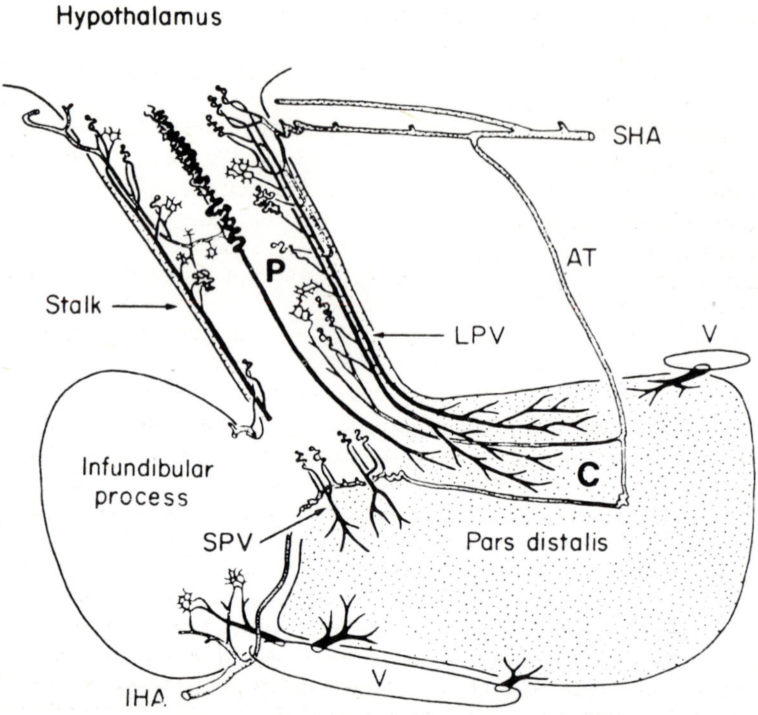

Figure 1 Diagram of relationship between the superior hypophysial artery (SHA), primary capillary bed (P) in the hypothalamus, long portal vessels (LPV) connecting P and the anterior pituitary gland, and the target cells (C) in the anterior pituitary gland. (Reprinted, by permission, from Adams, J. H., Daniel, P. M. and Prichard, M. M. L. (1965). *Neuroendocrinology,* **1,** 193–213.)

analogs are those which are resistant to endopeptidase cleavage and have receptor binding affinities higher than that of LHRH itself.

The structure of the LHRH is identical in the mammalian species studied but the LH/FSH-releasing hormones from chickens and fish are now known to differ from mammalian LHRH (Chapter 29). The ability of LHRH to control the fertility cycle and gonadal steroid production in domestic animals (Chapter 30) and fish (Chapter 29) are reviewed.

It was initially forecast that LHRH would be used for treatment of infertility and that competitive antagonists would comprise a new class of non-steroidal contraceptives. Results with LHRH were disappointing because a short period of pituitary stimulation was followed by a prolonged refractory state. More potent agonists were tried but they resulted in a more rapid suppression of pituitary LH secretion. It was then shown that LHRH must be administered in a pulsatile fashion to mimic the bursts of LHRH which normally occur at ~ 60 min intervals (Chapter 22). Continuous administration of LHRH or treatment with long acting agonists results in a paradoxical desensitization of pituitary gonadotropes by receptor down regulation and results in suppression of fertility.

The paradoxical antifertility effects of prolonged treatment with LHRH or agonistic analogs can be demonstrated at the receptor level by a sharp drop in the number of available receptors (Chapter 4). Direct gonadal effects of LHRH analogs have been documented in rats but not in any other species. For example, in cultured rat Leydig cells, the refractory state results in a blockade of testicular steroidogenesis through inhibition of the enzymes 17α-hydroxylase and 17,20 desmolase (Chapter 13). In female rats, LHRH inhibits hormone-stimulated ovarian steroidogenesis and gonadotropin receptor formation. From the most recent studies the parallelism of effects of LHRH analogs at the pituitary and gonad is almost complete. It has been demonstrated that the short term effects (3 or less hours) of agonists at the gonad are stimulatory of steroidogenesis, whereas the longer term exposure is inhibitory (Chapters 13 and 14). The significance of the short term effects to a paracrine role for an intragonadal LHRH-like material is still to be elucidated.

The paradoxical gonadal suppressive effects of LHRH agonists are the basis for most of the applications envisioned for these analogs (Table 1, sections 2, 3, 4). These applications may be broadly outlined as follows: in females – contraception, endometriosis, breast cancer, precocious puberty; in males – contraception, benign prostatic hypertrophy (BPH), prostatic cancer, precocious puberty. Profertility applications for LHRH in men such as for treatment of cryptorchidism and hypogonadotropic hypogonadism are also important. Chapters covering each of these topics (except endometriosis and

Table 1 Indications for LHRH analogs

1 *Profertility*
- (a) Through stimulation
  - Induction of puberty
  - Reversal of secondary hypogonadism
  - Treatment of cryptorchidism
- (b) Through suppression
  - Endometriosis
  - Protection against sterilization from chemotherapy

2 *Antifertility*
- Ovulation inhibition
- Luteolysis
- Inhibition of spermatogenesis

3 *Gonadal endocrinopathies*
- Precocious puberty (true, GH-induced)
- Short stature
- Prostatic cancer
- Breast cancer
- BPH
- Hirsutism

4 *Other*
- Gestational tumors
- Non-gestational tumors

BPH) are included in this book. An important application for LHRH and LHRH agonists is in the differential diagnosis of gonadal insufficiency. The LHRH challenge test (Chapter 28) is an important tool in the appropriate treatment of such disorders.

Very large increases in dosage are needed for LHRH analogs to be effective after oral administration (1000–10 000-fold). Consequently most studies have been performed by subcutaneous or nasal administration. The latter route requires a 20–100-fold increase in dosage relative to the former. The range of dosage routes for LHRH and its analogs is discussed and a new approach

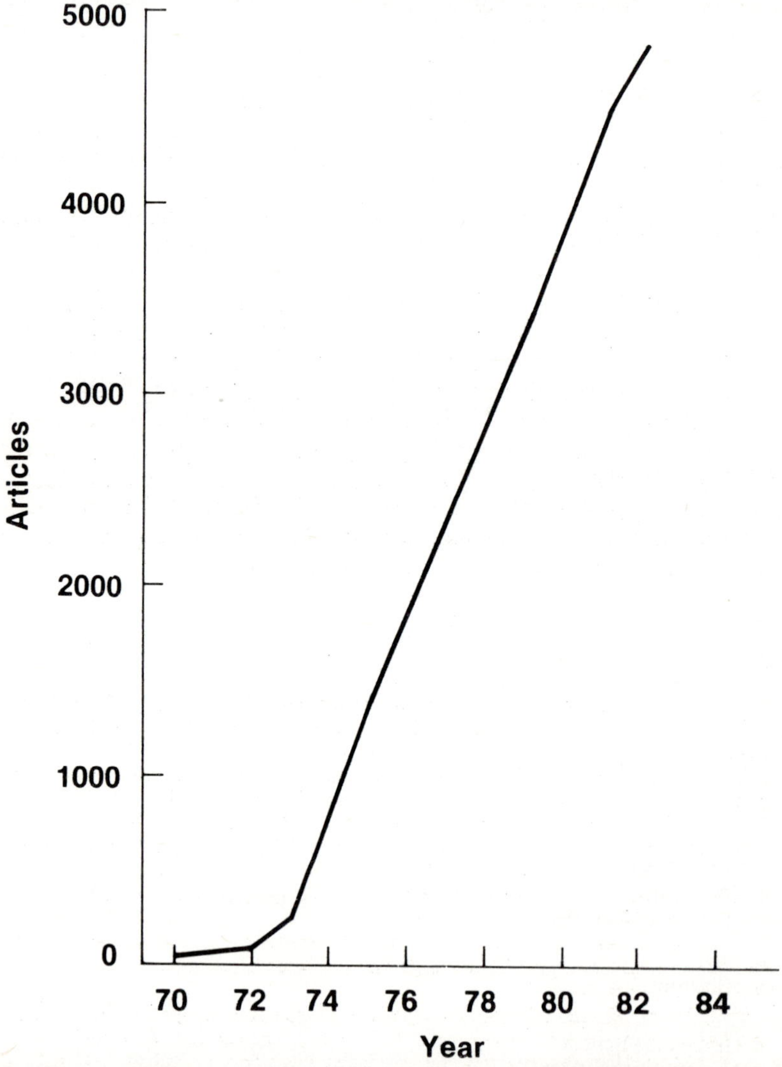

Figure 2 Cumulative number of publications on LHRH and analogs, 1970 to date.

using injectable, polymer-based depot formulations is described (Chapter 33).

The nomenclature used to denote the structures of the LHRH analogs in most instances follows the IUPAC-IUB recommendations, although the increasing use of unnatural amino acids has put some strains on this system. In this nomenclature system the superscript on the amino acid abbreviation in the brackets denotes the positions in the native LHRH structure which have been replaced by the substitutions cited. All other residues in the LHRH sequence are unchanged. The only significant deviations from past literature are in the cases of Pro-NHEt substitution in position 9 where it is felt that the additional designation of des-Gly^{10} is redundant. Thus buserelin is [D-Ser(tBu)^{6},Pro^{9}-NHEt]LHRH instead of des-Gly^{10}[D-Ser(TBU)^{6}]-LHRH ethylamide (or variations of the latter) as cited in some previous publications.

The past decade of research on LHRH and its analogs has been particularly impressive as it presents a very successful chemical and pharmacological research story. The chemical studies have resulted in the synthesis of well over a thousand LHRH agonists and antagonists, many of which are highly potent and long-lived, with receptor affinities greater than that of LHRH. The pharmacological investigations have uncovered an impressive list of clinical applications, several of which are currently being tested in patients. This field has been extremely active and rapidly growing, as evidenced by the steadily increasing number of literature citations (Figure 2). The decade which began with the hope that LHRH might offer a route to the induction or restoration of fertility has ended with a far broader perspective in which LHRH analogs may also contribute importantly to the treatment of cancer.

In order to present a state-of-the-art review, it has been our attempt to minimize the time from the invitation of contributions to publication. Additionally, the wide scope of this book has required that only the more recent and most pertinent references be cited. If this has led to inadvertent omissions or rigidity in style, it is the editors who bear the responsibility. We thank our contributors for their hard work and patience.

References

Burgus, R., Butcher, M., Amoss, M., Ling, N., Monahan, M. W., Rivier, J., Fellows, R., Blackwell, R., Vale, W. and Guillemin, R. (1972). Primary structure of the ovine hypothalamic luteinizing hormone-releasing factor (LRF). *Proc. Natl. Acad. Sci. USA*, **69,** 278

Bennett, H. P. J. and McMartin, C. (1979). Peptide hormones and their analogues: distribution, clearance from the circulation, and inactivation in vivo. *Pharmacol. Rev.*, **30,** 247

Harris, G. W. (1955). *Neural Control of the Pituitary Gland.* (London: Arnold)

Igarashi, M. and McCann, S. M. (1964). A hypothalamic follicle stimulating hormone-releasing factor. *Endocrinology*, **74,** 446

McCann, S. M., Taleisnik, S. and Friedman, H. M. (1960). LH-releasing activity in hypothalamic extracts. *Proc. Soc. Exp. Biol. Med.*, **104,** 432

Matsuo, H., Baba, Y., Nair, R. M., Arimura, A. and Schally, A. V. (1971*a*). Structure of the porcine LH- and FSH-releasing hormone. I. The proposed amino acid sequence. *Biochem. Biophys. Res. Commun.*, **43,** 1334

Matsuo, H., Arimura, A. and Schally, A. V. (1971*b*). Synthesis of the porcine LH- and FSH-releasing hormone by the solid-phase method. *Biochem. Biophys. Res. Commun.*, **45,** 822

Schally, A. V. (1979). Hypothalamic peptide hormones: basic and clinical studies. In Li, C.H. (ed.) *Hormonal Proteins and Peptides.* Vol. VII, pp. 1–54. (New York: Academic Press)

Schally, A. V., Arimura, A., Kastin, A. J. Matsuo, H., Baba, Y., Redding, T. W., Nair, R. M. G., Debeljuk, L. and White, W. F. (1971). Gonadotropin-releasing hormone; one polypeptide regulates secretion of luteinizing hormone and follicle stimulating hormones, *Science*, **173**, 1036

A retrospective
LHRH and its analogs: the first decade

A. V. SCHALLY

In 1971 our group isolated the luteinizing hormone and follicle stimulating hormone-releasing hormone (LHRH/FSH-RH) (Schally *et al.*, 1971*a*, *b*) from porcine hypothalami, determined the amino acid composition, elucidated its structure and synthesized it (Matsuo *et al.*, 1971*a*, *b*; Schally *et al.*, 1971*a*, *b*). Physiological and immunological studies established that LHRH is the main link between the brain and the pituitary gland insofar as reproductive function is concerned (Schally *et al.*, 1976, 1980). Various clinicians, including our collaborators, established clinical uses of LHRH (Schally *et al.*, 1976, 1980). Although the full potential of the diagnostic use of LHRH in differentiating between hypothalamic and pituitary causes of hypogonadism has not yet been reached, LHRH does seem to help elucidate the functional state of the pituitary. In 1971 we also postulated that LHRH or its derivatives might be useful for the control of fertility by disrupting the menstrual cycle and preventing the ovulatory LH surge (Schally and Kastin, 1971). We suggested that replacement or deletion of one or more amino acids in LHRH might result in analogs possessing features requisite for an effective binding, but lacking those that are necessary for a functional effect, i.e. the stimulating of LH and FSH release (Schally and Kastin, 1971). Since 1972 systematic work has been proceeding to design and synthesize agonistic and antagonistic analogs of LHRH. There is little doubt that in addition to scientific reasons for determining structure–function relationships for this hormone, a strong interest in possible veterinary and medical applications of LHRH derivatives stimulated this synthetic undertaking. In the past 10 years an estimated 1500 analogs of LHRH have been synthesized (Coy *et al.*, 1979*a*, *b*; Schally and Coy, 1983). Many agonistic analogs more potent than the parent hormone have been made. Some of these analogs were tested clinically.

Various investigators have determined that large doses of superactive stimulatory analogs of LHRH cause paradoxical antifertility effects in animals and human beings (Auclair *et al.*, 1977; Corbin *et al.*, 1978; Sandow *et al.*, 1978; Bergquist *et al.*, 1979). Extensive work is in progress to apply these effects to the development of new contraceptive methods. The phenomena of desensitization and inhibition of sex steroid levels by LHRH agonists are already being used for treatment of true idiopathic precocious puberty (Crowley *et al.*, 1981; Laron *et al.*, 1981). The paradoxical inhibitory effects induced by chronic administration of LHRH agonists have also been linked to the regression of endocrine dependent cancers (DeSombre *et al.*, 1976; Redding and Schally, 1981; Tolis *et al.*, 1982). We have shown an inhibition of prostate tumor growth in two rat models by chronic administration of [D-Trp^6]LHRH (Redding and Schally, 1981). We and others have also demonstrated tumor growth inhibition in patients with prostatic carcinoma after treatment with LHRH agonists (Glode, 1982; Tolis *et al.*, 1982).

Potent inhibitory analogs of LHRH which block ovulation in laboratory animals have also been synthesized (Coy *et al.*, 1979*a*, *b*; Schally *et al.*, 1976, 1980; Schally and Coy, 1983). Several antagonists of LHRH have been tested in men and women and shown to be active and powerful enough for practical use (Gonzalez-Barcena *et al.*, 1977; Zárate *et al.*, 1981). The synthetic approach based on inhibitory analogs of LHRH has clearly been proved feasible for the development of new methods of birth control, although the exact clinical regimens are still lacking (Schally and Coy, 1983). In addition, it is possible that the LHRH antagonists could be useful for treatment of precocious puberty, endometriosis, the symptoms of menopause, such as the hot flashes, and on the basis of recent experimental results also for management of breast and prostate carcinoma (Redding *et al.*, 1982). Thus, in addition to opening a new approach to birth control, it appears that analogs of LHRH may counter hormone sensitive prostate cancers and perhaps breast cancers.

Andrew V. Schally
New Orleans,
August 1982

References

Auclair, C., Kelly, P. A., Labrie, F., Coy, D. H. and Schally, A. V. (1977). *Biochem. Biophys. Res. Commun.*, **76,** 855

Bergquist, C., Nillius, S. J. and Wide, L. (1979). *Lancet,* **2,** 215

Corbin, A., Beattie, C. W., Tracy, J., Jones, R., Foell, T. J., Yardley, J. and Rees, R. W.A. (1978). *Int. J. Fertil.,* **23,** 81

Coy, D. H., Mezo, I., Pedroza, E., Nekola, M. V., Vilchez-Martinez, J. A., Piyachaturawata, P., Schally, A. V., Seprodi, J. and Teplan, I. (1979*a*). In Gross, E. and Meienhofer, J. (eds.) *Peptides – Structure and Biological Function. Proceedings of the Sixth American Peptide Symposium,* pp. 775–779. (Rockford, IL: Pierce Chem. Co.)

Coy, D. H., Seprodi, J., Vilchez-Martinez, J. A., Pedroza, E., Gardner, J. and Schally, A. V. (1979*b*). In Collu, R. (ed.) *Central Nervous System Effects of Hypothalamic Hormones and Other Peptides,* pp. 317–323. (New York: Raven Press)

Crowley, W. F., Comite, F., Vale, W., Rivier, J., Loriaux, D. L. and Cutler, G. B. Jr. (1981). *J. Clin. Endocrinol. Metab.,* **52,** 370

DeSombre, E. R., Johnson, E. S. and White, W. F. (1976). *Cancer Res.,* **36,** 3830

Glode, L. M. (1982). *Proceedings of the 18th Annual Meeting of the American Society of Clinical Oncology,* April 25–27, Abstract C-426, p. 110

Gonzalez-Barcena, D., Kastin, A. J., Coy, D. H., Trevino-Ortiz, H., Gordon, F., Nikolics, K. and Schally, A. V. (1977). *Lancet,* **2,** 997

Laron, Z., Kauli, R., Ben Zeev, Z., Comaru-Schally, A. M. and Schally, A. V. (1981). *Lancet,* **2,** 955

Matsuo, H., Arimura, A., Nari, R. M. G. and Schally, A. V. (1971*a*). *Biochem. Biophys. Res. Commun.,* **45,** 822

Matsuo, H., Baba, Y., Nair, R. M. G., Arimura, A. and Schally, A. V. (1971*b*). *Biochem. Biophys. Res. Commun.,* **43,** 1334

Redding, T. W. and Schally, A. V. (1981). *Proc. Natl. Acad. Sci. USA,* **78,** 6509

Redding, T. W., Coy, D. H. and Schally, A. V. (1982). *Proc. Natl. Acad. Sci. USA,* **79,** 1273

Sandow, J., von Rechenberg, W., Konig, W., Hahn, M., Jerzabek, G. and Fraser, H. (1978). In Gupta, D. and Voelter, W. (eds.) *Hypothalamic Hormones – Chemistry, Physiology and Clinical Applications,* pp. 307–326. (New York: Verlag Chemie)

Schally, A. V. and Kastin, A. J. (1971). *Drug. Ther.,* **1,** 29

Schally, A. V., Arimura, A., Baba, Y., Nair, R. M. G., Matsuo, H., Redding, T. W., Debeljuk, L. and White, W. F. (1971*a*). *Biochem. Biophys. Res. Commun.,* **43,** 393

Schally, A. V., Nair, R. M. G., Redding, T. W. and Arimura, A. (1971*b*). *J. Biol. Chem.,* **246,** 7230

Schally, A. V., Kastin, A. J. and Coy, D. H. (1976). *Int. J. Fertil.,* **21,** 1

Schally, A. V., Arimura, A. and Coy, D. H. (1980). *Vitam. Horm.,* **38,** 257

Schally, A. V. and Coy, D. H. (1983). In *The Role of Peptides and Proteins in Control of Reproduction.* Proceedings of the Workshop Sponsored by the Reproductive Biology Study Section of NIH, Feb. 15–16, 1982, Bethesda. (New York: Elsevier-North Holland) p. 89

Tolis, G., Ackman, D., Stellos, A., Mehta, A., Labrie, F., Fazekas, A. T. A., Comaru-Schally, A. M. and Schally, A. V. (1982). *Proc. Natl. Acad. Sci. USA,* **79,** 1658

Zárate, A., Canales, E., Schally, A. V., Coy, D. H. and Comaru-Schally, A. M. (1981). In Zatuchni, G. I., Shelton, J. D. and Sciarra, J. J. (eds.) *LH-RH Peptides as Female and Male Contraceptives,* pp. 227–236. (Philadelphia: Harper & Row)

SECTION I

CHEMISTRY AND BASIC REPRODUCTIVE PROPERTIES

1
Development of agonistic LHRH analogs

J. J. NESTOR Jr.

The varied and important potential clinical applications of LHRH stimulated active analog synthesis programs by several groups following the disclosure of its primary sequence (Matsuo *et al.*, 1971*a*; Burgus *et al.*, 1972). These efforts were directed at an understanding of the structural characteristics of the molecule required for action and at the synthesis of analogs with increased potency and prolonged action. This historical review outlines the development of the synthesis programs which have produced the highly potent LHRH agonistic analogs now under clinical development. Other detailed reviews are available (Schally *et al.*, 1981; Corbin, 1982).

STRUCTURE/ACTIVITY RELATIONSHIPS

Following the initial descriptions of the synthesis of LHRH (Matsuo *et al.*, 1971*b*; Monahan *et al.*, 1971), the first analog exhibiting a biological potency greater than LHRH itself ('superagonist') was reported (Fujino *et al.*, 1972). A study of numerous C-terminal amides of LHRH showed that, while decapeptide amides (e.g. LHRH-methylamide, LHRH-ethylamide, etc.) were only weakly active, nonapeptide alkyl amides were very potent. One of these analogs, [Pro^9-NHEt]LHRH, was six times more potent than LHRH. It was important that the chain length be similar to that of LHRH since longer (NHBu) or shorter (NHMe) analogs were less potent than the NHEt analog. Although 15 different linear and cyclic amines were investigated as C-terminal nonapeptide amides, the ethylamide was the most potent and has appeared frequently in further analogs.

The replacement of the other Gly residue in LHRH by D-amino acids yielded superagonist analogs. [D-Ala^6]LHRH has a potency five times that of LHRH in a dispersed pituitary cell assay, while the corresponding L-analog, [L-Ala^6]LHRH, has only 4 % of the activity of LHRH (Monahan *et al.*, 1973). The increased potency of the D-isomer was suggested to be due to its ability to stabilize the active conformation of the molecule, since a D-amino acid can stabilize a type IIβ-bend when it is in position i + 1 in the turn (Nemethy and

Printz, 1972). The demonstration that [N-MeLeu^{7}]LHRH was slightly more potent than LHRH (Ling and Vale, 1975) cast some doubt on this interpretation because in this analog the bend-stabilizing, i to i + 2 hydrogen bond would be absent. *In vitro* degradation studies with enzyme preparations obtained from brain homogenates determined that a major site of proteolytic cleavage is at position 6. Although initial work with impure homogenates indicated Gly–Leu cleavage (Koch *et al.*, 1974), and experiments with a purified hypothalamic protease showed Tyr–Gly cleavage (Horsthemke *et al.*, 1981), D-Ala^{6} substitution should impede either mode of proteolysis. While [D-Ala^{6}]LHRH and other superactive analogs are degraded more slowly than LHRH by these homogenates (Marks and Stern, 1974; Koch *et al.*, 1977; Horsthemke *et al.*, 1981), LHRH analogs may not be exposed to these enzymes *in vivo*.

The combination of these two modifications in [D-Ala^{6},Pro^{9}-NHEt]LHRH (Fujino *et al.*, 1974; Coy *et al.*, 1974; Rivier *et al.*, 1975) has synergistic effects on biological activity. This compound has an *in vitro* potency thirteenfold greater than LHRH. The incorporation of other D-amino acids into position 6 gave still more potent analogs (Table 1.1). For example, [D-Leu^{6},Pro^{9}-NHEt]LHRH (leuprolide) had a potency 15 times LHRH *in vitro*. A trend toward increased potency is associated with aromatic, hydrophobic side chains in position 6. In the disubstituted series, [D-Trp^{6},Pro^{9}-NHEt]LHRH was the most potent analog with an *in vitro* potency of 144 times LHRH (Rivier *et al.*, 1975).

A similar trend toward higher potency for aromatic, more hydrophobic D-amino acids in position 6 was found in the monosubstituted series (Coy *et al.*, 1976). Although [D-Trp^{6},Pro^{9}-NHEt]LHRH has one-half the *in vitro* potency of [D-Trp^{6}]LHRH, *in vivo* studies show them to be equipotent (Schally *et al.*, 1981; B. Vickery and G. McRae, unpublished). The Pro^{9}-NHEt modification heightens the potency of the less potent, more hydrophilic analogs but not that of the more hydrophobic analogs (Coy *et al.*, 1976; Nestor *et al.*, 1982).

The tertiary-butyl ether of D-serine was incorporated into position 6 of LHRH in combination with the C-terminal amide modification (Konig *et al.*, 1975). The resulting [D-Ser(tBu)^{6},Pro^{9}-NHEt]LHRH (buserelin), is 140 times as potent as LHRH for induction of ovulation in rats. In this acute *in vivo* assay, [D-Leu^{6},Pro^{9}-NHEt]LHRH had a potency of 80 times LHRH.

The incorporation of aza-Gly(-NHNHCO-) in position 10 also gave superagonist analogs (Dutta *et al.*, 1978). The aza-Gly modification was known to lead to resistance to proteolysis and, in combination with the D-Ser(tBu)^{6} substitution, it yielded an analog ([D-Ser(tBu)^{6},aza-Gly^{10}]LHRH) sevenfold more potent than buserelin ([D-Ser(tBu)^{6},Pro^{9}-NHEt]LHRH) (Dutta *et al.*, 1978). This substitution may confer high potency by protection of the analog from the highly active post-proline-cleaving-enzyme in rat plasma (Benuck and Marks, 1976). The relevance of this modification for analogs to be used in human therapy is less clear since a threefold to fivefold lower amount of this enzymatic activity is present in human plasma (Walter *et al.*, 1975).

More hydrophobic analogs have recently been reported. The His(Bzl) residue was introduced into position 6 in order to give an analog with

Table 1.1 Comparative potencies of LHRH analogs

Compound	*LH release*		*Ovulation induction*[c]	*Estrus suppression*[d]	*Dose in women*[e] (*μg; s.c. inj*)
	In vitro[a]	*Male rat*[b]			
LHRH	1	1	1	1	100–250
[D-Ala^6,Pro^9-NHEt]LHRH	13.5				
[D-Leu^6,Pro^9-NHEt]LHRH	15	15			5–25
[D-Trp^6,Pro^9-NHEt]LHRH	144	7		100	10
[D-Trp^6]LHRH	36(90[b])	13		100	10
[D-Trp^6,N-MeLeu^7,Pro^9-NHEt]LHRH					
[D-Ser(tBu)^6,Pro^9-NHEt]LHRH			15		
[D-Ser(tBu)^6,aza-Gly^{10}]LHRH			100	54	
[D-His(Bzl)^6,Pro^9-NHEt]LHRH	210			100	
[D-Nal(2)^6]LHRH				200	
[D-Nal(2)^6,Pro^9-NHEt]LHRH				90	
[D-Nal(2)^6,aza-GlyNH$_2^{10}$]LHRH				230	

[a] Rivier *et al.* (1975); [b] Coy *et al.* (1976); [c] Dutta *et al.* (1978); [d] Nestor *et al.* (1982); [e] Dose required for maximal LH release in women (Corbin, 1982)

increased water solubility at an acidic pH (where the imidazole function of His would be protonated), but which becomes less soluble at neutral pH in the body (Vale *et al.*, 1979). This type of modification provides a more soluble analog for purification and formulation work but behaves like a more hydrophobic compound *in vivo*. [D-His(Bzl)^6,Pro^9-NHEt]LHRH had a potency 200 times that of LHRH, when assayed *in vitro* in the dispersed pituitary cell assay.

The effect of still further increases in the hydrophobicity of the side chain of D-amino acids in position 6 was described recently (Nestor *et al.*, 1982), and has been extended to the antagonist series (Chapter 4). The most potent analogs in this series are 200 or more times as potent as LHRH when assayed in a rigorous, 2 week assay involving suppression of rat estrous cyclicity (Nestor *et al.*, 1982) (Table 1.2). From this series of analogs, [D-Nal(2)^6]LHRH was chosen for clinical development.

RECEPTOR BINDING AND METABOLISM

The increased *in vivo* potency of the analogs containing D-amino acid substitutions in position 6, with or without the Pro^9-NHEt modification, may be due to either increased receptor affinity and/or protection from enzymatic degradation (Marks and Stern, 1974). The major enzymes in rat hypophyseal extracts which are responsible for degrading LHRH are pyroglutamate aminopeptidase, LHRH degrading endopeptidase, and post-proline-cleaving-enzyme (Bauer *et al.*, 1979). The Pro^9-NHEt substitution decreases the rate of cleavage by the post-proline-cleaving-enzyme and D-amino acid substitution in position 6 blocks proteolysis by the LHRH cleaving endopeptidase. Such doubly modified analogs therefore have prolonged *in vivo* survival.

Receptor binding studies have shown that both the 6 and the 10 position modifications confer increased binding affinity on LHRH analogs using either pituitary membrane preparations (Heber and Odell, 1978; Perrin *et al.*, 1980) or whole cell preparations (Loumaye *et al.*, 1982). In addition, the more hydrophobic 6 position substitutions give analogs with still higher binding affinity. Since proteolytic activity may be associated with the membranes used in these receptor studies (Clayton *et al.*, 1979), part of this increased affinity may be due to protection from degradation in the assay. A peptide with high specific receptor affinity plus resistance to proteolysis should exhibit a higher *in vivo* potency.

The rate of clearance of a peptide hormone analog may be dependent on other factors in addition to resistance to enzymatic degradation. Very hydrophobic LHRH analogs (Chapter 3) may partition into hydrophobic regions in the body (plasma membranes, lipoprotein assemblies, hydrophobic carrier proteins etc.). Such a molecule would not be exposed continuously to the body's clearance mechanisms (proteolysis and glomerular filtration) and might partition back to the plasma to give a prolonged biological half-life (Chapters 33, 34).

Table 1.2 LHRH analogs in clinical development[a] or clinical studies[b]

Compound	*US adopted name*	*Indications*	*Dosage forms*	*Company[a]/sponsor[b]*
[D-Ala^{6},Pro^{9}-NHEt]LHRH		Prostate/breast cancer	inj	TAP Pharmaceuticals[c]/ Abbott
[D-Leu^{6},Pro^{9}-NHEt]LHRH	leuprolide/ leuprorelin	Prostate/breast cancer	inj	TAP Pharmaceuticals/ Abbott
[D-Trp^{6},Pro^{9}-NHEt]LHRH		Female/male contraception	inj	Salk Institute
[D-Trp^{6}]LHRH				Ayerst
[D-Trp^{6},N-MeLeu^{7},Pro^{9}-NHEt]LHRH		Pregnancy interruption/ prostate cancer	inj/nasal	Wyeth
[D-Ser(tBu)^{6},Pro^{9}-NHEt]LHRH	buserelin	Female/male contraception Prostate/breast cancer Endometriosis	inj/nasal	Hoechst
[D-Ser(tBu)^{6},aza-Gly^{10}]LHRH		Prostate/breast cancer	inj polymer release	ICI
[D-His(Bzl)^{6},Pro^{9}-NHEt]LHRH	nafarelin	Female/male contraception		Population Council
[D-Nal(2)^{6}]LHRH	acetate	Female/male contraception Prostate/breast cancer Endometriosis Precocious puberty	inj/nasal polymer release	Syntex

[a] Compounds undergoing toxicological, clinical and pharmacological development by a pharmaceutical company
[b] Compounds in clinical evaluation with academic or non-industrial sponsorship
[c] Takeda-Abbott Products (TAP)

RELATIVE POTENCIES

The analogs which are currently in clinical studies may be broken down into three classes (Table 1.1): (1) analogs with potencies in the 5–15 times LHRH range ([D-Ala^6,Pro^9-NHEt]LHRH; [D-Leu^6,Pro^9-NHEt]LHRH), (2) hydrophobic analogs with higher *in vivo* potency, in the range from 15 to 100 times LHRH ([D-Ser(tBu)^6,Pro^9-NHEt]LHRH; [D-Trp^6]LHRH; [D-Trp^6,Pro^9-NHEt]LHRH; [D-Trp^6,N-MeLeu^7,Pro^9-NHEt]LHRH) and (3) hydrophobic analogs of the highest potency, 200 or more times LHRH ([D-Nal(2)^6]LHRH; [D-His(Bzl)^6,Pro^9-NHEt]LHRH). In view of the low level of absorption of LHRH analogs by the nasal route (1–5%), physical and economic factors may prevent the utilization of nasal delivery systems for the less potent agonists.

COMPOUNDS IN CLINICAL DEVELOPMENT

Table 1.2 is a list of compounds which are undergoing evaluation in clinical pharmacology studies. Several of these analogs are in clinical development by pharmaceutical companies. Extensive clinical trials have been carried out with: [D-Leu^6,Pro^9-NHEt]LHRH; [D-Ser(tBu)^6,Pro^9-NHEt]LHRH; [D-Ser(tBu)^6,aza-Gly^{10}]LHRH; [D-Trp^6,Pro^9-NHEt]LHRH; and [D-Trp^6,N-MeLeu^7,Pro^9-NHEt]LHRH.

Two of the most potent LHRH analogs reported – [D-Nal(2)^6]LHRH and [D-His(Bzl)^6,Pro^9-NHEt]LHRH – are in Phase II clinical trials.

Detailed discussions of the clinical results with several of these compounds are found in later chapters.

CONCLUDING REMARKS

The development of the most potent LHRH agonist structures has followed a stepwise and, for the most part, empirical course. These analogs all contain a D-amino acid substitution in position 6, with the highest potencies (~200 times LHRH) reported for amino acids with hydrophobic, aromatic amino acid substitutions. Potency increases may be obtained by replacement of the Gly residue at position 10 by an ethylamide residue in the more hydrophilic analogs. Both modifications are known to provide resistance to enzymatic degradation in studies with tissue homogenates and both modifications cause increases in receptor binding affinities. Metabolic clearance studies in man with two hydrophobic superagonist analogs have shown them to have biological half-lives significantly longer than LHRH itself.

References

Bauer, K., Horsthemke, B., Knisatschek, H., Novak, P. and Kleinkauf, H. (1979). Degradation of luliberin (LH-RF) by brain and pituitary tissue enzymes. *Z. Physiol. Chem.*, **360**, 229

Benuck, N. and Marks, N. (1976). Differences in the degradation of hypothalamic releasing factors by rat and human serum. *Life Sci.*, **19**, 1271

Burgus, R., Butcher, M., Amoss, M., Ling, N., Monahan, M. W., Rivier, J., Fellows, R., Blackwell, R., Vale, W. and Guillemin, R. (1972). Primary structure of the ovine hypothalamic luteinizing hormone-releasing factor (LRF). *Proc. Natl. Acad. Sci. USA*, **69,** 278.

Clayton, R. N., Shakespear, R. A., Duncan, J. A. and Marshall, J. C. (1979). Luteinizing hormone-releasing hormone inactivation by purified pituitary plasma membrane: effects on receptor binding studies. *Endocrinology*, **104,** 1484

Corbin, A. (1982). From contraception to cancer: a review of the therapeutic applications of LHRH analogues as antitumor agents. *Yale J. Biol. Med.*, **55,** 27

Coy, D. H., Coy, E. J., Schally, A. V., Vilchez-Martinez, J. A., Hirotsu, Y. and Arimura, A. (1974). Synthesis and biological properties of [D-Ala-6,des-Gly-NH_2^{10}]-LHRH ethylamide, a peptide with greatly enhanced LH- and FSH-releasing activity. *Biochem. Biophys. Res. Commun.*, **57,** 335

Coy, D. H., Vilchez-Martinez, J. A., Coy, E. J. and Schally, A. V. (1976). Analogs of luteinizing hormone-releasing hormone with increased biological activity produced by D-amino acid substitutions in position 6. *J. Med. Chem.*, **19,** 423

Dutta, A. S., Furr, B. J. A., Giles, M. B., Valcaccia, B. and Walpole, A. L. (1978). Potent agonist and antagonist analogues of luliberin containing an azaglycine residue in position 10. *Biochem. Biophys. Res. Commun.*, **81,** 382.

Fujino, J., Kobayashi, S., Obayashi, M., Fukuda, T., Shinagawa, S., Yamazaki, I., Nakayama, R., White, W. F. and Rippel, R. H. (1972). Structure-activity relationships in the C-terminal part of luteinizing hormone-releasing hormone (LH-RH). *Biochem. Biophys. Res. Commun.*, **49,** 863

Fujino, M., Fukuda, T., Shinagawa, S., Kobayashi, S., Yamazaki, I., Nakayama, R., Seely, J. H., White, W. F. and Rippel, R. H. (1974). Synthetic analogs of luteinizing hormone-releasing hormone (LH-RH) substituted in position 6 and 10. *Biochem. Biophys. Res. Commun.*, **60,** 406

Heber, D. and Odell, W. D. (1978). Pituitary receptor binding activity of active, inactive, superactive and inhibitory analogs of gonadotropin-releasing hormone. *Biochem. Biophys. Res. Commun.*, **82,** 67

Horsthemke, B., Knisatschek, H., Rivier, J., Sandow, J. and Bauer, K. (1981). Degradation of luteinizing hormone-releasing hormone and analogs by adenohypophyseal peptidases. *Biochem. Biophys. Res. Commun.*, **100,** 753

Koch, Y., Baram, T., Chobsieng, P. and Fridkin, M. (1974). Enzymic degradation of luteinizing hormone-releasing-hormone (LHRH) by hypothalamic tissue. *Biochem. Biophys. Res. Commun.*, **61,** 95

Koch, Y., Baram, T., Hazum, E. and Fridkin, M. (1977). Resistance to enzymatic degradation of LHRH analogues possessing increased biological activity. *Biochem. Biophys. Res. Commun.*, **74,** 488

Konig, W., Sandow, J. and Geiger, R. (1975). Structure–function relationships of LH-RH/FSH-RH. In Walter, R. and Meienhofer, J. (eds.) *Peptides: Chemistry, Structure, Biology – Proceedings of the Fourth American Peptide Symposium*, pp. 883–888. (Ann Arbor: Ann Arbor Science)

Ling, N. and Vale, W. (1975). Analogs of luteinizing hormone releasing factor (LRF) – synthesis and biological activity of [(Nα-Me)Leu^7]LRF and [D-Ala^6, (Nα-Me)Leu^7]LRF. *Biochem. Biophys. Res. Commun.*, **63,** 801

Loumaye, E., Naor, Z. and Catt, K. J. (1982). Binding affinity and biological activity of gonadotropin-releasing hormone agonists in isolated pituitary cells. *Endocrinology*, **111,** 730

Marks, N. and Stern, F. (1974). Enzymatic mechanisms for the inactivation of luteinizing hormone-releasing hormone (LH-RH). *Biochem. Biophys. Res. Commun.*, **61,** 1458

Matsuo, H., Baba, Y., Nair, R. M., Arimura, A. and Schally, A. V. (1971*a*). Structure of the porcine LH- and FSH-releasing hormone. I. The proposed amino acid sequence. *Biochem. Biophys. Res. Commun.*, **43,** 1334

Matsuo, H., Arimura, A., Nair, R. M. G. and Schally, A. V. (1971*b*). Synthesis of the porcine LH- and FSH-releasing hormone by the solid-phase method. *Biochem. Biophys. Res. Commun.*, **45,** 822

Monahan, M., Rivier, J., Burgus, R., Amoss, M., Blackwell, R., Vale, W. and Guillemin, R. (1971). Synthèse totale par phase solide d'un décapeptide qui stimule la secrétion des gonadotropines hypophysaires LH et FSH. *Compt. Rend. Ser. D.*, **273,** 508

Monahan, M. W., Amoss, M. S., Anderson, H. A. and Vale, W. (1973). Synthetic analogs of the hypothalamic luteinizing hormone releasing factor with increased agonist or antagonist properties. *Biochemistry,* **12,** 4616

Nemethy, G. and Printz, M. P. (1972). The η-turn, a possible folded conformation of the polypeptide chain. Comparison with the β turn. *Macromolecules,* **5,** 775

Nestor, J. J. Jr., Ho, T. L., Simpson, R. A., Horner, B. L., Jones, G. H., McRae, G. I. and Vickery, B. H. (1982). Synthesis and biological activity of some very hydrophobic superagonist analogues of luteinizing hormone-releasing hormone. *J. Med. Chem.,* **25,** 795

Perrin, M. H., Rivier, J. E. and Vale, W. W. (1980). Radioligand assay for gonadotropin-releasing hormone: relative potencies of agonists and antagonists. *Endocrinology,* **106**, 1289

Rivier, J., Ling, N., Monahan, M., Rivier, C., Brown, M. and Vale, W. (1975). Luteinizing hormone releasing factor and somatostatin analogs. In Walter, R. and Meienhofer, J. (eds.) *Peptides: Chemistry, Structure and Biology – Proceedings of the Fourth American Peptide Symposium,* pp. 863–870. (Ann Arbor: Ann Arbor Science)

Schally, A. V., Arimura, A. and Coy, D. H. (1981). Recent approaches to fertility control based on derivatives of LH-RH. *Vitam. Horm.,* **38,** 257

Vale, W. W., Rivier, C., Perrin, M. and Rivier, J. (1979). LRF agonists and fertility regulation in the male. In Gross, E. and Meienhofer, J. (eds.) *Peptides – Structure and Biological Function, Proceedings of the Sixth American Peptide Symposium,* pp. 781–93. (Rockford, IL: Pierce Chem. Co.)

Walter, R., Neidle, A. and Marks, N. (1975). Significant differences in the degradation of Pro-Leu-Gly-NH_2 by human serum and that of other species. *Proc. Soc. Expl. Biol. Med.,* **148,** 98

2
LHRH analogs as antiovulatory agents

J. RIVIER, C. RIVIER, M. PERRIN, J. PORTER and W. VALE

While chronic treatment with LHRH agonists interferes with reproductive functions (Rivier *et al.*, 1978, 1979; Rivier and Vale, 1979, 1981*b*; Vale *et al.*, 1979), it is at first associated with an increase in gonadotropin and steroid secretion. This initial stimulation may be considered undesirable under some clinical circumstances. Additionally, LHRH agonists have a multiplicity of sites of action in rats which, if verified in humans, may also prove them unacceptable for human use.

In the female rat, an injection of LHRH antagonist at noon on the day of proestrus results in the inhibition of the LH surge and a blockade of ovulation (Rivier *et al.*, 1981*a,b*). When an antagonist is administered chronically to regularly cycling female rats, it results in irregular cycling throughout the treatment period. This acyclicity is accompanied by a high degree of infertility, though mating of such treated animals results in a limited number of pregnancies (Rivier *et al.*, 1981*a*). Cessation of antagonist treatment is followed by a resumption of normal reproductive functions. LHRH antagonists also interfere with pregnancy. The effectiveness of the analogs is highest during the second week of gestation, at a time when survival of the embryos is dependent upon LH and progesterone secretion, as illustrated by the ability of hCG or progesterone to counteract the antigestational effects of the antagonists (Rivier *et al.*, 1981*a,b*; Rivier and Vale, 1981*a*, 1982).

Daily treatment of adult male rats with LHRH antagonists abolishes mating behavior and disrupts spermatogenesis (Rivier *et al.*, 1978, 1980). This is accompanied by a sharp decrease in plasma testosterone levels and accessory organ weights. The concomitant administration of small amounts of androgen is capable of restoring sexual activity while the rats remain infertile (Rivier *et al.*, 1981*c*). Fertility is restored by administration of larger amounts of androgen (Rivier *et al.*, 1981*c*).

SYNTHETIC TECHNIQUES

Solid phase peptide synthesis (Barany and Merrifield, 1980) by standardized experimental protocols (Rivier *et al.*, 1973) was used to prepare protected peptido-resins. High performance reverse phase liquid chromatography (RP-

HPLC) is the preferred purification method for deprotected peptides because high resolution and reproducible separations are obtained directly from crude peptides. Different solvent systems often have altered selectivities for peptides and impurities (Rivier, 1978; Dunlap *et al.*, 1978). The rapid, reproducible separations which are obtained may ultimately be performed automatically. The reversed phase columns can be reused with no cross-contamination if proper clean-up procedures are followed (repeated washes with high concentrations of organic modifiers). The improved resolution obtained with RP-HPLC leads to better recovery since one does not have to sacrifice yield for purity. Preparative HPLC purifications were carried out on a preparative LC-500 (Waters Associates) using a gradient former (Eldex) and u.v. detection. Empty cartridges (Waters Associates) were dry packed with Vydac C_{18} end-capped silicas (30 nm pore size) having varying particle sizes (10, 15, 17 and 20 μm). The resolution and high recovery of peptides with these silicas is similar to that of analytical columns but loads of 1–3 g of crude product per run are used (Rivier *et al.*, 1982, 1983*c*).

STRUCTURE–ACTIVITY RELATIONSHIPS

The synthesis of analogs that probe positions 4 and 5 in a systematic manner following the Topliss manual method for applying the Hansch approach to drug design (Topliss, 1977) is in keeping with our earlier work on position 2 substitutions (Rivier *et al.*, 1981*d*). In the meantime high biological potency was reported for antagonists having a D-Arg substitution at position 6 in conjunction with an aromatic D-amino acid at position 1 and D-Ala at position 10 (Coy *et al.*, 1982). Another basic amino acid, D-Lys, can be introduced into the [N-Ac-Δ^3-Pro^1,D-pF-Phe^2,D-Trp^3] analog with retention of very high potency both *in vitro* (Rivier *et al.*, 1981*d*) and in the binding assay (Perrin *et al.*, 1983). A new concept has emerged whereby the introduction of a hydrophilic moiety at the 6th position is compatible with other modifications at the N- and C-termini, provided that these are fairly hydrophobic. A certain level of overall hydrophobicity may be required for tight binding to the receptor and possibly for resistance to degradative enzymes. The optimization of global hydrophilic/hydrophobic, electronic and steric effects may lead to extremely potent and long acting LHRH analogs.

The properties sought for in the design of analogs are high potency and duration of action in an *in vivo* system. Most results will therefore be discussed in terms of an analog's ability to interfere with ovulation in an antiovulatory assay (AOA) test (Corbin and Beattie, 1975). Results are expressed in terms of the ratio of LHRH antagonist-treated rats ovulating to vehicle-administered controls. The peptides were dissolved in corn oil and injected subcutaneously in a volume of 200 μl at noon on the day of proestrus. For evaluation of prolonged action in this system, the peptides were injected on the second day of diestrus. The peptides were also tested for their ability to inhibit LHRH-mediated luteinizing hormone secretion by cultured pituitary cells (Vale and Grant, 1974). Potencies of LHRH antagonists are expressed relative to the standard shown at the top of Tables 2.1 and 2.2. K_D values are a reflection of the peptide's affinity for its receptor. K_Ds of analogs were calculated from displacement data relative to the standard (Perrin *et al.*, 1983). Potencies determined in the tissue culture assay and receptor binding assay may be less influenced by distribution, degradation and elimination processes.

Position 4 substitutions

Table 2.1 lists a series of LHRH antagonists with substitutions for Ser at position 4, while positions 1,2,3 and 6 remain constant (Rivier *et al.*, 1981*d*). The very hydrophobic substituent D-Nal(2) at position 3 and 6 led to a peptide three times more potent than the corresponding standard, [N-Ac-Δ^3-Pro^1,D-pF-Phe^2,D-Trp^{3,6}]LHRH. Backbone modifications, caused by the introduction of the unrestrained glycine residue or highly constrained Pro, decreased potency. The more closely related Ala, which lacks the hydroxyl function of serine, is two to four times less potent than the standard, suggesting that the hydrophilic character of serine is important. The steric aspect at that position is less critical since the more bulky diamino propionic acid (Dap), Orn or even Arg (but not Lys) substitutions are not drastically detrimental. Since the Met analog (isosteric to Orn) in this series is less potent, the role of Ser may be to give the molecule a local hydrophilic character that can be mimicked by an Orn residue. Most noticeable, however, is the drastic negative effect of the introduction of Dap^4 or Orn^4 in one of the most potent analogs reported so far, i.e. [N-Ac-D-Nal(2)^1,D-pF-Phe^2,D-Trp^3,D-Arg^6]LHRH.

Position 5 substitutions

Table 2.2 lists a series of LHRH antagonists with substitutions for Tyr at position 5 of our standard. The first six peptides contain the initial aromatic substitutions suggested for the manual version of the Hansch approach (Topliss, 1977). The order of potency obtained, H=OH > p-Cl=p-Me =pMeO=m, p-Cl_2, in the AOA assay does not correlate with the order (OH > p-MeO > H > p-Cl > m, p-Cl_2 > p-Me) derived from K_D values. Neither result corresponds to that obtained when this approach was applied to D-Phe substitutions in position 2 (Rivier *et al.*, 1981*d*). Although *para* halogen substitutions led to more potent analogs in position 2, *ortho* or *meta* substitution of the aromatic ring is better tolerated in position 5. Steric hindrance resulting from the introduction of two bulky D-Nal(2) residues compared with two D-Trp residues may be responsible for the detrimental effect of both Phe or oF-Phe substitutions in [N-Ac-Δ^3-Pro^1,D-pF-Phe^2,D-Nal(2)^{3,6}]LHRH although the Nal(2) substitutions increased potency in the standard. Interestingly, substitution of oCl-Phe for Tyr in [N-Ac-D-Nal(2)^1,D-pF-Phe^2,D-Trp^3,oCl-Phe^5,D-Arg^6]LHRH is compatible with high potency *in vivo*. Further constraints on the backbone by introduction of an N$^\alpha$-MeLeu^7 ([N-Ac-D-Nal(2)^1, D-pF-Phe^2, D-Trp^3, oCl-Phe^5, D-Arg^6, N$^\alpha$-MeLeu^7]LHRH) results in significant lowering of potencies. Iodination of [N-Ac-D-Nal(2)^1,D-pF-Phe^2,D-Trp^3,D-Arg^6]-LHRH which results in the introduction of a bulky

Table 2.1 Position 4 substitutions

Compound	K_D[a] (nM)	*Potency* in vitro	*Antiovulatory assay* *Dose* (μg)	*% Inhibition*
[N-Ac-Δ^3-Pro^1,D-pF-Phe^2,D-Trp^{3,6}]LHRH	0.13	1.0	7.5	100
[N-Ac-Δ^3-Pro^1,D-pF-Phe^2,D-Nal(2)^{3,6}]LHRH	0.72	2.3	2.5	100
[N-Ac-Δ^3-Pro^1,D-pF-Phe^2,D-Nal(2)^{3,6},Gly^4]LHRH	2.8	0.64	10	70
[N-Ac-Δ^3-Pro^1,D-pF-Phe^2,D-Nal(2)^{3,6},Ala^4]LHRH	1.6	1.03	10	90
[N-Ac-Δ^3-Pro^1,D-pF-Phe^2,D-Nal(2)^{3,6},Met^4]LHRH	2.4	0.78	10	40
[N-Ac-Δ^3-Pro^1,D-pF-Phe^2,D-Nal(2)^{3,6},Orn^4]LHRH	1.3	0.29	1	20
[N-Ac-Δ^3-Pro^1,D-pF-Phe^2,D-Nal(2)^{3,6},Dap^4]LHRH	–	–	2.5	0
[N-Ac-Δ^3-Pro^1,D-pF-Phe^2,D-Nal(2)^{3,6},Lys^4]LHRH	3.2	–	10	20
[N-Ac-Δ^3-Pro^1,D-pF-Phe^2,D-Nal(2)^{3,6},Arg^4]LHRH	3.4	–	5	100
[N-Ac-Δ^3-Pro^1,D-pF-Phe^2,D-Trp^{3,6},Pro^4]LHRH	25	0.01	15	10
[N-Ac-D-Nal(2)^1,D-pF-Phe^2,D-Trp^3,Dap^4,D-Arg^6]LHRH	9.6	–	2.5	0
[N-Ac-D-Nal(2)^1,D-pF-Phe^2,D-Trp^3,Orn^4,D-Arg^6]LHRH	76	–	25	10

[a] K_D for [D-Ala^6,N$^\alpha$MeLeu^7,Pro^9-NHEt]LHRH (standard) (Scatchard analysis) is 0.3 nmol/l

Table 2.2 Position 5 substitutions

Compound	K_D[a] (nM)	*Potency* in vitro	*Antiovulatory assay*	
			Dose (μg)	*% Inhibition*
[N-Ac-Δ^3-Pro^1,D-pF-Phe^2,D-Trp^{3,6}]LHRH	0.13	1.00	7.5	100
[N-Ac-Δ^3-Pro^1,D-pF-Phe^2,D-Trp^{3,6},Phe^5]LHRH	0.48	0.77	5	70
[N-Ac-Δ^3-Pro^1,D-pF-Phe^2,D-Trp^{3,6},pCl-Phe^5]LHRH	0.57	0.27	10	20
[N-Ac-Δ^3-Pro^1,D-pF-Phe^2,D-Trp^{3,6},pMe-Phe^5]LHRH	2.3	0.22	10	20
[N-Ac-Δ^3-Pro^1,D-pF-Phe^2,D-Trp^{3,6},pMeO-Phe^5]LHRH	0.35	0.21	10	20
[N-Ac-Δ^3-Pro^1,D-pF-Phe^2,D-Trp^{3,6},mpCl$_2$-Phe^5]LHRH	1.3	1.46	20	20
[N-Ac-Δ^3-Pro^1,D-pF-Phe^2,D-Trp^{3,6},pF-Phe^5]LHRH	0.7	0.9	25	80
[N-Ac-Δ^3-Pro^1,D-pF-Phe^2,D-Trp^{3,6},mF-Phe^5]LHRH	0.4	0.45	5	90
[N-Ac-Δ^3-Pro^1,D-pF-Phe^2,D-Trp^{3,6},mCl-Phe^5]LHRH	0.32	1.02	5	70
[N-Ac-Δ^3-Pro^1,D-pF-Phe^2,D-Trp^{3,6},oF-Phe^5]LHRH	0.4	1.9	5	80
[N-Ac-Δ^3-Pro^1,D-pF-Phe^2,D-Trp^{3,6},oCl-Phe^5]LHRH	1.7	1.15	2.5	50
[N-Ac-Δ^3-Pro^1,D-pF-Phe^2,D-Nal(2)^{3,6}]LHRH	0.72	2.3	2.5	100
[N-Ac-Δ^3-Pro^1,D-pF-Phe^2,D-Nal(2)^{3,6},Phe^5]LHRH	6.8	0.82	7.5	60
[N-Ac-Δ^3-Pro^1,D-pF-Phe^2,D-Nal(2)^{3,6},oF-Phe^5]LHRH	3.2	–	15	30
[N-Ac-D-Nal(2)^1,D-pF-Phe^2,D-Trp^3,D-Arg^6]LHRH	0.57	0.50	0.5	62
[N-Ac-D-Nal(2)^1,D-pF-Phe^2,D-Trp^3,Phe^5,D-Arg^6]LHRH	1.2	–	1	67
[N-Ac-D-Nal(2)^1,D-pF-Phe^2,D-Trp^3,oCl-Phe^5,D-Arg^6]LHRH	1.6	0.51	0.5	50
[N-Ac-D-Nal(2)^1,D-pF-Phe^2,D-Trp^3,mF-Phe^5,D-Arg^6]LHRH	1.5	–	1	14

[a] See Table 2.1

iodine atom on the Tyr[5] in the *meta* position gave a potent analog. It is very fortunate since it can easily be generated with ^{125}I from the parent compound and can be used as a tracer in a multitude of assays.

Position 6 substitutions

Table 2.3 shows the results of replacement of Gly at position 6. The increased potency which resulted from substitution of the two D-Trp residues in our standard antagonist by the more hydrophobic D-Nal(2) residues led us to investigate the effect of introducing D-Me_5-Phe and D-pMe-Phe at the six positions. These two analogs have potencies that are intermediate between those of the D-Trp and D-Nal(2) substitutions at position 6.

While we were investigating the binding affinity of [N-Ac-Δ^3-Pro^1,D-pF-Phe^2,D-Trp^3,D-Lys^6]LHRH we were surprised to find out that it had a very high affinity for the LHRH receptor in several systems (Perrin *et al.*, 1983). Antagonists containing the hydrophilic D-Arg at position 6 and modified at the N-terminus by D-pCl-Phe^1 (i.e. [N-Ac-D-pCl-Phe^1,D-pCl-Phe^2,D-Trp^3,D-Arg^6]LHRH) have even more powerful antiovulatory activity (Coy *et al.*, 1982). Introduction of D-Arg at position 6 of our standard (i.e. [N-Ac-Δ^3-Pro^1,D-pF-Phe^2,D-Trp^3,D-Arg^6]LHRH) showed decreased potency. High potency could be restored and enhanced by the introduction at position 1 of a very hydrophobic residue (i.e. [N-Ac-D-Nal(2)^1,D-pF-Phe^2,D-Trp^3,D-Arg^6]LHRH). However N-Ac-D-Nal(1) and N-Ac-L-Nal(2) in the equivalent analog gave a less potent antagonist (Tables 2.3 and 2.4). It is apparent that, as a general concept, the receptor will tolerate either hydrophobic or hydrophilic residues at position 6 as long as they are concomitantly paired with a hydrophilic (N-Ac-Δ^3-Pro) or hydrophobic (N-Ac-D-Nal(2)) residue, respectively, at position 1. We are investigating the validity of this approach by substituting pairs of amino acid previously suggested to be in close proximity in the active conformation on the receptor.

Physicochemical studies on LHRH which were directed toward the elucidation of a putative tertiary conformation in solution have been reviewed by Donzel *et al.* (1977), who used intramolecular charge transfer complexes to support theoretical predictions of a stable type IIβ-bend. It is only with the introduction by Freidinger *et al.* (1980) of a fixed lactam ring at position 6 that additional support for a bioactive conformation containing a 'Tyr–Gly–Leu–Arg' type II′ β-turn was provided. Another type of constraint and peptide backbone can be brought about by cyclization. The synthesis of bioactive cyclic LHRH analogs (Seprodi *et al.*, 1978; Rivier *et al.*, 1980) suggests that the receptor bound LHRH or its analogs assume a folded conformation that brings N- and C-termini in close proximity (Grant and Vale, 1972).

Other D- basic amino acids that were introduced at the 6 position include D-pNH_2-Phe and D-His(Bzl). The more basic side chain substituents in position 6 result in more potent analogs (Table 2.3). This observation was also reported for the analogs having D-pCl-Phe substitutions at positions 1 and 2 (Coy *et al.*, 1982).

Table 2.3 Position 6 substitutions

Compound	K_D[a] (nM)	*Potency* in vitro	*Antiovulatory assay* *Dose* (μg)	*Antiovulatory assay* *% Inhibition*
[N-Ac-Δ^3-Pro^1,D-pF-Phe^2,D-Trp^3,D-Trp^6]LHRH	0.13	1.00	7.5	100
[N-Ac-Δ^3-Pro^1,D-pCl-pF-Phe^2,D-Trp^3,D-Me$_5$-Phe^6]LHRH	5.3	0.50	10	100
[N-Ac-Δ^3-Pro^1,D-pF-Phe^2,D-Trp^3,D-pMe-Phe^6]LHRH	0.89	0.67	2.5	40
[N-Ac-Δ^3-Pro^1,D-pF-Phe^2,D-Trp^3,D-Lys^6]LHRH	0.2	0.07	–	–
[N-Ac-Δ^3-Pro^1,D-pF-Phe^2,D-Trp^3,D-Arg^6]LHRH	0.31	0.06	20	60
[N-Ac-Δ^3-Pro^1,D-pF-Phe^2,D-Trp^3,D-pNH$_2$-Phe^6]LHRH	0.21	0.46	5	50
[N-Ac-D-Nal(2)^1,D-pF-Phe^2,D-Trp^3,D-Arg^6]LHRH	0.57	0.44	0.5	62
[N-Ac-D-Nal(2)^1,D-pF-Phe^2,D-Trp^3,D-Arg^6-N-MeLeu^7]LHRH	1.0	–	1	87
[N-Ac-D-Nal(2)^1,D-pCl-Phe^2,D-Trp^3,D-Arg^6]LHRH	0.8	–	0.5	60
[N-Ac-D-Nal(2)^1,D-pF-Phe^2,D-Trp^3,D-pNH$_2$-Phe^6]LHRH	0.25	1.37	5	50
[N-Ac-D-Nal(2)^1,D-pF-Phe^2,D-Trp^3,D-His^6(Bzl)]LHRH	1.7	0.55	10	0
[N-Ac-Δ^3-Pro^1,D-pF-Phe^2,D-5Br-Trp^{3,6}]LHRH	0.48	1.40	5	62

[a] See Table 2.1

Table 2.4 Multiple substitutions

Compound	K_D[a]	*Potency* in vitro	*Antiovulatory assay* *Dose* (μg)	*% Inhibition*
[N-Ac-D-Phe^1,D-pF-Phe^2,D-Trp^3,D-Arg^6,Pro^9-NHEt]LHRH	0.38	0.073	10	90
[N-Ac-D-Nal(2)^1,D-pF-Phe^2,D-Trp^3,D-Arg^6,Pro^9-NHEt]LHRH	0.32	0.44	5	67
[N-Ac-D-Nal(2)^1,D-pCl-Phe^2,D-Trp^3,D-Arg^6,Pro^9-NHEt]LHRH	–	0.38	1	50
[N-Ac-D-Nal(2)^1,D-pBr-Phe^2,D-Trp^3,D-Arg^6,Pro^9-NHEt]LHRH	–	0.46	2.5	10
[N-Ac-D-Nal(2)^1,D-pNO_2-Phe^2,D-Trp^3,D-Arg^6,Pro^9-NHEt]LHRH	–	0.20	5	60
[N-Ac-D-Nal(1)^1,D-pF-Phe^2,D-Trp^3,D-Arg^6,Pro^9-NHEt]LHRH	–	0.02	25	0
[N-Ac-D-Nal(2)^1,D-pF-Phe^2,D-Trp^3,D-Nal(2)^6,Pro^9-NHEt]LHRH	–	0.30	25	0
[N-Ac-D-Nal(2)^1,D-pF-Phe^2,D-Trp^3,D-Arg^6,Sar^{10}]LHRH	–	–	10	60
[N-Ac-D-Nal(2)^1,D-pF-Phe^2,D-Trp^3,D-Arg^6,D-Ala^{10}]LHRH	–	0.63	1	90

[a] See Table 2.1

Multiple substitutions

From the data reported in Table 2.4 we can conclude that introduction of the Pro^9-NHEt modification results in a slight, but significant, decrease in potency. The substitution at position 1 by the D-Nal(1) versus D-Nal(2) results in a considerable loss of potency, an observation also made by Horvath *et al.* (1982). The most drastic and negative effect is, however, observed when D-$Nal(2)^6$ substitutes D-Arg^6 in the very hydrophobic analog [N-Ac-D-$Nal(2)^1$,D-pF-Phe^2,D-Trp^3,D-$Nal(2)^6$,Pro^9-NHEt]LHRH.

DURATION OF ACTION

Data presented in Table 2.5 address the duration of action of two selected antagonists in the ovulation test. A 20- to 100-fold increase in dose is necessary to block ovulation when subcutaneous injection is done on diestrus II instead of proestrus. The need for a higher dose is not surprising since the peptide must be present for a period greater than 24 hours in order to inhibit the gonadotropin surge on the afternoon of proestrus. The effect of the diluent on biological potency does not seem to be significant in the case of [N-Ac-D-$Nal(2)^1$,D-pF-Phe^2,D-Trp^3,D-Arg^6]LHRH.

Table 2.5 Duration of action – antiovulatory assay

Compound	*Vehicle*	*Dose* (μg)	*Time*	*% Inhibition*
[N-Ac-Δ^3-Pro^1,D-pF-Phe^2,D-$Trp^{3,6}$]LHRH	corn oil	5	Pro	75
		7.5	Pro	100
		100	Di-2	71
		1000	Di-2	100
[N-Ac-D-$Nal(2)^1$,D-pF-Phe^2,D-Trp^3,D-Arg^6] LHRH	corn oil	0.5	Pro	82
		1.0	Pro	100
		10	Di-2	67
		100	Di-2	100
	Bacterio-	0.5	Pro	83
	static	1.0	Pro	100
	water	100	Di-2	100

ORAL ACTIVITY

Oral administration would be more acceptable for human use than daily or long-lasting depot injections. Complete inhibition of ovulation is achieved by administering 2.5 mg per rat of [N-Ac-D-$Nal(2)^1$,D-pF-Phe^2,D-Trp^3,D-Arg^6]LHRH by gavage, whereas 0.5 mg achieves partial blockade. Rats that ovulated at the lower dose were shown to have high plasma levels of LH

(12.5 ng/ml ± 1.9) (Rivier *et al.*, 1983*a,b*) in blood samples taken at 4:30 p.m. on the day of administration.

On the basis of the data obtained for this peptide after subcutaneous injection (Table 2.2), less than 1 % of the peptide enters the general circulation after oral administration. Degradative processes or poor adsorption may be responsible for this low efficacy. Similar data reported for [N-Ac-D-pCl-Phe^1,D-pCl-Phe^2,D-Trp^3,D-Arg^6,D-Ala^{10}]LHRH suggest that absorption by the gut may not be dependent on the peptide's structure (Nekola *et al.*, 1982). The administration of peptides, including LHRH agonists, by nasal spray also requires higher doses than injection (1–3 % of drug absorbed).

CONCLUDING REMARKS

A greater than 10 000-fold increase in biological potency has been achieved for LHRH antagonists over the past 10 years. Even more potent analogs can be anticipated, thus compensating for the inefficiency of the routes of administration presently available. The need for better ways to administer peptides is strongly felt and progress in the area of design of drug delivery systems is forthcoming. Demonstration, however, that these peptides can be effective under different modes of administration for contraceptive and therapeutic purposes, is the best incentive for further studies. New amino acids are therefore being synthesized. New hypotheses on the tertiary structure of the active conformer are generated *de novo* from molecular dynamic studies or through the analysis of structure activity relationships. There is strong evidence that LHRH and its antagonists interact with the receptor in a conformation that brings both N- and C-termini in close proximity. The next generation of LHRH analogs may well have a restricted conformation (possibly cyclic) that should render them enzymatically more stable.

Acknowledgements

This study was supported by NIH Grants HD-13527 and NO1-HD-0-2836, The Rockefeller Foundation, The Texas–Salk Institute Foundation, and The March of Dimes–Birth Defects Foundation. Research was conducted in part by The Clayton Foundation for Research, California Division. Drs C. Rivier, M. Perrin and W. Vale are Clayton Foundation Investigators. Most anti-ovulatory data were supplied by Drs R. Naqvi and C. Lindberg of The Mason Research Institute under contract NO1-HD-0-2846 with the Contraceptive Development Branch, NICHHD. The excellent technical assistance of S. Quijada, N. Keating, R. Kaiser, R. Galyean. R. McClintock, M. Newberry, A. Corrigan, G. Yamamoto, Y. Haas and P. Hernandez is acknowledged. L. Wheatley and D. Weigand are thanked for manuscript preparation.

References

Barany, G. and Merrifield, R. B. (1980). Solid-phase peptide synthesis. In Gross, E. and Meienhofer, J. (eds.) *The Peptides*. Vol. 2, pp. 1–284. (New York: Academic Press)

Corbin, A. and Beattie, C. W. (1975). Inhibition of the pre-ovulatory proestrus gonadotropin surge, ovulation and pregnancy with a peptide analogue of luteinizing hormone releasing hormone. *Endocr. Res. Commun.*, **2**, 1

Coy, D. H., Horvath, A., Nekola, M. V., Coy, E. J., Erchegyi, J. and Schally, A. V. (1982). Peptide antagonists of LH-RH: Large increases in antiovulatory activities produced by basic D-amino acids in the six position. *Endocrinology*, **110**, 1445

Donzel, B., Rivier, J. and Goodman, R. (1977). Study of the secondary structure of the luteinizing hormone releasing factor using intramolecular charge transfer complexes. *Biochemistry*, **16**, 2611

Dunlap, C. E. III, Gentleman, S. and Lowney, L. I. (1978). Use of trifluoroacetic acid in the separation of opiates and opioid peptides by reversed-phase high-performance liquid chromatography. *J. Chromatogr.*, **160**, 191

Freidinger, R. M., Veber, D. F. and Perlow, D. S. (1980). Bioactive conformation of luteinizing hormone-releasing hormone: Evidence from a conformationally constrained analog. *Science*, **210**, 656

Grant, G. and Vale, W. (1972). Speculations on structural relationships between the hypothalamic releasing factors of pituitary hormones. *Nature* (*Lond.*), **237**, 182

Horvath, A., Coy, D. H., Nekola, M. V., Coy, E. J., Schally, A. V. and Teplan, I. (1982). Synthesis and biological activity of LH-RH antagonists modified in position 1. *Peptides*, **3**, 969

Nekola, M. V., Horvath, A., Ge, L.-J., Coy, D. H. and Schally, A. V. (1982). Suppression of ovulation in the rat by an orally active antagonist of luteinizing hormone-releasing hormone. *Science*, **218**, 160

Perrin, M. H., Haas, Y., Rivier, J. E. and Vale, W. W. (1983). Gonadotropin-releasing hormone binding to rat anterior pituitary membrane homogenates: comparison of antagonists and agonists using radiolabeled antagonist and agonist. *Mol. Pharmacol.*, **23**, 44

Rivier, J., Vale, W., Burgus, R., Ling, N., Amoss, M., Blackwell, R. and Guillemin, R. (1973). Synthetic luteinizing hormone releasing factor analogs. Series of short chain amide LRF homologs converging to the amino terminus. *J. Med. Chem.*, **16**, 545

Rivier, J. (1978). Use of trialkyl ammonium phosphate (TAAP) buffers in reverse phase HPLC for high resolution and high recovery of peptides and proteins. *J. Liq. Chromatogr.*, **1**, 343

Rivier, C., Rivier, J. and Vale, W. (1978). Chronic effects of [DTrp^6-Pro^9-NEt] luteinizing hormone-releasing factor on reproductive processes in the female rat. *Endocrinology*, **103**, 2299

Rivier, C., Rivier, J. and Vale, W. (1979). Chronic effects of [DTrp^6,Pro^9-NEt]-LRF on reproductive processes in the male rat. *Endocrinology*, **105**, 1191

Rivier, C. and Vale, W. (1979). Hormonal secretion in male rats chronically treated with [DTrp^6,Pro^9-NEt]-LRF. *Life Sci.*, **25**, 1065.

Rivier, C., Rivier, J. and Vale, W. (1980). Anti-reproductive effects of potent GnRH antagonist in the male rat. *Science*, **210**, 93

Rivier, C., Rivier, J. and Vale, W. (1981*a*). GnRH antagonists: Physiologic and contraceptive applications in the female rat. In Zatuchni, G. I., Shelton, J. D. and Sciarra, J. J. (eds.) *LHRH Peptides as Female and Male Contraceptives*, pp. 140–150. (Philadelphia: Harper & Row)

Rivier, C., Rivier, J. and Vale, W. (1981*b*). Anti-reproductive effects of a potent GnRH antagonist in the female rat. *Endocrinology*, **108**, 1425

Rivier, C., Rivier, J. and Vale, W. (1981*c*). Effect of a potent GnRH antagonist and testosterone propionate on mating behavior and fertility in the male rat. *Endocrinology*, **108**, 1998

Rivier, J., Rivier, C., Perrin, M., Porter, J. and Vale, W. (1981*d*). GnRH analogs: Structure–activity relationships. In Zatuchni, G. I., Shelton, J. D. and Sciarra, J. J. (eds.) *LHRH Peptides as Female and Male Contraceptives*, pp. 13–23. (Philadelphia: Harper & Row)

Rivier, C. and Vale, W. (1981*a*). Temporal relationship between the abortifacient effects of GnRH antagonists and hormonal secretion. *Biol. Reprod.*, **24**, 1061

Rivier, C. and Vale, W. (1981*b*). Interaction of GnRH agonists, pituitary hormones and corticosteroids on progesterone secretion in the male rat. *Life Sci.*, **29**, 1523

Rivier, C. and Vale, W. (1982). Interaction of GnRH agonist and antagonist with progesterone. PRL or hCG during pregnancy in the rat. *Endocrinology*, **110**, 347

Rivier, C., Rivier, J., Perrin, M. and Vale, W. (1983*a*). Comparison of the effect of several GnRH antagonists on LH secretion, receptor binding and ovulation. *Biol. Reprod.*, **29**, 374

Rivier, C., Vale, W. and Rivier, J. (1983*b*). Effects of gonadotropin releasing hormone/agonists and antagonists on reproductive function. *J. Med. Chem.*, **26**, 1545

Rivier, J., Spiess, J., Thorner, M. and Vale, W. (1982*b*). Characterization of a growth hormone releasing factor from a human pancreatic islet tumor. *Nature* (*Lond.*), **300,** 276

Rivier, J., Rivier, C., Spiess, J. and Vale, W. (1982*c*). High-performance liquid chromatographic purification of peptide hormone: Ovine hypothalamic amunine (corticotropin releasing factor). *Anal. Biochem.*, **127,** 258

Seprodi, J., Coy, D. H., Vilchez-Martinez, J. A., Pedroza, E., Huang, W.-Y. and Schally, A. V. (1978). Cyclic analogues of luteinizing hormone-releasing hormone with significant biological activites. *J. Med. Chem.*, **21,** 993

Topliss, J. G. (1977). A manual method for applying the Hansch approach to drug design. *J. Med. Chem.*, **20,** 463

Vale, W. and Grant, G. (1974). In vitro pituitary hormone secretion for hypophysiotropic substances. In O'Malley, B. W. and Hardman, J. G. (eds.) *Methods in Enzymology, Hormones and Cyclic Nucleotides.* Vol. 37, pp. 82–93. (New York: Academic Press)

Vale, W., Rivier, C., Perrin, M. and Rivier, J. (1979). LRF agonists and fertility regulation in the male. In Gross, E. and Meienhofer, J. (eds.) *Peptides: Structure and Biological Function,* pp. 781–793. (Rockford, IL: Pierce Chem. Co.)

3
LHRH agonists and antagonists containing very hydrophobic amino acids

J. J. NESTOR Jr., T. L. HO, R. TAHILRAMANI, B. L. HORNER, R. A. SIMPSON, G. H. JONES, G. I. McRAE and B. H. VICKERY

LHRH agonists with potencies greater than 200 times that of the native hormone have resulted from structure/activity studies in many laboratories (see Chapter 1; Rivier *et al.*, 1975; Schally *et al.*, 1981). The ability of these agents to cause desensitization of target cells in the pituitary (Sandow *et al.*, 1978) and gonads (Hsueh and Erickson, 1979) upon prolonged treatment has caused increased interest in their potential as contraceptive and as anti-steroidal therapeutic agents (Corbin and Beattie, 1975; Vickery, 1981). The most potent agonists can block estrous cyclicity in the rat with doses less than 0.1 μg twice daily (Nestor *et al.*, 1982*a*).

Structure/activity studies in the LHRH antagonist field have resulted in a stepwise decrease in the effective antiovulatory dose in the rat from the multimilligram range to the nanogram range. The most potent LHRH antagonists now have binding affinities for the pituitary LHRH receptor which are substantially greater than that of LHRH itself (Perrin *et al.*, 1980, 1983).

Hydrophobic amino acid substitutions in LHRH analogs have resulted in major potency increases in both the agonist and antagonist fields. This chapter describes the synthesis of highly potent LHRH agonists and antagonists using very hydrophobic, unnatural amino acid substitutions.

LHRH AGONISTS

The primary sites for successful substitutions in the LHRH structure are at positions 3, 6, 7 and 10. The substitution of D-amino acids for the Gly residue in position 6 (Monahan *et al.*, 1973) gave an up to fortyfold increase in agonistic potency, with hydrophobic amino acids yielding the most active analogs. D-Trp in position 6 was the most effective substitution by a natural amino acid (Rivier *et al.*, 1977; Coy *et al.*, 1976). Substitution of N-MeLeu at position 7 gave a small increase in potency and increased resistance to enzymatic degradation (Ling and Vale, 1975). Replacement of the Gly residue in position 10 by NHEt (Fujino *et al.*, 1972), $NHCH_2CF_3$ (Coy *et al.*, 1975), or aza-Gly (Dutta *et al.*, 1978) yielded significantly more potent agonistic analogs. The replacement of the Trp residue in position 3 by 3-(1-naphthyl)alanine (Nal(1)), but not by 3-(2-naphthyl)alanine (Nal(2)) led to a doubling of agonistic potency relative to LHRH (Yabe *et al.*, 1976; Prasad *et al.*, 1976). The combination of substitutions at positions 6, 7 and 10 had cumulative effects on potency (Rivier *et al.*, 1975).

Hydrophobic agonists

Increased hydrophobicity at position 6 appeared to be responsible for higher biological potency. This could be due to increased receptor binding affinity, decreased enzymatic degradation, or both. The hydrophobicity of the amino acid side chain in this position therefore was substantially increased by incorporating very hydrophobic, unnatural D-amino acids. The most effective hydrophobic amino acid substitutions at position 6 also were combined with the modifications at positions 3, 7 and 10 described above.

More hydrophobic analogs could be expected to have a prolonged biological half-life, based on the hypothesis that the whole body could act as a depot due to binding of hydrophobic analogs to tissue membranes or hydrophobic plasma carrier proteins, with a later release of the analog to the circulation. Therefore, the normally rapid clearance which is seen after bolus administration of a polypeptide would be circumvented. Such analogs also should exhibit the favorable characteristic of slow release from hydrophobic depot formulations.

The 15 unnatural amino acids incorporated in position 6 have a range of structural types and varied hydrophobicities (Nestor *et al.*, 1982). Several of the analogs are arranged in Table 3.1 in order of increasing hydrophobicity, as represented by their k′ values ($k' = [{}^{t}retention - {}^{t}unretained]/{}^{t}unretained$) from reversed-phase high performance liquid chromatography (HPLC). The analogs were studied in a 2 week estrus suppression assay designed to show their paradoxical antifertility effects during chronic administration (Nestor *et al.*, 1982). The biological potencies were calculated relative to [D-Trp^6, Pro^9-NHEt]LHRH which has a potency 100 times that of LHRH. The structures of the D-amino acids range from the hydrophilic 3-(3,4,5-trimethoxyphenyl)alanine (Tmo), to the hydrophobic 3-(2-naphthyl)alanine [Nal(2)] and 3-(2,4,6-trimethylphenyl)alanine (Tmp), to the exceedingly hydrophobic 3-(dicyclohexylmethyl)Ala (Dca). Preliminary studies correlating biological potency with retention time in HPLC indicated that increased hydrophobicity led to higher potency (Rivier *et al.*, 1977), but more detailed studies did not uphold this interpretation (Rivier *et al.*, 1981*a*). However, a quantitative structure–activity relationship (QSAR) was reported between agonistic potency and the hydrophobicity (calculated from fragmental constants) of the side chain of the D-amino acid in position 6 for a series of monosubstituted LHRH analogs (Nadasdi and Medzihradszky, 1981). This

Table 3.1 LHRH analogs – estrus suppression activity[a]

Analog	*HPLC, k′*	*ED_{50} (μg/inj)*	*Potency*
[D-Tmo^6]LHRH	0.59	0.09	1.4
[D-Trp^6,Pro^9-NHEt]LHRH	1.29	0.13	1.0[b] (standard)
[D-Cha^6]LHRH	1.45	0.20	0.6
[D-Pfp^6]LHRH	1.73	0.12	1.1
[D-Nal(1)^6]LHRH	1.91	0.26	0.5
[D-Nal(2)^6]LHRH	1.95	0.07	1.9
[D-Mtf^6]LHRH	2.05	0.13	1.0
[D-Ptf^6]LHRH	2.14	0.11	1.2
[D-Tmp^6]LHRH	2.18	0.07	1.9
[D-Nal(2)^6,Pro^9-NHEt]LHRH	3.55	0.16	0.8
[D-Nal(2)^6,N-MeLeu^7]LHRH	3.73	0.08	1.6
[D-Tmp^6,N-MeLeu^7]LHRH	5.13	0.35	1.1
[D-Dca^6]LHRH	26.27	0.14	0.9

[a] Nestor *et al.*, 1982*a* [b] Potency of standard = 100 × LHRH

QSAR relationship also indicated that analogs more hydrophobic than those studied should be more potent.

The *in vivo* biological potencies for the very hydrophobic analogs described here, however, do not follow the strict correlation found with the more hydrophilic agonist analogs. For example, although [D-Tmo^6]LHRH has a k′ one-half that of [D-Trp^6, Pro^9-NHEt]LHRH, it has a relative potency of 1.4. The analog pair [D-Nal(1)^6]LHRH/[D-Nal(2)^6]LHRH also illustrates the inadequacy of using hydrophobicity alone as a prediction of potency. These analogs are isolipophilic, but there is a fourfold difference in relative potency (Table 3.1). A correlation of biological activity with hydrophobicity usually exhibits a parabolic relationship, with a sharp drop in potency as optimum hydrophobicity is exceeded (Hansch *et al.*, 1967). However, the most hydrophobic compound in this series, [D-Dca^6]LHRH, is as active as the standard, but has a more than tenfold larger k′.

Two substitutions which resulted in the highest potency analogs ([D-Nal(2)^6]LHRH and [D-Tmp^6]LHRH) were combined with the modifications which were previously shown to give multiplicative effects in the less hydrophobic analog series. The Pro^9-NHEt modification led to a potency decrease in [D-Nal(2)^6, Pro^9-NHEt]LHRH (Table 3.1). The N-Me Leu substitution had little effect on potency when combined with Nal(2) in [D-Nal(2)^6,N-MeLeu^7]LHRH but caused a decrease in potency in combination with a more sterically hindered amino acid ([D-Tmp^6,N-MeLeu^7]LHRH).

Heteroaromatic agonists

A new class of heteroaromatic amino acids was synthesized and incorporated into LHRH analogs (Nestor *et al.*, 1984). The novel amino acid structures

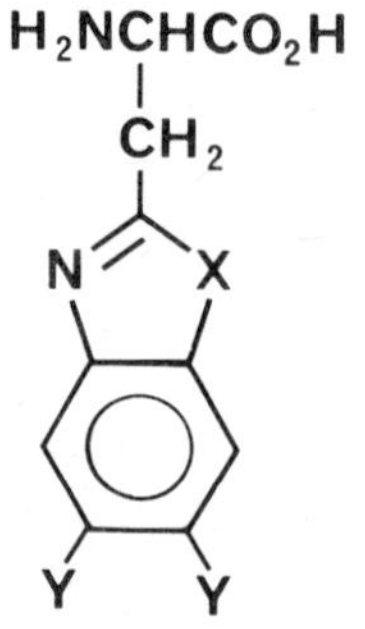

X = NH	; Y = H	Bia
	; Y = CH_3	Dmb
	; Y = Cl	Dcb
X = O	; Y = H	Boa
X = S	; Y = H	Bta

Figure 3.1 Heteroaromatic amino acid structures and abbreviations.

were prepared by chiral synthesis from D-aspartic acid and various *o*-substituted anilines. This led to a structurally homologous series of heteroaromatic amino acids (Figure 3.1) with a range of hydrophobicity and basicity but a steric bulk similar to Trp.

When incorporated into the 6 position of LHRH, these amino acids also gave an extremely potent series of agonistic analogs (Table 3.2). The most potent compounds in this series, [D-Tba^6,Pro^9-NHEt]LHRH and [D-Bia^6,Pro^9-NHEt]LHRH, were both less hydrophobic than the standard, [D-Trp^6,Pro^9-NHEt]LHRH. Moreover, the less hydrophobic of the pair ([D-Tba^6,Pro^9-NHEt]LHRH) was more potent than [D-Trp^6,Pro^9-NHEt]-LHRH. The dialkylimidazole side chain of this amino acid may have a protonated side chain at physiological pH and the enhanced potency of this compound may be related to the positive charge in this position. Similarly, a positively charged residue in position 6 gave increased LHRH antagonistic potency in another study (Coy *et al.*, 1982).

Aza-Gly analogs

One of the most useful substitutions in position 10 has been the aza-Gly residue. When the Pro^9-NHEt C-terminus of buserelin was substituted by an

Table 3.2 Heteroaromatic amino acid substitutions – estrus suppression activity[a]

Analog	*HPLC, k'*	*ED$_{50}$* (*μg/inj*)	*Potency*[b]
[D-Boa^6]LHRH	0.71	0.22	0.6
[D-Bta^6]LHRH	0.83	0.16	0.8
[D-Tba^6,Pro^9-NHEt]LHRH		0.10	1.3
[D-Bia^6,Pro^9-NHEt]LHRH	0.92	0.14	0.9
[D-Dmb^6]LHRH	0.96	0.20	0.6
[D-Dcb^6]LHRH	1.38	0.46	0.3

[a] Nestor *et al.*, 1984*b*

[b] Calculated relative to [D-Trp^6,Pro^9-NHEt]LHRH (potency = 1)

aza-Gly residue, the resultant analog ([D-Ser(tBu)^6,aza-Gly^{10}]LHRH, ICI 118630) was sevenfold more potent than the parent compound in an ovulation induction assay (Dutta *et al.*, 1978).

Those 6-position substituents conferring greatest potency were combined with the aza-Gly residue (Ho *et al.*, 1984). This hydrophilic 10-position substitution yields more potent analogs (Table 3.3) for the more hydrophobic 6-position substituents (Dmb, Nal(2)). For the more hydrophilic Bia substitution, a slight decrease in potency is observed. The most potent LHRH agonist reported (approximately 230 times the potency of LHRH) is [D-Nal(2)^6,aza-Gly^{10}]LHRH (Ho *et al.*, 1984).

The aza-Gly substitution may give increased potency by protecting against post-proline cleaving enzyme (Horsthemke *et al.*, 1981). The importance of this type of protection for human therapy may be overestimated, however, since it is known that the activity of this enzyme in humans is approximately one fifth that in rats (Benuck and Marks, 1976).

Table 3.3 Aza-Gly containing LHRH agonists – estrus suppression

Analog[a]	*HPLC, k′*	*ED_{50} (μg/inj)*	*Potency*[b]
[D-Bia^6,aza-Gly^{10}]LHRH	0.28	0.42	0.4
[D-Dmb^6,aza-Gly^{10}]LHRH	0.74	0.09	1.9
[D-Nal(2)^6,aza-Gly^{10}]LHRH	1.78	0.06	2.3

[a] Ho *et al.*, 1984
[b] Calculated relative to [D-Trp^6,Pro^9-NHEt]LHRH (potency = 1)

Metabolism

The biological half-life of LHRH agonists has been lengthened by increasing their hydrophobicity. This approach led to compounds which are amongst the most potent LHRH agonists yet reported, with *in vivo* potencies 200–230 times greater than that of LHRH. The extended biological half-life of [D-Nal(2)^6]LHRH, one of the most potent analogs, has been reported (Anik *et al.*, 1984). Women were treated subcutaneously with 5 μg or intranasally with 500 μg of [D-Nal(2)^6]LHRH. The metabolic clearance phase of the plasma decay curve indicated a biological half-life of 2 h for [D-Nal(2)^6]LHRH. The half-life for LHRH under similar conditions is 5–6 min.

LHRH ANTAGONISTS

Another approach to the regulation of reproductive functions is the use of competitive antagonists of LHRH. Initial successes in the search for antagonistic analogs of LHRH were reported quite soon after the structure of LHRH was disclosed (Monahan *et al.*, 1972, 1973). The development of potent LHRH antagonists followed a stepwise pattern of substitution similar to that in the agonist series (Schally *et al.*, 1981).

Hydrophobic antagonists

The necessity that LHRH antagonists be present continuously to block the binding of LHRH to receptors makes good pharmacokinetics essential. Our successful design of very hydrophobic agonistic analogs of LHRH with increased potency and biological half-life led to a similar approach with LHRH antagonists.

The initial series which served as a probe for this type of modification was: [D-Phe^2,D-Nal(2)^6]LHRH; [D-Phe^2,D-Trp^3,D-Nal(2)^6]LHRH; [D-Phe^2, D-Nal(2)^{3,6}]LHRH; [N-Ac-Pro^1,D-Phe^2,D-Trp^3,D-Nal(2)^6]LHRH; [N-Ac-Pro^1,D-pCl-Phe^2,D-Nal(2)^{3,6}]LHRH; [N-Ac-Pro^1,D-pF-Phe^2,D-Nal(2)^{3,6}] LHRH (Nestor *et al.*, 1983, 1984). The latter two analogs were the most potent antagonists (Table 3.4).

The substitution of positions 3 and 6 by D-Nal(2) confers extremely high potency. In addition, the N-Ac-Pro modification is consistent with very high potency, as was found in a different analog series (Humphries *et al.*, 1978). The potency difference between [N-Ac-Pro^1,D-pF-Phe^2,D-Nal(2)^{3,6}]LHRH and [N-Ac-Δ^3-Pro^1, D-pF-Phe^2, D-Nal(2)^{3,6}] LHRH (Rivier *et al.*, 1981*a*) is not statistically significant in these studies and the N-Ac-Δ^3-Pro substitution offers no advantage over the less expensive and simpler N-Ac-Pro modification.

The delivery vehicle used may affect the potency of antagonists. Studies

Table 3.4 LHRH antagonists – rat antiovulatory potency (noon proestrus)

Analog[a]	*HPLC*[b] *k'*	ED_{50} (μg/inj) 50% *PG/saline*	*Corn oil*
[N-Ac-Pro^1,D-pF-Phe^2,D-Nal(2)^3,D-pNH$_2$-Phe^6] LHRH	0.4	72	
[N-Ac-D-Ser^1,D-pF-Phe^2,D-Nal(2)^{3,6}]LHRH	0.5	4.3	1.4
[N-Ac-D-Thr^1,D-pF-Phe^2,D-Nal(2)^{3,6}]LHRH	0.6	7.0	4.5
[N-Ac-D-Phe^1,D-pCl-Phe^2,D-Trp^{3,6}]LHRH[c]	0.7	160	74
[N-Ac-Pro^1,D-pF-Phe^2,D-Phe^3,D-Nal(2)^6]LHRH	0.7	12.2	
[N-Ac-Pro^1,D-pCl-Phe^2,D-Phe^3,D-Nal(2)^6]LHRH	0.9	5.6	
[N-Ac-Pro^1,D-pF-Phe^2,D-Nal(2)^{3,6}]LHRH	1.03	2.2	3.3
[N-Ac-Δ^3-Pro^1,D-pF-Phe^2,D-Nal(2)^{3,6}]LHRH[d]	1.05		2.8
[N-Formyl-Pro^1,D-pF-Phe^2,D-Nal(2)^{3,6}]LHRH	1.06	3.0	4.4
[N-Ac-Pro^1,D-pCl-Phe^2,D-Nal(2)^{3,6}]LHRH	1.6	4.8	3.6
[N-Ac-Pro^1,D-pF-Phe^2,D-Nal(2)^{3,6},Pro^9-NHEt]LHRH	2.2	3.4	
[N-Ac-D-pCl-Phe^1,D-pCl-Phe^2,D-Nal(2)^{3,6}]LHRH	2.8	>400	
[Boc-Ser(OBzl)^1,D-pF-Phe^2,D-Nal(2)^{3,6}]LHRH	5.8	>400	

[a] Nestor *et al.*, 1983*b*
[b] Eluent 60% CH_3CN/40% H_2O (0.03 mol/l NH_4OAc, pH 7)
[c] Coy *et al.*, 1979
[d] Compound supplied by Dr J. Rivier (Rivier *et al.*, 1981*a*)

with less hydrophobic analogs demonstrated enhanced potency when corn oil was used instead of a saline-based vehicle (Coy *et al.*, 1979). Corn oil may act as a depot, causing the analog to partition between the oil and plasma phases and be more slowly released to the plasma. For the most hydrophobic analogs, however, the analog may not partition out of the oil at a rate sufficient for enough inhibitor to bind to receptors. The biological potency will then be lower for the antagonist in oil rather than in a saline-based vehicle. Hydrophobic analogs should therefore be tested in both oil and saline-based vehicles.

Use of a propylene glycol/saline vehicle enhanced the potency of [N-Ac-Pro^1,D-pF-Phe^2,D-$Nal(2)^{3,6}$]LHRH. This compound therefore exhibits the prolonged biological $t_{\frac{1}{2}}$ required in the rat antiovulatory assay, without an added depot agent. Human clinical applications are incompatible with continued administration of oil vehicle and this property may offer distinct advantages.

Further modifications to the [N-Ac-Pro^1,D-p-Halo-Phe^2,D-$Nal(2)^{3,6}$] LHRH structure were made to alter the hydrophobicity of these analogs (Nestor *et al.*, 1984*b*). The compounds are arranged in order of increasing hydrophobicity in Table 3.4. A modification which imparts greater hydrophobicity and protection from post-proline cleaving enzyme is Pro^9-NHEt. Although Pro^9-NHEt decreased potency in earlier antagonists (Vilchez-Martinez *et al.*, 1975), it does not decrease potency in the tetrasubstituted analog series. Thus, the potencies of [N-Ac-Pro^1,D-pF-Phe^2,D-$Nal(2)^{3,6}$]LHRH and of [N-Ac-Pro^1,D-pF-Phe^2,D-$Nal(2)^{3,6}$, Pro^9-NHEt] LHRH are not significantly different. This substitution was thought to decrease potency because of intrinsic agonistic activity (Vilchez-Martinez *et al.*, 1975). This may not be the case for analogs which incorporate a D-amino acid in position 3 since this modification removes residual agonistic activity (Coy *et al.*, 1977). In the N-Ac-Pro series, compounds with a k′ greater than 2.4 or less than 0.7 are of decreased potency.

Hydrophilic antagonists

This approach to potent LHRH antagonists emphasized very hydrophobic amino acid substitutions to achieve the desired pharmacokinetics. However, a D-Arg substitution in position 6 can also be effective (Coy *et al.*, 1982). Thus [N-Ac-D-pCl-Phe^1,D-pCl-Phe^2,D-Trp^3,D-Arg^6,D-Ala^{10}]LHRH has an antiovulatory ED_{50} of 2 μg. This more hydrophilic analog was more potent when administered in oil, suggesting that higher intrinsic hydrophobicity in this class of analog structure may give better pharmacokinetics and greater potency. We therefore coupled the hydrophilic D-Arg modification with our very hydrophobic amino acid substitutions (Nestor *et al.*, 1983*b*).

The incorporation of D-Arg into our most potent hydrophobic analog resulted in decreased potency ([N-Ac-Pro^1,D-pF-Phe^2,D-$Nal(2)^3$,D-Arg^6] LHRH, ED_{50} 21 μg). Combination with the hydrophobic Pro^9-NHEt modification led to a small further decrease in potency (Table 3.5). Incorporation of D-pCl-Phe with Pro^9-NHEt gave a slightly more hydro-

Table 3.5 LHRH antagonists containing D-Arg: antiovulatory assay[a]

Antagonist	*HPLC*[b] *k′*	ED_{50} (μg)
[N-Ac-Pro[1],D-pF-Phe[2],D-Nal(2)[3],D-Arg[6]]LHRH	0.25	21
[N-Ac-D-Nal(2)[1],D-pF-Phe[2],D-Trp[3],D-Arg[6]]LHRH[c]	0.39	2.4
[N-Ac-D-pCl-Phe[1],D-pCl-Phe[2],D-Trp[3],D-Arg[6],D-Ala[10]]LHRH[d]	0.43	1.8
[N-Ac-Pro[1],D-pF-Phe[2],D-Nal(2)[3],D-Arg[6],Pro[9]-NHEt]LHRH	0.45	32
[N-Ac-D-Nal(2)[1],D-pF-Phe[2],D-Nal(2)[3],D-Arg[6]]LHRH	0.57	16
[N-Ac-Pro[1],D-pCl-Phe[2],D-Nal(2)[3],D-Arg[6],Pro[9]-NHEt]LHRH	0.6	14

[a] Nestor *et al.*, 1984*b*
[b] Eluent 60% CH_3CN/H_2O (0.03 mol/l NH_4OAc, pH 7)
[c] See also Rivier *et al.*, 1984
[d] Coy *et al.*, 1982

phobic analog and an increase in potency (ED_{50} 14 μg), but all of the N-Ac-Pro[1] analogs were less potent than our most potent hydrophobic antagonist (Table 3.5). Combination of the D-Arg residue with an aromatic amino acid in position 1, as in the hydrophilic standard, was investigated but the incorporation of two D-Nal(2) residues (positions 1 and 3) is not effective (ED_{50} 16 μg). A D-Nal(2) in position 1 gives a potent analog when combined with D-Trp in position 3 ([N-Ac-D-Nal(2)[1],D-pF-Phe[2],D-Trp[3],D-Arg[6]]LHRH; ED_{50} 2.4 μg; PG/saline). Similar results with this combination of the very hydrophobic D-Nal(2) residue and D-Arg were reported recently (Horvath *et al.*, 1983; Rivier *et al.*, 1984).

The D-Arg containing analogs exhibit a prolonged duration of action in the antiovulatory assay when administered 24 h earlier, at noon on diestrus II (Nekola, 1984; Rivier *et al.*, 1984; Nestor *et al.*, 1984*b*). This may be due to their slightly higher receptor affinity, which may be caused by increased interaction of this positively charged residue with sialic acid in the receptor (Hazum *et al.*, 1982) or increased interaction with phospholipid membranes. We studied a new series of N,N′-dialkylguanido-D-homoArg analogs designed to enhance the latter interaction by a combination of charge and hydrophobic interaction. Several types of substitution were studied and the D-hArg (Et_2) analogs are collected in Table 3.6. All of these analogs are very potent antagonists and several exhibit prolonged action (dosage multiple of less than 5 for diestrus II treatment).

[N-Ac-D-Nal(2)[1],D-pCl-Phe[2],D-Trp[3],D-hArg(Et_2)[6]]LHRH is remarkable, with a dosage multiple less than two for diestrus II treatment. The observation that several of these analogs are not significantly improved by administration in corn oil is interesting since previous D-Arg containing analogs may be more than twice as potent in corn oil.

[N-Ac-D-Nal(2)[1],D-pCl-Phe[2],D-Trp[3],D-hArg(Et_2)[6],D-Ala[10]]LHRH appears to be the most potent LHRH antagonist reported (potency 3.6 times [N-Ac-D-Nal(2)[1],D-pF-Phe[2],D-Trp[3],D-Arg[6]]LHRH) when tested in PG/saline on proestrus.

Table 3.6 LHRH antagonists containing D-hArg(Et_2)[a]

Antagonist	*ED_{50} (μg) antiovulatory assay* Proestrus (PG/saline)	Proestrus (Corn oil)	Diestrus II (Corn oil)
[N-Ac-D-Nal(2)[1],D-pF-Phe[2],D-Trp[3],D-hArg(Et_2)[6]]LHRH	1.6	1.4	3.5
[N-Ac-D-pCl-Phe[1],D-pCl-Phe[2],D-Trp[3],D-hArg(Et_2)[6]]LHRH	2.0	2.4	16
[N-Ac-D-pCl-Phe[1],D-pCl-Phe[2],D-Trp[3],D-Arg(Et_2)[6], D-Ala[10]]LHRH	1.7	1.6	>8
[N-Ac-D-Nal(2)[1],D-pCl-Phe[2],D-Trp[3],D-hArg(Et_2)[6]]LHRH	2.0	1.0	1.7
[N-Ac-D-Nal(2)[1],D-pCl-Phe[2],D-Trp[3],D-hArg(Et_2)[6], D-Ala[10]]LHRH	0.67	0.5	2.5

[a] Nestor *et al.*, 1984*c*

CONCLUDING REMARKS

The biological potency of LHRH agonists and antagonists has been increased by altering their pharmacokinetics. This was achieved by the incorporation of very hydrophobic D-amino acids into positions in these structures where there is a known flexibility of substitution. It was expected that such very hydrophobic compounds might be protected from clearance by their partitioning into hydrophobic depot sites which would serve as a continuing source of drug. Agonistic LHRH analogs have resulted which are amongst the most potent yet reported (200–230 times that of LHRH). [D-Nal(2)[6]]LHRH has a biological half-life in women of 2 h, particularly noteworthy in comparison to the reported value of 6 min for LHRH.

Very hydrophobic LHRH antagonists (e.g., [N-Ac-Pro[1],D-pF-Phe[2], D-Nal(2)[3,6]]LHRH and [N-Ac-D-Ser[1],D-pF-Phe[2],D-Nal(2)[3,6]]LHRH) with high biological potencies also were synthesized. Synthesis of analogs containing novel dialkyl-guanido substituted homo-arginine analogs has resulted in [N-Ac-D-Nal(2)[1],D-pCl-Phe[2], D-Trp[3], D-hArg(Et_2)[6], D-Ala[10]]LHRH, the most potent LHRH antagonist reported.

References

Anik, S., Chaplin, M., Nerenberg, C., Kushinsky, S. and Sanders, L. (1983). Absorption and metabolism of LHRH and its analogs. This volume, Chapter 33

Benuck, N. and Marks, N. (1976). Differences in the degradation of hypothalamic releasing factors by rat and human serum. *Life Sci.*, **19,** 1271

Corbin, A. and Beattie, C. W. (1975). Inhibition of the preovulatory proestrous gonadotropin surge, ovulation, and pregnancy with a peptide analog of luteinizing hormone-releasing hormone. *Endocr. Res. Commun.*, **2,** 1

Coy, D. H., Vilchez-Martinez, J. A., Coy, E. J., Nishi, N., Arimura, A. and Schally, A. V. (1975). Polyfluoroalkylamine derivatives of luteinizing hormone-releasing hormone. *Biochemistry*, **14,** 1848

Coy, D. H., Vilchez-Martinez, J. A., Coy, E. J. and Schally, A. V. (1976). Analogs of luteinizing hormone-releasing hormone with increased biological activity produced by D-amino acid substitutions in position 6. *J. Med. Chem.*, **19,** 423

Coy, D. H., Vilchez-Martinez, J. A. and Schally, A. V. (1977). Structure function studies on LRF. In Loffet, A. (ed.) *Peptides 1976,* pp. 463–469. (Brussels: Editions de l'Université de Bruxelles)

Coy, D. H., Mezo, I., Pedroza, E., Nekola, M. V., Vilchez-Martinez, J. A., Piyachaturawat, P., Schally, A. V., Seprodi, J. and Teplan, I. (1979). LRF agonists and fertility regulation in the male. In Gross, E. and Meienhofer, J. (eds.) *Peptides, Proceedings of the 6th American Peptide Symposium,* pp. 775–779. (Rockville, IL: Pierce Chem. Co.)

Coy, D. H., Horvath, A., Nekola, M. V., Coy, E. J., Erchegyi, J. and Schally, A. V. (1982). Peptide antagonists of LH-RH: Large increases in antiovulatory activities produced by basic D-amino acids in the six position. *Endocrinology,* **110,** 1445

Dutta, A. S., Furr, B. J. A., Giles, M. B., Valcaccia, B. and Walpole, A. L. (1978). Potent agonist and antagonist analogues of luliberin containing an azaglycine residue in position 10. *Biochem. Biophys. Res. Commun.,* **81,** 382

Fujino, J., Kobayashi, S., Obayashi, M., Fukuda, T., Shinagawa, S., Yamazaki, I., Nakayama, R., White, W. F. and Rippel, R. H. (1972). Structure–activity relationships in the C-terminal part of luteinizing hormone-releasing hormone (LH-RH). *Biochem. Biophys. Res. Commun.,* **49,** 863

Hansch, C., Steward, A. R., Anderson, S. M. and Bentley, D. (1967). The parabolic dependence of drug action on lipophilic character as revealed by a study of hypnotics. *J. Med. Chem.,* **11,** 1

Hazum, E. (1982). GnRH-receptor of rat pituitary is a glycoprotein: differential effect of neuraminidase and lectins on agonists and antagonists binding. *Mol. Cell. Endocrinol.,* **26,** 217

Ho, T. L., Nestor, J. J. Jr., McRae, G. I. and Vickery, B. H. (1983). Hydrophobic Aza-Gly analogs of LHRH. *J. Med. Chem.* (In press)

Horsthemke, B., Knisatschek, H., Rivier, J., Sandow, J. and Bauer, K. (1981). Degradation of luteinizing hormone-releasing hormone and analogs by adenohypophyseal peptidases. *Biochem. Biophys. Res. Commun.,* **100,** 753

Horvath, A., Coy, D. H., Nekola, M. V., Coy, E. J., Schally, A. V. and Teplan, I. (1983). Synthesis and biological activity of LHRH antagonists modified in position 1. *Peptides,* **3,** 969

Hsueh, A. J. W. and Erickson, G. F. (1979). Extrapituitary action of gonadotropin-releasing hormone: direct inhibition of ovarian steroidogenesis. *Science,* **204,** 854

Humphries, J., Wasiak, T., Wan, Y.-P., Folkers, K. and Bowers, C. Y. (1978). An antiovulatory decapeptide of higher potency which has an L-amino acid (Ac-Pro) in position 1. *Biochem. Biophys. Res. Commun.,* **85,** 709

Ling, N. and Vale, W. (1975). Analogs of luteinizing hormone releasing factor (LRF) – synthesis and biological activity of (Nα-Me)Leu^{7}LRF and [D-Ala^6,(Nα-Me)Leu^7]LRF. *Biochem. Biophys. Res. Commun.,* **63,** 801

Monahan, M. W., Rivier, J., Vale, W. and Guillemin, R. (1972a). [Gly^2]LRF and des-His^2-LRF. The synthesis, purification, and characterization of two LRF analogues antagonistic to LRF. *Biochem. Biophys. Res. Commun.,* **47,** 551

Monahan, M. W., Amoss, M. S., Anderson, H. A. and Vale, W. (1973). Synthetic analogs of the hypothalamic luteinizing hormone releasing factor with increased agonist or antagonist properties. *Biochemistry,* **12,** 4616

Nadasdi, L. and Medzihradszky, K. (1981). A study of the applicability of QSAR calculation for peptide hormones. *Biochem. Biophys. Res. Commun.,* **99,** 451

Nekola, M. V. and Coy, D. H. (1984). LHRH antagonists in females: This volume Chapter 10

Nestor, J. J. Jr., Ho, T. L., Simpson, R. A., Horner, B. L., Jones, G. H., McRae, G. I. and Vickery, B. H. (1982). Synthesis and biological activity of some very hydrophobic superagonist analogues of luteinizing hormone-releasing hormone. *J. Med. Chem.,* **25,** 795

Nestor, J. J. Jr., Jones, G. H. and Vickery, B. H. (1983). Nonapeptide and decapeptide analogs of LHRH, useful as LHRH antagonists. U.S. Patent 4,419,347 (issued 12/6/83)

Nestor, J. J. Jr., Horner, B. L., Ho, T. L., Jones, G. H., McRae, G. I. and Vickery, B. H. (1984*a*). Synthesis of a novel class of heteroaromatic amino acids and their use in the preparation of analogues of luteinizing hormone-releasing hormone. *J. Med. Chem.* (In press)

Nestor, J. J. Jr., Tahilramani, R., Ho, T. L., McRae, G. I. and Vickery, B. H. (1984*b*). Luteinizing hormone-releasing hormone antagonists containing very hydrophobic amino acids. *J. Med. Chem.* (In press)

Nestor, J. J. Jr., Tahilramani, R., Ho, T. L., McRae, G. I. and Vickery, B. H. (1983*c*). New LHRH antagonists. In Hruby, V. J. (ed.) *Peptides – Proceedings of the Eighth American Peptide Symposium.* (In press)

Perrin, M. H., Rivier, J. E. and Vale, W. W. (1980). Radio-ligand assay for gonadotropin-releasing hormone: relative potencies of agonists and antagonists. *Endocrinology,* **106,** 1289

Perrin, M. H., Haas, Y., Rivier, J. E. and Vale, W. W. (1983). Gonadotropin-releasing hormone binding to rat anterior pituitary membrane homogenates: comparison of antagonists and agonists using radiolabeled antagonist and agonist. *Mol. Pharmacol.,* **23, 44**

Prasad, K. U., Roeske, R. W., Weitl, F. L., Vilchez-Martinez, J. A. and Schally, A. V. (1976). Structure–activity relationships in luteinizing hormone-releasing hormone. *J. Med. Chem.,* **19,** 492

Rivier, J., Ling, N., Monahan, M., Rivier, C., Brown, M. and Vale, W. (1975). Luteinizing hormone releasing factor and somatostatin analogs. In Walter, R. and Meienhofer, J. (eds.) *Peptides: Chemistry, Structure and Biology – Proceedings of the Fourth American Peptide Symposium,* pp. 863–870. (Ann Arbor: Ann Arbor Science)

Rivier, J., Brown, M., Rivier, C., Ling, N. and Vale, W. (1977). Hypothalamic hypophysiotropic hormones. In Loffet, A. (ed.) *Peptides 1976,* pp. 427–451. (Brussels: Editions de l'Université de Bruxelles)

Rivier, J., Rivier, C., Perrin, M., Porter, J. and Vale, W. W. (1981*a*). GnRH analogs: structure–activity relationships. In Zatuchni, G. I., Shelton, J. D. and Sciarra, J. J. (eds.) *LHRH Peptides as Female and Male Contraceptives,* pp. 13–23. (Philadelphia: Harper & Row)

Rivier, J., Rivier, C., Perrin, M., Porter, J. and Vale, W. (1981*b*). Application of the Hansch approach to design GnRH analogs using Topliss' manual method. In Brunfeldt, K. (ed.) *Peptides 1980 – Proceedings of the 16th European Peptide Symposium,* pp. 566–571. (Copenhagen: Scriptor)

Rivier, J., Rivier, C., Perrin, M., Porter, J. and Vale, W. (1984). LHRH analogs as antiovulatory agents. This volume, Chapter 2

Sandow, J., von Rechenberg, W., Jerzabek, G. and Stoll, W. (1978). Pituitary gonadotropin inhibition by a highly active analog of luteinizing hormone-releasing hormone. *Fertil. Steril.,* **30,** 205

Schally, A. V., Arimura, A. and Coy, D. H. (1981). Recent approaches to fertility control based on derivatives of LH-RH. *Vitam. Horm.,* **38,** 257

Vickery, B. H. (1981). Antigonadotropic, antisteroidogenic and antisteroidal activities of agonist analogs of luteinizing hormone-releasing hormone as revealed by their antireproductive activities. In Agarwal, M. K. (ed.) *Hormone Antagonists,* pp. 623–657. (New York: de Gruyter)

Vilchez-Martinez, J. A., Schally, A. V., Coy, D. H., Coy, E. J., Miller, C. M. and Arimura, A. (1975). An in vivo assay for anti-LH-RH and anti-FSH-RH activity of inhibitory analogues of LH-RH. *Endocrinology,* **96,** 1130

Yabe, Y., Miura, C., Horikoshi, H. and Baba, Y. (1976). Analogues of luteinizing hormone-releasing hormone with modification in position 3. *Chem. Pharm. Bull.,* **24,** 3149

4
Pharmacological regulation of pituitary LHRH receptors

R. N. CLAYTON

The tonic and pulsatile release of pituitary gonadotropic hormones is regulated by LHRH (Fink, 1976). In physiological circumstances, the secretion of LHRH is pulsatile rather than continuous. There is increasing evidence that modulation of pulse frequency, rather than the pulse amplitude, plays a critical role in the regulation of gonadotropin secretion, and hence the reproductive state of the organism (Knobil, 1980). In the physiological state, hypophysial portal plasma levels of LHRH may be altered by the hormonal milieu (e.g. steroids) and such regulation is the final integrated response arising from interaction of many feedback signals within the central nervous system.

When synthetic LHRH became available it was anticipated that it could be applied therapeutically to stimulate fertility. LHRH was administered parenterally as frequent large doses, but after an initial stimulation of gonadotropin secretion, the pituitary became progressively more refractory to each subsequent injection (Sandow, 1982). This refractoriness was thought to be due to the short biological half-life of native LHRH in the pituitary (Clayton and Catt, 1981*a*). However, enzyme resistant, long acting agonist analogs caused pituitary gonadotrope refractoriness even sooner than native LHRH. This phenomenon of pituitary refractoriness (desensitization), to frequent high doses of the stimulating hormone was only overcome when the early data concerning gonadotropin pulsatility were appreciated. Thus, in monkeys without endogenous LHRH, normal gonadotropin secretion could be restored only if LHRH replacement was given at intervals approximating the frequency of naturally occurring serum gonadotropin surges (Belchetz *et al.*, 1978). By analogy with the cellular desensitization observed with insulin and the gonadotropic hormones, the possibility that gonadotrope desensitization after frequent LHRH or LHRH agonist exposure involved receptor down regulation seemed high.

The initial interaction of LHRH with gonadotropes occurs with specific receptors located within the plasma membrane of the cells (Clayton and Catt, 1981*a*). Subsequently, a series of intracellular events is activated which ultimately results in secretion of stored gonadotropins, and probably leads to stimulation of their synthesis. Any or all of the steps in the stimulus–secretion pathway have the potential for regulation by LHRH itself, gonadal hormones, and possibly other intra- and extracellular signals.

LHRH RECEPTOR MEASUREMENT

Initial attempts to quantitate pituitary binding sites for LHRH employed radio-iodinated LHRH (^{125}I-LHRH) as the ligand with either crude rat pituitary membranes or enriched bovine plasma membrane fractions. These assays were unsatisfactory because of the presence of a high proportion (75 % of specific binding) of low-affinity (K_D† 1 μmol/l) LHRH binding sites of dubious physiological significance, and substantial (30–40 %) ligand degradation, even during 40 min incubations at 4°C (Clayton *et al.*, 1979*a*).

Degradation of ^{125}I-LHRH by bovine pituitary subcellular fractions is greatest in those containing plasma membrane elements and this degrading activity is co-enriched with specific ^{125}I-LHRH binding during purification (Clayton *et al.*, 1979*a*). Suppression of ^{125}I-LHRH degradation by certain enzyme inhibitors also reduced specific LHRH binding. The majority of specific binding of LHRH was to low-affinity sites, suggesting that the low-affinity receptor might be the degrading enzyme(s). This hypothesis is supported by the much reduced affinity of the metabolically hindered analog [D-Ser(tBu)^6,Pro^9-NHEt]LHRH (LHRH-A) for low affinity receptors (Clayton *et al.*, 1979*a,b*). This membrane-associated degrading activity may be an enzyme intrinsic to the cell membrane, or may merely represent contamination by peptidases contained within lysosomal membranes. Thus the binding of ^{125}I-LHRH to the low-affinity binding site masked any changes in high-affinity receptors.

The problems of ligand degradation and low-affinity binding were resolved with the availability for radio-labeling of superactive, slowly degradable, agonist analogs of LHRH (Clayton *et al.*, 1979*b*). ^{125}I-[D-Ser(tBu)^6,Pro^9-NHEt]LHRH (^{125}I-LHRH-A), or other analogs with D-amino acid substitutions in position 6 and glycinamide^{10} replaced by ethylamide, interact with a single class of high-affinity binding sites in pituitary membrane preparations and cultured anterior pituitary cells (Naor *et al.*, 1980). The apparent K_a ($5 \times 10^9 M^{-1}$) of LHRH receptors for LHRH-A is tenfold greater than that of LHRH ($K_a 3 \times 10^8 M^{-1}$). The receptor binding affinity of a series of LHRH analogs, both agonists and antagonists, has correlated well with biological activity (Clayton and Catt, 1980; Perrin *et al.*, 1980*a*; Loumaye *et al.*, 1982).

Although antagonists seem to bind to the same receptor site as agonists, the kinetics and effects of altered ionic environment on receptor interaction are different for an ^{125}I-LHRH antagonist versus the ^{125}I-LHRH agonist ligand (Meridan and Koch, 1981; Hazum, 1981). These differences suggest that different regions of the receptor domain are involved in the binding of antagonists.

For accurate quantitation of pituitary LHRH receptors (LHRH-R) in various physiological circumstances, and during pharmacological treatment with LHRH agonists and antagonists, radioreceptor assays (RRA) using agonist analogs as the radioligand are the method of choice. This methodology enables the quantitation of the LHRH receptor content in single rat pituitary glands, permitting their correlation with individual serum and pituitary hormone levels. Tissue specificity studies have identified LHRH-R only in those tissues in which the decapeptide has a biological effect. Even within the pituitary, LHRH-R are restricted to the gonadotropes (Naor *et al.*, 1982).

PHYSIOLOGICAL REGULATION OF LHRH RECEPTORS

Estrous cycle

LHRH-R values on proestrus are double those measured during estrus and early metestrus (Savoy-Moore *et al.*, 1980; Clayton *et al.*, 1980; Adams and Spies, 1981; Ferland *et al.*, 1981). LHRH-R increase between the evening of metestrus and diestrus II morning, prior to increased sensitivity of the pituitary to LHRH, and at a time when serum estradiol concentrations begin to rise (Savoy-Moore *et al.*, 1980). Estradiol, acting directly upon the pituitary, is capable of increasing LHRH-R by 60% and is accompanied by a decrease in the ED_{50} of LHRH-stimulated LH release (Loumaye and Forni, 1982). One consequence of this LHRH-R increase *in vivo* could be an increased sensitivity of the pituitary to the increased endogenous LHRH secretion which occurs on the afternoon of proestrus (Sarkar *et al.*, 1976).

LHRH-R decline rapidly to nadir values at the time of the serum LH rise (Savoy-Moore *et al.*, 1980; Clayton *et al.*, 1980). This was interpreted as loss of LHRH receptors due to increased occupancy during the LH surge. Endogenous LHRH secretion is maximal at this time in the cycle and blockade of the spontaneous LHRH and LH surges with pentobarbital (pentobarbitone) in the early afternoon of proestrus prevents this LHRH receptor fall (Barkan *et al.*, 1981). A reduction in LHRH-R was observed 30 min following 200 μg of LHRH intravenously, although this drop was 15 min after the serum LH peak (Savoy-Moore *et al.*, 1981). However, LHRH-R reduction was not achieved by administration of LHRH to pentobarbital blocked rats (Barkan *et al.*, 1981). Although direct evidence indicates that part of the dramatic decline in LHRH-R on proestrus can be accounted for by *in vivo* receptor occupancy (White and Ojeda, 1982), a decrease in endogenous opiate activity in the hypothalamus may play a role in the sudden decrease in LHRH-R on the afternoon of proestrus (Barkan *et al.*, 1983).

Postpartum/hyperprolactinemia

The postpartum and lactational periods are characterized by reduced fertility due to suppression of hypothalamic function by hyperprolactinemia. This physiological state is associated with reduced hypothalamic LHRH secretion and depressed responsiveness to exogenous LHRH. Pituitary LHRH-R in lactating rats were found to be 50% of those in metestrous females (Clayton *et al.*, 1980). Experimental hyperprolactinemia can attenuate the LHRH-R and serum LH increases following gonadectomy (Clayton and Bailey, 1982*d*; Marchetti and Labrie, 1982). Thus, diminished pituitary responsivity to LHRH is accompanied by reduced LHRH-R, supporting the concept of a positive correlation between LHRH-R, basal serum gonadotropin levels, and responsiveness of the gonadotroph to the releasing hormone.

Gonadectomy

LHRH-R are elevated by two to threefold following ovariectomy and orchidectomy, an increase prevented by concurrent treatment with appropriate gonadal steroids (Clayton and Catt, 1981*b*; Frager *et al.*, 1981). Although a direct action of androgens at the pituitary level to suppress gonadotropin secretion and LHRH-R levels has been reported (Giguere *et al.*, 1981), an additional level of negative steroid feedback at the hypothalamic level appears likely. Negative androgen feedback on LHRH-R is demonstrated during male sexual development, when high prepubertal LHRH-R values fall progressively with increasing testosterone secretion from the maturing testis (Chan *et al.*, 1981). A summary of pituitary LHRH-R changes in physiological states is presented in Table 4.1.

Table 4.1 Physiological regulation of pituitary LHRH receptors

Physiological change	*LHRH-R level change*	*Effect of steroids*[a]
Orchidectomy	Rapid (1 d) 2–3-fold increase, coincident with basal LH/FSH rise	Blocked by T, dihydro T, E, DES; attenuated by P
Ovariectomy	Slow (2–3 d) 2-fold increase, just prior to LH rise	Blocked by E, P, E and P
Estrous cycle (4 d)	Metestrus – increase from nadir Diestrus, proestrus – high level Steep fall to nadir, coincident with LH surge	Coincident with rising E
Puberty		
Male	Decrease from high level	Coincident with rising T
Female	Decrease from high level	Decreases after drop in LH/FSH and E levels
Lactation	50% decrease from estrus nadir	

[a] Testosterone (T), estradiol (E), diethylstilbestrol (DES), progesterone (P)

AUTOREGULATION OF LHRH RECEPTORS

There is a positive correlation between the pituitary LHRH-R content and hypothalamic LHRH secretory activity. This led to the hypothesis that LHRH-R are regulated by LHRH itself (Clayton *et al.*, 1982*a,b*; Pieper *et al.*, 1982).

Effect of hypothalamic lesions

The stereotactic placement of a destructive lesion in the floor of the 3rd ventricle (median eminence lesion, MEL), prior to orchidectomy, completely prevents the LHRH-R and serum LH increases after castration. When MEL-bearing, orchidectomized rats were administered LHRH three times daily, castration-like responses were restored (Clayton *et al.*, 1982*a*). Removal of endogenous LHRH rapidly reduced LHRH-R following their elevation 10 d postcastration. LHRH-R values in MEL animals were 30 % lower than those of intact controls, similar to the situation in animals treated with LHRH antiserum (Clayton *et al.*, 1982*b*).

PASSIVE TRANSFER OF LHRH ANTIBODY

Immunoneutralization of endogenous LHRH by daily subcutaneous injection of a high-affinity antiserum also prevents the postorchidectomy LH responses, and further reduces LHRH-R values in chronically orchidectomized animals. An LHRH agonist analog which does not cross-react with this antiserum can induce LHRH-R. The recovery of LHRH-R following cessation of antiserum administration coincided with the disappearance of LHRH binding capacity in the serum (Clayton *et al.*, 1982*b*).

Blockade of receptor with antagonist

When the potent LHRH antagonist analog [N-Ac-L-Ala^{1},D-Phe^{2},D-Trp^{3,6}] LHRH is infused continuously to orchidectomized rats, it prevents the postcastration LHRH-R and serum LH increase. The antagonist-induced reduction in measurable LHRH-R is dose dependent, with LHRH-R values at highest doses being only 25 % of those of intact animals. LHRH-R values from antagonist infused orchidectomized animals are indistinguishable from those of antagonist infused intact controls, though the postcastration rise in LHRH-R has been prevented (Clayton *et al.*, 1982*a*). LHRH antagonists act as 'receptor blocking' agents without inducing pituitary receptor down regulation. These conclusions are supported by finding a normal increment in LH release following exogenous LHRH in animals infused with high doses of antagonist (Clayton *et al.*, 1982*a*). Clearly the unoccupied LHRH receptors are functional, in contrast to the situation when LHRH-R are occupied to a similar degree by LHRH agonists (Clayton, 1982). These experiments show that LHRH interaction with its receptors is a prerequisite for the post-orchidectomy LHRH-R increase.

Antibodies against the antagonist, which cross-link receptors occupied by antagonist molecules, convert the antagonist to an agonist (Conn *et al.*, 1982*a*). Microaggregation of LHRH-R is therefore an important early consequence of LHRH agonist interaction with its receptor. Although LHRH agonist activity is achieved by cross-linking receptors (Conn *et al.*, 1982*b*), macroscopic clustering and internalization of LHRH-R is not essential for agonist activity (Conn and Hazum, 1981).

Endogenous LHRH is required for the maintenance of a normal complement of its own receptors. In this manner the hypothalamus can exercise control over the sensitivity and maximum responsiveness of pituitary gonadotroph function.

BIPHASIC REGULATION OF LHRH RECEPTORS

Infrequent LHRH treatment

The increased pituitary responsiveness occurring on proestrus might be due to self-priming by autoinduction of LHRH-R (Fink, 1976). LHRH receptors are induced in adult male rats following either subcutaneous injections of LHRH three times daily (Frager *et al.*, 1979) or injection of an LHRH agonist analog once daily (Clayton *et al.*, 1980; Marchetti *et al.*, 1982). The number of LHRH receptors induced is slightly less than that following orchidectomy, suggesting that increased androgen secretion, resulting from the exogenous LHRH, might limit the receptor rise. A direct inhibitory effect of androgen on LHRH receptors and LH release in pituitary cells incubated with the steroid *in vitro* has been noted (Giguere *et al.*, 1981).

A similar up-regulation of LHRH-R exists in cultured pituitary cells exposed to LHRH (Loumaye and Catt, 1982). The magnitude of the LHRH-R increase (60 %) is similar to that produced by LHRH *in vivo*. LHRH agonist analogs share this property, which is blocked in a dose dependent fashion by LHRH antagonists. LHRH-R up regulation is dose dependent at concentrations effective at releasing LH, but high concentrations (10^{-8} mol/l analog, 10^{-6} mol/l LHRH) caused receptor 'down regulation' or occupancy. Depolarizing stimuli (50 mmol/l K^+), which induced LH release, also increased LHRH-R (Loumaye and Catt 1983). Immunocytochemical studies suggest the existence of LHRH-R on secretory granules of gonadotrophs (Sternberger and Petrali, 1975; Wagner and von Zur Mohlen, 1982). These data suggest insertion of LHRH receptors into the plasma membrane from secretory granules following stimulated LH release.

Pharmacological LHRH treatment

The method by which LHRH is administered determines pituitary gonadotrope responsiveness (Belchetz *et al.*, 1978). Continuous infusion of LHRH causes an initial abrupt rise in serum LH, which then declines progressively as the infusion continues. During the infusion period, additional increments of LHRH fail to elicit an LH response, although administration of other secretagogs is effective in this regard (Smith and Vale, 1981). The pituitary desensitization induced by LHRH therefore is not due to exhaustion of pituitary gonadotropin stores, and a defect in the LHRH-stimulated LH release mechanism is indicated. LHRH-induced receptor loss (down regulation) resulting from increased processing of occupied receptors (Catt *et al.*, 1979) or uncoupling of occupied hormone receptors from the intracellular events leading to gonadotropin release may be implicated.

Pituitary refractoriness was investigated in adult male rats by continuous infusion of either LHRH or an agonist analog. Initially, LHRH-R increased by 30–40 %, and serum LHRH values of about 40 pg/ml were achieved during LHRH infusion. These LHRH values are similar to those measured in rat pituitary stalk plasma (Eskay *et al.*, 1979; Sarkar and Fink, 1979). Basal serum LH values were unchanged by these levels of serum LHRH. Low doses of LHRH-agonist (serum levels of LHRH-A < 50 pg/ml) induced larger (~ 70 %) LHRH-R increases in intact (but not castrated animals) (Clayton, 1982), and basal serum LH levels were doubled in the intact animals with LHRH-R increases. Although an increase in pituitary LHRH-R was found 4 h after beginning a continuous LHRH infusion, continuation of the infusion reduced LHRH-R by 12 h, suggesting either receptor occupancy or down regulation (Nett *et al.*, 1981).

Different regimens of LHRH or agonist analog administration cause different effects on LHRH receptors (Table 4.2). In castrates, doses of the peptides which stimulate LHRH-R in intact rats produce a profound reduction in measurable LHRH-R (Clayton, 1982). Since LHRH secretion is high postcastration, the addition of exogenous ligand would result in greater receptor occupancy at lower concentrations of the infused peptide.

Increasing the infusion dose of LHRH or LHRH-A to orchidectomized rats caused a dose dependent reduction in LHRH-R and basal serum LH levels. Receptor occupancy accounted for about 65 % of the measured reduction in LHRH-R, with net receptor loss contributing the remainder (Clayton, 1982). Despite this high degree of receptor occupancy, both basal serum LH and pituitary LH content fell in the castrated animals. This suggests that the occupied receptors were functionally uncoupled from the intracellular mechanisms for normal hormone release and synthesis. Thus, high doses of LHRH (10 μg s.c.) given towards the end of the LHRH or LHRH-A infusion

Table 4.2 Regulation of pituitary LHRH-R in intact male rats

LHRH treatment	*LHRH-R level*[a]	*[D-Ser(tBu)⁶,Pro⁹-NHEt]LHRH Treatment*	*LHRH-R level*[a]
Injection – 240 ng t.i.d., 4 d[b]	170 %	Injection	
		40 ng t.i.d., 4 d[e]	140–200 %
		100 ng/d, 8 d[f]	150 %
		200 ng/d, 14 d[g]	200 %
Infusion, 7 d[c]		Infusion, 7 d[c]	
low dose (serum LHRH 40 pg/ml)	130 %	low dose (serum level < 50 pg/ml)	170 %
med. dose (serum LHRH 250 pg/ml)	100 %	med. dose (serum level ~ 100 pg/ml)	100 %
high dose (serum LHRH 1500 pg/ml)	sharp decrease	high dose (serum level ~ 1000 pg/ml)	sharp decrease
2.5 μg/h[d]: 4 h	200 %		
12 h	70 %		
24 h	50 %		

[a] Normal basal level is 100 %; [b] Frager *et al.*, 1979; [c] Clayton, 1982; [d] Nett *et al.*, 1981; [e] Frager *et al.*, 1981; [f] Clayton *et al.*, 1980: [g] Marchetti *et al.*, 1982

failed to raise serum LH values. However, such an LHRH injection, to animals with about 75% of receptors occupied by an LHRH antagonist, produced a brisk serum LH increase. Thus, the gonadotrope's intracellular release mechanism can distinguish between receptors occupied by an LHRH agonist or antagonist analog.

Desensitization by 'uncoupling' of receptors might arise from conformational changes in the gonadotrope surface membrane. LHRH receptors in cultured gonadotrophs aggregate into clusters, are internalized, and then migrate to the pole of the cell within a very short time of exposure to the ligand (Naor *et al.*, 1981; Hazum *et al.*, 1980). Such processing of hormone-receptor complexes might account for receptor loss when the cells are exposed to pharmacological ligand concentrations.

At the extremes of circulating LHRH concentrations pituitary receptors can be either induced (low LHRH) or markedly reduced (high LHRH). It is likely that the LHRH receptor number is maintained *in vivo* within a narrow range, and depends on a balance between occupancy-induced processing and the rate of reappearance of vacant receptors on the cell surface. Processing of hormone-receptor complexes and desensitization may represent a generalized mechanism by which target cells protect themselves from excessive stimulation.

While receptor 'down regulation' is one factor in pituitary refractoriness to LHRH, the pituitary LH content also falls. Although this might be caused by the two to threefold higher serum LH values, serum LH values are tenfold greater 6 d after orchidectomy and the pituitary LH content is not reduced. The reduced gonadotropin stores may result from receptor loss and/or uncoupling. This implies that LHRH is required for gonadotropin synthesis as well as release, and that both actions of LHRH are mediated through the same receptors.

GONADAL LHRH RECEPTORS

The direct antigonadal actions of LHRH, both *in vivo* and in cultured granulosa, luteal, and Leydig cells *in vitro*, has been well established in the rat (Chapters 13 and 14). Such actions are mediated through specific high-affinity LHRH receptors in the respective steroidogenic cells (for review, see Clayton and Catt, 1981*a*). These receptors exhibit the same LHRH analog specificity as LHRH receptors in rat pituitary. The direct antigonadal actions of LHRH do not apply to all species. LHRH fails to antagonize gonadotropic hormone action in cultured granulosa cells from human follicles (Caspar *et al.*, 1982) or in monkey luteal cells (Asch *et al.*, 1981*a*). LHRH is also without effect on mouse Leydig cell function *in vitro* (Hunter *et al.*, 1982). In monkey corpora lutea cells and mouse Leydig cells, no high-affinity LHRH receptors can be detected by assay systems giving positive results for rat tissues (Asch *et al.*, 1981*b*; Hunter *et al.*, 1982). No ^{125}I-LHRH-A binding in membrane preparations from mouse ovaries was detected (Naik and Clayton, unpublished), while ovarian membranes from rats were always positive. High-affinity LHRH receptors were not found in human corpora lutea, obtained from the luteal phase of the menstrual cycle (Clayton and Huhtaniemi, 1982). Human and monkey testicular membrane preparations were negative for LHRH receptors. LHRH-R could not be detected in corpora lutea from cows, sheep or pigs (J. J. Reeves, personal communication). It is possible that LHRH-R are present in these species, but in such low concentrations as to be undetectable by the most sensitive methods available. However, it appears unlikely that LHRH has any role in direct regulation of gonadal function in species other than the rat.

CONCLUDING REMARKS

Superagonist analogs of LHRH have made possible the development of accurate and reproducible radioreceptor assays for LHRH. LHRH receptors can now be determined in single pituitary glands. LHRH receptor numbers change in many physiological circumstances, without alteration in their affinity. A positive correlation exists between pituitary LHRH receptors, basal gonadotropin secretion, and the levels of LHRH present in hypophysial portal plasma. The concentration of pituitary LHRH receptors is regulated by LHRH itself, and thus their measurement reflects the degree of prior exposure of the pituitary to LHRH. Positive regulation of LHRH-R by low concentrations of LHRH may contribute to the self-priming effect observed during the estrus cycle. Conversely, gonadotroph desensitization following repeated exposure to pharmacological concentrations of LHRH results from uncoupling of occupied receptors from the release machinery, depletion of pituitary LH available for release and net receptor loss. The receptor regulation by pharmacological concentrations of LHRH and LHRH-A may be used for the therapeutic manipulation of fertility and for medical gonadectomy where indicated.

Acknowledgements

This work was supported, in part, by grants from the Medical Research Council, UK. I am grateful to Miss L. C. Bailey and Mr K. Schumacher for hormone assays.

References

Adams, T. E. and Spies, H. G. (1981). Binding characteristics of gonadotrophin-releasing hormone receptors throughout the estrous cycle of the hamster. *Endocrinology*, **108**, 2245

Asch, R. A., Smith, C. G., Eddy, C. A., Siler-Khodr, T. and Schally, A. V. (1981*a*). Luteolytic effect of luteinizing hormone releasing hormone (LHRH) analog (D-Trp^6 LHRH) in the nonhuman primate: its mechanism of action. *Fertil. Steril.*, **36**, 271

Asch, R. A., van Sickle, M., Rettori, V., Balmaceda, J. P., Eddy, C. A., Coy, D. H. and Schally, A. V. (1981*b*). Absence of LHRH binding sites in corpora lutea from rhesus monkeys. *J. Clin. Endocrinol. Metab.*, **53**, 215

Barkan, A., Regiani, S., Duncan, J. A. and Marshall, J. C. (1981). Pituitary GnRH receptors during the LH surge in female rats: effects of pentobarbital blockage and GnRH injections.

Abstr. No. 820, *Program of the 63rd Meeting of the Endocrine Society,* 17–19 June, *Cincinnati, Ohio*

Barkan, A., Regiani, S., Duncan, J., Paparasilou, S. and Marshall, J. C. (1983). Opioids modulate pituitary receptors for gonadotrophin releasing hormone. *Endocrinology,* **112,** 387

Belchetz, P. E., Plant, T. M., Nakai, Y., Keogh, E. J. and Knobil, E. (1978). Hypophysial responses to continuous and intermittent delivery of hypothalamic gonadotrophin-releasing hormone. *Science,* **202,** 631

Caspar, R. F., Erickson, G. F., Rebar, R. W. and Yen, S. S. C. (1982). The effect of luteinizing hormone releasing factor and its agonist on cultured human granulosa cells. *Fertil. Steril.,* **37,** 406

Catt, K. J., Harwood, J. P., Aquilera, G. and Dufau, M. L. (1979). Hormonal regulation of peptide receptors and target cell responses. *Nature* (*Lond.*), **280,** 109

Chan, V., Clayton, R. N., Knox, G. and Catt, K. J. (1981). Ontogeny of pituitary GnRH receptors in the rat. *Endocrinology,* **108,** 2086

Clayton, R. N. (1982). Gonadotrophin releasing hormone modulation of its own pituitary receptors: evidence for biphasic regulation. *Endocrinology,* **111,** 152

Clayton, R. N., Shakespear, R. A., Duncan, J. A. and Marshall, J. C. (1979*a*). Luteinizing hormone-releasing hormone inactivation by purified pituitary plasma membrane: effects on receptor binding studies. *Endocrinology,* **104,** 1484

Clayton, R. N., Shakespear, R. A., Duncan, J. A. and Marshall, J. C. with Appendix by Munson, P. J. and Rodbard, D. (1979*b*). Radioiodinated nondegradable gonadotrophin releasing hormone analogs: new probes for the investigation of pituitary gonadotrophin releasing hormone receptors. *Endocrinology,* **105,** 1369

Clayton, R. N. and Catt, K. J. (1980). Receptor-binding affinity of gonadotrophin-releasing hormone analogs: analysis by radioligand-receptor assay. *Endocrinology,* **106,** 1154

Clayton, R. N., Solano, A. R., Garcia-Vela, A., Dufau, M. L. and Catt, K. J. (1980). Regulation of pituitary receptors for gonadotrophin releasing hormone during the rat estrous cycle. *Endocrinology,* **107,** 699

Clayton, R. N. and Catt, K. J. (1981*a*). Gonadotrophin releasing hormone receptors: characterization, physiological regulation and relationship to reproductive function. *Endocr. Rev,* **2,** 186

Clayton, R. N. and Catt, K. J. (1981*b*). Regulation of pituitary gonadotrophin releasing hormone receptors by gonadal hormones. *Endocrinology,* **108,** 887

Clayton, R. N. and Huhtaniemi, I. T. (1982). Absence of gonadotrophin-releasing hormone receptors in human gonadal tissue. *Nature* (*Lond.*), **299,** 56

Clayton, R. N., Channabasavaiah, K., Stewart, J. M. and Catt, K. J. (1982*a*). Hypothalamic regulation of pituitary gonadotrophin-releasing hormone receptors I: effects of hypothalamic lesions and a gonadotrophin releasing hormone antagonist. *Endocrinology,* **110,** 1108

Clayton, R. N., Popkin, R. M. and Fraser, H. M. (1982*b*). Hypothalamic regulation of pituitary GnRH receptors II: effects of gonadotrophin-releasing hormone immuno-neutralization. *Endocrinology,* **110,** 1116

Clayton, R. N. and Bailey, L. C. (1982). Hyperprolactinaemia attenuates the gonadotrophin releasing hormone receptors response to gonadectomy. *J. Endocrinol.,* **95,** 267

Conn, P. M. and Hazum, E. (1981). Luteinizing hormone release and gonadotrophin releasing hormone (GnRH) receptor internalization: independent actions of GnRH. *Endocrinology,* **109,** 2040

Conn, P. M., Rogers, D. C., Stewart, J. M., Niedel, J. and Sheffield, T. (1982*a*). Conversion of a gonadotrophin-releasing hormone antagonist to an agonist. *Nature* (*Lond.*), **296,** 653

Conn, P. M., Rogers, D. C. and McNeil, R. (1982*b*). Potency enhancement of a GnRH agonist: GnRH-receptor microaggregation stimulates gonadotrophin release. *Endocrinology,* **111,** 335

Eskay, D. L., Mical, R. S. and Porter, J. C. (1979). Relationship between luteinizing hormone releasing hormone concentration in hypophysial portal blood and luteinizing hormone release in intact castrated and electrochemically-stimulated rats. *Endocrinology,* **100,** 263

Ferland, L., Marchetti, B., Seguin, C., Lefebvre, F. A., Reeves, J. J. and Labrie, F. (1981). Dissociated changes of pituitary luteinizing hormone releasing hormone (LHRH) receptors and responsiveness to the neurohormone induced by 17β estradiol and LHRH in vivo in the rat. *Endocrinology,* **109,** 87

Fink, G. (1976). The development of the releasing factor concept. *Clin. Endocrinol.*, **5** (Suppl.), 245s

Frager, M., Duncan, J., Pieper, D., Tonetta, S. and Marshall, J. C. (1979). Induction of pituitary membrane GnRH receptors by GnRH and a superagonist analog. Abstr. No. 432, *61st Meeting of the Endocrine Society*

Frager, M. S., Pieper, D. R., Tonetta, S., Duncan, J. A. and Marshall, J. C. (1981). Pituitary gonadotrophin-releasing hormone receptors: effects of castration, steroid replacement and the role of GnRH in modulating receptors in the rat. *J. Clin. Invest.*, **67**, 615

Giguere, V., Lefebvre, F. A. and Labrie, F. (1981). Androgens decrease LHRH binding sites in rat anterior pituitary cells in culture. *Endocrinology*, **108**, 350

Hazum, E. (1981). Some characteristics of GnRH-receptors in rat pituitary membranes: differences between an agonist and an antagonist. *Mol. Cell. Endocrinol.*, **23**, 275

Hazum, E., Cuatrecasas, P., Marian, J. and Conn, P. M. (1980). Receptor mediated internalization of fluorescent gonadotrophin releasing hormone by pituitary gonadotrophs. *Proc. Natl. Acad. Sci. U.S.A.*, **77**, 6692

Hunter, M. G., Sullivan, M. H. I., Dix, C. J., Aldred, L. F. and Cooke, B. A. (1982). Stimulation and inhibition by LHRH analogues of cultured rat Leydig cell function and lack of effect on mouse Leydig cells. *Mol. Cell. Endocrinol.*, **27**, 31

Knobil, E. (1980). The neuroendocrine control of the menstrual cycle. *Recent Prog. Horm. Res.*, **36**, 53

Loumaye, E. and Catt, K. J. (1982*a*). Homologous regulation of gonadotrophin releasing hormone receptors in cultured pituitary cells. *Science*, **215**, 983

Loumaye, E. and Catt, K. J. (1983). Agonist-induced regulation of pituitary receptors for gonadotropin releasing hormone. *J. Biol. Chem.*, **258**, 12002

Loumaye, E. and Forni, L. (1982). Regulatory actions of 17β estradiol and progesterone upon pituitary GnRH receptors in vitro. Abstr. No. 825, *64th Annual Meeting of the Endocrine Society*, June, San Francisco

Loumaye, E., Naor, Z. and Catt, K. J. (1982). Binding affinity and biological activity of gonadotrophin-releasing hormone agonists in isolated pituitary cells. *Endocrinology*, **111**, 730

Marchetti, B. and Labrie, F. (1982). Prolactin inhibits pituitary LHRH receptors in the rat. *Endocrinology*, **111**, 1209

Marchetti, B., Reeves, J. J., Pelletier, G. and Labrie, F. (1982). Modulation of pituitary luteinizing hormone releasing hormone receptors by sex steroids and LHRH in the rat. *Biol. Reprod.*, **27**, 133

Meridan, R. and Koch, Y. (1981). Binding of luteinizing hormone-releasing hormone analogues to dispersed rat pituitary cells. *Life Sci.*, **28**, 1961

Naor, Z., Clayton, R. N. and Catt, K. J. (1980). Characterization of gonadotrophin-releasing hormone receptors in cultured rat pituitary cells. *Endocrinology*, **107**, 1144

Naor, Z., Atlas, D., Clayton, R. N., Forman, D. S., Amsterdam, A. and Catt, K. J. (1981). Interaction of fluorescent gonadotrophin-releasing hormone with receptors in cultured pituitary cells. *J. Biol. Chem.*, **256**, 3049

Naor, Z., Childes, G. V., Leifer, A. M., Clayton, R. N., Amsterdam, A. and Catt, K. J. (1982). Gonadotrophin releasing hormone binding and activation of enriched population of pituitary gonadotrophs. *Mol. Cell. Endocrinol.*, **25**, 85

Nett, T. M., Crowder, M. E., Moss, G. E. and Duello, T. M. (1981). GnRH-Receptor interaction. V. Down-regulation of pituitary receptors for GnRH in ovariectomized ewes by infusion of homologous hormone. *Biol. Reprod.*, **24**, 1145

Perrin, M. H., Rivier, J. E. and Vale, W. W. (1980). Radioligand assay for gonadotrophin-releasing hormone: relative potencies of agonists and antagonists. *Endocrinology*, **106**, 1289

Pieper, D. R., Gala, R. R., Regiani, S. R. and Marshall, J. C. (1982). Dependence of pituitary gonadotrophin releasing hormone receptors on GnRH secretion from the hypothalamus. *Endocrinology*, **110**, 749

Sandow, J. (1983). Clinical applications of LHRH analogues. *Clin. Endocrinol.* (In press)

Sarkar, D. K. and Fink (1979). Effects of gonadal steroids on output of luteinizing hormone releasing factor into pituitary stalk blood in the female rat. *J. Endocrinol.*, **80**, 303

Sarkar, D. K., Chiappa, S. A. and Fink, G. (1976). Gonadotrophin releasing hormone surge in proestrus rats. *Nature* (*Lond.*), **264**, 461

Savoy-Moore, R., Schwartz, N. B., Duncan, J. A. and Marshall, J. C. (1980). Pituitary gonadotrophin releasing hormone receptors during the rat estrous cycle. *Science*, **209**, 942

Savoy-Moore, R. T., Schwartz, N. B., Duncan, J. A. and Marshall, J. C. (1981). Pituitary GnRH receptors on proestrus: effect of pentobarbital blockade of ovulation in the rat. *Endocrinology,* **109,** 1360

Smith, M. A. and Vale, W. W. (1981). Desensitization to gonadotrophin releasing hormone observed in superfused pituitary cells on cytodex beads. *Endocrinology,* **108,** 752

Sternberger, L. A. and Petrali, J. P. (1975). Quantitative immunocytochemistry of pituitary receptors for luteinizing hormone releasing hormone. *Cell Tiss. Res.,* **162,** 141

Wagner, T. O. F. and von Zur Mohlen, A. (1982). Interaction of gonadotrophin releasing hormone (GnRH) and GnRH analogue with the anterior pituitary gonadotroph. In Motta, M., Zanisi, M. and Piva, F. (eds.) *Pituitary Hormones and related Peptides, Serono Symposia No. 49,* pp. 171–81. (London: Academic Press)

White, S. S. and Ojeda, S. R. (1982). Pituitary LHRH receptors during puberty in the female rat: is the pro-estrous decline in receptor content due to occupancy? *Endocrinology,* **111,** 353

SECTION II

REPRODUCTIVE PHYSIOLOGY AND PHARMACOLOGY IN LABORATORY ANIMALS

5
Biological assays utilized to characterize LHRH and its analogs

D. W. HAHN, J. L. McGUIRE, W. VALE and J. RIVIER

Many methods for assaying the activity and potency of LHRH agonists and antagonists in the female have been developed. Considerably fewer assays have been done in males. Although several good comparisons of LHRH and its analogs have been conducted in male laboratory animals (Labrie *et al.*, 1980), extensive potency studies on the reproductive effects of these peptides have been more conveniently assessed in females because the dosing schedules have been shorter and the endpoints more easily determined. Although the number and variations of the assays used to evaluate LHRH analogs have proliferated, they can be conveniently divided for ease of review into *in vitro* and *in vivo* assays.

IN VITRO ASSAYS

In vitro assays have been especially useful in the initial characterization of newly synthesized analogs. Requiring only very small quantities of peptide, they quickly provide information about the activity analogs possess and, in a relative sense, how potent they might be. Two types of *in vitro* assays have been used to evaluate analogs.

The first utilizes the secretion of LH or FSH or both by cultures of pituitary fragments, dispersed pituitary cells or pituitary cell monolayers. Both agonists and antagonists have been evaluated with these assays. In general, activities of agonists are assessed by their ability to release gonadotropins, and antagonists are assessed by their ability to inhibit LHRH-induced gonadotropin release. The earliest culture technique involved the use of pituitary halves or quarters (Saffran and Schally, 1955). Although these cultures were simple to construct, they yielded results with considerable variability due to variations in individual pituitary responses (Guillemin and Vale, 1970). This problem was circumvented by culturing several fragments, each from different animals, in each incubation flask (Schally *et al.*, 1970). The problem of pituitary gland heterogenicity, however, is best overcome by enzymatic dispersion of the pituitary cells (Vale *et al.*, 1972). In this technique, multiple aliquots of cells are withdrawn from a single pool of dispersed pituitary cells, resulting in many subcultures which are challenged with various analogs in multiple doses. Although acutely dispersed cells have been used they do not always respond well to extrinsic hypothalamic factors (Vale *et al.*, 1972). Pituitary cells which have been cultured for 3–4 days, and have formed a monolayer, seemed to be most sensitive to LHRH and to yield consistent results. The secretion of LH from such cells after a 2.5 h exposure to 10^{-8} mol/l synthetic LHRH was elevated approximately 15-fold over unexposed cells and the culture to culture variation was small (Vale *et al.*, 1972). The consistency of this response has made this procedure an important assay in analog evaluation.

The second type of *in vitro* assay which has been used to evaluate analog potency is a receptor binding assay. As with other peptide hormones, LHRH produces its effects by first binding to specific receptor sites on target cells. Following the demonstration of specific LHRH receptors on pituitary cells (Spona, 1973*a*,*b*; Grant *et al.*, 1973), the binding affinities of analogs for purified membrane fractions were used to estimate the potencies of newly synthesized peptides (Vale *et al.*, 1981). In this technique, radioactively labeled analog is incubated with a pituitary membrane fraction purified by centrifugation (Clayton and Catt, 1980; Perrin *et al.*, 1980). The system is incubated for approximately an hour at 4 °C. After isolating the bound hormone, the radioactivity is quantitated and the competition between analogs assessed. Since specific receptors for LHRH exist in the gonads these experiments were also performed with ovarian and testicular membrane preparations (Vale *et al.*, 1981). Pituitary, ovary and testis membranes contain 400, 40 and 17 fmol of binding sites per mg membrane protein, respectively, while their respective K_D values for binding to [^{125}I-Tyr^5,D-Ala^6,N-MeLeu^7,Pro^9-NHEt]LHRH were 0.32, 0.27 and 0.26 nmol/l (Vale *et al.*, 1981). Because the membrane assay measures only binding affinity, it does not distinguish agonistic from antagonistic activities.

The binding assay yielded lower potencies for super agonists relative to LHRH than did the pituitary cell culture assay. [D-Trp^6,Pro^9-NHEt]LHRH and [D-His(Bzl)^6,Pro^9-NHEt]LHRH were 144 and 210 times more potent than LHRH in the pituitary cell culture assay. In the membrane binding assay, however, these peptides were only 50 and 55 times more potent than LHRH. The increased potencies of the super agonists may result from factors other than greater binding affinities for pituitary cell receptors. It has been suggested that the increased hydrophobicity of these molecules may provide them with an advantage in the culture assay which uses intact cells but not in the receptor assay which uses membranes (Vale *et al.*, 1981). Furthermore, since the agonists are incubated for several hours at 37 °C in the culture assay but only for 30 min at 0 °C in the receptor assay, their increased resistance to degradation (Koch *et al.*, 1977) may also explain their higher potencies in the pituitary culture system (Vale *et al.*, 1981).

These assays do provide relative *in vitro* potencies of new analogs, but do not yield information about the rate and extent of absorption or the rate of clearance of analogs, all of which contribute to the biological response.

IN VIVO ASSAYS

To understand the various *in vivo* biological assays which have been utilized in various laboratories to characterize LHRH analogs, one must consider our current understanding of the role of LHRH. LHRH is important in all reproductive functions including normal cyclicity and pregnancy. Loss of LHRH results in interruption of normal estrous cycles, gonadal atrophy, suppression of secretion of gonadal steroids and blockade of gestation in mammalian species.

Although the same bioassays can be utilized to study agonists and antagonists of LHRH, for convenience in describing the use of these assays, we have separated agonist and antagonist assays in the following discussion.

Agonists

Induction of ovulation

The most widely used animal models for the induction of ovulation by LHRH and the agonists have been the proestrous rat or hamster whose spontaneous ovulatory mechanism has been blocked with pentobarbital (Corbin and Bex, 1980*a*; Corbin *et al.*, 1978), the diestrous rat or hamster (Hahn *et al.*, 1981*a*; Bex *et al.*, 1982), and the androgen-sterilized rat (Hahn *et al.*, 1981*b*; Hahn and McGuire, 1978).

The first assay procedure stems from the work of Everett and Sawyer (1950), who first demonstrated that administration of a moderate dose of Nembutal to 4-day cyclic rats at 2:00 p.m. during proestrus consistently blocked LH release. The second assay is the induction of ovulation in diestrous rats. The third assay, induction of ovulation in androgen-sterilized rats, is based on the finding that androgen treatment of newborn female rats produces a hypothalamic disorder resulting in persistent vaginal cornification, anovulation and subsequent alteration of cyclic release of LH from the pituitary. LHRH and its agonists will stimulate LH release and induce ovulation in these three animal models.

These three animal models for the induction of ovulation exhibit different sensitivities to LHRH and its agonists (Hahn *et al.*, 1983). In studies evaluating LHRH and [D-His(Bzl)^6,Pro^9-NHEt]LHRH in these test systems, the nembutalized proestrous rat responded to low doses of the agonist (ED_{50} = 0.06 μg/kg) and was the most sensitive model (Table 5.1). The androgen-sterilized rat was the next most sensitive animal and the diestrous rat was the least sensitive of the three models tested.

There are also differences between species. In a comparison of the sensitivities of three species (Figure 5.1), the diestrous rat was most sensitive to the induction of ovulation with [D-His(Bzl)^6,Pro^9-NHEt]LHRH, the diestrous hamster was intermediate in sensitivity, and the diestrous mouse was the least sensitive species tested (Hahn *et al.*, 1983; Bex *et al.*, 1982). Hormone patterns in the three species may vary during the estrous cycle, accounting for some of the differences in sensitivities.

Table 5.1 The induction of ovulation with [D-His(Bzl)^6,Pro^9-NHEt]LHRH in three animal models

Ovulation induction model	*LHRH*	*ED*$_{50}$ (μg/kg)[a] [*D-His(Bzl)*^{6},*Pro*^{9}-*NHEt*]*LHRH*	*Ratio LHRH/Agonist*
Nembutalized proestrous rat	0.19	0.06	3.2
Androgen-sterilized rat	1.76	0.36	4.9
Diestrous rat	5.17	0.56	9.2

[a] Dose which induced ovulation in 50% of the animals

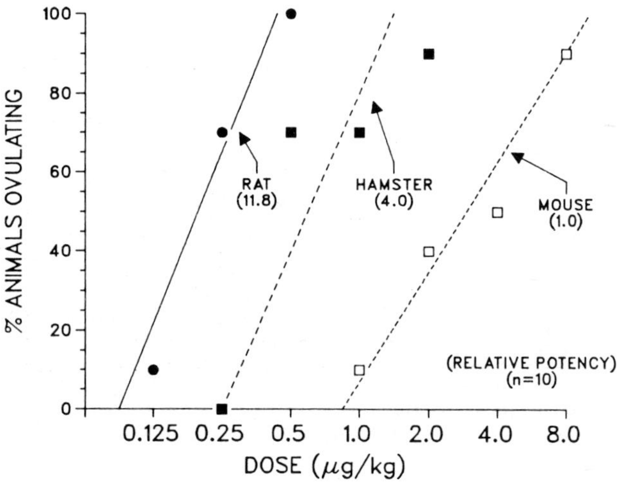

Figure 5.1 Induction of ovulation with [D-His(Bzl)^6,Pro^9-NHEt]LHRH in diestrous rats, hamsters and mice. All animals treated on diestrus, subcutaneously with saline vehicle (Hahn *et al.*, 1983).

Disruption of the estrous cycle

Less commonly used, but none the less important, for identifying the paradoxical antireproductive effect of LHRH agonists is a bioassay based on disruption of the estrous cycle. Prolonged treatment with superagonists leads to ovarian and uterine regression, accompanied by decreased sex steroid levels and a state of constant diestrus (Johnson *et al.*, 1976). Regular cyclicity and normal reproductive function return quickly (Johnson *et al.*, 1976) and both disruption of the cycle (Nestor *et al.*, 1982) and recovery (Corbin and Bex, 1980*b*) appear dose related.

The antifertility effects of LHRH analogs are evaluated by monitoring the rat estrous cycle during chronic treatment. The most commonly used regimen involves injections twice daily for 14 days (Nestor *et al.*, 1982) while monitoring vaginal cytology. Other parameters such as the delay of mating (Beattie and Corbin, 1977) and the return to fertility (Corbin and Bex, 1980*b*) after the cessation of treatment have also been evaluated. Although this test system is less sensitive than the ovulation–induction systems, dose responses have been shown (Corbin and Bex, 1980*b*) and relative potencies comparing agonists have been estimated (Nestor *et al.*, 1982).

As an example, [D-His(Bzl)^6,Pro^9-NHEt]LHRH was evaluated in the rat during 14 days of treatment for effects on cyclicity, subsequent mating and pregnancy after cessation of treatment. This agonist caused a delay in the occurrence of estrus as determined by vaginal cytology (Table 5.2). When these same rats were cohabited with males after treatment had ended, control animals mated in 2 days, whereas treated rats mated in 3–4 days. In addition, the mean number of implants was reduced in a dose-related manner in the treated animals.

Table 5.2 Effect of [D-His(Bzl)^6,Pro^9-NHEt]LHRH on cyclicity, subsequent mating and pregnancy in the rat

Dose μg/kg[a]	*Mean no. days ± SE* *Estrus delayed*	*Mean no. days ± SE* *Mating occurred after treatment*	*Mean no. (± SE) uterine implants*
0	0	2.0±0	11.8±1.9
0.156	0.5±0.2	2.7±0.2	11.2±1.6
0.625	6.2±1.5	3.7±0.4	10.1±2.3
1.25	11.0±0	3.6±0.2	5.7±2.0

[a] Rats treated subcutaneously, once daily (saline vehicle) for 14 days beginning on diestrus I

Effects on pregnancy

A third parameter which is routinely examined when studying LHRH agonists is effects on pregnancy. Agonistic analogs of LHRH interfere with established pregnancy in the rabbit (Hilliard *et al.*, 1976), hamster (Windsor *et al.*, 1977) and rat (Corbin *et al.*, 1979; Rivier *et al.*, 1978). The mouse, however, appears to be resistant to the antifertility effects of the agonists (Bex *et al.*, 1982). The relative potencies of the agonists in affecting pregnancy in the rat correspond to the potencies generated by the induction of ovulation (Corbin *et al.*, 1978). The agonists are active by various routes of administration (Corbin and Bex, 1980*a*) and in various vehicles (Rivier *et al.*, 1978). It appears that vehicles which afford slow, sustained release (e.g. corn oil) or aqueous vehicle in divided doses result in greater activity (Rivier *et al.*, 1978) than a single daily administration in an aqueous vehicle. Agonists inhibit pregnancy when administered either before or after implantation (Rivier *et al.*, 1978) and a return to normal cyclicity and fertility occurs quickly (Corbin *et al.*, 1979). Preimplantation treatment with LHRH causes a distortion of LH and FSH patterns, an inhibition of prolactin and progesterone and a delay and reduction of estradiol secretion (Corbin *et al.*, 1979). The inhibition and delay of implantation is partially attributable to a premature rise in serum LH which is luteolytic during early pregnancy, and a delay in the serum estrogen rise which is required for normal implantation. The action of the agonists on gestation involves an increased secretion of LH which results in a decrease of ovarian LH receptor concentration (Kledzik *et al.*, 1978). These changes are associated with luteolysis and a decrease in serum progesterone. The contragestational effects of the agonists are related to their ability to inhibit progesterone and can be reversed by concomitant treatment with progesterone (Jones, 1979; Rivier and Vale, 1982).

The major mechanism of action appears to be at the level of the pituitary–gonadal axis. Since the pituitary is not necessary for maintenance of pregnancy in the rat after day 12, data showing that agonists can terminate pregnancy in the hypophysectomized rat (Bex and Corbin, 1981) suggest an extrapituitary site of action (i.e. ovary or placenta).

Effect on uterine growth

Although chronic treatment with LHRH or agonistic analogs causes a regression of the reproductive tract in mature and immature female rats (Johnson *et al.*, 1976), short term administration for 3 days produces a dose-related increase in uterine growth in immature mice (Corbin *et al.*, 1979; Hahn *et al.*, 1981*b*). This animal model provides a system which has been used to compare analog potencies. In studies evaluating two LHRH agonists, [D-Trp^6,Pro^9-NHEt]LHRH and [D-His(Bzl)^6,Pro^9-NHEt]LHRH were 55 and 57 times more potent than LHRH, respectively (Figure 5.2). Both peptides

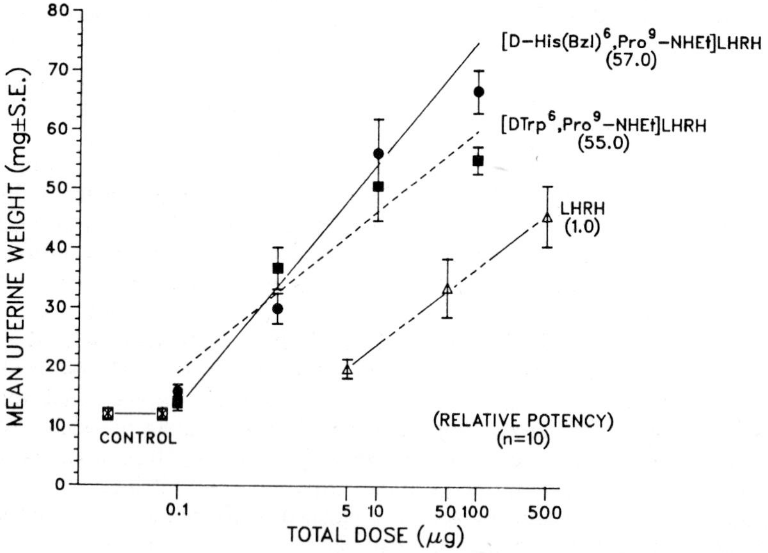

Figure 5.2 The uterotropic activity of LHRH and two agonists in the immature mouse. Mice treated subcutaneously (sesame oil), once daily for 3 consecutive days. Uteri recovered and weighed on day 4. (Hahn *et al.*, 1983).

exhibited dose response curves which were statistically parallel to the curve obtained for LHRH.

This animal model has also been used to illustrate the importance of the vehicle used in administering these peptides. When LHRH or the agonists were administered in a daily s.c. injection in sesame oil, a dose-related increase in uterine weight was induced. When saline was used instead of the oil, little or no uterine growth was induced. However, if the same daily dose in saline was spread over five injections, significant uterine growth occurred (Hahn *et al.*, 1981*b*). It appears that this animal model, as has been reported for other animal models (Rivier *et al.*, 1978), may require a vehicle which provides a slow, sustained release to obtain maximum activity.

Antagonists

Inhibition of ovulation

Antagonistic analogs of LHRH inhibit ovulation in rats, hamsters and rabbits (Nishi *et al.*, 1976; Reel *et al.*, 1980). The blockade of ovulation is due to inhibition of the preovulatory LH surge (Pedroza *et al.*, 1978). Proper timing of antagonist treatment is critical (Hahn *et al.*, 1983; Beattie *et al.*, 1975). Although treatment with inhibitory analogs has caused a disruption of hormone levels in several species of monkey, success in inhibition of ovulation has been limited (Balmaceda *et al.*, 1981). This may be due to the timing of the LH surge of the monkey which is more difficult to predict than that of the rat.

The rat antiovulatory model has become the standard assay for evaluating new antagonistic analogs of LHRH (Corbin and Bex, 1980*b*) especially since *in vitro* activities do not always correlate with *in vivo* activities (Corbin and Bex, 1980*b*; Humphries *et al.*, 1978). Proper timing of antagonist treatment depends on the lighting schedule of the animal colony. Various dosing regimens have been tested under one lighting schedule (Corbin and Beattie, 1975) and it was found that 1200–1230 *h* was the most sensitive time for treatment in the rat when an antagonist was given subcutaneously in corn oil, while 0900 h was the most sensitive time when intramuscular administration was used. This regimen has been widely used for analog screening (Erchegyi *et al.*, 1981; Rivier *et al.*, 1981*a*). Our own studies (12 h light/dark, lights on at 6:00 a.m.) have indicated that 1400–1500 h in the rat and 1000 h in the hamster were the most sensitive periods for treatment in our laboratory (Hahn *et al.*, 1983).

Different species also exhibit varying sensitivities to the inhibition of ovulation with LHRH antagonists. A study which examined the ability of [N-Ac-Δ^3-Pro^1,D-pF-Phe^2,D-Trp^{3,6}]LHRH to inhibit spontaneous ovulation in hamsters and rats has shown the rat to be more sensitive to this antagonist than the hamster. Approximately 14 times more antagonist was needed in the hamster as compared to the rat to achieve the same response (Hahn *et al.*, 1983).

It is clear that many factors, including time of treatment, species treated, vehicle, route of administration and rate of metabolism, play important roles in determining the effects of the antagonists on ovulation.

Disruption of the estrous cycle

There have been few reports involving the disruption of the rat estrous cycle with antagonists. [N-Ac-Δ^3-Pro^1,D-pF-Phe^2,D-Trp^{3,6},Pro^9-NHEt]LHRH has been shown to interfere with the cyclicity of 50 % of the rats treated with a single 200 μg injection. One 200 μg injection every fourth day altered cyclicity in all treated rats (Rivier *et al.*, 1981*b*). These changes in cyclicity were characterized by vaginal smears exhibiting alternate patterns of leukocytic and cornified cells with periods of prolonged estrus. Antagonists also may cause periods of prolonged diestrus (Reel *et al.*, 1980).

Effect on pregnancy

Whereas many studies have been reported involving the effects of LHRH agonists on pregnancy, relatively few have been reported using the antagonists. [D-pGlu^1,D-Phe^2,D-Trp^{3,6}]LHRH has been shown to inhibit pregnancy in 100 % of the rats treated twice daily (2.5 mg × 2) on days 1–7 (inclusive) of gestation (Rivier *et al.*, 1979). Lower doses caused a delay of parturition. In studies in which [N-Ac-Δ^3-Pro^1,D-pCl-Phe^2,D-Trp^{3,6},N-MeLeu^7]LHRH or [N-Ac-Δ^3-Pro^1,D-pF-Phe^2,D-Trp^{3,6}]LHRH was administered to rats at various stages of pregnancy it was shown that postimplantation treatment was more effective in terminating pregnancy than was preimplantation treatment (Rivier and Vale, 1981). Concomitant treatment with progesterone reversed the contragestational effects of the antagonists given either pre- or postimplantation (Rivier and Vale, 1981).

Serum gonadotropin levels

Potency determinations of agonists can be made by measuring the release of LH and FSH into the peripheral circulation, and of antagonists, by measuring the inhibition of LHRH induced gonadotropin release. Serum gonadotropin levels have been studied in several different animal models, including ovariectomized, estrogen and progesterone treated rats (Ramirez and McCann, 1963), immature male rats (Gupta *et al.*, 1975), androgen-sterilized female rats (Uilenbroek and Gribling-Hegge, 1977), intact male and female mice (Bex *et al.*, 1982) and rats (Cao *et al.*, 1982), hypophysectomized rats (Cao *et al.*, 1982), chimpanzees (Sundaram *et al.*, 1982), rabbits (Rippel *et al.*, 1975) and the ram (Bremner *et al.*, 1980). The rat has become the animal model of choice, largely because it is small, responds well to surgical manipulation and has a well-characterized hypothalamic–pituitary–gonadal axis. The ovariectomized, estrogen and progesterone treated female rat is an especially sensitive model for assessing LH-releasing activity of agonists (Ramirez and McCann, 1963).

To measure the integrated release of gonadotropins, two approaches have been used. In one, several groups of animals were given the analog and each group was killed and bled at different times (Moger, 1982). This procedure, however, required many animals and a sizable amount of peptide. A second approach has been to collect serial blood samples from a single group of animals. These samples were procured by venipuncture (Rippel *et al.*, 1975), but the number obtained from each animal was limited and stress-related effects were possible. Alternatively, a catheter implanted in the jugular vein permits several samples to be collected over several hours. A possible shortcoming of this procedure is that the effects of surgery and anesthesia on gonadotropin release are not completely understood. Pentobarbital (Gupta *et al.*, 1975) and urethane (Arimura *et al.*, 1972) have been used in the male rat, and reportedly have no significant effect on LH levels (Ondo and Pass, 1980). To circumvent anesthesia or other surgical effects, animals have been implanted with indwelling catheters and permitted to recover a day or more before testing. An added advantage of this method is that data may be collected over several days if necessary. The catheters, however, must be kept patent, accomplished with heparin and silastic tubing material (Ondo and Pass, 1980).

CONCLUDING REMARKS

There are many *in vitro* and *in vivo* assays available which are used to characterize the multitude of LHRH-analogs synthesized. *In vitro* potencies are most commonly quoted, but ultimately these analogs will be used *in vivo*. Therefore, it is important that *in vivo* data be obtained relatively early as a means of guiding synthetic efforts. Although the activity and potency of LHRH analogs have been reported by many investigators, comparisons of *in vivo* data by different groups are valid only if the same bioassays are utilized in precisely the same manner.

The pharmaceutical properties of a compound (such as particle size, crystalline form, solubility characteristics and partition coefficient), its vehicle and its route of administration can all influence the rate and extent of absorption of a compound and the biologic response. Reported studies with LHRH and its analogs routinely use different vehicles. Various studies have also used different routes of administration and have measured different biologic endpoints which can produce markedly different results with LHRH. Care must be taken in comparing results from different assays in which these variables are not controlled.

References

Arimura, A., Debeljuk, L. E. and Schally, A. V. (1972). Stimulation of FSH release *in vivo* by prolonged infusion of synthetic LHRH. *Endocrinology*, **91**, 529

Balmaceda, J. P., Schally, A. V., Coy, D. and Asch, R. H. (1981). The effects of an LHRH antagonist ([N-Ac-D-Trp^{1,3},D-p-Cl-Phe^{2}, D-Phe^{6},D-Ala^{10}]-LHRH) during the preovulatory period of the rhesus monkey. *Contraception*, **24**, 275

Beattie, C. W. and Corbin, A. (1977). Pre- and postcoital contraceptive activity of LHRH in the rat. *Biol. Reprod.*, **16**, 333

Beattie, C. W., Corbin, A., Foell, T. J., Garsky, V., McKinley, W. A., Rees, R. W. A., Sarantakis, D. and Yardley, J. P. (1975). Luteinizing hormone-releasing hormone. Antiovulatory activity of analogs substituted in positions 2 and 6. *J. Med. Chem.*, **18**, 1247

Bex, T. J. and Corbin, A. (1981). Luteinizing hormone-releasing hormone (LHRH) and LHRH agonist termination of pregnancy in hypophysectomized rats: Extrapituitary site of action. *Endocrinology*, **108**, 273

Bex, T. J., Corbin, A. and France, E. (1982). Resistance of the mouse to the antifertility effects of LHRH agonists. *Life Sci.*, **30,** 1263

Bremner, W. J., Findlay, J. K., Lee, W. K., de Kretser, D. M. and Cumming, I. A. (1980). Feedback effects of the testis on pituitary responsiveness to luteinizing-hormone releasing hormone infusions in the ram. *Endocrinology,* **106,** 329

Cao, Y., Sundaram, K., Bardin, C. W., Rivier, J. and Vale, W. (1982). Direct inhibition of testicular steroidogenesis and gonadotrophin receptor levels by [(imBzl)-D-His^6,Pro^9-NEt]-GnRH and [D-Trp^6,Pro^9-NEt]-GnRH, potent agonists of GnRH. *Int. J. Androl.*, **5,** 158

Clayton, R. N. and Catt, K. J. (1980). Receptor-binding affinity of gonadotropin-releasing hormone analogs: analysis by radioligand-receptor assay. *Endocrinology,* **106,** 1154

Corbin, A. and Beattie, C. W. (1975). Inhibition of the pre-ovulatory proestrous gonadotropin surge, ovulation and pregnancy with a peptide analogue of luteinizing hormone releasing hormone. *Endocr. Res. Commun.*, **2,** 1

Corbin, A., Beattie, C. W., Tracy, J., Jones, R., Foell, T. J., Yardley, J. and Rees, R. W. A. (1978). The anti-reproductive pharmacology of LHRH and agonistic analogues. *Int. J. Fertil.*, **23,** 81

Corbin, A., Beattie, C. W., Jones, R. and Bex, F. (1979). Peptide contraception: Antifertility properties of LHRH analogues. *Int. J. Gynaecol. Obstet.*, **16,** 359

Corbin, A. and Bex, T. J. (1980*a*). Reproductive pharmacology of LHRH and agonists in females and males. *Acta Eur. Fertil.*, **11,** 113

Corbin, A. and Bex, T. J. (1980*b*). Luteinizing hormone releasing hormone and analogues: Conceptive and contraceptive potential. In Briggs, M. and Corbin, A. (eds.) *Progress in Hormone Biochemistry and Pharmacology*. Vol. 1, pp. 227–297. (St Albans, VT: Eden Medical Research)

Erchegyi, J., Coy, D. H., Nekola, M. V., Coy, E. J., Schally, A. V., Mezo, I. and Teplan, I. (1981). Luteinizing hormone-releasing hormone analogs with increased anti-ovulatory activity. *Biochem. Biophys. Res. Commun.*, **100,** 915

Everett, J. W. and Sawyer, C. H. (1950). A 24-hour periodicity in the 'LH-release apparatus' of female rats, disclosed by barbiturate sedation. *Endocrinology,* **47,** 198

Grant, G., Vale, W. and Rivier, J. (1973). Pituitary binding sites for [^{3}H]-labelled luteinizing hormone releasing factor (LRF). *Biochem. Biophys. Res. Commun.*, **50,** 771

Guillemin, R. and Vale, W. (1970). Bioassays of the hypophysiotropic hormones: *in vitro* systems. In Meites, J. (ed.) *Hypophysiotropic Hormones of the Hypothalamus,* pp. 21–31. (Baltimore: Williams & Wilkins)

Gupta, D., Rager, K., Eichner, M., Zech, K., Fuchs, S. and Voelter, W. (1975). Pituitary gonadotrophins and androgen release induced by a synthetic tetrapeptide in male prepubertal and adult rats. *J. Endocrinol.*, **64,** 391

Hahn, D. W. and McGuire, J. L. (1978). The androgen-sterilized rat: Induction of ovulation and implantation by luteinizing hormone-releasing hormone. *Endocrinology,* **102,** 1741

Hahn, D. W., Phillips, A. and McGuire, J. L. (1981*a*). The need for controlling variables involved in biologic assays of LHRH. In Zatuchni, G. I., Shelton, J. D. and Schiarra, J. J. (eds.) *LHRH Peptides as Female and Male Contraceptives,* pp. 366–373. (Philadelphia: Harper & Row)

Hahn, D. W., Phillips-Probst, A. and McGuire, J. L. (1981*b*). The importance of biopharmaceutic considerations in biological assays of LHRH and its analogs. *Endocr. Res. Commun.*, **8,** 273

Hahn, D. W., Lai, M. T., Klimek, S., Ericson, E. W., Phillips, A. and McGuire, J. L. (1983). In vivo pharmacological evaluation of LHRH agonists and antagonists. *Endocr. Res. Commun.*, (In press)

Hilliard, J., Pang, C. and Sawyer, C. H. (1976). Effects of luteinizing hormone-releasing hormone on fetal survival in pregnant rabbits. *Fertil. Steril.*, **27,** 421

Humphries, J., Wan, Y. P., Folkers, K., and Bowers, C. Y. (1978). Inhibitory analogues of the luteinizing hormone-releasing hormone having D-aromatic residues in positions 2 and 6 and variation in position 3. *J. Med. Chem.*, **21,** 120

Johnson, E. S., Gendrich, R. L. and White, W. F. (1976). Delay of puberty and inhibition of reproductive processes in the rat by a gonadotropin-releasing hormone agonist analog. *Fertil. Steril.*, **27,** 853

Jones, R. C. (1979). Reversal of the anti-implantational effect of luteinizing hormone-releasing hormone (LHRH) by estradiol-17β and progesterone, alone and in sequence. *Contraception,* **19,** 239

Kledzik, G. S., Cusan, L., Auclair, C., Kelly, P. A. and Labrie, F. (1978). Inhibitory effect of luteinizing hormone (LH)-releasing hormone agonist on rat ovarian LH and follicle-stimulating hormone receptor level during pregnancy. *Fertil. Steril.*, **29,** 560

Koch, Y., Baram, T., Hazum, E. and Fridkin, M. (1977). Resistance to enzymic degradation of LHRH analogues possessing increased biological activity. *Biochem. Biophys. Res. Commun.*, **74,** 488

Labrie, F., Bélanger, A., Cusan, L., Séguin, C., Pelletier, G., Kelly, P. A., Reeves, J. J., Lefebvre, F.-A., Lemay, A., Gourdeau, Y. and Raynaud, J.-P. (1980). Antifertility effects of LHRH agonists in the male. *J. Androl.* **1,** 209

Moger, W. H. (1982). Impact of pulsatile administration of gonadotropin-releasing hormone on the pituitary testicular axis of the immature rat. *J. Androl.*, **3,** 256

Nestor, J. J. Jr., Ho, T. L., Simpson, R. A., Horner, B. L., Jones, G. H., McRae, G. I. and Vickery, B. H. (1982). Synthesis and biological activity of some very hydrophobic superagonist analogues of luteinizing hormone-releasing hormone. *J. Med. Chem.*, **25,** 795

Nishi, N., Coy, D. H., Coy, E. J., Arimura, A. and Schally, A. V. (1976). Suppression of LHRH-induced ovulation in hamsters and rats by synthetic analogues of LHRH. *J. Reprod. Fertil.*, **48,** 119

Ondo, J. G. and Pass, K. A. (1980). Pituitary LH response to LHRH in male rats following pentobarbital anesthesia. *Life Sci.*, **27,** 2071

Pedroza, E., Vilchez-Martinez, J. A., Coy, D. H., Arimura, A. and Schally, A. V. (1978). Correlation between *in vivo* inhibition of gonadotropin release induced by LHRH and the blockade of ovulation by synthetic analogues of LHRH. *Int. J. Fertil.*, **23,** 294

Perrin, M. H., Rivier, J. E. and Vale, W. W. (1980). Radioligand assay for gonadotropin-releasing hormone: relative potencies of agonists and antagonists. *Endocrinology*, **106,** 1289

Ramirez, V. D. and McCann, S. M. (1963). A highly sensitive test for LH-releasing activity: the ovariectomized, estrogen, progesterone-blocked rat. *Endocrinology*, **73,** 193

Reel, J. R., Humphrey, R. R., Jones, D. C., Jordan, J. H., Pastushok, C. A., Sakowski, R., Windsor, B. L. and Edgren, R. A. (1980). The biological effect of two antagonistic analogues of luteinizing hormone releasing hormone. *Contraception*, **22,** 39

Rippel, R. H., Johnson, E. S., White, W. F., Fujino, M., Fukuda, T. and Kobayashi, S. (1975). Ovulation and gonadotropin-releasing activity of [D-Leu^6,Des-Gly NH_2^{10},Pro-ethylamide^9]-GnRH. *Proc. Soc. Exp. Biol. Med.*, **148,** 1193

Rivier, C., Rivier, J. and Vale, W. (1978). Chronic effects of [D-Trp^6-Pro^9-NEt] luteinizing hormone-releasing factor on reproductive processes in the female rat. *Endocrinology*, **103,** 2299

Rivier, C., Rivier, J. and Vale, W. (1979). Effect of the LRF-antagonist [D-pGlu^1,D-Phe^2, D-Trp^{3,6}]-LRF on pregnancy in the rat. *Contraception*, **19,** 185

Rivier, C. and Vale, W. (1981). Temporal relationships between the abortifacient effects of GNRH antagonists and hormonal secretion. *Biol. Reprod.*, **24,** 1061

Rivier, J., Rivier, C., Perrin, M., Porter, J. and Vale, W. W. (1981*a*). GnRH analogs: Structure–activity relationships. In Zatuchni, G. I., Shelton, J. D. and Sciarra, J. J. (eds.) *Contraceptives*, pp. 13–23. (Philadelphia: Harper & Row)

Rivier, C., Rivier, J. and Vale, W. W. (1981*b*). GnRH antagonists: Physiologic and contraceptive applications in the female rat. In Zatuchni, G. I., Shelton, J. D. and Sciarra, J. J. (eds.) *Contraceptives*, pp. 140–150. (Philadelphia: Harper & Row)

Rivier, C. and Vale, W. (1982). Interaction of gonadotropin-releasing hormone agonist and antagonist with progesterone, prolactin, or human chorionic gonadotropin during pregnancy in the rat. *Endocrinology*, **110,** 347

Saffran, M. and Schally, A. V. (1955). The release of corticotrophin by anterior pituitary tissue in vitro. *Can. J. Biochem. Physiol.*, **33,** 408

Schally, A. V., Mittler, J. C. and White, W. F. (1970). Failure of putrescine and other polyamines to promote FSH release in vitro. *Endocrinology*, **86,** 903

Spona, J. (1973*a*). LHRH interaction with pituitary plasma membrane. *FEBS Lett.*, **34,** 24

Spona, J. (1973*b*). LHRH-stimulated gonadotropin release mediated by two distinct pituitary receptors. *FEBS Lett.*, **35,** 50

Sundaram, K., Connell, K. G., Bardin, C. W., Samojlik, E. and Schally, A. V. (1982). Inhibition of pituitary-testicular function with [D-Trp^6]-luteinizing hormone-releasing hormone in rhesus monkeys. *Endocrinology*, **110,** 1308

Uilenbroek, J. T. J. and Gribling-Hegge, L. A. (1977). Pituitary responsiveness to LH-RH in intact and ovariectomized androgen-sterilized rats. *Neuroendocrinology*, **23,** 43

Vale, W., Grant, G., Amoss, M., Blackwell, R. and Guillemin, R. (1972). Culture of enzymatically dispersed anterior pituitary cells: functional validation of a method. *Endocrinology*, **91,** 562

Vale, W. W., Rivier, C., Perrin, M., Smith, M. and Rivier, J. (1981). Pharmacology of gonadotropin releasing hormone: a model regulatory peptide. In Martin, J. B., Reichlin, J. and Bick, K. L. (eds.) *Neurosecretion and Brain Peptides*, pp. 609–625. (New York: Raven Press)

Windsor, B. L., Humphrey, R. R., Reel, J. R. and Edgren, R. A. (1977). Postnidatory effects of luteinizing hormone releasing hormone (LHRH) in hamsters. *Int. J. Fertil.*, **22,** 184

6
Male contraceptive potential of nafarelin acetate assessed in the dog

B. H. VICKERY and G. I. McRAE

It was originally expected that LHRH and its agonist analogs would achieve therapeutic utility as profertility agents and conversely that antagonist analogs would find their niche as contraceptive agents (Schally and Kastin, 1971). Early findings, however, dramatically affected our thoughts, strategy and progress with these peptide agents. Firstly, it was found that agonist potency was particularly responsive to minor structural modification, e.g. substitution of D-amino acids in place of the sixth amino acid, glycine (Monahan *et al.*, 1973), and replacement of the C-terminal glycinamide by alkylamide (Fujino *et al.*, 1972). By virtue of increases in receptor binding affinity (Perrin *et al.*, 1980) and in protection from metabolic degradation (Koch *et al.*, 1977), extraordinarily potent analogs (superagonists) with potencies more than 200-fold greater than that of the natural hormone were achieved (Nestor *et al.*, 1982). The second finding was that LHRH is required to act in a pulsatile, but low frequency, fashion for normal reproductive functioning or for profertility effects (Belchetz *et al.*, 1978). Thus the fact that continuous infusion of LHRH (McNeil *et al.*, 1979) or even once daily administration of 'superagonists' (Laron *et al.*, 1981) (because of their longevity *in vivo*) results in 'paradoxical' antisteroidogenic and antireproductive effects could be explained as due to a desensitization of target cells in the pituitary (Heber *et al.*, 1982) and possibly also at peripheral sites including the gonad (Hsueh and Jones, 1981).

Emphasis was therefore placed on the identification of highly potent agonist analogs of LHRH to be evaluated as potential contraceptives. One of the most potent of these analogs to be identified was [6-D-3(2-naphthyl)-alanine]LHRH, ([D-Nal(2)^6]LHRH) which, using a screening procedure in rats designed to assay antireproductive activity, was originally assigned a potency of 190–230 times LHRH (Nestor *et al.*, 1982). More recent data suggest a greater rate of metabolism of this compound in rats than in primates including man and that the relative potency of [D-Nal(2)^6]LHRH may be even greater in the latter species.

RATIONALE FOR THE USE OF DOGS

Early studies with LHRH demonstrated that as little as 0.5 μg per rat per day could delay the onset of spermatogenesis and affect testicular steroidogenesis (Oshima *et al.*, 1975). This report went largely unnoticed until, 3–4 years later, antispermatogenic effects of LHRH agonist analogs in mature rats were described (Bex and Corbin, 1978; Labrie *et al.*, 1978). There are now numerous reports describing the effects of these agents in male rats and attempting to use the male rat in elucidating mechanism(s) of activity (Labrie *et al.*, 1980, 1981).

Suppressive effects can be obtained in male rats *in vivo* using either intact (Bélanger *et al.*, 1980) or hypophysectomized states (Bex and Corbin, 1981) and even *in vitro* (Hsueh *et al.*, 1981). The latter two effects are apparently mediated via specific LHRH receptors (Lefebvre *et al.*, 1980). However, long term chronic administration of LHRH agonists to intact male rats results in chronically elevated levels of gonadotropins (Vickery and McRae, 1979). This is at variance with findings in men where lowered, or at least non-responsive, levels of LH are observed (Davies *et al.*, 1977). While there has been considerable debate as to whether the mechanism of action of these agents involves down regulation of homologous testicular gonadotropin receptors or direct testicular effects of LHRH analogs (Seguin *et al.*, 1981), neither mechanism may be critical in men. The search for testicular LHRH receptors in men has so far gone unrewarded (Huhtaniemi and Clayton, 1982).

The rat further differs from man in the unique and inexplicable calcification of the testes which occurs following LHRH agonist treatment (Vickery, 1981); this, together with the incompleteness of spermatogenic inhibition that is achievable (Vickery, 1981; Heber and Swerdloff, 1981), made a more relevant animal model necessary. Of commonly available laboratory species, only dogs and baboons responded to LHRH agonist administration with clear depression of circulating levels of testosterone. Mice, cynomolgus and rhesus (Vickery and McRae, 1980; Bex *et al.*, 1982) (except via special circumstances (Akhtar *et al.*, 1982)) did not respond in such a fashion. Inhibition of spermatogenesis was rapid in dogs (Vickery *et al.*, 1982) and appeared comparable to early reports of the effects of these agents in men (Linde *et al.*, 1981).

EFFECTS ON TESTOSTERONE AND ON ANDROGEN DEPENDENT FUNCTIONS

The earliest studies on the effects of LHRH agonist analogs on sexual function in male dogs were performed with compacted cholesterol pellets containing [D-Trp^6,Pro^9-NHEt]LHRH. After implantation, circulating levels of testosterone were elevated for about a week, then fell to one twentieth of normal. This formulation was a useful tool to evaluate the effects of such analogs with a minimal amount of handling or trauma to the test subjects and made possible the evaluation of effects upon cystic hyperplasia of the prostate in geriatric dogs (Vickery *et al.*, 1982). However, the exponential decay in release

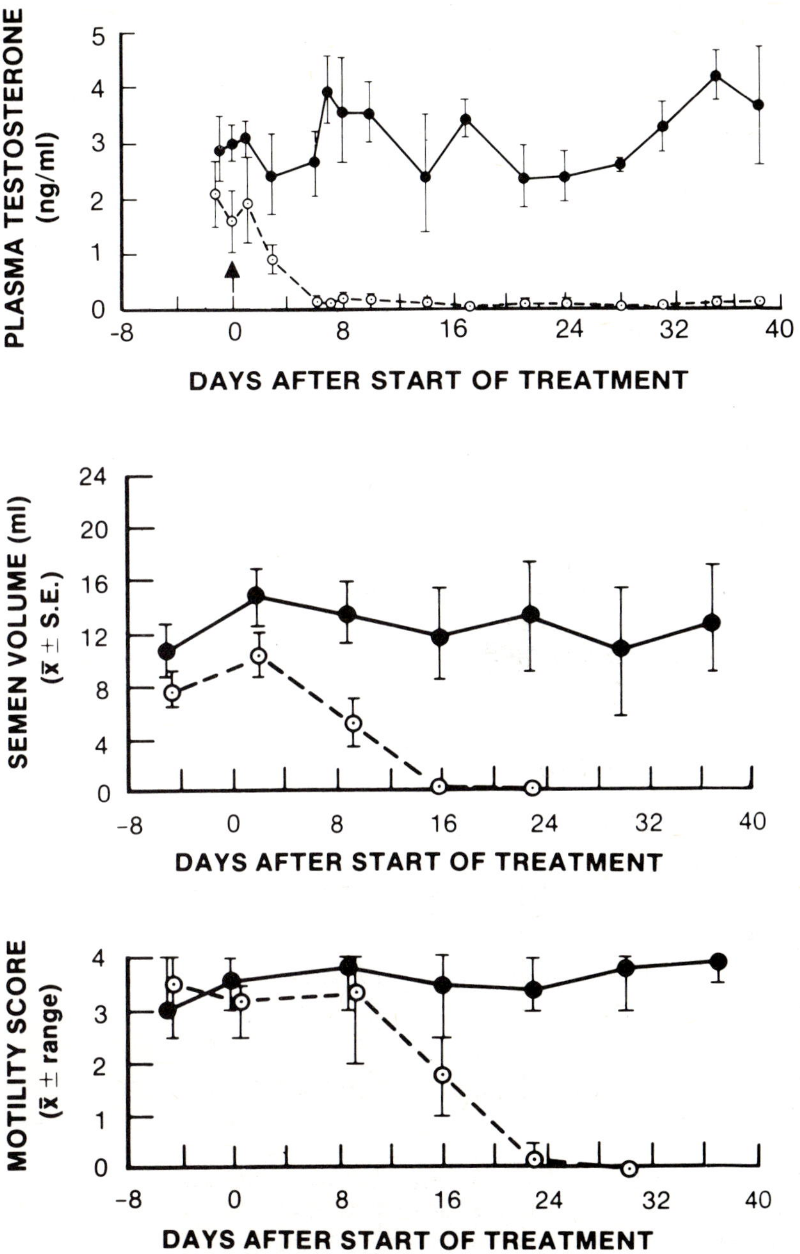

Figure 6.1 Plasma testosterone levels (upper panel), ejaculate volumes (middle panel) and spermatozoal motility (lower panel) of male beagle dogs injected subcutaneously for 38 consecutive days with either vehicle (●———●, $n = 4$) or 10 μg/kg per day of [D-Nal(2)[6]]LHRH (⊙– – –⊙, $n = 2$).

rate from such a matrix or channeling formulation, with attendant variability in duration of action encouraged the switch to daily injectable dosing. Short term (10 d) subcutaneous administration of 10 μg/kg per day of [D-Nal(2)^6]LHRH caused only transient elevation in circulating levels of testosterone with a day by day declining response. Within 3 days the basal, preinjection values of testosterone were markedly suppressed. No effects on sexual function were noted in response to such short term treatment in dogs, consistent with the findings for short duration treatment in men (Bhasin *et al.*, 1982).

Six weeks of treatment in dogs is associated with a disappearance of the acute testosterone response to daily injection by the 4th week of treatment. The testosterone withdrawal results in progressive decline in ejaculate volume and in sperm motility (Figure 6.1). Presumably in response to testosterone withdrawal, a decline in sperm maturity (evidenced by increasing frequency of cytoplasmic droplets) and some lowering of libido (duration of erection) is also noted. At the end of 6 weeks of treatment prostate weight is reduced to 36% of normal.

Administration of lower doses of [D-Nal(2)^6]LHRH on this daily basis is consistent with a more slowly evolving down regulation. By 3 weeks of treatment with 0.5 μg/kg per day, basal testosterone levels are maximally suppressed to levels less than 10% of normal values. Acute responses diminished over a period of weeks. Ejaculatory volume also declined at a slower rate than at higher doses. After 6 weeks of treatment prostate weight is reduced to a lesser degree than at higher doses, presumably in response to a shorter period of testosterone deprivation (Figure 6.2). These data resemble

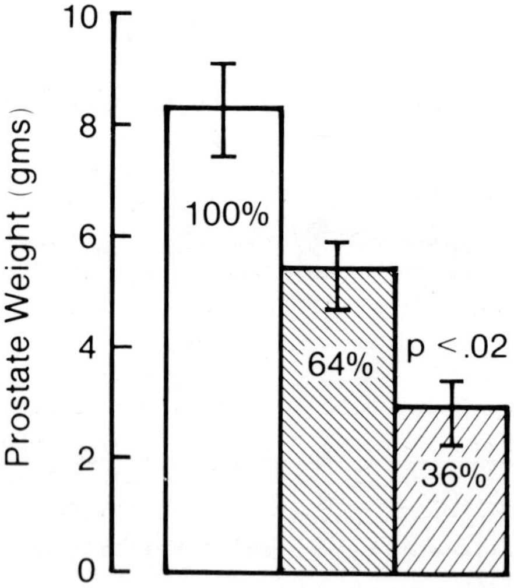

Figure 6.2 Prostate weights from male beagle dogs injected once daily, subcutaneously with vehicle for 10–42 d (□, n = 7) or with [D-Nal(2)^6]LHRH at 0.5 μg/kg per day for 42 d (▧, n = 3) or 10 μg/kg per day for 38 d (▨, n = 2). Vertical bars indicate mean ± SE for n = 3 or more, mean ± range for n < 3. Statistical comparisons are against vehicle control using Student's t-test.

the findings in men, in whom the time to down regulation, judged by integrated response, was inversely related to dose (Bhasin *et al.*, 1982).

EFFECTS ON SPERMATOGENESIS

Inhibition of spermatogenesis in response to daily injection of [D-Nal(2)^6]LHRH is rapid. After only 10 days of treatment with 10 μg/kg per day of [D-Nal(2)^6]LHRH, testicular sections show obvious signs of spermatogenic suppression. Sloughing of germinal cells into the lumina of seminiferous tubules and passage of these cells into the epididymides has been noted (Vickery, 1981). By 38 consecutive days of treatment spermatogenesis is absent, with only Sertoli cells and a few germinal elements remaining. These testicular changes are reflected by a progressive decline in testicular volume, which makes it possible to follow effects week by week. Using testicular volume as an index it can be seen that, as is the case for effects on testosterone levels and ejaculate volume, the effects on testis dimensions are dose related. The suppression of testicular volume obtained with 0.5 μg/kg per day of [D-Nal(2)^6]LHRH parallels that obtained with 10 μg/kg per day, but lags by about 2 weeks (Figure 6.3). Complete suppression of spermatogenesis is still achieved, over the dose range of [D-Nal(2)^6]LHRH studied, after 6 weeks of treatment, as judged by testicular histology and by absence of sperm from the epididymides (Figure 6.4).

The effects on spermatogenesis can also be followed by sperm counts on the ejaculates, although this is complicated by the severe decline in ejaculate volume. Severe oligospermia occurs before ejaculate volumes reach zero (Figure 6.5).

REVERSIBILITY AFTER CESSATION OF TREATMENT

Studies on the reversibility of effects of chronic treatment with [D-Nal(2)^6]LHRH in dogs have so far evaluated only differing duration of treatment at 10 μg/kg per day. Figure 6.6 presents testosterone levels, ejaculate volumes and sperm counts following 13 d or 42 d of treatment. There may be an interaction between duration of treatment and time to recovery, although this may be confounded by achievement of only partial suppression with the shorter duration of treatment. After a short treatment period, basal circulating testosterone levels had returned to pretreatment levels by 4 d after cessation of treatment. In response to this restoration of testosterone, ejaculate volumes increased by 10 d after end of treatment. Sperm count continued to decline following cessation of treatment, for a further 24 d, reaching a nadir of 2 % of pretreatment values. Normal values were regained after a further 3 weeks.

After a longer treatment period, 3 weeks were required before basal plasma testosterone levels returned to pretreatment values. A further lag of 3 weeks was observed before measurable ejaculates were obtained. These ejaculates and those obtained for 2 further weeks were azoospermic. During the next 4–6

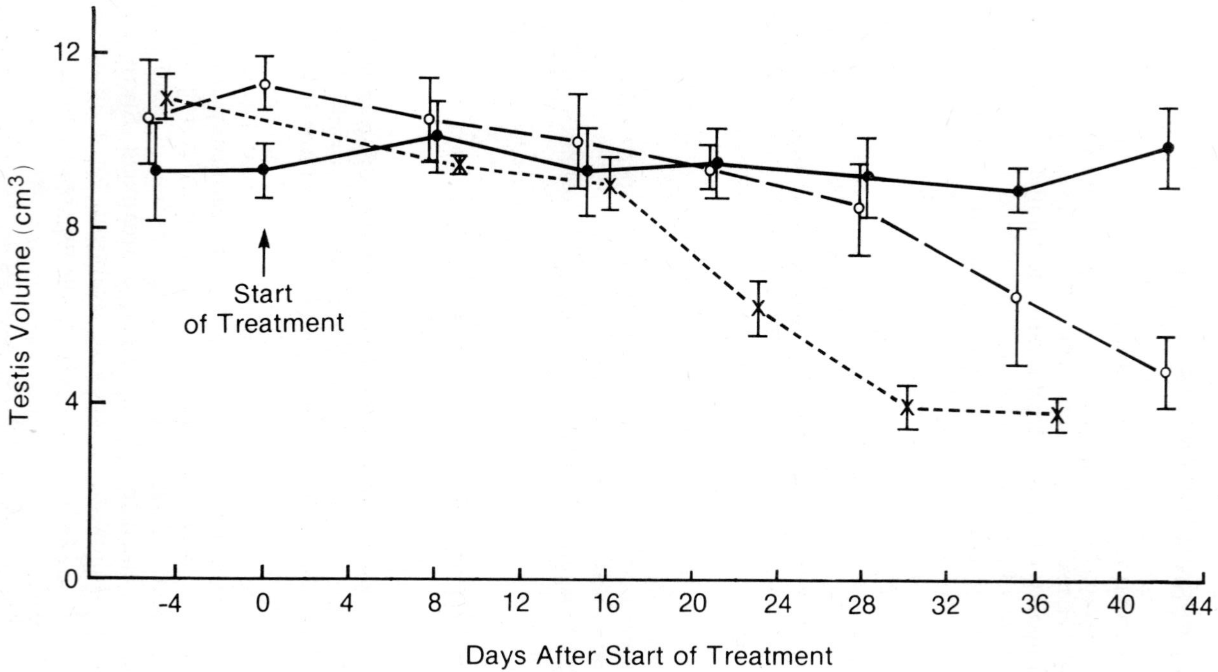

Figure 6.3 Testis volume of male beagle dogs during once daily subcutaneous injection of vehicle (●——●, $n = 3$) or of [D-Nal(2)[6]]LHRH at 0.5 μg/kg per day (○– – –○, $n = 3$) or 10 μg/kg per day (x – – – x , $n = 2$). Vertical bars indicate mean ± SE for $n = 3$, mean ± range for $n = 2$).

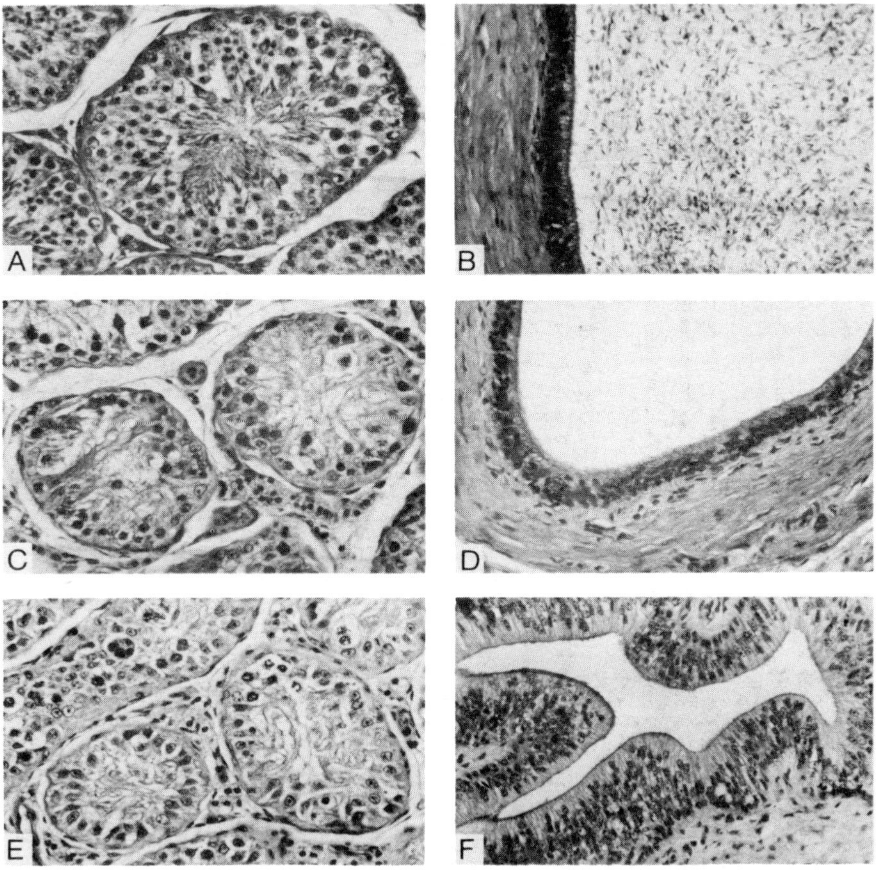

Figure 6.4 Histology of sections of testis and epididymis from male beagle dogs after receiving 42 consecutive subcutaneous daily injections of vehicle (**A** and **B**), 0.5 μg/kg per day of [D-Nal(2)^6]LHRH (**C** and **D**) or 10 μg/kg per day of [D-Nal(2)^6]LHRH (**E** and **F**).

weeks, sperm counts progressively increased to reach normal values. The elapsed time of 9 weeks from cessation of treatment until first appearance of sperm in the ejaculate indicates essentially an immediate re-establishment of spermatogenesis, as the spermatogenic cycle in dogs is approximately 54 d (Foote *et al.*, 1972). The oligospermia in the reversal phase was, unlike that in the suppression phase, associated with good motility and no persistent cytoplasmic droplets, as might be expected in the presence of normal circulating levels of testosterone.

Histology of the reproductive tract 126 d after cessation of treatment in these dogs was normal.

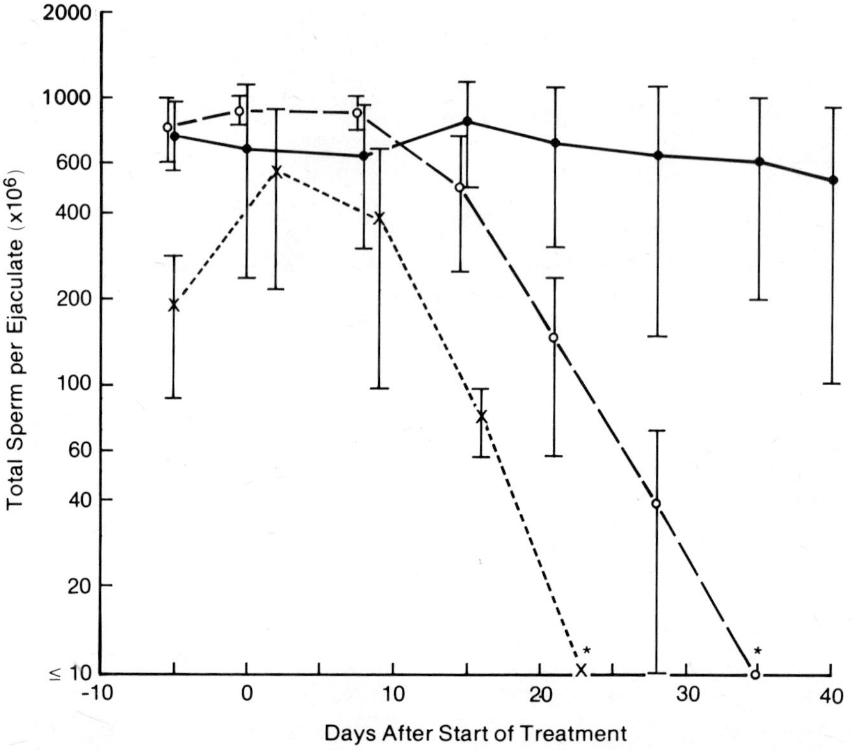

Figure 6.5 Total ejaculated spermatozoa obtained from male beagle dogs injected once daily, subcutaneously with vehicle (●——●, $n = 3$) or [D-Nal(2)^6]LHRH at 0.5 μg/kg per day (○– – –○, $n = 3$) or at 10 μg/kg per day (x – – – x, $n = 2$). Vertical bars indicate mean ± SE for $n = 3$, mean ± range for $n = 2$.

EFFECTS OF TESTOSTERONE SUPPLEMENTATION

On the day of first injection of 10 μg/kg per day of [D-Nal(2)^6]LHRH, either 20 or 40 cm per dog of Silastic tubing packed with crystalline testosterone was implanted subcutaneously (Vickery *et al.*, 1983). Basal plasma testosterone levels, during [D-Nal(2)^6]LHRH treatment, were maintained at 1.5 and 3.0 ng/ml respectively, i.e. at the low and middle regions of the normal range for these dogs. The progressive decline in acute response to [D-Nal(2)^6]LHRH was unaffected in all cases, showing the evolution of down regulation to be unchanged by testosterone supplementation. Either level of testosterone was sufficient to maintain the duration of erection in the normal range. However, only the higher level was capable of maintaining prostatic secretory function (on the basis of ejaculate volume) or prostatic weight. Both parameters declined at the lower level of testosterone supplementation. The restoration of potentia while prostate size is decreased, could have widespread application for treatment of benign prostatic hyperplasia in men. Both levels of

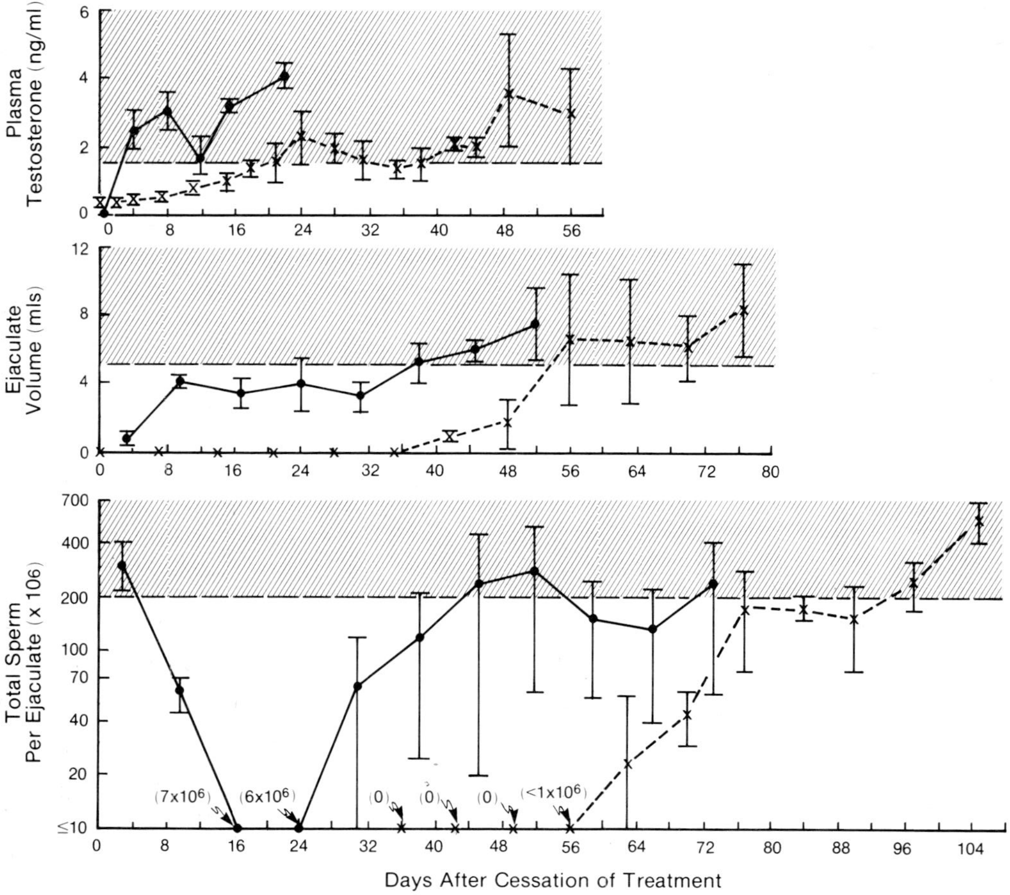

Figure 6.6 Plasma testosterone levels (upper panel), ejaculate volume (middle panel) and spermatozoal count (lower panel) of male beagle dogs following cessation of treatment with either 13 (●——●, $n = 2$) or 42 (x - - - x, $n = 3$) consecutive daily subcutaneous injections of 10 μg/kg per day of [D-Nal(2)^6]LHRH. Vertical bars indicate mean + SE for $n = 3$, mean ± range for $n = 2$.

testosterone maintained epididymal function, as judged by the recovery of highly motile, mature sperm from the ejaculates. Testicular size was equally suppressed by LHRH analog alone or when supplemented with either level of testosterone. Severe oligospermia was achieved. Testosterone, at these levels, did not appear to exert a protective effect against the testicular suppression due to [D-Nal(2)^6]LHRH. Although epididymal function and cell morphology were maintained by testosterone supplementation, epididymal weights still fell to those noted for LHRH analog treatment alone, possibly reflecting the absence of spermatozoa from the epididymal lumina.

The requirement for higher testosterone levels to maintain prostatic function and weight than to maintain epididymal function or potentia may be a real physiological difference. This difference could possibly result from a direct prostatic effect of the LHRH analog, as has been noted in the rat (Wright *et al.*, 1982). There was no evidence from these studies in the dog that testosterone was synergizing with the LHRH analogs to bring about a more rapid or severe suppression of spermatogenesis as suggested for rat and for man (Heber and Swerdloff, 1981; Bhasin *et al.*, 1982).

MECHANISM OF ACTION

There is ample evidence that LHRH and its analogs can act at multiple sites in the rat but there is no evidence for any but a pituitary site of action of LHRH analogs in men. Direct actions of these agents on human ovarian components have been documented recently (Tureck *et al.*, 1982; Lamberts *et al.*, 1982). Testicular LHRH receptors in men have not been found (Huhtaniemi and Clayton, 1982) and the ability of high levels of exogenous gonadotropin to down regulate testicular function in men is open to question. The response to chronic LHRH agonist treatment in normal or hypogonadotropic men (Bergquist *et al.*, 1979; Mortimer *et al.*, 1974) is the suppression of gonadotropin response to challenge. In such suppressed subjects a gonadotropin challenge is capable of eliciting a testicular steroidogenic response (Bhasin *et al.*, 1982).

It appears unnecessary at the present time to postulate direct testicular effects of LHRH analogs in dogs. The decline in testicular steroidogenesis appears, as in men, to be attributable to a declining pituitary response. A steroidogenic response to exogenous hCG challenge has been obtained in the face of chronic treatment with [D-Nal(2)^6]LHRH (Table 6.1).

CONTRACEPTIVE POTENTIAL

The results in dogs using [D-Nal(2)^6]LHRH support the further investigation of this agent as a male contraceptive. Suppression of spermatogenesis is rapid, complete and quantitatively reversible. Administration of the agent alone results in inhibition of testicular steroidogenesis giving rise in turn to adjunctive contraceptive effects such as interference with sperm maturation and motility. However, the testosterone withdrawal also leads to undesirable

Table 6.1 Change in plasma testosterone from 0 to 24 h after an intramuscular injection of 100 iu hCG in male beagles receiving once daily subcutaneous injections of 10 μg RS-94991/kg or vehicle

			Change in plasma testosterone	
Treatment group	*Injection*	*Dog*	ng/ml *Increase*	% *Increase*
1	Vehicle	SB19	6.34	459
		LL19	10.60	635
2	RS-94991	PX09	>2.11 and <2.31	1055[a]
		NF09	>1.11 and <1.30	550[a]

[a] The lower limit of the ng/ml increase was assumed for calculation of the % increase

effects including loss of potentia and of ejaculate volume. Upon cessation of treatment, testosterone levels and potentia return to normal well before sperm appear in the ejaculate – leading to the suggestion that episodic, perhaps 1 month out of 3, treatment might obviate the need for androgen replacement (Vickery *et al.*, 1981). However, in addition to the above effects of testosterone withdrawal, a high proportion of men rapidly experience 'hot flashes' (Linde *et al.*, 1981). Therefore for LHRH agonist treatment to be a viable contraceptive method, testosterone supplementation will be required.

These data indicate that it is possible to supplement with testosterone sufficiently to restore libido, potentia and ejaculate volume without preventing the antispermatogenic effects of [D-Nal(2)^6]LHRH. Such supplementation will likely maintain sperm motility and maturity through the progressive oligospermia until azoospermia is achieved and this time may be a period of weeks. Thus an additional contraceptive technique such as barrier contraception will be necessary during this induction phase.

The probable need to administer two different non-orally active agents, a steroid and an oligopeptide, will require advanced formulation techniques. The biodegradable polymers may be applicable to the delivery of both types of drug.

THERAPEUTIC POTENTIAL

The benefit:side-effect ratio will probably determine the acceptability of treatment with LHRH analog alone in andrological pathologies. In a life-threatening situation such as prostatic cancer, which in 80% of cases is dependent on testicular steroidogenesis, there are only benefits with LHRH analog treatment (Jàcobi and Wenderoth, 1982). The side effects resulting from testosterone withdrawal may not be tolerated by patients with benign prostatic hypertrophy, however. The studies in dogs suggest that titration of testosterone supplementation may allow potentia to be maintained while prostate size decreases.

LHRH analogs might be able to protect against the sterilant effects of cancer chemotherapy (Globe *et al.*, 1981). This would have particular relevance to Hodgkin's disease, which has a relatively high incidence in young adult men and in which a high remission rate is being achieved, with chemotherapy (Sutcliffe *et al.*, 1978). There is a high incidence of sterility resulting from chemotherapy, persisting often for years after treatment (Chapman *et al.*, 1979; Whitehead *et al.*, 1982). Semen cryopreservation banking has been advised; however, due to the disease, low sperm counts and motility are often present even prior to chemotherapy. The alkylating agents used in chemotherapy act during cell division (Jackson, 1970, 1972). Regression of spermatogenesis to stem cells by LHRH analog treatment offers an excellent chance of protection. On the basis of the dog studies, androgen supplementation would not affect the antispermatogenic action of LHRH analogs, and so could probably be employed to increase the quality of life for these patients further.

CONCLUDING REMARKS

Azoospermia can be achieved in dogs with agonistic analogs of LHRH, but this has yet to be proven in man. For contraceptive use, testosterone supplementation will be required. In dogs, such supplementation does not interfere with the antispermatogenic action of LHRH agonists. Fertility during the oligospermia of induction and recovery phases must be studied. The interference with sperm maturity and motility during the oligospermia induced with [D-Nal(2)^6]LHRH treatment alone would probably result in infertility. However, the maintained sperm motility observed during testosterone supplementation would suggest the need for adjunctive contraception during periods of oligospermia. While sperm counts of less than 10 million per ml have been associated with infertility (Eliasson, 1981), it is now believed that additional factors are involved as treatment of hypogonadal men results in pregnancies at sperm counts of 1–2 million per ml (W. F. Crowley Jr., personal communication, 1982).

The advantages of LHRH agonist plus testosterone over other combination regimens such as danazol/testosterone or progestogen/testosterone are not clear. However, the steroid combinations do not reliably induce azoospermia, and unexplained ‘escapes’ from therapy also occur. If LHRH agonist plus testosterone were able to result in reliable induction of azoospermia in men, then that would be the advantage we are seeking. Reversibility of long term treatment with LHRH agonists will await further study. The potential of LHRH analogs is exciting. The first commercial utility will be in the therapeutic area, no doubt for treatment of prostatic carcinoma. There is, however, an unfulfilled need for a male contraceptive to occupy a niche equivalent to combination oral contraceptives for women. LHRH analogs are presently the leading candidates to fulfill that need.

Acknowledgement

This research was supported in part by Prime Contract No. NO1-HD-0-2811 to Syntex from the U.S. National Institutes of Health, Department of Health and Social Services.

References

Akhtar, F. B., Marshall, G. R., Wickings, E. J. and Nieschlag, E. (1982). Antifertility effects of chronic LHRH agonist infusion by osmotic pumps in adult male monkeys. Abstr. No. 17, *Programme of the 1st Joint Meeting of British Endocrine Societies*, May 1982, London

Bélanger, A., Cusan, L., Auclair, C. Séguin, C., Caron, S. and Labrie, F. (1980). Effect of an LHRH agonist and hCG on testicular steroidogenesis in the adult rat. *Biol. Reprod.*, **22,** 1094

Belchetz, P. E., Plant, T. M., Nakai, Y., Keogh, E. J. and Knobil, E. (1978). Hypophysial responses to continuous and intermittent delivery of hypothalamic gonadotropin-releasing hormone. *Science,* **202,** 631

Bergquist, C., Nillius, S. J., Berg, T., Skarin, G. and Wide, L. (1979). Inhibitory effects on gonadotrophin secretion and gonadal function in men during chronic treatment with a potent stimulatory luteinizing hormone-releasing hormone analogue. *Acta Endocrinol.*, **91,** 601

Bex, F. J. and Corbin, A. (1978). Inhibition of reproductive processes in the immature and mature male rat with an LHRH agonist. Abstract No. 6, *3rd Annual Meeting*, *Am. Soc. Androl.*, Nashville

Bex, F. J. and Corbin, A. (1981). In vivo and in vitro investigation of the extrapituitary antireproductive effects of a potent LHRH agonist in immature and adult male rats. *J. Androl.*, **2,** 152

Bex, F. J., Corbin, A. and France, E. (1982). Resistance of the mouse to the antifertility effects of LHRH agonists. *Life Sci.*, **30,** 1263

Bhasin, S., Heber, D., Steiner, B., Peterson, M. and Swerdloff, R. S. (1982). Enhanced inhibition of gonadotropin secretion in man by combined GnRH agonist and testosterone. *Endocrinology,* **111,** 193A

Chapman, R. M., Sutcliffe, S. B., Rees., L. H., Edwards, C. R. W. and Malpas, J. S. (1979). Cyclical combination chemotherapy and gonadal function. *Lancet,* **1,** 285

Davies, T. F., Gomez-Pan, A., Watson, M. J., Mountjoy, C. Q., Hanker, J. P., Besser, G. M. and Hall, R. (1977). Reduced 'gonadotrophin response to releasing hormone' after chronic administration to impotent men. *Clin. Endocrinol.*, **6,** 213

Eliasson, R. (1981). Sperm count and fertility: Facts and myths. In Frajese, G., Hafez, E. S. E., Conti, C. and Fabbrini, A. (eds.) *Oligozoospermia: Recent Progress in Andrology*, pp. 1–8. (New York: Raven Press)

Foote, R. H., Swierstra, E. E. and Hunt, W. L. (1972). Spermatogenesis in the dog. *Anat. Rec.*, **173,** 341

Fujino, M., Kobayashi, S., Obayashi, M., Shinagawa, S., Fukuda, T., Kitada, C., Nakayama, R., Yamazaki, I., White, W. F. and Rippel, R. H. (1972). Structure–activity relationships in the C-terminal part of luteinizing hormone-releasing hormone (LH-RH). *Biochem. Biophys. Res. Commun.*, **49,** 863

Glode, L. M., Robinson, J. and Gould, S. F. (1981). Protection from cyclophosphamide-induced testicular damage with an analogue of gonadotropin-releasing hormone. *Lancet,* **1,** 1132

Heber, D. and Swerdloff, R. S. (1981). Gonadotropin-releasing hormone analog and testosterone synergistically inhibit spermatogenesis. *Endocrinology,* **108,** 2019

Heber, D., Dodson, R., Stoskopf, C., Peterson, M. and Swerdloff, R. S. (1982). Pituitary desensitization and the regulation of pituitary gonadotropin-releasing hormone (GnRH) receptors following chronic administration of a superactive GnRH analog and testosterone. *Life Sci.*, **30,** 2301

Hsueh, A. J. W. and Jones, P. B. C. (1981). Extrapituitary actions of gonadotropin-releasing hormone. *Endocr. Rev.*, **2,** 437

Hsueh, A. J. W., Schreiber, J. R. and Erickson, G. F. (1981). Inhibitory effect of gonadotropin releasing hormone upon cultured testicular cells. *Mol. Cell. Endocrinol.*, **21,** 43

Huhtaniemi, I. and Clayton, R. N. (1982). Absence of gonadotrophin-releasing hormone receptors in human gonads. Abstr. No. 22, *Programme of the 1st joint Meeting of British Endocrine Societies,* May 1982, London

Jackson, H. (1970). Antispermatogenic agents. *Br. Med. Bull.*, **26,** 79

Jackson, H. (1972). Chemical methods of male contraception. In Austin, C. R. and Short, R. V. (eds.) *Reproduction in Mammals.* Vol. 5, pp. 67–86. (Cambridge: Cambridge UP)

Jacobi, G. H. and Wenderoth, U. K. (1982). Gonadotropin-releasing hormone analogues for prostate cancer: untoward side effects of high-dose regimens acquire a therapeutical dimension. *Eur. Urol.*, **8,** 129

Koch, Y., Baram, T., Hazum, E. and Fridkin, M. (1977). Resistance to enzymic degradation of LH-RH analogues possessing increased biological activity. *Biochem. Biophys. Res. Commun.*, **74,** 488

Laron, Z., Dickerman, Z., Ben Zeev, Z., Prager-Lewin, R., Comaru-Schally, A. M. and Schally, A. V. (1981). Long-term effect of D-Trp^6-luteinizing hormone-releasing hormone on testicular size and luteinizing hormone, follicle-stimulating hormone, and testosterone levels in hypothalamic hypogonadotropic males. *Fertil. Steril.*, **35,** 328

Labrie, F., Auclair, C., Cusan, L., Kelly, P. A., Pelletier, G. and Ferland, L. (1978). Inhibiting effects of LHRH and its agonists on testicular gonadotropin receptors and spermatogenesis in the rat. *Int. J. Androl.* (Suppl.) **2,** 303

Labrie, F., Bélanger, A., Cusan, L., Séguin, C., Pelletier, G., Kelly, P. A., Reeves, J. J., Lefebvre, F. A., Lemay, A., Gomdeau, Y. and Reynaud, J. P. (1980). Antifertility effects of LHRH agonists in the male. *J. Androl.*, **1,** 209

Labrie, F., Bélanger, A., Séguin, C., Cusan, L., Pelletier, G., Lefebvre, F. A., Kelly, P. A., Berland, L., Reeves, J. J., Lemay, A. and Raynaud, J. P. (1981). Inhibition of testicular and ovarian functions by LHRH agonists. In Jagiello, G. and Vogel, H. J. (eds.) *Bioregulators of Reproduction (P and S Biomed. Sci. Symp. Ser.)*, pp. 305–341. (New York: Academic Press)

Lamberts, S. W. J., Timmens, J. M., Oosterom, R., Verleun, T., Rommerts, F. G. and de Jong, F. H. (1982). Testosterone secretion by cultured arrhenoblastoma cells: Suppression by a luteinizing hormone-releasing hormone agonist. *J. Clin. Endocrinol. Metab.*, **54,** 450

Lefebvre, F. A., Reeves, J. J., Séguin, C., Massicotte, J. and Labrie, F. (1980). Specific binding of a potent LHRH agonist in rat testis. *Mol. Cell. Endocrinol.*, **20,** 127

Linde, R., Doelle, G. C., Alexander, N., Kirchner, F., Vale, W., Rivier, J. and Rabin, D. (1981). Reversible inhibition of testicular steroidogenesis and spermatogenesis by a potent gonadotropin-releasing hormone agonist in normal men. *N. Engl. J. Med.*, **305,** 663

McNeil, L. W., McKenna, T. J., Lacroix, A., Benveniste, R. and Rabin, D. (1979). Seventy-two hour infusions of LHRH in normal men: gonadotropin and testicular steroid responses. *J. Clin. Endocrinol. Metab.*, **49,** 149

Monahan, M., Amoss, M. S., Anderson, H. A. and Vale, W. (1973). Synthetic analogs of the hypothalamic luteinizing hormone-releasing factor with increased agonist or antagonist properties. *Biochemistry*, **12,** 4616

Mortimer, C. H., McNeilly, A. S., Fisher, R. A., Murray, M. A. F. and Besser, G. M. (1974). Gonadotrophin-releasing hormone therapy in hypogonadal males with hypothalamic or pituitary dysfunction. *Br. Med. J.*, **4,** 617

Nestor, J. J. Jr., Ho, T. L., Simpson, R. A., Horner, B. L., Jones, G. H., McRae, G. I. and Vickery, B. H. (1982). The synthesis and biological activity of some very hydrophobic analogs of luteinizing hormone-releasing hormone. *J. Med. Chem.*, **25,** 795

Oshima, H., Nankin, H. R., Fan, D. F., Yanaihara, T., Niizato, N., Yoshida, K. I. and Ochiai, K. I. (1975). Delay in sexual maturation of rats caused by synthetic LH-releasing hormone: enhancement of steroid Ω4-5α-hydrogenase in testes. *Biol. Reprod.*, **12,** 491

Perrin, M. H., Rivier, J. E. and Vale, W. (1980). Radioligand assay for gonadotropin-releasing hormone: relative potencies of agonists and antagonists. *Endocrinology*, **106,** 1289

Schally, A. V. and Kastin, A. J. (1971). *Drug Ther.*, **1,** 29

Schally, A. V., Kastin, A. J., Coy, D. H., (1976). Edward Tyler Prize Oration. LH-releasing hormone and its analogs: Recent basic and clinical investigations. *Int. J. Fertil.*, **21,** 1

Séguin, C., Bélanger, A., Cusan, L., Pelletier, G., Reeves, J. J., Lefebvre, F. A., Kelly, P. A. and Labrie, F. (1981). Relative importance of the adenohypophysial and gonadal sites of inhibitory action of LHRH agonists. *Biol. Reprod.*, **24,** 889

Sutcliffe, S. B., Wrigley, P. F. M., Peto, J. *et al.* (1978). MVPP chemotherapy regimen for advanced Hodgkin's disease. *Br. Med. J.*, **1,** 679

Tureck, R. W., Mastroianni, L. Jr., Blasco, L., Strauss, J. F. III (1982). Inhibition of human granulosa cell progesterone secretion by a gonadotropin-releasing hormone agonist. *J. Clin. Endocrinol. Metab.*, **54,** 1078

Vickery, B. H. (1981). Physiology and antifertility effects of LHRH and agonist analogs in male animals. In Zatuchni, G. I., Shelton, J. D. and Sciarra, J. J. (eds.) *LHRH Peptides as Female and Male Contraceptives*, pp. 275–290. (Philadelphia: Harper & Row)

Vickery, B. H. and McRae, G. I. (1979). Effects on male rats of continuous treatment with DesGly DAla^{10}Pro^{6}NHEt-LHRH (LHRH-A). *Endocrinology*, **104,** 183A

Vickery, B. H. and McRae, G. (1980). Responses of the males of different laboratory species to continuous administration of an LHRH agonist. *J. Androl.*, **1,** 62

Vickery, B., McRae, G., Bergstrom, K., Briones, W., Seidenberg, R. and Worden, A. (1981). Suppression of sexual function in male dogs with a new agonistic analogue of LHRH: Potential for male contraception without need for androgen replacement? *J. Androl.*, **2,** 30

Vickery, B. H., McRae, G. I. and Bonasch, H. (1982). Effect of chronic administration of a highly potent LHRH agonist on prostate size and secretory function in geriatric dogs. *The Prostate*, **3,** 123

Vickery, B. H., McRae, G. I., Briones, W., Worden, A., Seidenberg, R., Schanbacher, B. D. and Falvo, R. (1984). Effect of [D-Nal(2)^6]LHRH upon sexual function in male dogs: suppression, reversibility and effect of testosterone replacement. *J. Androl.* (In press)

Whitehead, E., Shalet, S. M., Blackledge, G., Todd, I., Crowther, D. and Beardwell, C. G. (1982). The effects of Hodgkin's disease and combination chemotherapy on gonadal function in the adult male. *Cancer*, **49,** 418

Wright, W., Chan, K., Sundaram, K. and Bardin, C. W. (1982). New observation on androgen action: Androgen receptor stabilization and antisteroid effects of LHRH agonists. *Adv. Exp. Med. Biol.*, **138,** 325

7
Male fertility control with an LHRH agonist: primate studies

F. BINT AKHTAR, E. J. WICKINGS and E. NIESCHLAG

The pulsatile administration of LHRH, mimicking its endogenous pattern of release stimulates the pituitary–gonadal axis enhancing fertility (Carmel *et al.*, 1976; Knobil, 1980; Wickings *et al.*, 1981*a*). However, continuous administration of identical doses of LHRH or more potent agonists leads to pituitary desensitization and paradoxical antifertility effects (Belchetz *et al.*, 1978; Sandow *et al.*, 1978). The initial hypersecretion of pituitary gonadotropins following high dose LHRH administration causes a down regulation of gonadal gonadotropin receptors. Chronic administration of LHRH agonists then leads to pituitary refractoriness. These effects are accompanied by decreased ovarian and testicular steroidogenesis which results in a regression of steroid dependent accessory reproductive organs.

Such effects in the male include a loss of testicular LH and prolactin receptors, a decrease in testis and accessory reproductive organ weights, pituitary desensitization, inhibition of androgen production and the disruption of spermatogenesis (Labrie *et al.*, 1980; Sandow, 1982a). Although these effects with LHRH agonists have mainly been attributed to pituitary desensitization, direct inhibition of gonadal functions by these agents has been shown in rats (Hsueh and Jones, 1981; Sharpe, 1982).

High dose LHRH agonist treatment suppresses testicular function in men (Linde *et al.*, 1981; Faure *et al.*, 1982; Tolis *et al.*, 1982). Such treatment is associated with decreased potency and libido and the occurrence of hot flashes, thus rendering concomitant testosterone supplementation inevitable for contraceptive application. The inhibition of ovulation in the female can be achieved by daily injections or intranasal administration of LHRH but the situation in the male is more difficult. Long term treatment is required to disrupt spermatogenesis. Much work is still needed on an appropriate mode of administration, adequate androgen substitution and the reversibility of azoospermia if an LHRH-based method for male fertility control is to be developed.

Characterization of the male rhesus monkey has shown that it provides a suitable model for the study of human testicular functions (Nieschlag and Wickings, 1980). Male rhesus monkeys have been found to be relatively

Table 7.1 The doses, modes of administration and effects of LHRH agonists on pituitary and testicular functions in adult rhesus monkeys during pre-clinical trials

Analog	*Dose* (μg/d)	*Mode*	*Duration* (weeks)	*Physiological effects* *Endocr. parameters*	*Seminal parameters*	*Reference*
[D-Ser(tBu^6,Pro^9-NHEt]LHRH	4	Daily s.c.	8	Uninfluenced	Uninfluenced	Wickings *et al.*, 1981
	20 (2 × 10)	Twice daily s.c.	4	Partial inhibition of pit. function	Uninfluenced	
	100 (2 × 50)	Twice daily s.c.	10	Partial inhibition of pit. function	Uninfluenced	Bint Akhtar *et al.*, 1982
	25	Daily s.c.	7	Partial inhibition of pit. function	Uninfluenced	Resko *et al.*, 1982
	48	Constant infusion	13 and 7 with T suppl.	Complete inhibition of pituitary and gonadal function	Suppressed in all animals	Bint Akhtar *et al.*, 1983
[D-Trp^6,Pro^9-NHEt]LHRH	500	Twice weekly	12	Uninfluenced	Uninfluenced	Sundaram *et al.*, 1982
	500	Daily s.c.	2	Uninfluenced	Uninfluenced	
	500	Daily s.c.	12	Marked inhibition of pituitary and gonadal function	Loss of ejac. behavior and suppression of spermatogenesis in 4 animals	

insensitive to the antifertility effects of an LHRH agonist ([D-Ser(tBu)^6,Pro^9-NHEt]LHRH; buserelin; Hoe 766) administered as daily or twice daily injections (Wickings *et al.*, 1981*b*; Bint Akhtar *et al.*, 1982). We consequently studied the effects of constant infusion of the LHRH agonist in these animals (Bint Akhtar *et al.*, 1983). The latter mode of application of the agonist overcame the resistance of this species and testicular functions in the monkey were suppressed. Effects of testosterone replacement therapy were then studied, in order to simulate the physiological testosterone status necessary to maintain all androgen dependent functions except spermatogenesis. To date, only few other studies describing the effects of chronic high dose LHRH agonist treatment in male non-human primates have been reported (Table 7.1).

TREATMENT BY DAILY OR TWICE DAILY INJECTIONS

Basal LH and testosterone levels

In an initial study, treatment of four male rhesus monkeys with 4 μg per day of buserelin for 8 weeks followed by 20 μg/day for 4 more weeks did not alter basal LH levels compared to normal in-season values (Wickings and Nieschlag, 1980). Serum testosterone was significantly suppressed during the first 2 weeks, followed by a return to initial values. During weeks 8–12, testosterone concentrations were again decreased (Wickings *et al.*, 1981*b*).

As no suppression of spermatogenesis was evident in this experiment, we then administered 100 μg/day buserelin s.c. as injections of 50 μg each at 09:00 and 18:00. Treatment for 10 weeks caused a significant suppression of basal serum LH levels. These levels, however, were not depressed below the normal out-of-season range. There was a corresponding suppression of serum testosterone levels (Bint Akhtar *et al.*, 1982). Comparing this dose to that first used in men, where a marked suppression of endocrine function was seen with only 5 μg/day buserelin (Bergquist *et al.*, 1979), reveals the relative insensitivity of the rhesus monkey.

Treatment of six male rhesus monkeys by daily s.c. injections of 25 μg buserelin resulted in a slight decrease in basal serum LH and a corresponding reduction in serum testosterone levels after 1 week of treatment. The levels remained suppressed over the entire 7 week treatment period. Large fluctuations in sperm counts and motility were seen in both the treated and control groups and as such were unattributable to buserelin treatment (Resko *et al.*, 1982).

Acute pituitary stimulation tests

The pituitary capacity to respond to challenges of 50 μg of LHRH or 4 μg of agonist remained unaffected during the agonist treatment in our first study. However, the sensitivity of the pituitary to a low dose of LHRH (5 μg) or the agonist (0.08 μg) was reduced at the end of the treatment period. These observations in primates are contrary to those seen in hamsters and rats, in which high dose treatment with LHRH agonist causes a direct inhibition of the pituitary, both in basal LH secretion and response to stimulation (Sandow *et al.*, 1978).

When the animals in our second study were challenged with 4 μg buserelin intravenously there was a reduced pituitary response after 9 weeks of treatment but not at earlier times. This dose of buserelin elicits a maximal gonadotropin response in untreated animals.

Pituitary and testicular responses

Serum LH levels measured at 30 and 60 min after the administration of 4 μg buserelin did not change over the entire treatment period of 12 weeks. Before chronic treatment of the rhesus monkeys in our second study, a single subcutaneous injection of 50 μg buserelin resulted in a sharp increase in serum LH levels, which remained markedly elevated during the entire observation period of 8 h. There was a corresponding increase in serum testosterone over this time period. Hence it was decided that twice daily injections should be sufficient to maintain elevated LH levels in the rhesus monkeys.

During the 5th and 10th weeks of LHRH agonist treatment, the prolonged elevation of circulating LH in response to challenge evident before starting treatment no longer existed. Serum LH levels were not significantly different from basal values 4 h after the injection and serum testosterone returned to basal levels within 5 h. The period of elevated LH and testosterone levels was short and allowed time between the morning and evening injections for the pituitary to partially overcome the down regulatory effects of the agonist resulting in inadequate suppression of testicular functions.

The decrease in pituitary responsiveness to LHRH agonists may be due to a loss of pituitary LHRH receptors (Sandow, 1982*b*) and/or a depletion of the pituitary gonadotropin stores (Rivier *et al.*, 1979). As there was no change in the gonadotropin response to the treatment dose of LHRH agonists, it seems unlikely that the pituitary stores had been depleted. LHRH exerts an autoregulatory effect on its receptors in the pituitary (Clayton, 1982). Physiological levels of LHRH maintain receptor numbers whereas higher levels cause down regulation (Nett *et al.*, 1981). This latter observation would explain the findings in the rhesus monkeys.

Similar results were noted in the study using 25 μg buserelin daily where initially bioactive serum LH levels remained elevated over the next 12 h. After 1 week of daily treatment, the LH increment over basal levels was diminished and LH levels returned to basal values at 7 h (Resko *et al.*, 1982).

Administration of 500 μg of [D-Trp^6,Pro^9-NHEt]LHRH to four rhesus monkeys resulted in a maximum pituitary response (50-fold preinjection) after 4 h, thereafter LH levels declined slowly and returned to basal after 24–48 h (Sundaram *et al.*, 1982). When the animals were treated with 500 μg of the agonist twice weekly, there was a significant reduction in peak LH levels, and the maximum LH levels attained at weeks 3 and 11 were 25 % of those attained at week 0. As a biweekly regimen of 500 μg for 19 weeks failed to inhibit testicular functions in this group of monkeys, they were treated daily with the same dose for a period of 3 months. This treatment caused a further decrease in the maximum LH responses, which were only 5% of the initial response towards the end of the treatment period. The two monkeys which showed the greatest decrease in LH response no longer showed any increase in serum testosterone levels following agonist injection, whereas this response was only slightly decreased in the remaining two monkeys.

The preservation of the testosterone response in all the monkeys receiving chronic treatments of 4–100 μg buserelin per day and in two of the four monkeys receiving 500 μg [D-Trp^6,Pro^9-NHEt]LHRH shows that the responsiveness of the Leydig cells is not impaired under chronic LHRH agonist treatment. The partial inhibition of basal, as well as stimulated, testosterone can always be correlated to the diminished LH levels and is hence a consequence of the pituitary desensitization. The failure of prolonged treatment with high doses of LHRH agonists to suppress the testicular response indicates that the rhesus monkey is more resistant to such down regulation as compared to laboratory rodents and men (Labrie *et al.*, 1980; Bergquist *et al.*, 1979). In rats and men loss of testicular LH receptors is accompanied by lesions in the steroidogenic biosynthetic pathways, namely at the 17α-hydroxylase and the 17, 20 desmolase steps (Belanger *et al.*, 1980; Faure *et al.*, 1982). Lesions in the steroidogenic pathways in the monkey have not been demonstrated (Resko *et al.*, 1982).

Chronic treatment with high doses of LHRH agonists suppresses steroidogenesis (Sharpe, 1982). High affinity LHRH receptors were demonstrated in the gonads of both sexes of the rat (Magoffin and Erickson, 1982; Sharpe and Fraser, 1980). LHRH receptors in monkey and human gonadal tissue were not found, whereas rat gonads and human pituitaries gave positive results in the same assays (Clayton and Huhtaniemi, 1982). However, the presence of an LHRH-like substance has been reported in macaque testis (Sharpe *et al.*, 1981).

Testicular volumes

Administration of 4 μg buserelin per day to four monkeys for 8 weeks and increasing the dose to 20 μg/d for a period of 4 more weeks caused a significant decrease in testicular volumes after 3 weeks of treatment (Figure 7.1). A further small decrease was observed under continuing treatment. The volumes, however, remained within the in-season range (20–25 ml), as compared to out-of-season volumes of 10–15 ml (Wickings and Nieschlag, 1980).

100 μg/d for 10 weeks of buserelin had a similar effect on testicular volumes, i.e. a marked decrease occurred after 3 weeks of treatment and a further gradual decrease over the rest of the treatment period (Figure 7.1).

Ejaculatory behavior

The male rhesus monkey offers advantages over smaller laboratory animals as an experimental model for testicular functions because of the relative ease of

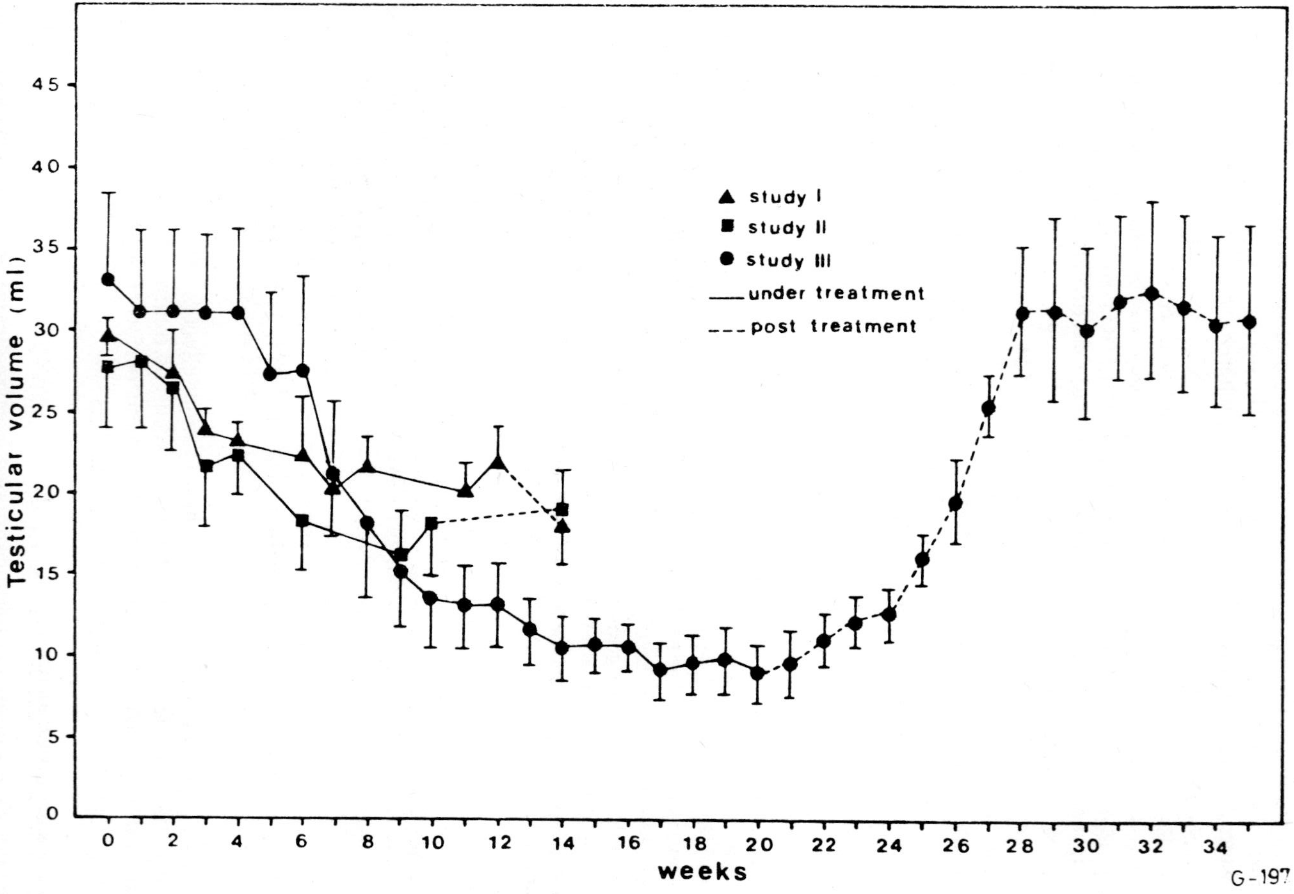

Figure 7.1 Comparison of effects of three chronic [D-Ser(tBu)[6],Pro[9]-NHEt]LHRH treatment regimens on testicular volumes in rhesus monkeys. Study I: 4 μg/d for 8 weeks followed by 20 μg/d for 4 weeks; s.c. injections. Study II: 2 × 50 μg/d for 10 weeks; s.c. injections. Study III: 48 μg/d for 20 weeks with

obtaining ejaculates by electrostimulation. The ejaculates thus obtained provide evidence about the functional state of the testis and also of the accessory reproductive organs. The frequency of spontaneous ejaculations, determined by counting the ejaculatory plugs under the monkeys' cages each morning, gives further insight into the reproductive status of the animals.

Ejaculatory behavior was uninfluenced by daily buserelin injections of up to 100 μg. Although occasional failures to produce ejaculates on electrostimulation were observed during the two treatment periods, all monkeys continued to ejaculate spontaneously at the normal frequency. There was also no effect on ejaculatory behavior when monkeys were treated with 500 μg [D-Trp^6,Pro^9-NHEt]LHRH twice weekly for 19 weeks (Sundaram *et al.*, 1982). When the same animals were treated with 500 μg/d of the same agonist for a period of a further 3 months, two of the four monkeys stopped ejaculating. This loss was associated with a fully abolished testosterone response to the analog administration in these two animals. The other two animals in the same study maintained normal ejaculatory behavior, in the presence of a reduced testosterone response, despite chronic treatment with an extremely high dose of the LHRH agonist.

Seminal parameters

Daily treatment with buserelin failed to suppress sperm counts below the normal range of 100–1100 × 10^6 sperm/ejaculate (Wickings and Nieschlag, 1980). There was no significant change either in sperm motility or in the percentage of normally formed spermatozoa. There was a tendency for ejaculate weights to decrease towards the end of both treatments. The ejaculates failed to coagulate normally towards the end of the second study, indicating an impaired functioning of the accessory reproductive organs.

Treatment of rhesus monkeys with 25 μg/day of buserelin for 7 weeks failed to affect seminal parameters evaluated during the 3rd and 7th weeks of treatment (Resko *et al.*, 1982). Treatment with [D-Trp^6,Pro^9-NHEt]LHRH twice weekly for 19 weeks did not influence sperm count or motility in any of the monkeys studied. When the same animals were put on a daily regimen of 500 μg agonist for 3 more months, two of the four monkeys stopped producing ejaculates, in association with their loss of testosterone response to the LHRH agonist. After the cessation of LHRH agonist treatment these two monkeys produced azoospermic ejaculates for 4–8 weeks. When sperm first reappeared in subsequent ejaculates, motility was low. Both the animals produced ejaculates with normal sperm counts and motility 12–14 weeks after the cessation of agonist treatment (Sundaram *et al.*, 1982).

TREATMENT BY CONSTANT INFUSION

Basal LH and testosterone levels

Continuous administration of 48 μg/day buserelin via subcutaneously implanted Alzet^R osmotic minipumps resulted in an initial transitory rise of serum and testosterone levels. Twenty-four hours after the implantation of the first pump, serum LH levels were elevated fivefold above the basal levels and then declined to below pretreatment levels during the next 7 days of LHRH agonist infusion (Figure 7.2). Levels were undetectable by the 3rd week of agonist treatment, and LH remained suppressed until treatment was discontinued. There was a close correlation between serum LH and testosterone concentrations. Serum testosterone also showed an initial increase, followed by a gradual decline. The levels remained between 8 and 15% of pretreatment values until week 13 of the treatment, when testosterone-containing Silastic capsules were implanted to obtain a prolonged elevation of serum testosterone. Serum levels of LH and testosterone increased 1 week after the cessation of agonist treatment, and rose above the pretreatment levels before falling again to normal values (Figure 7.2).

Acute pituitary stimulation tests

Before starting buserelin treatment, administration of a 50 μg bolus intravenous injection of LHRH resulted in an LH peak occurring at 15 min (sixfold increase) and a corresponding testosterone peak at 60 min. Both responses were abolished after 3 weeks of LHRH agonist infusion and reappeared only after the treatment was discontinued. A maximal pituitary and gonadal response was observed during the 4th week of the recovery phase.

Although there is no evidence for the loss of pituitary LHRH receptors in the monkeys under constant buserelin treatment, comparable studies in the castrated male rat have shown that the LH response to exogenous LHRH is also abolished and that there is a net loss of pituitary LHRH receptors (Clayton, 1982).

Testicular volumes

Continuous administration of LHRH agonist resulted in a significant decrease in testicular volumes (Figure 7.1). Volumes decreased dramatically after 6 weeks of treatment and were in out-of-season range by 10 weeks. A further decrease occurred over the next 5 weeks of treatment and volumes in two monkeys were comparable to those seen in stalk-sectioned animals (Marshall *et al.*, 1983).

Ejaculatory behavior

All monkeys maintained normal ejaculatory behavior during the first 5 weeks of buserelin infusion. Occasional failures to produce an ejaculate in response to ejaculatory stimulation were observed from week 6 onwards. The impairment of ejaculatory behavior was associated with the sharp decrease in testicular volumes, evident after 6 weeks of treatment, rather than with the suppression in testosterone levels already evident after 3 weeks. Frequency of spontaneous ejaculation also decreased markedly after 5–6 weeks of the agonist treatment. No monkey ejaculated spontaneously after 8 weeks of

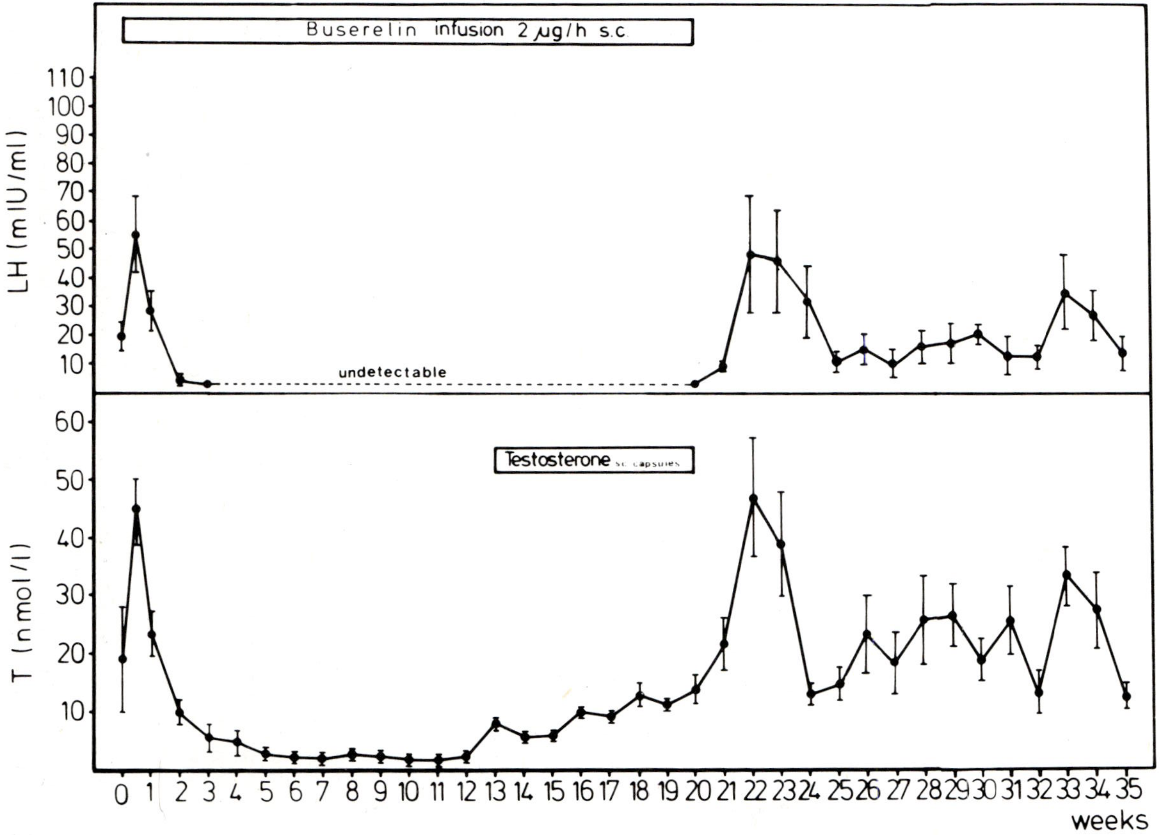

Figure 7.2 Mean serum levels of LH and testosterone in 4 male rhesus monkeys before and during constant minipump infusion of buserelin (48 μg/d), and during a 15 week recovering period. Week 0 represents mean of several basal values from each animal. Bars indicate SE (Reproduced, with permission, from Bint Akhtar *et al.*, 1983. Copyright, 1983, The Endocrine Society.)

treatment. A normal mean frequency of 11 spontaneous ejaculations per monkey per month was achieved for each animal in the first month following termination of LHRH agonist treatment.

Seminal parameters

Sperm count and motility were not affected during the first 5 weeks of agonist treatment (Figure 7.3). One of the four animals showed extreme oligozoospermia accompanied by low spermatozoal motility on week 7 of treatment. The same monkey became azoospermic after 8 weeks of treatment, and remained so for the rest of the treatment period. Two other monkeys which had sperm counts within the normal range until week 9 and 10 respectively showed decreased sperm motility at this stage and, subsequently, either they failed to respond to electrostimulation or ejaculates produced were azoospermic. The fourth monkey had normal sperm counts and motility until week 10, and then showed a marked decrease in ejaculate weight and sperm motility before it stopped responding to electrostimulation at week 13. Sperm morphology was not affected by LHRH agonist treatment.

From week 8 onwards the ejaculates that were obtained failed to coagulate. There was a gradual decrease in ejaculate weight under LHRH agonist infusion. These changes are attributable to the malfunctioning of the accessory reproductive organs resulting from very low circulating androgens. In any clinical application of constant, high dose LHRH agonist administration, the loss of ejaculatory behavior such as that seen in the rhesus monkey would be considered highly undesirable. Men receiving 50 μg [D-Trp^6,Pro^9-NHEt]LHRH per day reported loss of libido and potency, and the occurrence of hot flashes, causing five of the eight men to withdraw from the study (Linde *et al.*, 1981). The three remaining subjects had very low circulating testosterone levels and sperm counts below 5×10^6/ml.

Effects of testosterone replacement in monkeys receiving constant buserelin infusions

Testosterone-containing Silastic capsules were implanted subcutaneously in the monkeys during week 13 of the LHRH agonist treatment. The resulting serum testosterone levels were in the lower physiological range, and ejaculatory behavior was re-established. Three of the four monkeys produced azoospermic ejaculates until after treatment was discontinued. The fourth animal had very few sperm in its ejaculates under testosterone therapy, but also produced azoospermic ejaculates during weeks 2–7 of the recovery phase.

There was some increase in ejaculate weight during testosterone supplementation but normal weights were not re-established. The ejaculates obtained during testosterone supplementation coagulated normally. Spontaneous ejaculatory behavior also improved under testosterone supplementation and a mean frequency of six ejaculates per month for each animal was achieved under substitution. The mean pretreatment frequency for each animal was

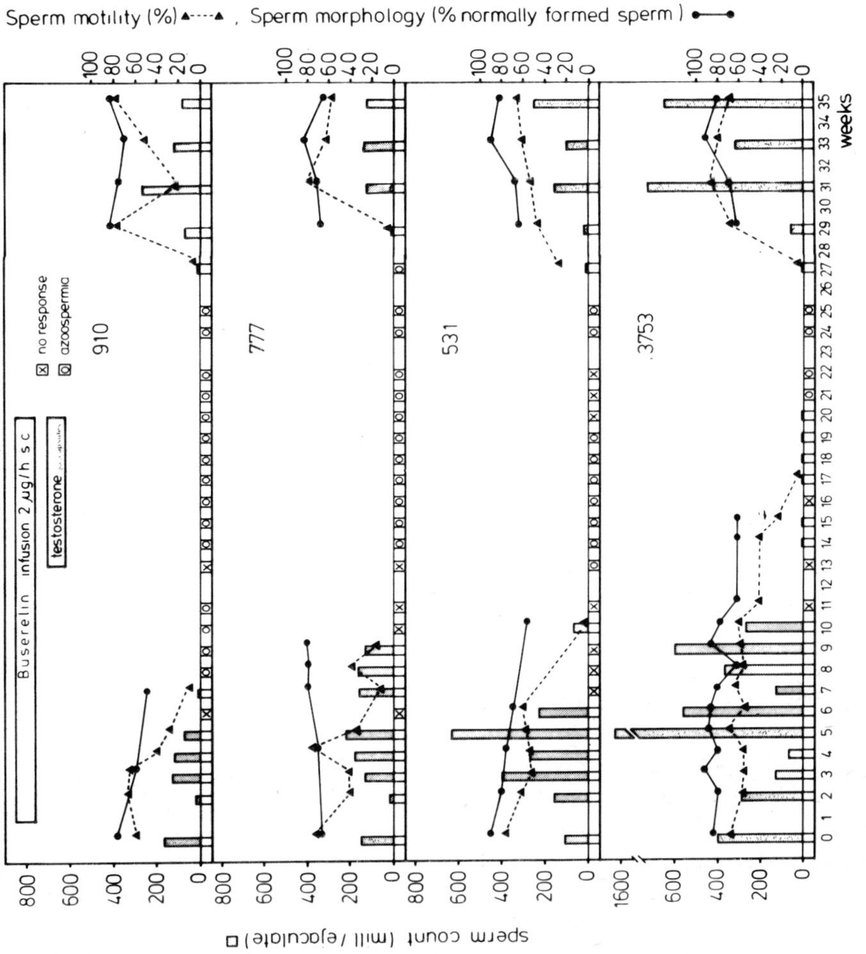

Figure 7.3 Sperm count, motility and percentage of normally formed sperm in four rhesus monkeys before and during buserelin infusion (20 weeks), and during the recovery period (15 weeks). Week 0 represents mean of at least two basal values from each animal (Reproduced, with permission, from Bint Akhtar *et al.*, 1983. Copyright, 1983, The Endocrine Society.)

13 ejaculates per month. Testicular volumes were not influenced by these levels of testosterone.

Recovery of testicular functions

Testicular volumes increased rapidly during the recovery phase, were in the in-season-range by the 6th post-treatment week and had fully recovered 8 weeks after LHRH agonist treatment was terminated.

Like the endocrine parameters and testicular volumes, seminal parameters also recovered fully after the cessation of LHRH agonist treatment. A normal frequency of spontaneous ejaculations prevailed within 1 month of discontinuing treatment. There was a gradual increase in ejaculate weight during the recovery phase. All monkeys started producing ejaculates of normal size within 4–7 weeks after stopping the treatment. Sperm reappeared in the ejaculates of all monkeys by the 7th–9th post-treatment weeks. All animals showed low sperm motility when sperm first reappeared in the ejaculates, but all four animals had normal sperm counts and motility 11 weeks after the cessation of treatment, as well as during the 4 subsequent weeks.

CONCLUDING REMARKS

These preclinical trials in rhesus monkeys showed that LHRH agonist administration, with concomitant androgen supplementation, provides a feasible approach to male fertility control. The induction of and complete reversibility from azoospermia fulfils one of the major prerequisites for acceptance. It remains to be determined if testosterone administration synergizes the suppressive effects of the LHRH agonist as in the rat (Heber and Swerdloff, 1980, 1981) or even antagonizes them. Rhesus monkeys have a very low androgen threshold for ejaculatory response (Zumpe *et al.*, 1980) and high doses of testosterone alone are capable of maintaining spermatogenesis (Marshall *et al.*, 1983). If the same applies to men, much care must be taken in determining testosterone substitution doses. Two other major drawbacks in the use of LHRH agonists for male fertility control, which may prohibit acceptance, are decreased testicular volumes and the long time-frame needed to achieve azoospermia.

Acknowledgements

Buserelin used in all our studies was the gift of Dr J. Sandow, Hoechst AG, Frankfurt, F. R. Germany. F. Bint Akhtar is the recipient of a fellowship from the Deutscher Akademischer Austauschdienst.

References

Bélanger, A., Auclair, C., Ferland, L., Caron, S. and Labrie, F. (1980). Time-course of the effect of treatment with a potent LHRH agonist on testicular steroidogenesis and gonadotropin receptor levels in the adult rat. *J. Steroid Biochem.*, **13**, 191

Belchetz, P. E., Plant, T. M., Nakai, Y., Keogh, E. J. and Knobil, E. (1978). Hypophyseal responses to continuous and intermittent delivery of hypothalamic gonadotropin releasing hormone. *Science,* **202,** 631

Bergquist, C., Nillius, S. J., Bergh, T., Skarin, G. and Wide, L. (1979). Inhibitory effects on gonadotrophin secretion and gonadal functions in men during treatment with a potent stimulatory luteinizing hormone-releasing hormone analogue. *Acta Endocrinol.,* **91,** 601

Bint Akhtar, F., Wickings, E. J., Zaidi, P. and Nieschlag, E. (1982). Pituitary and testicular functions in sexually mature rhesus monkeys under high dose LRH agonist treatment. *Acta Endocrinol.,* **101,** 113

Bint Akhtar, F., Marshall, G. R., Wickings, E. J. and Nieschlag, E. (1983). Reversible induction of azoospermia in rhesus monkeys by constant infusion of a GnRH agonist using osmotic minipumps. *J. Clin. Endocrinol. Metab.* **56,** 534

Carmel, P. W., Araki, S. and Ferin, M. (1976). Pituitary stalk blood collection in rhesus monkeys: evidence for pulsatile release of gonadotropin releasing hormone (GnRH). *Endocrinology,* **99,** 243

Clayton, R. N. (1982). Gonadotropin-releasing hormone modulation of its own pituitary receptors: evidence for biphasic regulation. *Endocrinology,* **111,** 152

Clayton, R. N. and Huhtaniemi, I. P. (1982). Absence of gonadotropin releasing hormone receptors in human gonadal tissue. *Nature (Lond.),* **299,** 56

Faure, N., Labrie, F., Lemay, A., Bélanger, A., Gourdeau, Y., Laroche, B. and Robert, G. (1982). Inhibition of serum androgen levels by chronic intranasal and subcutaneous administration of a potent luteinizing hormone-releasing hormone (LHRH) agonist in adult men. *Fertil. Steril.,* **37,** 416

Heber, D. and Swerdloff, R. S. (1980). Male contraception: Synergism of gonadotropin-releasing hormone analog and testosterone in suppressing gonadotropin. *Science,* **209,** 936

Heber, D. and Swerdloff, R. S. (1981). Gonadotropin-releasing hormone analog and testosterone synergistically inhibit spermatogenesis. *Endocrinology,* **108,** 2019

Hsueh, A. J. W. and Jones, P. B. C. (1981). Extrapituitary actions of gonadotropin-releasing hormone. *Endocr. Rev.,* **2,** 437

Knobil, E. (1980). The neuroendocrine control of the menstrual cycle. *Rec. Progr. Horm. Res.,* **36,** 53

Labrie, F., Bélanger, A., Cusan, L., Séguin, C., Pelletier, G., Kelly, P. A., Reeves, J. J., Lefebvre, F. A., Lemay, A., Gourdeau, Y. and Raynaud, J. P. (1980). Antifertility effects of LHRH agonists in the male. *J. Androl.,* **1,** 209

Linde, R., Doelle, G. C., Alexander, N., Kirchner, F., Vale, W., Rivier, J. and Rabin, D. (1981). Reversible inhibition of testicular steroidogenesis and spermatogenesis by a potent gonadotropin-releasing hormone agonist in normal men. *N. Engl. J. Med.,* **305,** 663

Magoffin, D. A. and Erickson, G. F. (1982). Mechanism by which GnRH inhibits androgen synthesis directly in ovarian interstitial cells. *Mol. Cell. Endocrinol.,* **27,** 191

Marshall, G. M., Wickings, E. J., Lüdecke, D. K. and Nieschlag, E. (1983). Stimulation of spermatogenesis in stalk-sectioned rhesus monkeys by testosterone alone. *J. Clin. Endocrinol. Metab.,* **57,** 152

Nett, T. M., Crowder, M. E., Moss, G. E. and Duello, T. M. (1981). GnRH-receptor interaction. V. Down-regulation of pituitary receptors for GnRH in ovariectomized ewes by infusion of homologous hormone. *Biol. Reprod.,* **24,** 1145

Nieschlag, E. and Wickings, E. J. (1980). Does the rhesus monkey provide a suitable model for human testicular functions? In Serio, M. and Martini, L. (eds.) *Animal Models in Human Reproduction,* pp. 103–119. (New York: Raven Press)

Resko, J. A., Bélanger, A. and Labrie, F. (1982). Effects of chronic treatment with a potent luteinizing hormone releasing hormone agonist on serum luteinizing hormone and steroid levels in male rhesus monkeys. *Biol. Reprod.,* **26,** 378

Rivier, C., Rivier, J. and Vale, W. (1979). Chronic effects of (D-Trp^6,Pro^9-NEt) luteinizing hormone-releasing factor on reproductive processes in the male rat. *Endocrinology,* **105,** 1191

Sandow, J. (1982*a*). Inhibition of pituitary and testicular function by LH-RH analogues. In Jeffcoate, S. L. (ed.) *Progress Towards a Male Contraceptive,* pp. 19–39. (Chichester: Wiley)

Sandow, J. (1982*b*). Gonadotropic and antigonadotropic actions of LH-RH analogues. In Müller, E. E. and Macleod, R. M. (eds.) *Neuroendocrine Perspectives.* Vol. 1, pp. 339–395. (Amsterdam: Elsevier Biomedical Press)

Sandow, J., von Rechenberg, W., Jerzabek, G. and Stoll, W. (1978). Pituitary inhibition by a highly active analog of luteinizing hormone-releasing hormone. *Fertil. Steril.*, **30**, 205

Sharpe, R. M. (1982). Cellular aspects of the inhibitory actions of LH-RH on the ovary and testis. *J. Reprod. Fertil.*, **64**, 517

Sharpe, R. M. and Fraser, H. M. (1980). Inhibition of maturational changes in Leydig cell function by treatment of rats with an agonist of LHRH. *J. Reprod. Fertil.*, **60**, 359

Sharpe, R. M., Fraser, H. M., Cooper, J. and Rommerts, F. F. G. (1981). Sertoli–Leydig cell communication via an LHRH-like factor. *Nature (Lond.)*, **290**, 785

Sundaram, K., Connell, K. G., Bardin, C. W., Samojlik, E. and Schally, A. V. (1982). Inhibition of pituitary-testicular function with (D-Trp^6) luteinizing hormone-releasing hormone in rhesus monkeys. *Endocrinology*, **110**, 1308

Tolis, G., Ackman, D., Stellos, A., Mehta, A., Labrie, F., Fazekas, A. T. A., Comaru-Schally, A. M. and Schally, A. V. (1982). Tumor growth inhibition in patients with prostatic carcinoma treated with luteinizing hormone-releasing hormone agonists. *Proc. Natl. Acad. Sci. USA*, **79**, 1658

Wickings, E. J. and Nieschlag, E. (1980). Seasonality in endocrine and exocrine testicular function of the adult rhesus monkey (Macaca mulatta) maintained in a controlled laboratory environment. *Int. J. Androl.*, **3**, 87

Wickings, E. J., Zaidi, P. and Nieschlag, E. (1981*a*). Stimulation of pituitary and testicular functions with LH-RH agonist or pulsatile LHRH treatment in the rhesus monkey during the non-breeding season. *J. Reprod. Fertil.*, **63**, 129

Wickings, E. J., Zaidi, P. and Nieschlag, E. (1981*b*). Effect of chronic, high-dose LHRH-agonist treatment on pituitary and testicular functions in rhesus monkeys. *J. Androl.*, **2**, 72

Zumpe, D., Bonsall, R. W. and Michael, R. P. (1981). Low androgen threshold for ejaculatory responses in male rhesus monkeys. *Am. J. Primatol.*, **1**, 351

8
LHRH agonists for control of female fertility: primate studies

B. H. VICKERY and G. I. McRAE

Following the extraction, sequencing and synthesis of LHRH, it was forecast that agonistic and antagonistic analogs would be synthesized and would warrant evaluation for profertility and antifertility uses, respectively (Schally and Kastin, 1971). Early studies with LHRH itself proved disappointing in regard to induction of fertility and this status continued in spite of the identification and testing of highly potent agonist (superagonist) analogs. The ease of generating highly potent agonist analogs was not reflected in the case of antagonist congeners. Beginning in 1975, literature began to appear on effects of LHRH agonists which was at odds with the accepted profertility functions of LHRH. These paradoxical effects, as they were termed, included delay of puberty, inhibition of ovulation and luteal function, interruption of pregnancy and suppression of ovarian steroidogenesis (Johnson *et al.*, 1976; Corbin and Beattie, 1975). In the normal physiological state LHRH is required to be secreted in a pulsatile fashion (Belchetz *et al.*, 1978). Chronic administration, by infusion of LHRH (Rabin and McNeil, 1980) or by administration – as infrequently as once daily – of the highly potent agonist analogs, results in a desensitization of the pituitary gonadotropes (Clayton and Catt, 1981). This effect is sufficient to account for the paradoxical effects of LHRH analogs. However, the detection of LHRH-like materials in extrahypothalamic tissues such as the gonad (Ying and Guillemin, 1979; Ying *et al.*, 1981), placenta (Khodr and Siler-Khodr, 1980) and breast (Sarda and Nair, 1981) raises the possibility of direct peripheral tissue effects. In rats, there are complex interreactions between LHRH and gonadotropin receptors (Labrie *et al.*, 1981) and between LHRH and steroid receptors (Singh and Muldoon, 1982). Effects have been noted upon steroidogenic and steroid metabolic enzyme systems in rats (Jones and Hsueh, 1981; Hillier *et al.*, 1981). While most of these studies have not been duplicated with human tissues one must allow for the greater difficulty in conducting such studies. Early confirmatory studies of direct effects of LHRH upon human granulosa cell aromatase activity (Tureck *et al.*, 1982), arrhenoblastoma culture (Lamberts *et al.*, 1982) and placental explants (Khodr and Siler-Khodr, 1978) or cell cultures (Butzow, 1982), may be just the beginning of a flood of new information. The discovery of multiple sites of action for LHRH or like peptides, now accepted for the rat and perhaps lower vertebrates, may yet be repeated in man.

This chapter will describe studies, in infra-human primates, which were designed to assess the potential of LHRH agonists for contraception in women, and will relate them to available clinical data in women.

OVULATION INHIBITION

Chronic administration

Following the initial demonstrations in rats of the ability of an LHRH analog, [D-Leu^6,Pro^9-NHEt]LHRH, to inhibit estrous cyclicity and cause reversible atrophy of the ovaries and uterus of the adult rat (Johnson *et al.*, 1976) reports of short term administration of other analogs to women began to appear. The preliminary report of efficacy of [D-Ser(tBu)^6,Pro^9-NHEt]LHRH (Nillius *et al.*, 1978) was followed by a study with LHRH itself, using only ten times the dose (Lambe *et al.*, 1979). Longer term ovulation suppression in monkeys was then reported. Continuous delivery of agonist was achieved by use of a pelleted formulation of [D-Trp^6,Pro^9-NHEt]LHRH, delivering compound continuously over 7 months (Vickery *et al.*, 1980). Comparison of the gonadotropin levels in these animals with those in other rhesus treated by daily administration of LHRH analog (the regimen used in all other reported studies) reveals some important differences. LH values in the animals receiving pellets declined to undetectable levels by 4 days after onset of treatment (Figure 8.1) and continued at undetectable levels until 4 days after cessation of treatment (7 months later). Animals receiving a completely effective ovulation inhibiting dose by once daily administration, on the other hand, continued to show acute responsivity of LH release to each daily administration of agonist, although this tended to decrease with time (Figure 8.2). Basal levels of LH measured immediately prior to each injection were always within the range of pretreatment levels (Figure 8.3). The gonadotropin suppression achieved by continuous administration may have been duplicated by the recent attempts at 'medical oophorectomy' reported by Meldrum *et al.* (1982), who used daily administration of [D-Trp^6,Pro^9-NHEt]LHRH to women, but at 40 times the dose necessary to inhibit ovulation (Sheehan and Yen, 1981). Certainly, the castration levels of estrogens reported by Meldrum and co-workers are at variance with the body of the literature which has evaluated optimal or suboptimal ovulation inhibiting dose levels of LHRH agonists. Similar disparate findings are being reported for daily versus continuous administration of an LHRH agonist in male rhesus monkeys (Wickings *et al.*, 1981; Akhtar *et al.*, 1982). Any question of the effects of unopposed estrogen, and the occurrence of endometrial hyperplasia during treatment with LHRH agonists, should await characterization of the different endocrine responses to daily versus continuous administration of these agents in women. Down regulation at both pituitary and ovary seems likely in women, as neither estrogen challenge (Fraser, 1981*a*; Bergquist *et al.*, 1982) nor

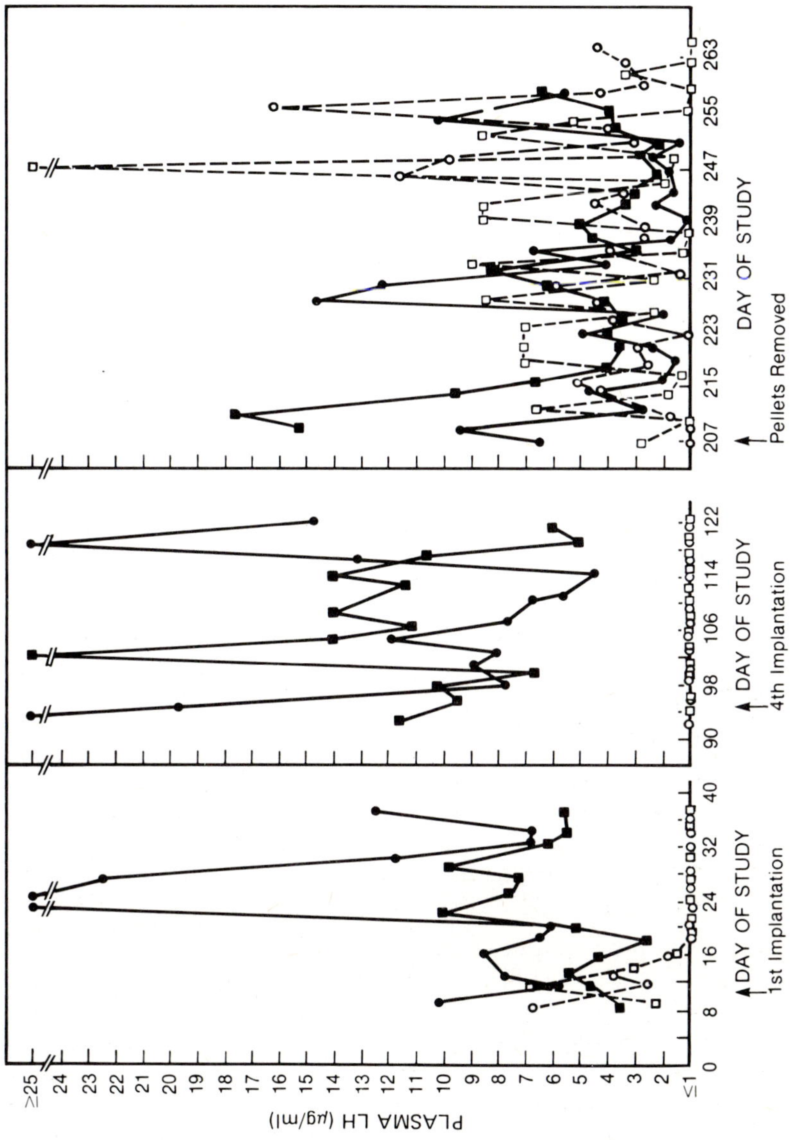

Figure 8.1 Plasma LH in rhesus monkeys either sham implanted (●, ■) or implanted every 4 weeks with 1 mg of pelleted [D-Trp⁶]LHRH ethylamide (□).

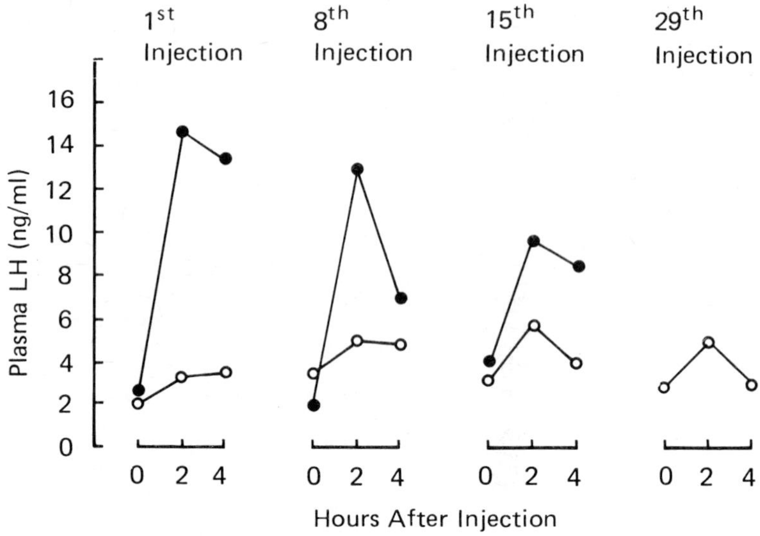

Figure 8.2 Acute responses of plasma LH following daily intramuscular injection of 5 μg [D-Nal(2)^6]LHRH in two female monkeys.

exogenous gonadotropin challenge (Vickery, 1981) bring about their expected responses.

Effects on folliculogenesis and subsequent luteal function

Administration of 'inhibin' (porcine follicular fluid) to rhesus monkeys during the early follicular phase caused an inadequate luteal phase (Stouffer and Hodgen, 1980; DiZerega *et al.*, 1981). It was postulated that a similar timing of LHRH agonist administration might effectively disrupt the menstrual cycle. Studies in women using [D-Trp^6,Pro^9-NHEt]LHRH resulted in a delay of ovulation, followed by a shortened luteal phase which was associated with lower peak levels of progesterone (Sheehan *et al.*, 1982*a*). Similar treatment of rhesus monkeys with [D-Nal(2)^6]LHRH resulted in a similar delay of ovulation, but the luteal phase appeared normal both for duration and integrated levels of progesterone (Figure 8.4). Treatment of women with [D-Ser(tBu)^6,Pro^9-NHEt]LHRH did not cause luteal inadequacy (Skarin *et al.*, 1982). These discrepancies may result from inadequately-understood dose–response relationships and further study will be required to resolve this question.

Interrupted administration

The finding that early follicular phase administration of LHRH agonists could delay ovulation by 7–9 days led to the evaluation of once weekly administration as a contraceptive regimen. Once weekly injection of 50 μg of

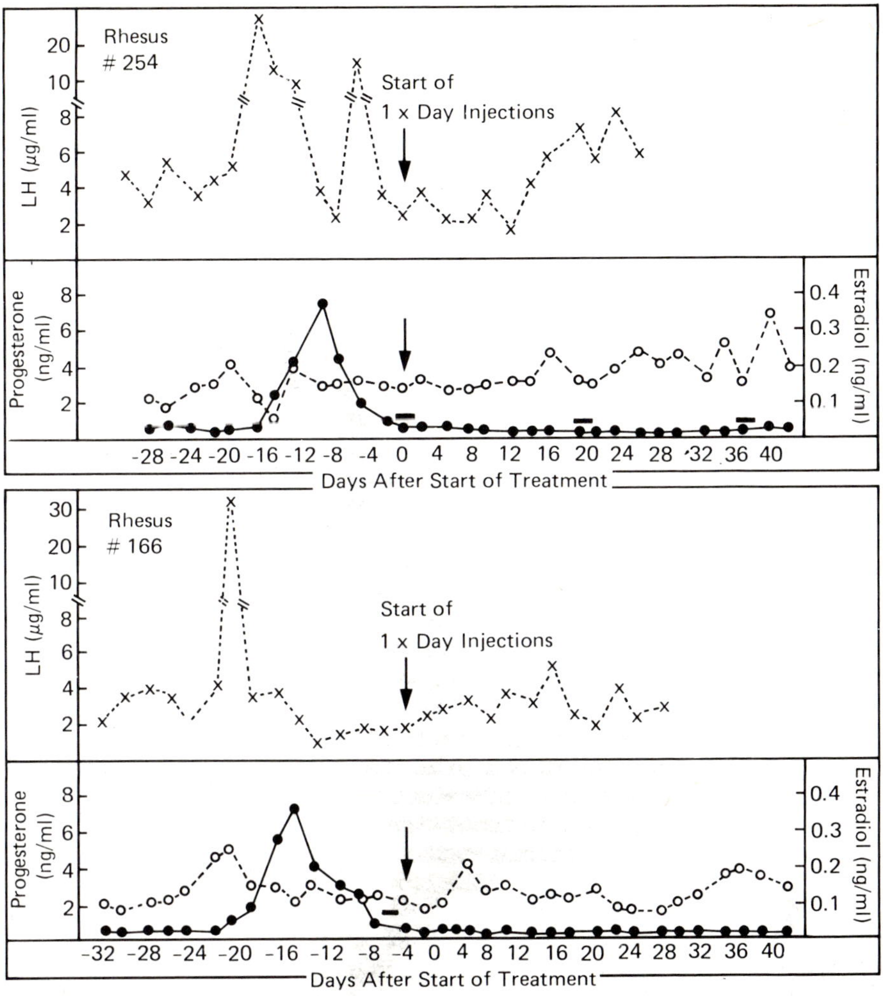

Figure 8.3 Effect of daily intramuscular injection of 5 μg [D-Nal(2)^6]LHRH in rhesus monkeys on LH (x--x), progesterone (●———●) and estradiol (○---○) levels.

[D-Nal(2)^6]LHRH to rhesus monkeys, starting during menstruation, blocked ovulation in only one of three. As the daily dose for ovulation inhibition in rhesus monkeys with [D-Nal(2)^6]LHRH is 5 μg, it is felt unlikely that once weekly administration is economically viable.

LUTEAL SUPPRESSION

Multiple doses of either LHRH (Koyama *et al.*, 1978) or [D-Ser(tBu)^6,Pro^9-NHEt]LHRH (Lemay *et al.*, 1979) to women during the luteal phase result in

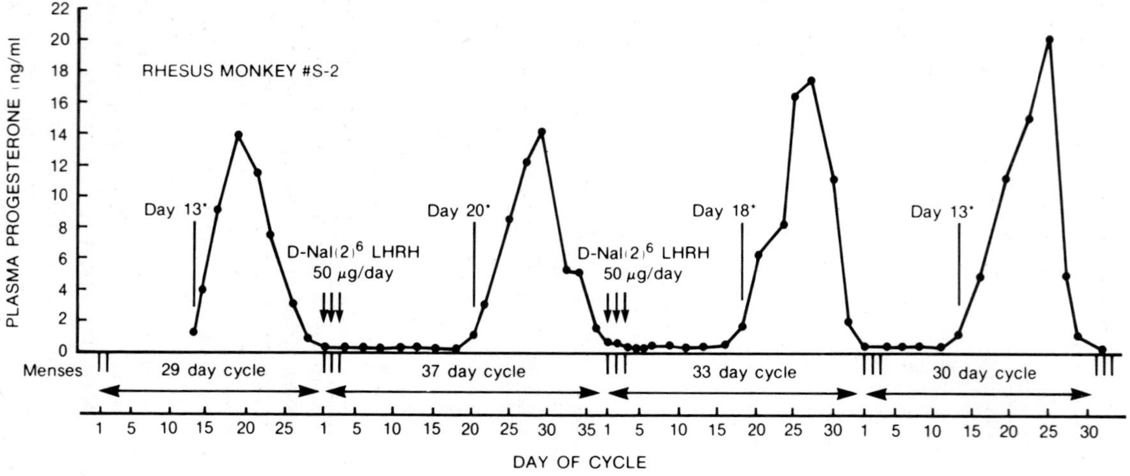

Figure 8.4 Effect of three consecutive daily intramuscular injections of 50 μg [D-Nal(2)^6]LHRH at the onset of each of two consecutive menstrual cycles in a female rhesus monkey.

luteolysis. This effect was also obtained with as few as two daily doses either by injection (Casper and Yen, 1979) or intranasally (Lemay *et al.*, 1979, 1984). Optimal results were obtained when the doses were given 5 or more days after ovulation (Sheehan *et al.*, 1982*b*). The original observations, of a shortening of cycle by 2 days and reduction of integrated levels of progesterone by 30 %, were not bettered in these later studies. Two daily injections of [D-Nal(2)^6]LHRH to female baboons were not luteolytic even at doses as high as 50 μg per injection. Previously, implantation of pelleted [D-Trp^6,Pro^9-NHEt]LHRH during the luteal phase of baboons had caused luteal suppression and premature onset of menstruation (Vickery and McRae, 1980*a*). In the latter study the animals had received continuous dosing. The effect of ten daily injections of [D-Nal(2)^6]LHRH starting 3 days after ovulation was then evaluated (Vickery, 1981; Vickery *et al.*, 1981*a*). A dose related suppression of luteal phase progesterone was obtained. However, even with suppression of progesterone by more than 40 %, as obtained with the highest dose level, no statistically significant changes in either menstrual cycle or luteal phase duration were obtained. A study of two other analogs in *Macaca fascicularis* gave similar results (Raynaud *et al.*, 1980). Consistent induction of shortened luteal phases has been found in rhesus monkeys when 10 μg/animal of [D-Trp^6,Pro^9-NHEt]LHRH was administered on day 3 or 5 but not on day 7 after ovulation (Asch *et al.*, 1981*a*). [D-Nal(2)^6]LHRH was administered as 50 μg per injection either once or twice daily for either 10 consecutive days or until onset of menstruation in baboons (Vickery *et al.*, 1982). Suppression of integrated levels of progesterone was obtained and was associated with a significant shortening of the duration of the luteal phase, amounting to as much as 8 days in one case. Similar findings have been noted with baboons treated with [D-Leu^6,Pro^9-NHEt]LHRH (Vickery, 1981). Similarly impressive effects have been recently reported for [D-Ser(tBu)^6,Pro^9-NHEt]LHRH administered intranasally to women starting 1–2 days after ovulation and continuing until onset of menstruation (Bergquist *et al.*, 1980). It is not known what mechanism is involved in luteal suppression due to LHRH agonist administration or even whether the mechanism is the same for effects of two doses or for more chronic administration. In the baboon studies, at least, acute rises in LH, FSH and progesterone routinely follow injections of agonist (Figure 8.5) which suggests that the pituitary is not suppressed. Seven consecutive daily injections of [D-Leu^6,Pro^9-NHEt]LHRH during the luteal phase of baboons caused estrone levels to rise to a peak 2–3 days after onset of dosing, regardless of the timing of start of injections (Vickery, 1981). This finding may implicate the luteolytic potential of estrogens (Schoonmaker *et al.*, 1981) in the mechanism of action of LHRH agonists as luteolytic agents. Whether estrogens are luteolytic in women is open to question (Gore *et al.*, 1973).

Suppression of the response of the corpus luteum to exogenous gonadotropin has followed implantation of pelleted [D-Trp^6,Pro^9-NHEt]LHRH during the luteal phase in rhesus monkeys (Vickery and McRae, 1980*b*). [D-Trp^6,Pro^9-NHEt]LHRH (Casper *et al.*, 1980) and [D-Ser(tBu)^6,Pro^9-NHEt]LHRH (Bergquist *et al.*, 1980) are reportedly unable to suppress luteal function in the face of exogenous hCG administration in women, although in

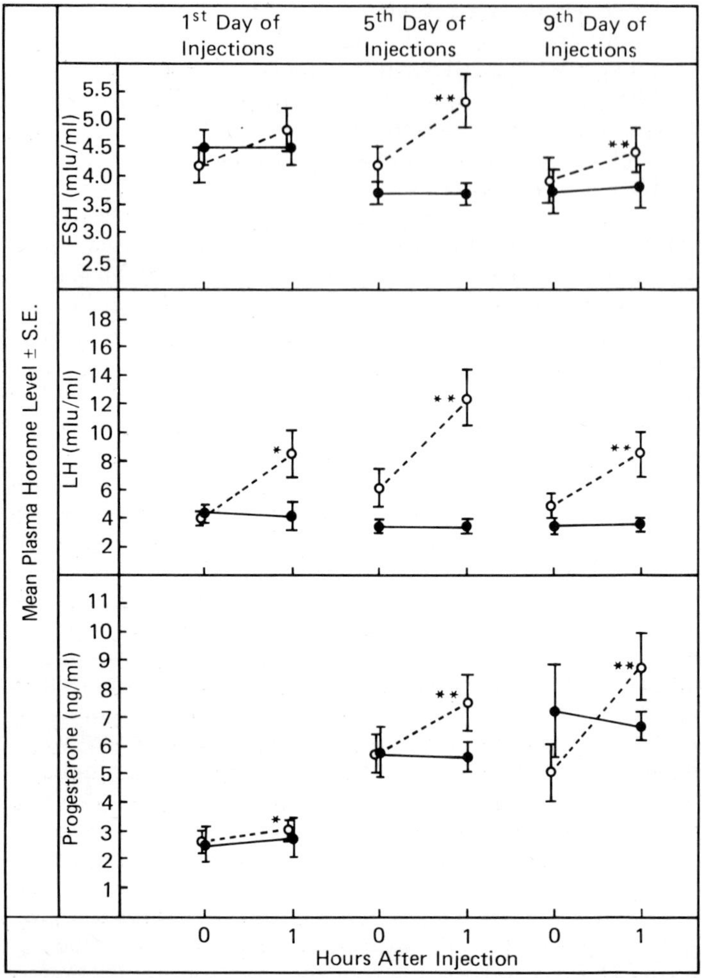

Figure 8.5 Effect of once- or twice-daily intramuscular injections of 50 μg [D-Nal(2)^6]LHRH into female baboons during the luteal phase of plasma FSH (upper panel), LH (middle panel) and progesterone levels (lower panel). Vehicle (●——●, $n = 3$) and [D-Nal(2)^6]LHRH-treated animals (○– – –○, $n = 9$). * $p < 0.05$ and ** $p < 0.01$ compared to respective T^0 value.

each case only two doses of agonist were given to combat 10 doses of hCG. Similarly, five daily doses of hCG were able to counteract the luteolytic effect of a single dose of [D-Trp^6,Pro^9-NHEt]LHRH in rhesus monkeys (Asch *et al.*, 1981*a*). Resolution of the discrepancies between results in monkeys and in women will probably await more careful evaluation of dosage and duration of treatment requirements in the latter. Specific luteal receptors for LHRH tissue such as have been identified in rat ovarian tissue (Pieper *et al.*, 1981) have not been demonstrated in monkeys or women (Asch *et al.*, 1981*b*; Clayton and Huhtaniemi, 1982).

PREGNANCY INTERRUPTION

Attempts to terminate pregnancy in women with [D-Trp^6,Pro^9-NHEt]LHRH or [D-Trp^6]LHRH have been unsuccessful (Casper *et al.*, 1980; Tolis *et al.*, 1981); the range of doses and the number of subjects studied was limited. As was the case for luteal suppression, studies on baboons seem to hold more promise. Thus, antagonism of the steroidogenic response to endogenous chorionic gonadotropin has been demonstrated for [D-Nal(2)^6]LHRH and [D-Trp^6,Pro^9-NHEt]LHRH (Vickery *et al.*, 1980), [D-Leu^6,Pro^6-NHEt] LHRH (Vickery, 1981) and even LHRH itself (R. A. Edgren, personal communication, 1980). In each case circulating levels of progesterone failed to respond to rising levels of chorionic gonadotropin. Pregnancy terminations have resulted in baboons (Vickery *et al.*, 1981*b*; D. Castracane and J. Goldzieher, personal communication, 1981; G. P. Talwar, personal communication, 1982). In addition to the luteolytic effects of the agonists, an interesting and unexpected effect on chorionic gonadotropin was observed (Vickery *et al.*, 1981*b*; G. P. Talwar, personal communication, 1982). The normal profile of chorionic gonadotropin was truncated and fell to undetectable levels by the 37th day of gestation. Whether this would have interfered with the progress of late pregnancy is unknown, as pregnancy was surgically terminated at 70–80 days of gestation in animals which had not already aborted. Fetuses were normal for size and weight at surgical delivery. The suppressive effect on chorionic gonadotropin production *in vivo* and on progesterone from human trophoblast *in vitro* (Wilson and Jawad, 1980) may be a parallel to the other 'paradoxical' effects of these agents. There does appear to be an LHRH-like material present in human placental tissue (DePalatis *et al.*, 1978; Khodr and Siler-Khodr, 1978, 1980; Siler-Khodr and Khodr, 1979) and in certain gestational tumors (Seppala and Wahlstrom, 1980) whose normal function may be to modulate chorionic gonadotropin synthesis and release (Khodr and Siler-Khodr, 1978; Nakano *et al.*, 1978) in turn controlling luteal/placental steroidogenesis. There are reports of the presence of LHRH receptors in human placental tissue (Currie *et al.*, 1981). No effects on hormonal levels were detected in response to 1 mg LHRH injected into six women at 5–7 weeks gestation (Tsai *et al.*, 1982). It has been suggested that the differences in response to LHRH agonists in pregnant baboons and women may be due to differences in placentation (C. W. Bardin, personal communication, 1982).

CONTRACEPTIVE POTENTIAL

Studies in monkeys and in women support the high potential of LHRH agonists as ovulation suppressive agents. Concern has been expressed over the effects of estrogen withdrawal or, alternatively, endometrial hyperplasia resulting from continued unopposed estrogen levels. In most studies low, early follicular phase estrogen levels persist, although estrogen deficiency symptoms do result from high multiples of the minimal ovulation inhibiting dose (Meldrum *et al.*, 1982). Endometrial biopsies obtained over the course of long

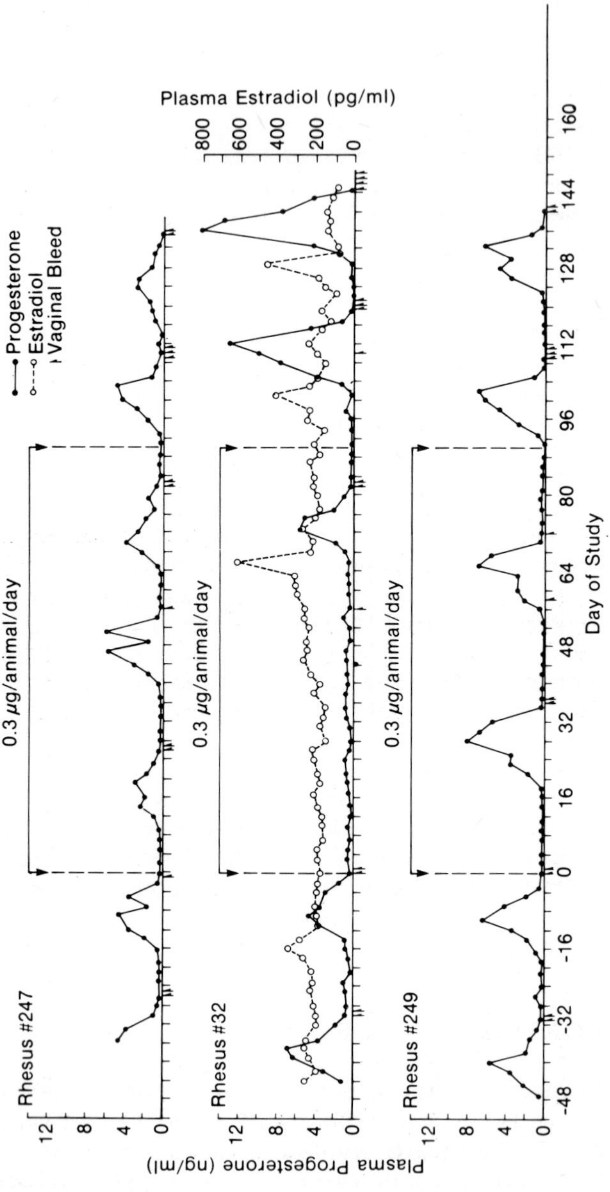
Progesterone
Estradiol
Vaginal Bleed
0.3 μg/animal/day
0.3 μg/animal/day
0.3 μg/animal/day
Rhesus #247
Rhesus #32
Rhesus #249
Plasma Estradiol (pg/ml)
Plasma Progesterone (ng/ml)
Day of Study

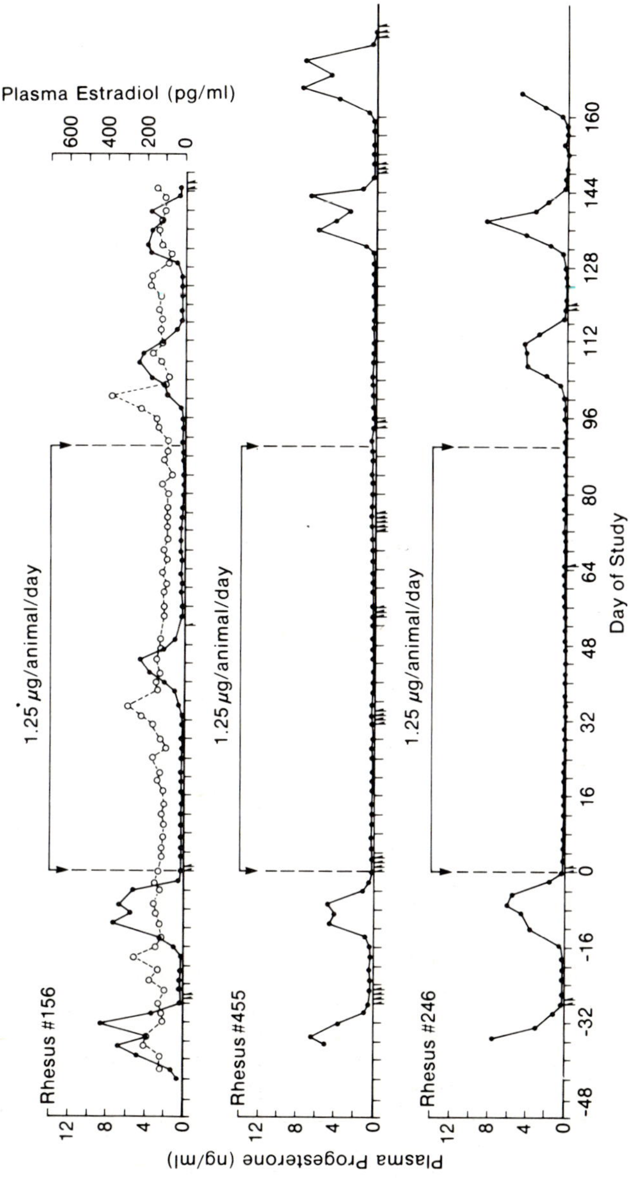

Figure 8.6 Effect of once daily administration of 0.3 or 1.25 μg per day subcutaneously of [D-Nal(2)[6]]LHRH into female rhesus monkeys on plasma estradiol (○- - - -○), plasma progesterone (●——●) levels. Days of menstruation are indicated by

term treatment in both stumptailed macaques (Fraser, 1981*b*) and women (Schmidt-Gollwitzer *et al.*, 1981) revealed that the majority of the endometria resembled the early phase of the follicular cycle or were atrophic. Hyperplasia continues to concern some investigators and has prompted the evaluation of discontinuous therapy with or without progestogen supplementation (Hardt *et al.*, 1984). When an adequate dose level is used, contraceptive efficacy is high. No pregnancies were reported in a long term study in rhesus monkeys with implanted [D-Trp^6,Pro^9-NHEt]LHRH (Vickery *et al.*, 1980) or in unprotected women taking nasal buserelin, daily (Bergquist *et al.*, 1979; Schmidt-Gollwitzer *et al.*, 1981). Suboptimal dose levels of LHRH agonists may allow a percentage of ovulatory cycles. These ovulations tend to be followed by inadequate luteal phases (Figure 8.6). Whether these luteal phases are rescuable by chorionic gonadotropin and thus compatible with pregnancy is being evaluated (Lemay *et al.*, 1984). Reversibility of ovulation suppression even after long term treatment is rapid, usually taking place within a normal follicular phase length (Fraser, 1982). The first return cycle is compatible with pregnancy (Vickery *et al.*, 1980).

The use of once weekly administration of the LHRH agonists does not appear to be economically feasible. Short term, early follicular phase administration initially appeared promising for [D-Trp^6,Pro^9-NHEt]LHRH and even appeared to approximate normal menstrual cyclicity since the induced delay in ovulation was followed by an almost equivalent shortening of the luteal phase (Sheehan *et al.*, 1982*a*). More recent studies in monkeys with [D-Nal(2)^6]LHRH (Vickery, 1981) and women with buserelin (Bergquist *et al.*, 1980) are not so encouraging.

The potential of LHRH agonists for interception has had a varied history. Initial studies in monkeys and women indicated luteolysis in the non-pregnant state to be feasible. Small scale studies in women then suggested that the induced luteolysis was overridden by chorionic gonadotropin. Our studies in rhesus and baboons indicated that there might be a differing and progressively higher dosage requirement for ovulation inhibition, for luteolysis and for pregnancy interception. Again, more work is required before the potential utility of LHRH agonists in this indication may be decided.

THERAPEUTIC POTENTIAL

The interference with ovarian steroidogenesis consequent upon chronic administration of LHRH agonists, whether mediated only at the pituitary or additionally at the ovary, has stimulated interest in their use as therapeutic agents in reproductive endocrine pathologies. Endometriosis, polycystic ovarian disease, and breast tumors are presently under investigation. The rationale for the use in breast cancer and the animal studies which have been performed are the subject of a recent review by Corbin (1982). The results so far reported for women are equivocal (Klijn and de Jong, 1982; Harvey *et al.*, 1981).

The potential connection between LHRH and chorionic gonadotropin in placental tissue, gestational tumors and even non-gestational tumors is intriguing. If LHRH-like materials govern the synthesis and release of CG in the same way that LHRH governs the synthesis and release of pituitary gonadotropins, it is possible that the paradoxical effect of agonists or the direct effect of antagonists may be of broader use in antitumor therapy. Chorionic gonadotropin or its subunits are produced by a wide variety of tumors, and may be ubiquitous to tumors (Braunstein, 1979). It is thought that chorionic gonadotropin may subserve an immunosuppressive or antigen-masking role in tumors. HCG suppresses the mixed lymphocyte response. An agent which could suppress chorionic gonadotropin release, as LHRH agonists suppress placental CG, might have use in a variety of metastatic tumors.

Cancer chemotherapy frequently results in amenorrhea and irreversible sterility in women. The alylating agents used in chemotherapy exert their effects on rapidly dividing tissue. Suppression of folliculogenesis by LHRH or its analogs may exert a protective effect against chemotherapy.

CONCLUDING REMARKS

Studies in primates indicate far-ranging potential utility for LHRH analogs, stretching from control of fertility to cancer therapy. A major obstacle facing development of these agents is their relative lack of oral activity. Formulations suitable for nasal administration appear to be economically feasible for use in ovulation inhibition, even with only 2% absorption. However, it is questionable that the higher doses which will be required for the other indications can be physically or economically feasible by the nasal route. Major emphasis is therefore expected to be placed on the development of depot injectable or implantable formulations. Although this is breaking new ground for relatively hydrophilic agents such as these, early reports are encouraging (Kent *et al.*, 1982; Sanders *et al.*, 1982).

Acknowledgement

This research was supported in part by Prime Contract No. NO1-HD-0-2811 to Syntex from the U.S. National Institutes of Health, Department of Health and Social Services.

References

Akhtar, F. B., Marshall, G. R., Wickings, E. J. and Nieschlag, E. (1982). Antifertility effects of chronic LHRH agonist infusion by osmotic pumps in adult male monkeys. Abstr. No. 17, *Programme of 1st Joint Meeting of British Endocrine Societies*, May 1982, London

Asch, R. H., Siler-Khodr, T. M., Smith, C. G. and Schally, A. V. (1981*a*). Luteolytic effect of D-Trp^6-luteinizing hormone-releasing hormone in the rhesus monkey (Macaca mulatta). *J. Clin. Endocrinol. Metab.*, **52,** 565

Asch, R. H., Sickle, M. van, Rettori, V., Balmaceda, J. P., Eddy, C. A., Coy, D. H. and Schally, A. V. (1981*b*). Absence of LH-RH binding sites in corpora lutea from rhesus monkeys (*Macaca mulatta*). *J. Clin. Endocrinol. Metab.*, **53,** 215

Belchetz, P. E., Plant, T. M., Nakai, Y., Keogh, E. J. and Knobil, E. (1978). Hypophyseal responses to continuous and intermittent delivery of hypothalamic gonadotropin-releasing hormone. *Science,* **202,** 631

Bergquist, C., Nillius, S. J. and Wide, L. (1979). Intranasal gonadotropin-releasing hormone agonist as a contraceptive agent. *Lancet,* **2,** 215

Bergquist, C., Nillius, S. J. and Wide, L. (1980). Luteolysis induced by a luteinizing hormone-releasing hormone agonist is prevented by human chorionic gonadotropin. *Contraception,* **22,** 341

Bergquist, C., Nillius, S. J. and Wide, L. (1982). Failure of positive feedback of oestradiol during chronic intranasal luteinizing hormone-releasing hormone agonist treatment. *Clin. Endocrinol.,* **16,** 147

Braunstein, G. D. (1979). Human chorionic gonadotropin in nontrophoblastic tumors and tissues. In Talwar, G. P. (ed.) *Recent Advances in Reproduction and Regulation of Fertility,* pp. 389–397. (Amsterdam: Elsevier/North Holland)

Butzow, R. (1982). Luteinizing hormone-releasing factor increases release of human chorionic gonadotropin in isolated cell columns of normal and malignant trophoblasts. *Int. J. Cancer,* **29,** 9

Casper, R. F. and Yen, S. S. C. (1979). Induction of luteolysis in the human with a long-acting analog of luteinizing hormone-releasing factor. *Science,* **205,** 408

Casper, R. F., Sheehan, K. L. and Yen, S. S. C. (1980). Chorionic gonadotropin prevents LRF-agonist-induced luteolysis in the human. *Contraception,* **21,** 471

Clayton, R. N. and Catt, K. J. (1981). Gonadotropin-releasing hormone receptors: Characterization, physiological regulation, and relationship to reproductive function. *Endocr. Rev.,* **2,** 196

Clayton, R. N. and Huhtaniemi, I. T. (1982). Absence of gonadotropin-releasing hormone receptors in human gonadal tissue. *Nature (Lond.),* **299,** 56

Corbin, A. (1982). From contraception to cancer: a review of the therapeutic applications of LHRH analogues as antitumor agents. *Yale J. Biol. Med.,* **55,** 27

Corbin, A. and Beattie, C. W. (1975). Post-coital contraceptive and uterotrophic effects of luteinizing hormone releasing hormone. *Endocr. Res. Commun.,* **2,** 445

Currie, A. J., Fraser, H. M. and Sharpe, R. M. (1981). Human placental receptors for luteinizing hormone releasing hormone. *Biochem. Biophys. Res. Commun.,* **99,** 332

DePalatis, L. R., Ho, R. H., Riorindo, R. P. and Elde, R. (1978). *Physiologist,* **21,** 27

DiZerega, G. S., Turner, C. K., Stouffer, R. L., Anderson, L. D., Channing, C. P. and Hodgen, G. D. (1981). Suppression of follicle-stimulating hormone-dependent folliculogenesis during the primate ovarian cycle. *J. Clin. Endocrinol. Metab.,* **52,** 451

Fraser, H. M. (1981*a*). Effect of oestrogen on gonadotropin release in stumptailed monkeys (Macaca arctoides) treated chronically with an agonist analogue of luteinizing hormone-releasing hormone. *J. Endocrinol.,* **91,** 525

Fraser, H. M. (1981*b*). Luteinizing hormone-releasing hormone and fertility control. In Finn, C. A. (ed.) *Oxford Reviews of Reproductive Biology.* Vol. 3, pp. 1–49. (Oxford: Oxford UP)

Fraser, H. M. (1982). Antifertility effects of GnRH. *J. Reprod. Fertil.,* **64,** 503

Gore, B. A., Caldwell, B. V. and Speroff, L. (1973). Estrogen-induced human luteolysis. *J. Clin. Endocrinol. Metab.,* **36,** 615

Hardt, W., Genz, T. and Schmidt-Gollwitzer, M. (1983). Antifertility by discontinuous treatment with buserelin in women. This volume, Chapter 18

Harvey, H. A., Lipton, A., Santen, R. J., Esher, G. C., Hardy, M. A., Glode, L. M., Segaloff, A., Landau, R. L., Schneir, H. and Max, D. T. (1981). Phase II study of a gonadotropin-releasing hormone analogue (Leuprolide) in postmenopausal advanced breast cancer patients. *Proc. Am. Assoc. Cancer Res./Am. Soc. Clin. Oncol.,* **22,** 444

Hillier, S. G., Reichert L. E. Jr. and van Hall, E. V. (1981). Modulation of FSH-controlled steroidogenesis in rat granulosa cells: Direct in vitro effects of LHRH and ICI-118630. *Mol. Cell. Endocrinol.,* **23,** 193

Johnson, E. S., Gendrich, R. L. and White, W. F. (1976). Delay of puberty and inhibition of reproductive processes in the rat by a gonadotropin-releasing hormone agonist analog. *Fertil. Steril.,* **27,** 853

Jones, P. B. C. and Hsueh, A. J. W. (1981). Regulation of ovarian 20αhydroxysteroid dehydrogenase by gonadotropin-releasing hormone and its antagonist in vitro and in vivo. *J. Steroid Biochem.,* **14,** 1169

Kent, J. S., Sanders, L. M., McRae, G. I., Vickery, B. H., Tice, T. R. and Lewis, D. H. (1982). In vivo controlled release of an LH-RH analog from injected polymeric microcapsules. *Contracept. Deliv. Syst.,* **3,** 58

Khodr, G. and Siler-Khodr, T. M. (1978). The effect of luteinizing hormone-releasing factor on human chorionic gonadotropin secretion. *Fertil. Steril.,* **30,** 301

Khodr, G. and Siler-Khodr, T. M. (1980). Placental luteinizing hormone-releasing factor and its synthesis. *Science,* **207,** 315

Klijn, J. G. and de Jong, F. H. (1982). Treatment with a luteinizing hormone-releasing hormone analogue (Buserelin) in premenopausal patients with metastatic breast cancer. *Lancet,* May 29, 1213

Koyama, T., Ohkura, T., Kumasaka, T. and Saito, M. (1978). Effect of postovulatory treatment with luteinizing hormone-releasing hormone on the plasma levels of progesterone in women. *Fertil. Steril.,* **30,** 549

Labrie, F., Bélanger, A., Séguin, C., Cusan, L., Pelletier, G., Lefebvre, F.-A., Kelly, P. A., Ferland, L., Reeves, J. J., Lemay, A. and Raynaud, J.-P. (1981). Inhibition of testicular and ovarian functions by LHRH agonists. In Jagiello, G. and Vogel, H. J. (eds.) *Bioregulators of Reproduction,* pp. 305–341. (New York: Academic Press)

Lambe, R. F., Werner-Zodrow, I., Darragh, A. and Mall-Hafeli, M. (1979). Contraceptive properties of luteinizing hormone releasing hormone. *Lancet,* October 13, 801

Lamberts, S. W. J., Timmers, J. M., Oosterom, R., Verleun, T., Rommerts, F. G. and de Jong, F. H. (1982). Testosterone secretion by cultured arrhenoblastoma cells: suppression by a luteinizing hormone-releasing hormone agonist. *J. Clin. Endocrinol. Metab.,* **54,** 450

Lemay, A., Labrie, F., Ferland, L. and Raynaud, J. P. (1979). Possible luteolytic effects of luteinizing hormone-releasing hormone in normal women. *Fertil. Steril.,* **31,** 29

Lemay, A., Faure, N., Labrie, F. and Fazekas, A. T. A. (1983). Postcoital contraception with intranasal buserelin. This volume, Chapter 17

Meldrum, D. R., Chang, R. J., Lu, J., Vale, W., Rivier, J. and Judd, H. L. (1982). 'Medical oophorectomy' using a long-acting GnRH agonist – a possible new approach to the treatment of endometriosis. *J. Clin. Endocrinol. Metab.,* **54,** 1081

Nakano, T., Okamato, S., Ishimaru, T., Miura, S. and Yamanabe, T. (1978). *Acta Obstet. Gynaecol. Jpn.,* **30,** 1361

Nillius, S. J., Bergquist, C. and Wide, L. (1978). Inhibition of ovulation in women by chronic treatment with a stimulatory LRH analogue – a new approach to birth control? *Contraception,* **17,** 537

Pieper, D. R., Richards, J. S. and Marshall, J. C. (1981). Ovarian gonadotropin-releasing hormone (GnRH) receptors: characterization, distribution, and induction by GnRH. *Endocrinology,* **108,** 1148

Rabin, D. and McNeil, L. W. (1980). Pituitary and gonadal desensitization after continuous luteinizing hormone-releasing hormone infusion in normal females. *J. Clin. Endocrinol. Metab.,* **51,** 873

Raynaud, J. P., Mary, I., Moguilewsky, M., Mouren, M. and Labrie, F. (1980). Inhibition of progesterone secretion during the luteal phase by two luteinizing hormone-releasing hormone agonists in Macaca fascicularis. *Fertil. Steril.,* **34,** 593

Sanders, L. M., Kent, J. S., McRae, G. I., Vickery, B. H., Tice, T. R. and Lewis, D. H. (1982). Controlled release of an LH-RH analog from injected polymeric microcapsules: formulation characteristics. *Contracept. Deliv. Syst.,* **3,** 60

Sarda, A. K. and Nair, R. M. G. (1981). Elevated levels of LRH in human milk. *J. Clin. Endocrinol. Metab.,* **52,** 826

Schally, A. V. and Kastin, A. J. (1971). *Drug Ther.,* **1,** 29

Schmidt-Gollwitzer, M., Hardt, W., Schmidt-Gollwitzer, K. and Nevinny-Stickel, L. (1981). Influence of the LH-RH analogue Buserelin on cyclic ovarian function and on the endometrium. A new approach to fertility control? *Contraception,* **23,** 187

Schoonmaker, G. N., Victery, W. and Karsch, F. J. (1981). A receptive period for estradiol-induced luteolysis in the rhesus monkey. *Endocrinology,* **108,** 1874

Seppala, M. and Wahlstrom, T. (1980). Identification of luteinizing hormone-releasing factor and alpha subunit of glycoprotein hormones in ductal carcinoma of the mammary gland. *Int. J. Cancer,* **26,** 267

Sheehan, K. L. and Yen, S. S. C. (1981). Clinical studies with LHRH agonists. In Zatuchni, G. I.,

Shelton, J. D. and Sciarra, J. J. (eds.) *LHRH Peptides as Female and Male Contraceptives*, pp. 237–241. (Philadelphia: Harper & Row)

Sheehan, K. L., Casper, R. F. and Yen, S. S. C. (1982*a*). Luteal phase defects induced by an agonist of luteinizing hormone-releasing factor: a model for fertility control. *Science*, **215**, 170

Sheehan, K. L., Casper, R. F. and Yen, S. S. C. (1982*b*). Induction of luteolysis by luteinizing hormone-releasing factor (LRF) agonist: sensitivity, reproducibility, and reversibility. *Fertil. Steril.*, **37**, 209

Siler-Khodr, T. M. and Khodr, G. S. (1979). Extrahypothalamic luteinizing hormone releasing factor (LRF): Release of immunoreactive LRF by the human placenta in vitro. *Fertil. Steril.*, **32**, 294

Singh, P. and Muldoon, T. G. (1982). A direct effect of LHRH on anterior pituitary estrogen receptors in the female rat. *J. Steroid Biochem.*, **16**, 31

Skarin, G., Nillius, S. J. and Wide, L. (1982). Early follicular phase luteinizing hormone-releasing hormone agonist administration – effects on follicular maturation and corpus luteum function in women. *Contraception*, **25**, 31

Stouffer, R. L. and Hodgen, G. D. (1980). Induction of luteal phase defects in rhesus monkeys by follicular phase administration at the onset of the menstrual cycle. *J. Clin. Endocrinol. Metab.*, **51**, 669

Tolis, G., Comaru-Schally, A. M., Mehta, A. E. and Schally, A. V. (1981). Failure to interrupt established pregnancy in humans by D-tryptophan-6-luteinizing hormone-releasing hormone. *Fertil. Steril.*, **36**, 241

Tsai, C. C., Mathur, R. S., Baker, E. R. and Nair, R. M. G. (1982). Lack of hormonal changes in response to 1 mg luteinizing hormone-releasing hormone injection during early human gestation. *Neuroendocr. Lett.*, **4**, 51

Tureck, R. W., Mastroianni L. Jr., Blasco, L. and Strauss J. F. III. (1982). Inhibition of human granulosa cell progesterone secretion by a gonadotropin-releasing hormone agonist. *J. Clin. Endocrinol. Metab.*, **54**, 1078

Vickery, B. H. (1981). Female contraceptive potential of superagonists of LHRH as assessed in infra human primates. In Zatuchni, G. I., Shelton, J. D. and Sciarra, J. J. (eds.) *LHRH Peptides as Female and Male Contraceptives*, pp. 109–125. (Philadelphia: Harper & Row)

Vickery, B. H. and McRae, G. I. (1980*a*). Effects of continuous treatment with superagonists of LHRH when initiated at different times of the menstrual cycle in female baboons. *Int. J. Fertil.*, **25**, 171

Vickery, B. H. and McRae, G. I. (1980*b*). Antagonism by an LHRH agonist of the steroidogenic effects of exogenous human chorionic gonadotrophin in the female primate. *Life Sci.*, **27**, 1409

Vickery, B. H., McRae, G. I. and Rowland, J. (1980). Effect of continuous long-term treatment with [Des-Gly^{10},D-Trp^{6},Pro-NHEt^{9}]LHRH on mating, ovulation and fertility in female rhesus monkeys. Abstr. No. 345, *VI Int. Congr. Endocr.*, Melbourne, Australia

Vickery, B. H., McRae, G. I., Briones, W., Powell, J. E. and Stevens, V. C. (1981*a*). Suppression of luteal function in baboons by an agonist analog of LHRH. Abstract No. 101, *Program of the 14th Annual Meeting, Society for Study of Reproduction*, Corvallis, Oregon

Vickery, B. H., McRae, G. I. and Stevens, V. C. (1981*b*). Suppression of luteal and placental function in pregnant baboons by an agonist analog of LHRH. *Fertil. Steril.*, **36, 664**

Vickery, B. H., McRae, G. I., Briones, W., Powell, J. E. and Stevens, V. C. (1982). Effects of [DNal(2)^{6}]LHRH (LHRH-A) upon pituitary and luteal function in cycling baboons. Abstr. No. 246, *Program of Annual Meeting of Society for Gynecologic Investigation*, Dallas, Texas

Wickings, E. J., Zaidi, P. and Nieschlag, E. (1981). Effects of chronic, high-dose LHRH agonist treatment on pituitary and testicular functions in rhesus monkeys. *J. Androl.*, **2**, 72

Wilson, E. A. and Jawad, M. J. (1980). Luteinizing hormone-releasing hormone suppression of human placental progesterone production. *Fertil. Steril.*, **33**, 91

Ying, S. Y. and Guillemin, R. (1979). Gonadostatine et gonadocrinine, polypeptides d'origine ovarienne à activités hypophysiotropes. *C.R. Acad. Sci. Paris Ser. D*, **289**, 943

Ying, S.-Y., Ling, N., Bohlen, P. and Guillemin, R. (1981). Gonadostatins and gonadocrinin: Peptides from the gonads regulating the secretion of gonadotropins. In Jagiello, G. and Vogel, H. J. (eds.) *Bioregulators of Reproduction*, pp. 389–402. (New York: Academic Press)

9
LHRH antagonists in rhesus and cynomolgus monkeys

R. H. ASCH, J. P. BALMACEDA and M. BORGHI

Kastin and Schally proposed the possibility of the synthesis of inhibitory analogs of LHRH (Kastin *et al.*, 1972). This hypothesis was shown to be correct and polypeptides capable of competing with LHRH for binding in the pituitary and decreasing the secretion of LH and FSH have been synthesized [Pedroza *et al.*, 1977; Coy *et al.*, 1979). Thus, dosages of [D-Phe^2,D-Trp^3,D-Phe^6]LHRH in the range of 1.5 mg per animal completely suppressed spontaneous ovulation in proestrous rats (de la Cruz *et al.*, 1976). These analogs were also found to be effective in inhibiting ovulation in hamsters and rabbits (de la Cruz *et al.*, 1975; Phelps *et al.*, 1977) and decreasing the response to LHRH in some non-human primates including baboons and chimpanzees (Hagino *et al.*, 1977; Gosselin *et al.*, 1979). Clinical studies performed in men with the antagonist [D-Phe^2,D-Trp^3,D-Phe^6]LHRH showed that a 90 mg dose could suppress the LH and FSH release in response to 25 μg of LHRH for up to 24 h (Gonzales-Barcena *et al.*, 1977). An antiovulatory effect was shown in women with the same dose of this antagonist (Canales *et al.*, 1980).

For the more potent analogs reported recently, the dose necessary to completely block ovulation in rats has been reduced to less than 62 μg (Coy *et al.*, 1979). The studies reported here for a more potent series of analogs were designed to determine the antigonadotropin and antireproductive properties of different LHRH inhibitory analogs in female non-human primates.

ANTAGONIST EFFECTS ON SERUM GONADOTROPIN LEVELS IN OOPHORECTOMIZED MONKEYS

Serum concentrations of FSH and LH decreased significantly in four oophorectomized rhesus monkeys after the administration of 1 mg of [N-Ac-D-Trp^1,D-pCl-Phe^2,D-Trp^3,D-Phe^6,D-Ala^{10}]LHRH (Balmaceda *et al.*, 1983*c*). Mean FSH serum concentrations decreased to 70 % by 4 h and to 80 % by 24 h and remained significantly lower than baseline values for up to 72 h following the administration of the antagonist.

Serum levels of LH also dropped significantly, but followed a different pattern. Concentrations of LH were significantly lower than the baseline levels as early as 2 h after the injection of the antagonist (44 %) and continued to decrease to 64 % by 24 h. However, in three of the four animals, serum LH levels increased to values markedly higher than the baseline 48 h after the antagonist administration. The fourth monkey presented a similar elevation 72 h after the injection of the antagonist.

In the control animals, serum FSH and LH increased to levels significantly higher than baseline 10 min after LHRH was administered (Figure 9.1). Maximum mean serum levels for both gonadotropins were reached 20 min after the injection of LHRH and they returned to baseline concentrations at approximately 120 min.

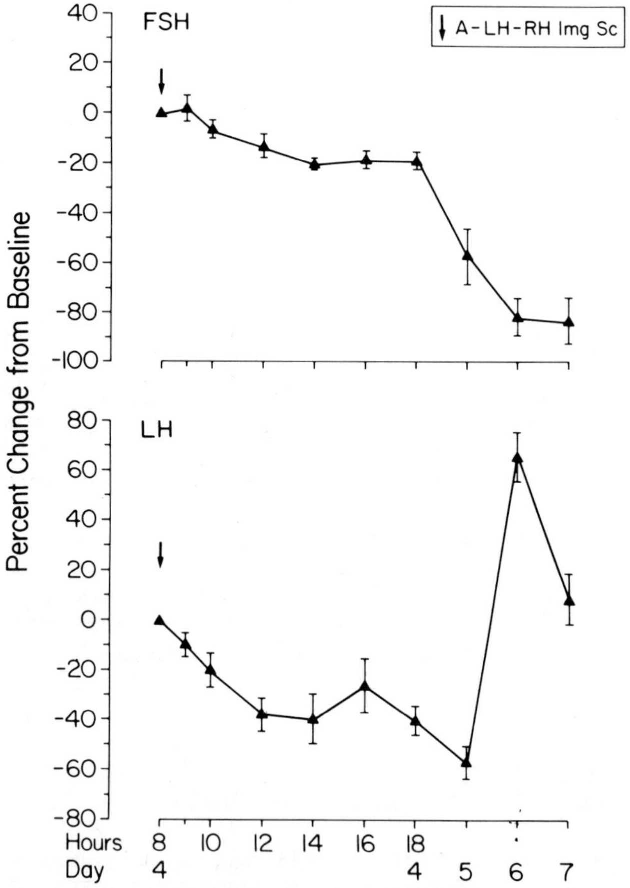

Figure 9.1 Serum concentrations of FSH and LH in oophorectomized rhesus monkeys before and after the administration of the LHRH antagonist [N-Ac-D-Trp^1,D-pCl-Phe^2,D-Trp^3,D-Phe^6,D-Ala^{10}]LHRH at the dose of 1 mg i.m. Significant depressions of FSH and LH occurred as early as 2 h after the administration of the antagonist, and lasted for 24 h. A rebound effect on LH levels to values higher than baseline was observed in three animals at 48 h, and in one animal at 72 h after the injection of the LHRH inhibitory analog.

When the monkeys received LHRH 2 h after the injection of the antagonist, the increase in serum concentrations of FSH and LH was not significantly different from that observed in the control group. Both gonadotropins were elevated significantly 10 min after the administration of LHRH and returned to baseline levels by 120 min (Figure 9.1). However, when LHRH was administered 18 h after the antagonist, serum concentrations of FSH and LH presented a significantly smaller and delayed response to LHRH, compared to

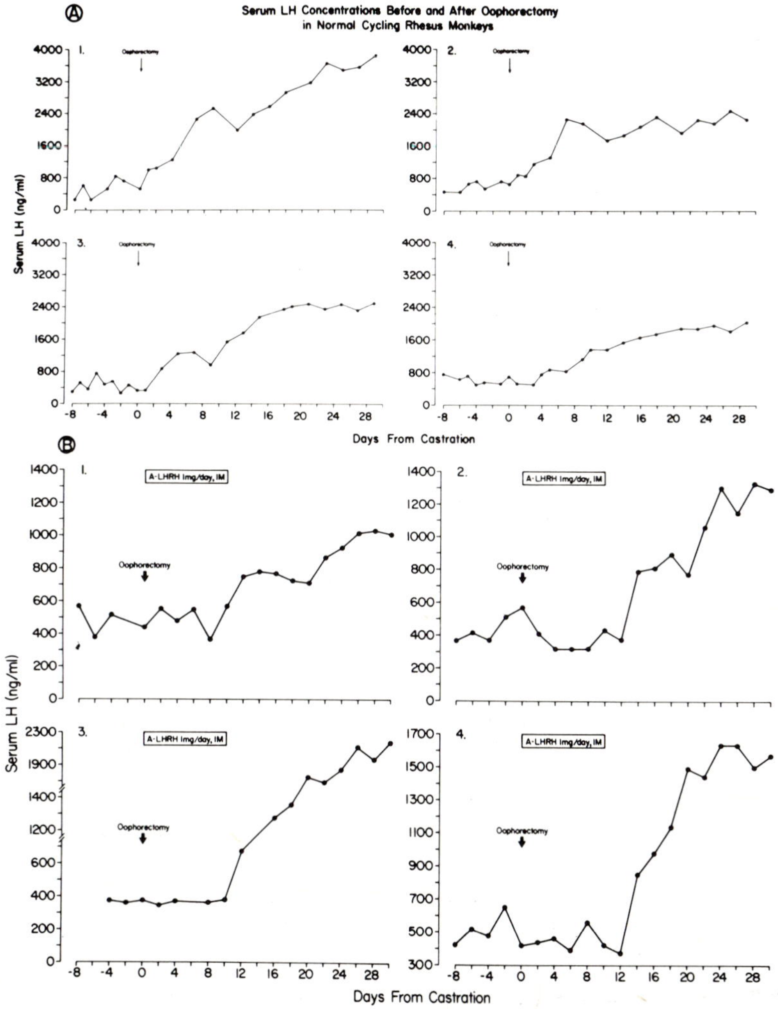

Figure 9.2 Peripheral serum concentrations of LH (LER-M0907D) in (A) control (vehicle-treated) and (B) experimental ([N-Ac-D-Trp^1,D-pCl-Phe^2,D-Trp^3,D-Phe^6,D-Ala^{10}]LHRH-treated) rhesus monkeys before and after bilateral oophorectomy (Asch *et al.*, 1981, reproduced with permission of the publisher, The American Fertility Society).

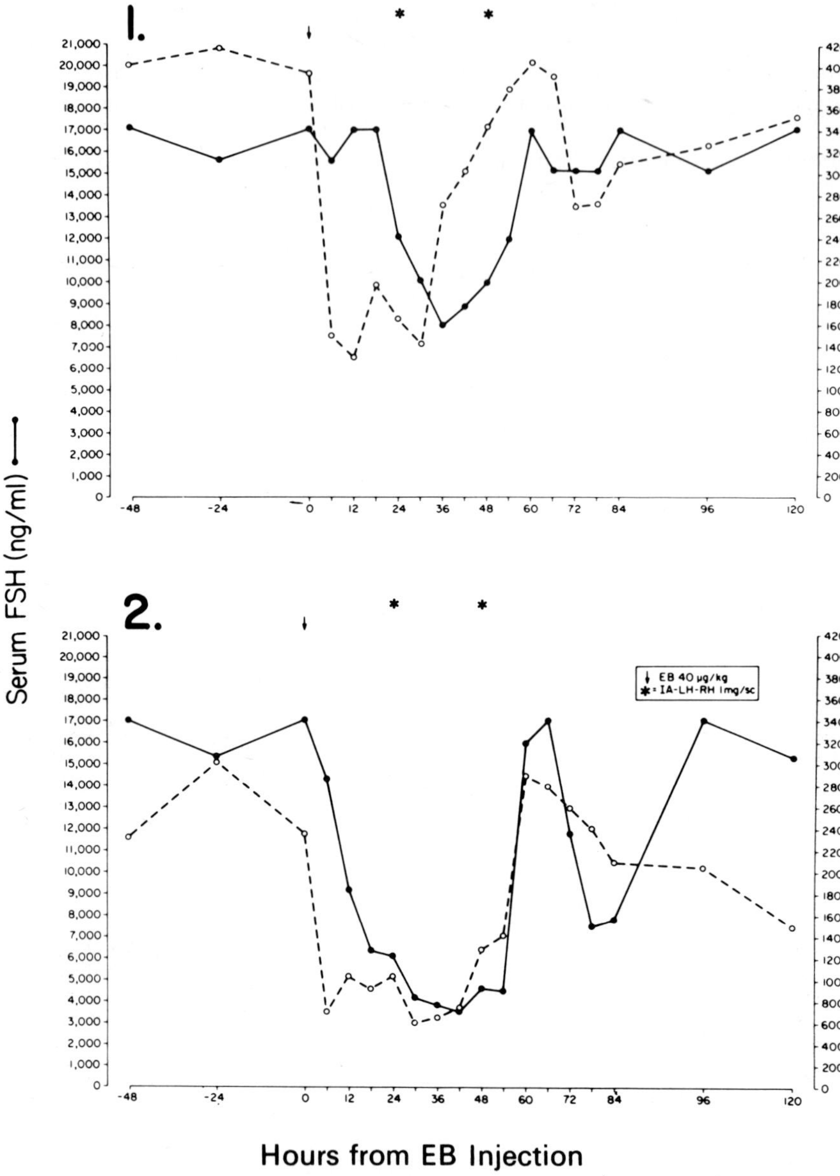

Figure 9.3 Effect of 40 µg/kg of estradiol benzoate (EB) on serum FSH and LH concentrations in oophorectomized rhesus monkeys which received an inhibitory analog of LHRH ([N-Ac-D-Trp^1,D-pCl-Phe^2,D-Trp^3,D-Phe^6,D-Ala^{10}]LHRH) at a dose of 200 µg daily from 24 to 48 h following EB injection (Group 4) (*Asch et al.*, 1983, reproduced by permission of the Editor-in-chief, *Journal of Clinical Endocrinology and Metabolism*).

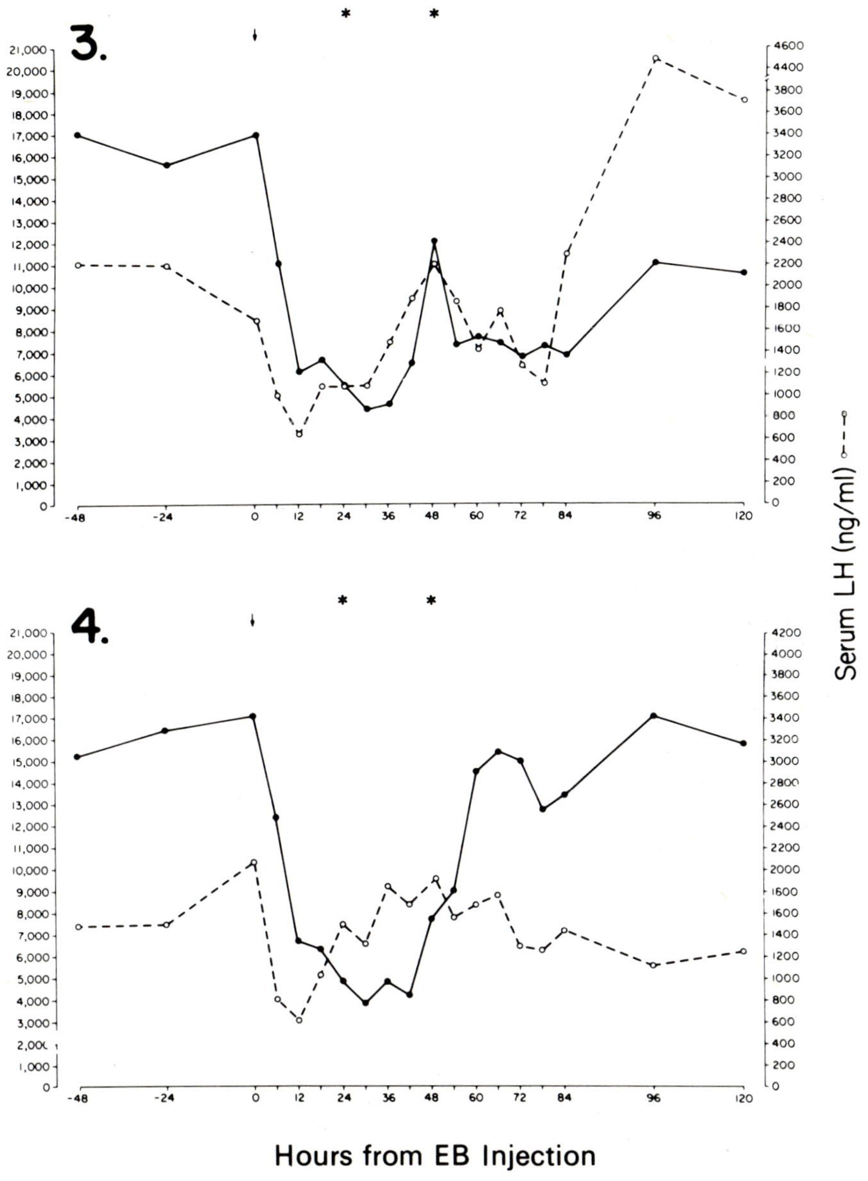

controls (Figure 9.1). In none of the animals did FSH or LH reach levels within the normal range, even during the LHRH challenge test. These studies revealed the ability of antagonists of LHRH to markedly suppress levels of pituitary gonadotropins, and to prevent the response to the LHRH challenge test in rhesus monkeys. These data opened a new area of research, which was investigated in the experiments shown in the next parts of this chapter, in order to prove biological applications of the antigonadotropic properties.

ANTAGONISTIC EFFECT ON POSTCASTRATION LH AND FSH LEVELS IN FEMALE RHESUS MONKEYS

The ability of an antagonist to affect the postoophorectomy rise of FSH and LH in rhesus monkeys was examined. Figure 9.2 shows the serum concentrations of FSH and LH before and after castration in rhesus monkeys from both groups, control animals and experimental animals. In control animals, LH and FSH consistently rose from precastration levels as soon as 3–4 days after surgery ($p<0.01$). Gonadotropins continued to rise until a plateau was reached, three to seven times baseline levels, between days 8 and 22 after oophorectomy. A similar trend was observed for both LH and FSH concentrations. The course of gonadotropin increase in this group was identical to that observed previously in non-treated regularly cycling rhesus monkeys after bilateral oophorectomy. In contrast, the release of gonadotropins after castration was profoundly altered by the daily administration of [D-Phe^2,D-Trp^3,D-Phe^6]LHRH. Two to four days following the discontinuation of the LHRH antagonist administration, FSH and LH concentrations were significantly higher than the baseline levels ($p < 0.05$). Gonadotropin levels continued to rise, reaching a plateau between 22 and 28 days after castration (12–18 days after the discontinuation of the LHRH antagonist administration). This magnitude was similar to that observed in control animals (two to six times baseline levels). The ability of LHRH antagonists to prevent the rise of pituitary gonadotropins following castration may have important clinical application in cases where it is desirable to decrease elevated levels of gonadotropins, as in precocious puberty and the menopause.

ANTAGONIST EFFECTS ON ESTRADIOL FEEDBACK ON GONADOTROPINS

Estrogens cause a biphasic effect on gonadotropin (FSH and LH) secretion in human and non-human primates. Current knowledge suggests that estrogens induce a negative as well as a positive feedback on gonadotropins by a direct action at the pituitary gland. Oophorectomized rhesus monkeys were injected with estradiol benzoate (EB) at a dose of 40 μg/kg s.c. at 0 time (controls). Three groups of animals received, additionally, the antagonist [N-Ac-D-pCl-Phe^1,D-pCl-Phe^2,D-Trp^3,D-Arg^6,D-Ala^{10}]LHRH, 200 μg s.c. daily at (1) -48 to 48 h, (2) 0 to 48 h and (3) 24 to 48 h from EB, respectively (Asch *et al.*, 1983). FSH and LH levels were measured by RIA from frequent blood samples (Figure 9.3).

Control animals revealed a 70–80% decrease in baseline FSH and LH levels during the first 24 h after EB injection, followed by a sharp rise to 60–80% above basal levels at 42–48 h post-EB. In contrast, animals that received the inhibitory analog of LHRH in different regimens showed a more pronounced and prolonged negative feedback of EB on gonadotropin concentrations (Figure 9.3). The positive feedback release of FSH and LH was significantly diminished or delayed when compared to controls.

These results indicate that this antagonist potentiates the negative feedback and suppresses the positive feedback of EB on gonadotropins, suggesting that estrogens induce the secretion of FSH and LH through a mechanism that involves the action of LHRH at the gonadotrope.

This basic study suggests that, if administered at the appropriate time, antagonists of LHRH would be able to suppress the midcycle surge of LH and consequently inhibit ovulation, opening a new approach for midcycle fertility control.

ANOVULATION AFTER AGONISTIC AND ANTAGONISTIC ANALOGS

The effects of [N-Ac-D-Trp^1,D-pCl-Phe^2,D-Trp^3,D-Phe^6,D-Ala^{10}]LHRH, an inhibitory analog, and [D-Trp^6]LHRH, an agonist of LHRH, were compared when administered to normally cycling cynomolgus monkeys. Animals were divided into three groups ($n = 5$ each) according to the drug administration: (1) 20 μg of [D-Trp^6]LHRH daily, (2) 1 mg of the antagonist and (3) vehicle, daily during the first 25 days of the menstrual cycle. Ovulation was established by serial laparoscopies and serum estradiol (Borghi *et al.*, 1983*b*).

There was no significant delay or change in the length of the luteal phase in the control group as a result of vehicle administration. However, ovulation was either suppressed or delayed markedly in the animals treated with either analog of LHRH (Table 9.1). All animals treated with the LHRH agonist or antagonist remained anovulatory during drug administration and ovulated 28,

Table 9.1 Cycle disruption by LHRH agonist and antagonist

	Vehicle ($n = 5$)	*[D-Trp^6]LHRH (agonist)* ($n = 5$)	*[N-Ac-D-Trp^1, D-pCl-Phe^2, D-Trp^3,D-Phe^6, D-Ala^{10}]LHRH (antagonist)* ($n = 5$)[a]
Follicular phase length (days)	12, 11, 15, 13, 14 (13 ± 1.4)[b]	22, 23, 18, 19, 20 (20.4 ± 1.8)[c]	22, 22, 24, 20 (22 ± 1.4)[c]
Luteal phase length (days)	14, 14, 14, 15, 13 (14 ± 0.6)	15, 15, 16, 14, 15 (15 ± 0.6)[d]	15, 16, 16, 13 (15 ± 1.2)[d]
Cycle length (days)			
Control cycles			
1	25, 26, 28, 30, 31 (28 ± 2.2)	27, 29, 28, 30, 28 (28.4 ± 1.0)[d]	29, 30, 31, 29, 28 (29.4 ± 1.0)[d]
2	27, 30, 31, 28, 29 (29 ± 1.4)	29, 28, 26, 27, 31 (28.2 ± 1.1)[d]	28, 30, 33, 29, 28 (29.6 ± 1.8)[d]
Treatment cycle	26, 25, 29, 28, 27 (27 ± 1.4)	37, 38, 34, 33, 35 (35.4 ± 1.8)[b]	37, 38, 40, 33 (37 ± 2.5)[b]
Post-treatment cycle	33, 28, 30, 28, 31 (30 ± 1.8)	29, 27, 29, 31, 30 (29.2 ± 1.3)[d]	30, 31, 33, 28 (30.5 ± 1.8)[d]

[a] One animal remained anovulatory for 65 days
[b] Values in parentheses are $\bar{x} \pm SD$
[c] $p < 0.01$ from controls
[d] n.s. = no statistical significance

18, 54, 20, and 28 days and 7, 8, 15, 13 and 125 days, respectively, following discontinuation of the drugs. Lengths of the follicular and the luteal phase of the cycles following treatment were not significantly different from those observed in the control cycles. Even though LH levels tended to be depressed in both groups during administration of LHRH analogs, individual responses were erratic and variable (Figures 9.4 and 9.5). Serum levels of estradiol were, in general, below 100 pg/ml during administration of either LHRH analog, indicating a lack of follicular development. The preovulatory estradiol and LH peaks that occurred after discontinuation of both LHRH analogs were similar in amplitude to those observed in the controls.

Prior to documentation by laparoscopic visualization, serum progesterone concentrations remained within preovulatory ranges. When ovulation occurred after discontinuation of analogs, serum progesterone rose to levels similar to those observed in controls and in our non-treated colony. This study clearly reveals the ability of both agonists and antagonists of LHRH, when administered in a continuous fashion from the onset of the menstrual cycle, to prevent ovulation in the non-human primate. Based on our observations, it would seem that antagonists cause fewer untoward effects, such as irregular bleeding or spotting and recovery of ovulatory function.

PREOVULATORY ADMINISTRATION OF ANTAGONIST

The effects of the potent antagonist [N-Ac-D-Trp^1,D-pCl-Phe^2,D-Trp^3,D-Phe^6,D-Ala^{10}]LHRH during the immediate preovulatory period of regularly cycling rhesus monkeys was studied (Balmaceda *et al.*, 1981). Seven regularly cycling rhesus monkeys were used in this experiment. The animals were followed during two consecutive cycles. During the first cycle (control), the animals did not receive any treatment and the date of ovulation was determined by using daily total serum estrogens and serial laparoscopies. In the second cycle, the animals received 1 mg daily of the antagonist by intramuscular injection from days 10 to 14. The date of ovulation was determined by using the same methodology as the control cycle. Blood samples were drawn daily from day 8 of the cycle until onset of menses, and the serum was used to measure total estrogens, progesterone and LH. A significant delay of the preovulatory LH peak and ovulation occurred in five of the seven animals resulting in a proportional increase in cycle length as compared to the control cycle (Table 9.2). No changes in cycle length or date of LH peak occurred in the other two animals (Figure 9.6). One of them did not present signs of ovulation as determined by laparoscopy (no recognizable stigma or corpus luteum). Progesterone production and length of the luteal phases were not affected by the treatment.

DELAY OF OVULATION BY LHRH ANALOGS ADMINISTERED DURING THE EARLY FOLLICULAR PHASE

It was reported that administration of LHRH agonists during the early follicular phase of the menstrual cycle disrupts the normal gonadotropin

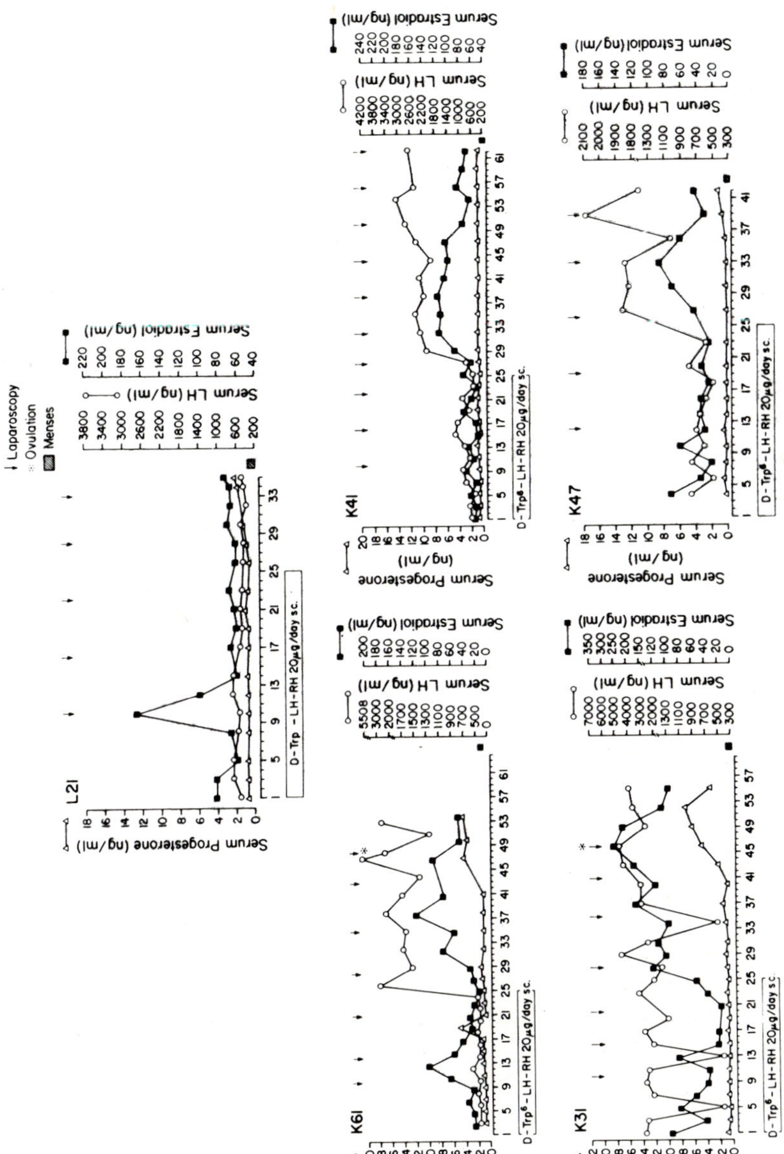

Figure 9.4 Serum concentrations of estradiol, progesterone and LH in animals treated with an agonistic analog of LHRH ([D-Trp[6]]LHRH) at a dose of 20 µg/day s.c. from day 1 to 25 of the menstrual cycle (Borghi *et al.*, 1983*b*, reproduced by permission of the Editor, *Contraception*).

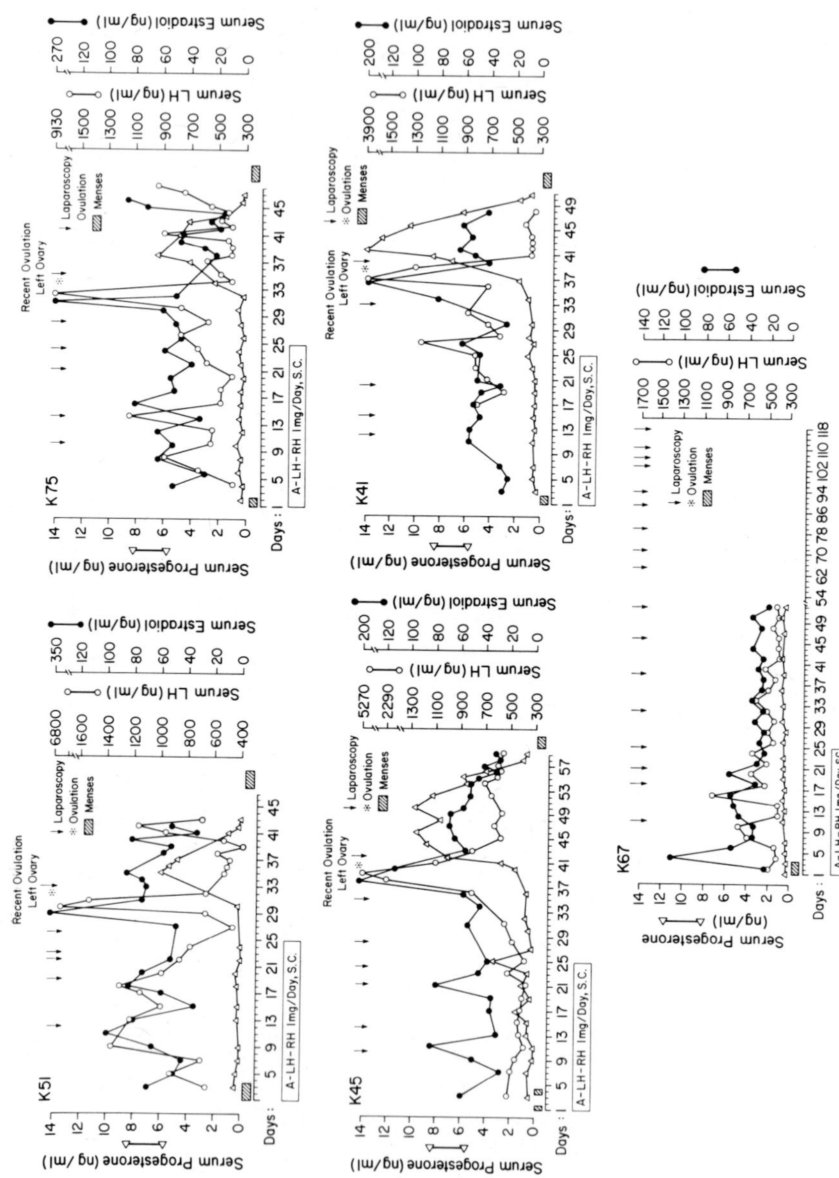

Figure 9.5 Serum concentration of estradiol, progesterone and LH in animals treated with an antagonist (A-LHRH = [N-Ac-D-Trp^1,D-pCl-Phe^2,D-Trp^3,D-Phe^6,D-Ala^{10}]LHRH), at a dose of 1 mg/day s.c. from day 1 to 25 of the menstrual cycle (Borghi *et al.*, 1983*b*, reproduced by permission of the Editor, *Contraception*).

Table 9.2 Prolongation of cycle by preovulatory administration of [N-Ac-D-Trp[1],D-pCl-Phe[2],D- Phe[6],D-Ala[10]]LHRH

	Day of ovulation		*Length of cycle*		*Length of luteal phase*	
Animal	*Control*	*Treated*	*Control*	*Treated*	*Control*	*Treated*
1	12	19	28	33	16	14
2	13	24	25	39	12	15
3	13	20	28	36	–	–
4	13	a	28	30	17	15
5	14	20	31	35	17	15
6	–	27	32	42	–	15
7	12	13	29	28	17	15

[a] Luteinized upruptured follicle

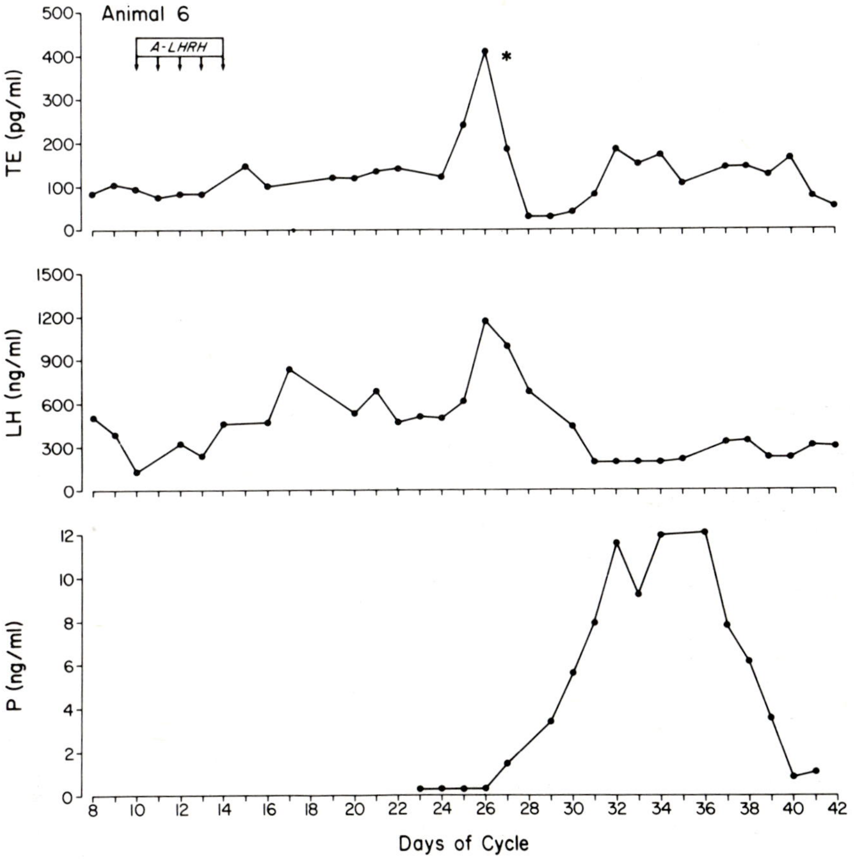

Figure 9.6 Serum concentrations of total estrogens (pg/ml), LH (ng/ml) and progesterone (ng/ml) of the treatment cycles ↓↓↓↓ indicates day of injection. * indicates day of ovulation (Balmaceda *et al.*, 1981, reproduced by permission of the Editor, *Contraception*).

secretion and induces inadequate luteal phases (Sheehan *et al.*, 1982). Other laboratories have not been able to confirm these observations (Sharin *et al.*, 1982). A similar study was therefore performed in rhesus monkeys. Regularly cycling rhesus monkeys received either (1) a potent LHRH agonist [D-Trp^{6}]LHRH, 20 μg/day ($n = 5$), (2) a potent LHRH antagonist [N-Ac-D-Trp^{1},D-pCl-Phe^{2},D-Trp^{3},D-Phe^{6},D-Ala^{10}]LHRH, 1 mg/day ($n = 5$) or (3) vehicle, from day 1 to 6 of the menstrual cycle. While controls showed normal cycles by dates of ovulation, length of luteal phases and hormonal profiles, animals treated with either analog had disrupted menstrual cycles. Animals from both groups presented delayed ovulations (LHRH agonist = days 22, 23, 17, 19, 20 of the cycle; LHRH agonist = 22, 22, 24 and 20 days of the cycle and one animal remained anovulatory for 65 days). Monkeys treated with either analog presented normal serum progesterone concentrations and luteal phase lengths (15, 15, 16, 14, 15 days and 15, 16, 16 and 13 days respectively). Thus, the administration of LHRH analogs during the early follicular phase disrupts gonadotropin secretion and delays ovulation without inducing luteal phase defects.

EFFECT OF POSTOVULATORY GONADOTROPIN LEVELS ON CORPUS LUTEUM

It is not clear what factors maintain the corpus luteum function in non-pregnant primates. The possible role of luteinizing hormone (LH) was evaluated in cycling rhesus monkeys (Balmaceda, 1983*b*). Ovulation was determined with an accuracy of ± 12 h by serial laparoscopies and daily serum estradiol (Pauerstein *et al.*, 1978). Starting on day 1, postovulatory animals received either a daily administration of a potent antagonist, [N-Ac-D-Trp^{1}, D-pCl-Phe^{2},D-Trp^{3},D-Phe^{6},D-Ala^{10}]LHRH, or vehicle (propylene glycol 20%, saline 80%) ($n = 5$) until the onset of menses. Daily measurements of serum FSH, LH, progesterone and estradiol were performed by RIA. Concentrations of FSH and LH diminished to levels near the sensitivity limit of the assay in animals treated with the antagonist (concentrations of approximately 50% of controls) (Figure 9.7). However, estradiol and progesterone levels were not

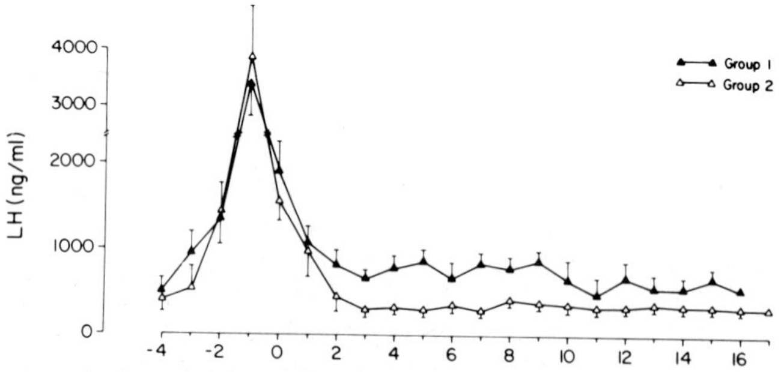

Figure 9.7 Serum concentrations of LH in monkeys treated continuously with potent LHRH inhibitory analogs during the luteal phase of the menstrual cycle.

different between the two groups. Luteal phase lengths of animals treated with vehicle or with the antagonist were normal (14–16 days and 14–17 days, respectively). Thus, the marked decrease of gonadotropin levels during the postovulatory period induced by an antagonist does not alter the luteal phase in rhesus monkeys. This supports the studies (Asch *et al.*, 1982) which show that the primate corpus luteum functions independently of postovulatory LH levels.

EFFECT OF LHRH ANALOGS ON RHESUS ENDOMETRIUM

Agonistic and antagonistic analogs of LHRH inhibit ovulation in several animal species, including primates. However, some concern has been expressed about these possible new approaches to fertility control due to reports that showed the occurrence of endometrial hyperplasia in humans and non-human primates (Schmidt-Gollwitzer *et al.*, 1981; Kerr-Wilson *et al.*, 1981). In order to study this possibility, we administered (1) vehicle ($n = 5$), (2) LHRH agonist ([D-Trp^6]LHRH, 20 μg/day) ($n = 5$) or (3) LHRH antagonist ([N-Ac-D-Trp^1,D-pCl-Phe^2,D-Trp^3,D-Phe^6,D-Ala^{10}]LHRH, 200 μg/day ($n = 5$) subcutaneously for 90 days to rhesus monkeys. Endometrial biopsies were obtained at days 1, 40, 90 and 120 and processed for histology and determination of estrogen and progesterone cytosol receptors. While agonist-treated animals had different degrees of endometrial hyperplasia during treatment (Figure 9.8), animals that received the LHRH antagonist showed either resting or atrophic endometrium (Table 9.3). LHRH agonist administration produced a marked increase in estrogen and progesterone endometrial receptors, while the antagonist induced a decrease in progesterone receptors (Figure 9.9). In both instances, reversal of the effects was observed 30 days after discontinuation of drug administration. Animals from both groups remained anovulatory during the course of drug administration.

We concluded from this study that, even though both agonistic and antagonistic analogs of LHRH are potent ovulation inhibitors in rhesus monkeys, the latter seem to be more promising, since they do not induce endometrial hyperplasia. Because of this, their clinical use, not only in fertility control, but also in cases of endometriosis and endometrial hyperplasia and neoplasm, seems to warrant investigation.

CONCLUDING REMARKS

The studies reported here demonstrate that LHRH antagonists are potent suppressors of pituitary gonadotropins in non-human primates. This antigonadotropic effect clearly results in anovulation when administered chronically to regularly cycling animals. The blockade of the preovulatory surge of FSH and LH is a consistent, reproducible phenomenon that presents very few side-effects. The studies of endometrial histology and steroid receptors showed that the antagonists may be superior to agonists of LHRH, since they do not induce endometrial hyperplasia. LHRH inhibitory analogs are not effective

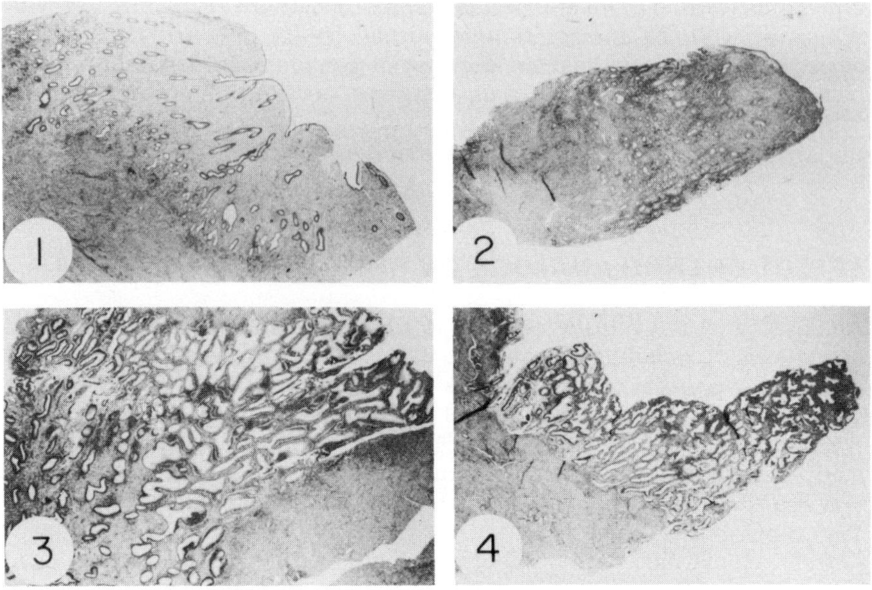

Figure 9.8 Photomicrographs of endometrial biopsies performed during chronic administration of LHRH agonist to regularly cycling rhesus monkeys. Numbers 1, 2, 3, and 4 show the histology at days 1, 40, 90, and 120 of the experiment, respectively. Note the marked hyperplasia in number 3 and the return to normal histology at 30 days after discontinuation of drug administration (4).

Table 9.3 Endometrial biopsies

	Animal no.	*1*	*2*	*3*	*4*
Group 1 (Control)	E01	P	P	P	S (16–17)
	E17	P	P	P	P
	E21	P	P	P	P
	E27	P	P	P	P
	A01	P	S (15–16)	P	P
Group 2 (Agonist)	137	P	P	H	P
	C17	P	P	R	S (19–20)
	E29	P	P	H	S (16)
	J45	P	P	P	P
	K61	P	R	H	S (17)
Group 3 (Antagonist)	195	P	P	R	P
	312	P	P	P	S (15–16)
	881	P	R	A	P
	973	P	R	R	P
	F09	P	P	R	S (17)

P = Proliferative; S = Secretory; H = Hyperplasia; R = Resting; A = Atrophic

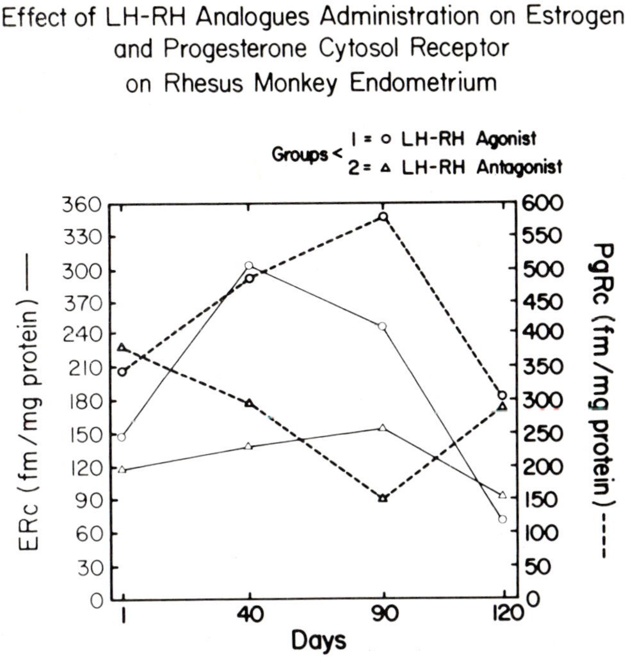

Figure 9.9 Concentrations of estrogen and progesterone receptors of rhesus monkey endometrium. The LHRH analogs were administered from days 1 to 90, inclusive, of the study.

when used during the luteal phase or early follicular phase of the cycle with regard to inducing luteal phase deficiencies.

The potent antigonadotropic effect of antagonists not only presents a new and interesting non-steroidal hormonal birth control method, but also opens the possibility for new therapeutic regimens in cases in which the inhibition of FSH and LH is desired, such as precocious puberty, endometriosis, menopause and hormonally dependent tumors. Current studies are in progress in our laboratories in order to test new routes of administration of LHRH antagonists, such as nasal, vaginal and long term, sustained-release forms (microcapsules and pellets).

Acknowledgements

We are grateful for the generous supply of LHRH analogs from Dr Andrew V. Schally and Dr David H. Coy. This work was supported in part by grants from the Ford Foundation [RHA], the Program for Applied Research on Fertility Regulation (PARFR), Northwestern University, and Subagreement PARFR 302 (DPE-0546-A-00-1003-00) [RHA], and the National Institute of Health (SP30HD 10202, Radioimmunoassay and Bioassay Cores).

References

Asch, R. H., Balmaceda, J. P., Eddy, C. A., Siler-Khodr, T. M., Coy, D. H. and Schally, A. V. (1981). Inhibition of the postcastration rise of LH and FSH in female rhesus monkeys (Macaca mulatta) by the administration of an LH-RH inhibitory analogue ([N-Ac-D-Trp^{1,3},D-p-Cl-Phe^{2},D-Phe^{6},D-Ala^{10}]-LH-RH). *Fertil. Steril.*, **36,** 388

Asch, R. H., Abou-Samra, M., Braunstein, G. and Pauerstein, C. J. (1982). Luteal function in hypophysectomized rhesus monkeys. *J. Clin. Endocrinol. Metab.*, **55,** 154

Asch, R. H., Balmaceda, J. P., Borghi, M. R., Niesvisky, R., Coy, D. H. and Schally, A. V. (1983). Suppression of the positive feedback of estradiol benzoate on gonadotropin secretion by an inhibitory analogue of LH-RH in oophorectomized rhesus monkeys. Evidence for a necessary synergism between LH-RH and estrogens. *J. Clin. Endocrinol. Metab.*, **57,** 367

Balmaceda, J. P., Schally, A. V., Coy, D. and Asch, R. H. (1981). The effects of an LH-RH antagonist ([N-Ac-D-Trp^{1,3},D-p-Cl-Phe^{2},D-Phe^{6},D-Ala^{10}]-LH-RH) during the preovulatory period of the rhesus monkey. *Contraception,* **24,** 275

Balmaceda, J. P., Borghi, M. R., Burgos, L., Pauerstein, C. J. and Asch, R. H. (1983*a*). Studies on the effects of LH-RH analogues in the histology and steroid receptors of the rhesus monkey endometrium. Presented at the *30th Annual Meeting of the Society for Gynecologic Investigation,* March 17–20, Washington, D.C., Abstract No. 99

Balmaceda, J. P., Borghi, M. R., Coy, D. H., Schally, A. V. and Asch, R. H. (1983*b*). Suppression of postovulatory gonadotropin levels does not affect corpus luteum function in rhesus monkeys. Presented at the *30th Annual Meeting of the Society for Gynecologic Investigation,* March 17–20, Washington, D.C., Abstract No. 454

Borghi, M. R., Niesvisky, R., Balmaceda, J. P. and Asch, R. H. (1983*a*). Administration of LH-RH analogues during the early follicular phase of the rhesus monkey menstrual cycle delayed ovulation without affecting the subsequent luteal phases. *Fertil. Steril.,* **40,** 678

Borghi, M. R., Niesvisky, R., Coy, D. H., Balmaceda, J. P., Schally, A. V. and Asch, R. H. (1983*b*). Administration of agonistic and antagonistic analogues of luteinizing hormone-releasing hormone anovulation in macaca fascicularis. *Contraception,* **27,** 619

Canales, E. S., Monvelinsky, H., Zárate, A., Kastin, A. J., Coy, D. H. and Schally, A. V. (1980). Suppressive effect of inhibitory LH-RH analog on the gonadotropin response to LH-RH in normal women. *Int. J. Fertil.,* **25,** 190

Coy, D. H., Mezo, I., Pedroza, E., Nekola, M. V., Vilchez, J., Piyachaturawat, P. and Schally, A. V. (1979). LH-RH antagonists with potent antiovulatory activity. In Gross, E. and Meienhofer, J. (eds.) *Peptides: Structure and Biological Function. Proceedings of the Sixth American Peptide Symposium,* pp. 775–779. (Rockford, IL: Pierce Chemical Company)

de la Cruz, A., Coy, D. H., Schally, A. V., Coy, E., de la Cruz, K. F. and Arimura, A. (1975). Blockage of the preovulatory LH surge in hamsters by an inhibitory analogue of LH-RH. *Proc. Soc. Exp. Biol. Med.,* **149,** 576

de la Cruz, A., Coy, D. H., Velchez-Martinez, J. A., Arimura, A. and Schally, A. V. (1976). Blockade of ovulation in rats by inhibitory analogs of luteinizing hormone releasing hormone. *Science,* **191,** 195

Gonzales-Barcena, D., Kastin, A. J., Coy, D. H., Nikolics, K. and Schally, A. V. (1977). Suppression of gonadotropin release in man by an inhibitory analogue of luteinizing hormone-releasing hormone. *Lancet,* **2,** 997

Gosselin, R. E., Fuller, B. G., Coy, D. H., Schally, A. V. and Hobson, W. C. (1979). Inhibition of gonadotropin release in chimpanzees by the LH-RH antagonist (D-Phe^{2},D-Trp^{3},D-Phe^{6})-LH-RH. *Proc. Soc. Exp. Biol. Med.,* **161,** 21

Hagino, N., Coy, D. H., Schally, A. V. and Arimura, A. (1977). Inhibition of LH release in the baboon by inhibitory analogs of luteinizing hormone releasing hormone. *Horm. Metab. Res.,* **9,** 247

Kastin, A. J., Schally, A. V., Gual, C. and Arimura, A. (1972). Release of LH and FSH after administration of synthetic LH-releasing hormone. *J. Clin. Endocrinol. Metab.,* **34,** 753

Kerr-Wilson, R. H. J., MacKenzie, L. and Fraser, H. M. (1981). Effects of chronic LHRH agonist treatment on the endometrium and ovaries of the stumptailed macaque. *Contraception,* **24,** 647

Pauerstein, C. J., Eddy, C. A., Croxatto, H. D., Hess, R., Siler-Khodr, T. M. and Croxatto, H. B. (1978). Temporal relationships of estrogen, progesterone, and luteinizing hormone levels to ovulation in women and infrahuman primates. *Am. J. Obstet. Gynecol.,* **130,** 876

Pedroza, E., Vilchez-Martinez, J. A., Fishback, J., Arimura, A. and Schally, A. V. (1977). Binding capacity of LH-RH and its analogs for pituitary receptor sites. *Biochem. Biophys. Res. Commun.*, **79,** 234

Phelps, C. P., Coy, D. H., Schally, A. V. and Sawyer, C. H. (1977). Blockage of LH release and ovulation in rabbits with inhibitory analogues of luteinizing hormone releasing hormone. *Endocrinology,* **100,** 1526

Schmidt-Gollwitzer, M., Hardt, W., Schmidt-Gollwitzer, K., von der Ohe, M. and Nevinny-Stickel, J. (1981). Influence of the LH-RH analogue buserelin on cyclic ovarian function and on endometrium. A new approach to fertility control? *Contraception,* **23,** 187

Sharin, G., Nillius, S. J. and Wide, L. (1982). Early follicular phase luteinizing hormone-releasing hormone agonist administration – effects of follicular maturation and corpus luteum function in women. *Contraception,* **25,** 31

Sheehan, K. L., Casper, R. F. and Yen, S. S. C. (1982). Luteal phase defects induced by an agonist of luteinizing hormone-releasing factor: A model for fertility control. *Science,* **215,** 170

10
LHRH antagonists in females

M. V. NEKOLA and D. H. COY

Chronic treatment with agonists of LHRH elicits first an increase in gonadotropins followed by desensitization of the pituitary to further agonist stimulation (Rivier *et al.*, 1978; Fraser *et al.*, 1980; Sandow, 1982). The initial high circulating levels of gonadotropins cause a reduction in the number of gonadal LH receptors and steroidogenesis decreases (Auclair *et al.*, 1977; Sandow, 1982). The agonists are potential contraceptives by virtue of their ability to lower hormone levels when given frequently. The difficulty is that reduced steroid levels can induce symptoms of gonadal insufficiency, such as impotency in males (Rabin *et al.*, 1981). Low doses of steroids are given concurrently in some trials (Heber and Swerdloff, 1980). The necessity for frequent administration and for steroid replacement may negate the clinical usefulness of the agonists.

Since the antagonists function by preventing the release of gonadotropins and not by depleting the pituitary of hormonal stores, it should be easier to block ovulation with the antagonists than with the agonists. Until recently, the antagonists have had low antiovulatory potencies. In the last few years, several hundredfold increases in potency were achieved (Coy *et al.*, 1982). These more potent antagonists exert prolonged biological activity and are active orally (Nekola *et al.*, 1982*b*).

RECENT ADVANCES IN THE DEVELOPMENT OF LHRH ANTAGONISTS

Medicinal chemistry studies with LHRH analogs developed into two major categories. The first was the development of more potent and long-acting agonist analogs and the second the synthesis of competitive antagonists of sufficient potency to be used as contraceptive compounds. The two endeavors were linked together since certain modifications to the peptide chain which gave improved gonadotropin-releasing activity could also be utilized to improve the antiovulatory activities of antagonist analogs. The use of agonist modifications in antagonists has since become a standard approach in structure–activity studies with other families of peptides.

In the case of LHRH, the observation that D-Ala substituted for Gly in position 6 gave much increased LH-releasing activity was used to improve the weak antagonist activity of [des-His^2]LHRH (Monahan *et al.*, 1973). Even more active were des-His^2-antagonists containing D-Phe^6 or D-Trp^6 (Coy *et al.*, 1976*a*) modifications which produced more potent superagonists than D-Ala^6 or D-Leu^6 (Coy *et al.*, 1976*b*).

A key modification which enabled analogs to be made which were potent enough to block ovulation in cycling rats was the D-Phe^2-substitution (Rees *et al.*, 1974) which was superior to the initial des-His^2-modification. Analogs such as [D-Phe^2,D-Leu^6]LHRH were able to block the proestrous surge of LH and FSH levels in cycling rats and to completely block ovulation when examined on the following day (Beattie *et al.*, 1976). However, repetitive injections were necessary to accomplish this. The first analogs to be effective after a single injection were [D-Phe^2,D-Phe^3]LHRH and [D-Phe^2,D-Trp^3] LHRH which gave 100% blockade of ovulation when administered at 12 noon on proestrus at doses of about 6 mg per rat (de la Cruz *et al.*, 1976).

D-Trp in position 3 of LHRH has been extensively used to increase the activities of antagonists. D-Trp^3-analogs were found to be approximately twice as effective as their L-Trp counterparts (Coy *et al.*, 1977) and D-Trp^3 is still utilized with a variety of other substituents. Antiovulatory activity was further increased by replacing pGlu in position 1 by its D-isomer (Rivier and Vale, 1978). Acylated D-amino acids, particularly D-Phe in position 1, gave even better results with full blockade of ovulation achieved by a 0.25 mg dose (Channabasavaiah and Stewart, 1979).

Of great importance in further lowering minimum effective dose levels was the discovery that a pCl-substituent on the aromatic ring of D-Phe in position 2 resulted in a tenfold increase in antiovulatory potency in rats as long as an acylated D-aromatic amino acid was present in the first position (Coy *et al.*, 1979). [N-Ac-D-Phe^1,D-pCl-Phe^2,D-$Trp^{3,6}$]LHRH gave good blockade of ovulation at a 31 μg dose level. This effective dose was then lowered to 15 μg per animal with the inclusion of N-Ac-D-pCl-Phe in position 1 (Erchegyi *et al.*, 1981*a*) and still further to 7.5 μg by replacement of Gly^{10} by D-Ala (Erchegyi *et al.*, 1981*b*).

The next improvement emanated from a study designed to improve the solubility of the antagonists. With so many aromatic amino acids present in the decapeptide chain, analogs at this stage were extremely lipophilic and had to be administered either in propylene glycol-saline solution or as a suspension in corn oil. Neither of these methods is ideal for clinical application. One way to improve water solubility would be to use basic D-amino acids rather than the standard D-aromatic amino acid replacements in the 6 position. It was assumed that this would cause some concomitant loss of acitivity. However, when the first analog of the series, [N-Ac-D-pCl-Phe^1,D-pCl-Phe^2,D-Trp^3, D-Lys^6,D-Ala^{10}]LHRH, was tested a significant increase in antiovulatory activity was actually obtained (Coy *et al.*, 1982). [N-Ac-D-pCl-Phe^1,D-pCl-Phe^2,D-Trp^3,D-Arg^6,D-Ala^{10}]LHRH was even more active and was effective at a dose of 1.5 μg. The latter analog is soluble in water at 2 mg per ml.

Improvements in potency have resulted from analogs containing N-Ac-D-Trp, N-Ac-D-Nal(2) or N-Ac-D-pBr-Phe in position 1 in conjunction with D-Arg^6 (Table 10.1). In addition to high potency, the current class of antagonists

Table 10.1 Increased antiovulatory activity of LHRH antagonists over the past 8 years

Antagonist	*Dose*[a] (mg)	*Blockade of ovulation* (%)
[D-Phe^{2},D-Leu^{6}]LHRH	2 (× 3)	82
[D-Phe^{2},Phe^{3},D-Trp^{6}]LHRH	1	40
[D-Phe^{2},D-Trp^{3},D-Phe^{6}]LHRH	0.5	80
[N-Ac-D-Phe^{1},D-Phe^{2},D-Trp^{3,6}]LHRH	0.25	78
[N-Ac-D-Phe^{1},D-pCl-Phe^{2},D-Trp^{3,6}]LHRH	0.031	64
[N-Ac-D-Phe^{1},D-pCl-Phe^{2},D-Trp^{3,6},D-Ala^{10}]LHRH	0.015	66
[N-Ac-D-pCl-Phe^{1},D-pCl-Phe^{2},D-Trp^{3,6},D-Ala^{10}]LHRH	0.008	90
[N-Ac-D-pCl-Phe^{1},D-pCl-Phe^{2},D-Trp^{3},D-Arg^{6},D-Ala^{10}]LHRH	0.003	78
[N-Ac-D-Trp^{1},D-pCl-Phe^{2},D-Trp^{3},D-Arg^{6},D-Ala^{10}]LHRH	0.003	91
[N-Ac-D-pBr-Phe^{1},D-pCl-Phe^{2},	0.003	100
D-Trp^{3},D-Arg^{6},D-Ala^{10}]LHRH	0.001	22
[N-Ac-D-Nal(2)^{1},D-pCl-Phe^{2},D-Trp^{3},D-Arg^{6},D-Ala^{10}]LHRH	0.001	50

[a] Antagonists injected once at 12 noon on proestrus in 40% propylene glycol and saline

exerts prolonged effects at low doses which appear to be related to D-Arg in position 6. Structure-function studies are underway to determine the chemical basis for the prolonged activities of the D-Arg^{6} compounds.

BIOLOGICAL EFFECTS OF THE ANTAGONISTS

Effect of vehicles

The antiovulatory activities of the antagonists are dependent on their chemistry and, to some extent, on their method of administration. This was demonstrated when the same antagonist had varying antiovulatory potencies in different vehicles (Table 10.2). The four tested vehicles are all pharmaceutically acceptable. For instance, Cremophor EL (glycerol-polyethyleneglycolricinoleate) is a solubilizer and emulsifier in producing medicines for oral application of hydrophobic substances (BASF Wynadotte Corporation). Propylene glycol, polyethylene glycol 400 and corn oil have low toxicities and are used as solvents in pharmaceuticals (Merck Index, 1976).

The analogs did not have the same inhibitory effect in all vehicles under the assay conditions. The best results were obtained with 40% propylene glycol in saline. Although corn oil can, in some cases, increase the potency of LHRH analogs (Rivier *et al.*, 1978), corn oil and the other two vehicles did not enhance the antiovulatory activities of these antagonists. The analogs dissolved fairly readily in propylene glycol, polyethylene glycol 400 and Cremophor EL but were given as a fine suspension in corn oil. The differences in results obtained with the four vehicles may depend on the solubility characteristics of the antagonists in the vehicles and on differences in absorption. There is no clear indication of what structural features are

Table 10.2 Effect of vehicle on the blockade of ovulation by potent antagonists

Antagonist	*Dose* (*μg/rat*)	*% of animals ovulating* Vehicle[a] 1	2	3	4
Vehicle control	0	100	100	100	100
[N-Ac-D-Phe[1],D-pCl-Phe[2],D-Trp[3,6]]LHRH	30	43	33	43	67
[N-Ac-D-pCl-Phe[1,2],D-Trp[3,6]]LHRH	30	0	0	100	100
[N-Ac-D-Phe[1],D-pCl-Phe[2],D-Trp[3,6],D-Ala[10]]LHRH	15	33	83	83	100
[N-Ac-D-Trp[1],D-pCl-Phe[2],D-Trp[3,6]]LHRH	15	13	50	100	ND[b]
[N-Ac-D-Trp[1],D-pCl-Phe[2],D-Trp[3],D-Phe[6],D-Ala[10]]LHRH	10	29	100	100	100
[N-Ac-D-pCl-Phe[1],D-pCl-Phe[2],D-Trp[3],D-Phe[6],D-Ala[10]] LHRH	10	0	67	100	ND

[a] 1, 40% propylene glycol in saline; 2, 40% polyethylene glycol 400 in saline; 3, 25% Cremophor EL in saline; 4, corn oil
[b] ND = not determined

necessary for increased activity in a particular vehicle. The search for a vehicle which is both tolerated by humans and potentiates the activity of the antagonists continues; however, water may eventually prove the ideal vehicle for more hydrophilic antagonists such as those containing D-Arg in position 6.

Prolonged activity

Suppression of gonadotropins

Another means of improving potency is to extend the action of the antagonists. The current antagonists exhibit prolonged antireproductive activity. A single injection of antagonist causes an immediate and sharp drop in serum gonadotropins in ovariectomized rats (Rivier *et al.*, 1981; Rivier and Vale, 1981; Nekola *et al.*, 1982*b*) which persists for over 24 hours, depending on the dose and the antagonist (Figures 10.1 and 10.2). A 100 μg dose of [N-Ac-D-Nal(2)[1],D-pCl-Phe[2],D-Trp[3],D-Arg[6],D-Ala[10]]LHRH reduced LH for 30 h with no sign of a return to baseline levels even 30 h postinjection (Figure 10.1). After a several-hour delay, the antagonist inhibited serum FSH as well as LH in these animals (Figure 10.2). The ability of the antagonists to suppress the postcastration rise in gonadotropins extends to primates. Thus, [N-Ac-D-Trp[1,3],D-pCl-Phe[2],D-Phe[6],D-Ala[10]]LHRH inhibited LH and FSH following oophorectomy in rhesus monkeys (Asch *et al.*, 1981). Antagonists should be selected for clinical use based on prolonged activity as well as increased potency and [N-Ac-D-Nal(2)[1],D-pCl-Phe[2],D-Trp[3],D-Arg[6],D-Ala[10]]LHRH is a prime candidate for trials in humans.

Blockade of ovulation

The prolonged biological activity of the antagonists seen in ovariectomized rats can also be demonstrated in cycling animals. In the standard anti-

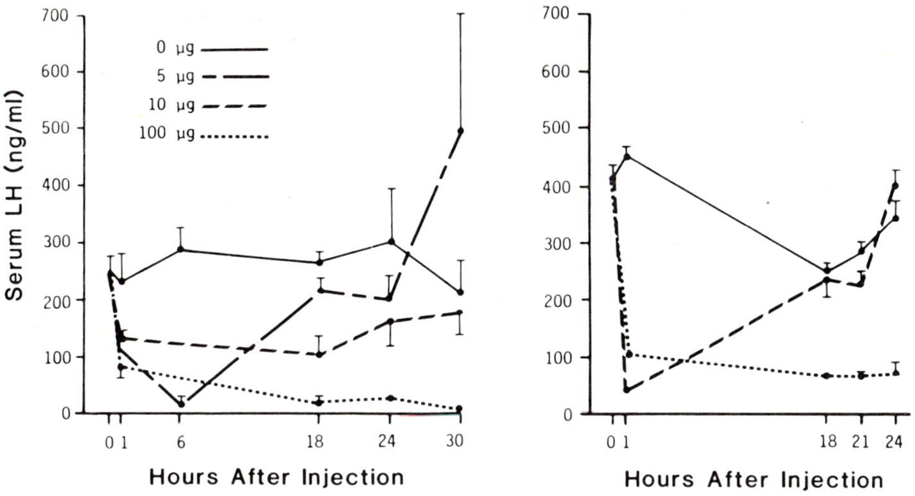

Figure 10.1 Suppression of LH in ovariectomized rats injected subcutaneously with [N-Ac-D-Nal(2)[1], D-pCl-Phe[2], D-Trp[3], D-Arg[6], D-Ala[10]]LHRH (left) or [N-Ac-D-pBr-Phe[1],D-pCl-Phe[2], D-Trp[3],D-Arg[6],D-Ala[10]]LHRH (right) in 40% propylene glycol and saline. The animals were decapitated at the times specified and their trunk blood analyzed for LH content by radioimmunoassay.

ovulatory assay, the antagonist is injected at noon on proestrus and the oviducts examined on the morning of estrus for the presence of ova. To demonstrate prolonged antiovulatory activity, 1.5 or 15 times the minimum effective antiovulatory dose of [N-Ac-D-pCl-Phe[1],D-pCl-Phe[2],D-Trp[3], D-Phe[6],D-Ala[10]]LHRH was injected on one of the days of the 4-day estrous cycle and the oviducts examined 1–4 days postinjection (Table 10.3). The antagonist blocked ovulation at 15 μg only when given on proestrus and delayed ovulation only for 1 day. The antagonist inhibited ovulation at 150 μg when given as early as 2 days before the preovulatory surge of gonadotropins and delayed ovulation for 3 days when given on proestrus. The prolonged antiovulatory activity of the antagonists suggests they could be administered on a flexible schedule because they can be given at various times before the preovulatory surge of gonadotropins and still inhibit ovulation. If this should prove true in humans, ovulation could be inhibited without daily antagonist treatment, thereby increasing the potential clinical value of the antagonists. It is unlikely that the antagonist itself is present for the entire period in which ovulation is inhibited. A more reasonable alternative is that the antagonist induces changes in pituitary and/or ovarian function which result in the delay.

Site of action

Pituitary

The inhibition of ovulation on estrus following injection on proestrus can be readily explained by suppression of the preovulatory peak of gonadotropins

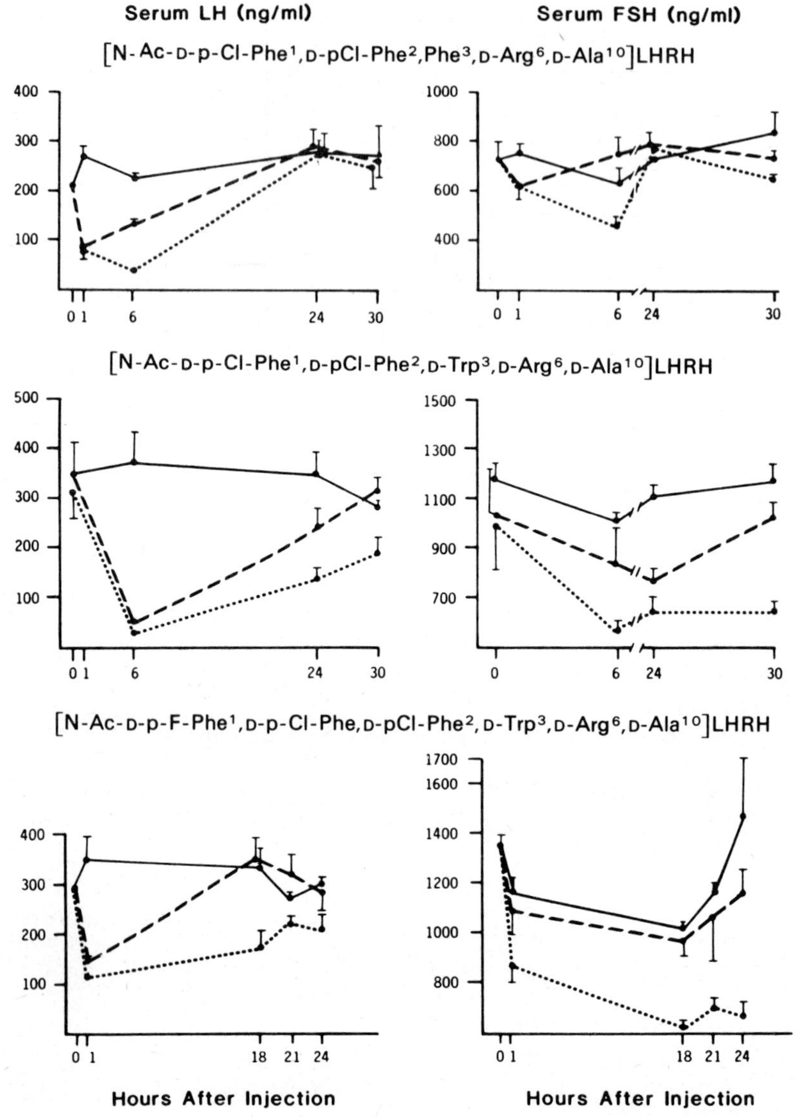

Figure 10.2 Suppression of LH and FSH in ovariectomized rats injected subcutaneously with LHRH antagonists (0 μg ———; 10 μg ----; 100 μg • • •).

by the antagonist. Presumably, the surge is delayed for 1–3 days in the 150 μg groups since most of the animals ovulate 1–3 days after estrus when given 150 μg of antagonist on diestrus I, II or proestrus.

It has been postulated that the antagonist has to suppress both tonic and surge levels of gonadotropins to inhibit ovulation when the antagonist is given on days other than proestrus (Rivier *et al.*, 1981). Morning LH, FSH,

Table 10.3 Delay in ovulation after a single injection of [N-Ac-D-pCl-Phe[1],D-pCl-Phe[2],D-Trp[3],D-Phe[6],D-Ala[10]]LHRH during the estrous cycle

		% of injected animals which ovulated			
Day of injection	*Dose (μg/rat)*	*Day of sacrifice: expected stage of cycle following injection* E	*DI*	*DII*	*P*
Estrus (E)	0	100[a]			
	15	100			
	150	100			
Diestrus I (DI)	0	100	0		
	15	100	0		
	150	17	80		
Diestrus II (DII)	0	100	0	0	
	15	88	25	0	
	150	6	60	0	
Proestrus (P)	0	100	0	0	0
	15	0	69	17	0
	150	0	0	14	33

[a] Each group represents 4–18 animals

estradiol and progesterone serum levels determined on the day of sacrifice were not affected by any treatment with the antagonist. More frequent sampling is required to verify that hormone levels were not transiently suppressed in animals when ovulation is blocked for an extended period. The use of the antagonists as contraceptives is more likely to be acceptable if some degree of ovarian steroidogenesis is maintained.

The antagonists probably inhibit gonadotropin secretion by occupying the pituitary LHRH receptors and interfering with endogenous LHRH (Clayton and Catt, 1981). This is supported by the fact that the affinity of a standard agonist ligand for pituitary LHRH receptors was not changed by antagonist treatment but the number of available binding sites was lowered (Figure 10.3). Antagonists of LHRH may bind to the receptors for 24 h (Heber *et al.*, 1982), but whether antagonists can occupy receptors and thereby cause antagonism for 2 or more days is unknown. Down regulation of gonadal receptors by homologous hormones occurs readily (Richards and Bogovich, 1980). The antagonists may bind to receptors for hours and also decrease the actual number of LHRH receptors in the pituitary. This phenomenon could explain the prolonged activity of the antagonists.

Ovary

In addition to the pituitary, rat gonads contain receptors for LHRH (Clayton *et al.*, 1980; Clayton and Catt, 1981; Hsueh and Jones, 1981). The direct action of LHRH and its agonists on the gonads is mainly inhibitory in nature (Clayton *et al.*, 1980; Clayton and Catt, 1981; Hsueh and Jones, 1981). To examine the possible direct effect of the antagonists on the ovaries in inhibiting ovulation, rats were given 10 or 100 μg of [N-Ac-D-pCl-Phe[1], D-pCl-Phe[2],D-Trp[3],D-Arg[6],D-Ala[10]]LHRH at noon and hCG at 4:00 p.m.,

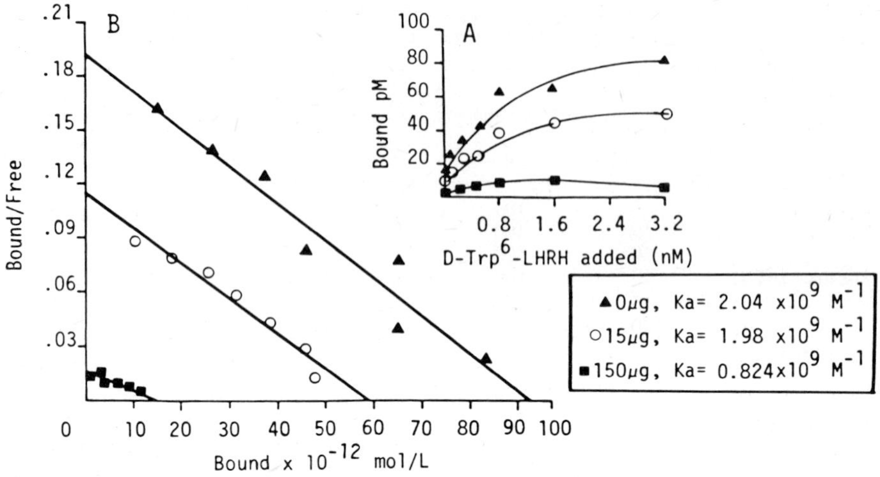

Figure 10.3 Saturation (A) and Scatchard (B) plots of [D-Trp^{6}]LHRH binding to pituitary homogenates of rats injected with different doses of [N-Ac-D-pCl-Phe^{1},D-pCl-Phe^{2},D-Trp^{3}, D-Phe^{6},D-Ala^{10}]LHRH on proestrus and sacrificed on estrus. The pituitaries from 12–15 similarly treated animals were pooled and homogenized.

the time when LH normally begins to rise in our colony (Nekola *et al.*, 1982*a*). HCG did induce ovulation in animals given inhibitory doses of the antagonist. Since hCG replaced the blocked surge of LH and overcame the inhibition of ovulation, the antagonist acted primarily at the level of the pituitary and not peripherally. However, twice as much hCG was required to induce ovulation in animals blocked with 100 μg antagonist than in those given only 10 μg. Hormone levels were similar between the two antagonist-treated groups, indicating that differences in hormones could not explain the increased hCG needed to induce ovulation in animals injected with 100 μg antagonist. Consequently, antagonists may have a secondary, but minor, direct effect on the ovary in the rat. A direct ovarian effect in other species is questionable since some, such as the human, do not possess gonadal LHRH receptors (Clayton and Huhtaniemi, 1982).

ORAL ACTIVITIES OF ANTAGONISTS

The data described above were obtained by injection. This method of administration is inappropriate for a contraceptive and alternative methods of administration were investigated. The first demonstration that an antagonist could block ovulation when given by mouth was recently reported (Nekola *et al.*, 1982*b*).

Degradation of the peptides by gastrointestinal enzymes and/or poor absorption from the gut could prevent demonstration of oral antiovulatory activity. We tried to minimize these possible effects in two ways. The antagonists were dissolved in 40 % propylene glycol, 10 % Trasylol (1000 iu/ml of gavage) in saline. Trasylol (a protease inhibitor) was added to retard degradation of the antagonist (Saffran *et al.*, 1979). In addition, all animals were deprived of food, but not water, from 10:00 a.m. to 3:30 p.m. on the day of assay. One milliter of vehicle containing antagonist was administered by gavage to conscious rats at 2:00 p.m. on proestrus. The oviducts were examined on the morning of estrus for the presence of ova.

The activities of three antagonists of similar structure were compared when given by mouth or by injection (Table 10.4). All control animals ovulated and all three antagonists were antiovulatory by injection. [N-Ac-D-pCl-Phe^{1}, D-pCl-Phe^{2},D-Trp^{3},D-Arg^{6},D-Ala^{10}]LHRH was the only antagonist to inhibit ovulation when given orally. Ovulation was blocked in all animals given 2 mg of this antagonist by gavage and in most of the animals treated with 1 mg. Even at 500 μg the antagonist induced a partial blockade of ovulation. Since the antagonist can inhibit the peak of LH (Figure 10.4) and block ovulation when given as late as 2:00 p.m. on proestrus, it appears to be quickly absorbed and fast acting. By extrapolation from the dose needed to inhibit ovulation by injection, less than 1 % of this compound was absorbed when given orally. It may be possible to facilitate absorption by changing the conditions of oral administration, such as by encapsulating the peptide in liposomes (Patel and Ryman, 1976).

The other two antagonists were only slightly less potent by injection, but they were completely inactive when given orally under the conditions of assay. Based on its activity by injection, we had anticipated that [N-Ac-D-pCl-Phe^{1},D-pCl-Phe^{2},Phe^{3},D-Arg^{6},D-Ala^{10}]LHRH would have induced a partial blockade of ovulation when given by gavage since [N-Ac-D-pCl-Phe^{1},D-pCl-Phe^{2},D-Trp^{3},D-Arg^{6},D-Ala^{10}]LHRH showed activity over a relatively wide dose range. The fact that it did not, suggests that the oral activities of the antagonists are not solely correlated with their ability to block ovulation by injection. Additional structure/oral activity studies are required to determine

Table 10.4 Antiovulatory potencies of LHRH antagonists given by gavage and injection

	Antiovulatory activity			
	Injection		*Gavage*	
Antagonist	*Dose* (μg)	*% Blockade of ovulation*	*Dose* (mg)	*% Blockade of ovulation*
[N-Ac-D-pCl-Phe^{1},D-pCl-Phe^{2},D-Trp^{3}, D-Phe^{6},D-Ala^{10}]LHRH	15	100 (0/10)[a]	2	0 (8/8)[a]
	7.5	86 (1/8)	1	0 (4/4)
[N-Ac-D-pCl-Phe^{1},D-pCl-Phe^{2},Phe^{3}, D-Arg^{6},D-Ala^{10}]LHRH	7.5	100 (0/6)	2	0 (9/9)
	5	0 (0/6)	1	0 (8/8)
[N-Ac-D-pCl-Phe^{1},D-pCl-Phe^{2},D-Trp^{3}, D-Arg^{6},D-Ala^{10}]LHRH[b]	5	100 (0/5)	2	100 (0/11)
	3	78 (2/9)	1	64 (4/11)
	1.5	10 (9/10)	0.5	18 (9/11)

[a] Number of animals ovulating/number of animals treated
[b] Nekola *et al.*, 1982*b*; copyright 1982 by the American Association for the Advancement of Science

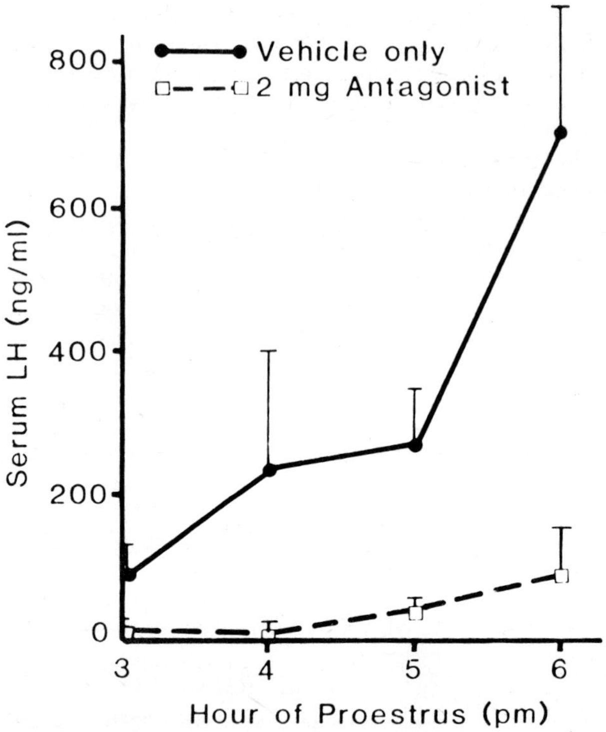

Figure 10.4 Blockade of preovulatory surge of LH in proestrous rats by oral administration of 2 mg of [N-Ac-D-pCl-Phe^1,D-pCl-Phe^2,D-Trp^3,D-Arg^6,D-Ala^{10}]LHRH at 14:00 hours (Nekola *et al.*, 1982*b*; copyright 1982 by the American Association for the Advancement of Science).

which modifications of LHRH yield antagonists of greater oral potency, and to determine if differences in degradation by gastrointestinal enzymes may account for varying oral antiovulatory activities.

CONCLUDING REMARKS

Multiple substitutions into positions 1, 2, 3, 6, and 10 of the sequence of LHRH have greatly increased the potencies of recent antagonists. Of particular interest is the insertion of D-Arg into position 6, which increased antiovulatory activity as well as the solubility of the antagonists in water. The new antagonists are also extremely long acting. They suppress gonadotropins in ovariectomized animals for more than 1 day and can block ovulation in cycling rats for 1–3 days. The antagonists probably exert their prolonged activity through the pituitary, perhaps by decreasing the number of available LHRH binding sites. In the rat, the antagonists may have a secondary, direct effect on the ovaries. The antagonist, [N-Ac-D-pCl-Phe^1,D-pCl-Phe^2,

D-Trp[3],D-Arg[6],D-Ala[10]]LHRH, is active in blocking ovulation when given orally. The higher potencies of the new antagonists, coupled with their extended activity, greatly increase the potential clinical value of the antagonists.

Acknowledgements

The research was supported by NIH contract NO1-HD-2-2809, and the Mellon Foundation.

References

Asch, R. H., Balmaceda, J. P., Eddy, C. A., Siler-Khodr, T., Coy, D. H. and Schally, A. V. (1981). Inhibition of the post-castration rise of luteinizing hormone and follicle-stimulating hormone in female rhesus monkeys (Macaca mulatta) by the administration of a luteinizing hormone-releasing hormone inhibitory analog ([N-Ac-D-Trp[1,3],D-p-Cl-Phe[2],D-Phe[6],D-Ala[10]]LH-RH). *Fertil. Steril.*, **36,** 388

Auclair, C., Kelly, P. A., Labrie, F., Coy, D. H. and Schally, A. V. (1977). Inhibition of testicular luteinizing hormone receptor level by treatment with a potent luteinizing hormone-releasing hormone agonist or human chorionic gonadotropin. *Biochem. Biophys. Res. Commun.*, **76,** 855

Beattie, C. W., Corbin, A., Foell, T. J., Garsky, V., Rees, R. W. A. and Yardley, J. (1976). Anti-ovulatory/anti-pregnancy effects of [D-Phe[2]]-LRH analogs administered early in the rat oestrous cycle. *Contraception,* **13,** 341

Channabasavaiah, K. and Stewart, J. M. (1979). New analogs of luliberin which inhibit ovulation in the rat. *Biochem. Biophys. Res. Commun.*, **86,** 1266

Clayton, R. N., Katikineni, M., Chan, V., Dufau, M. L. and Catt, K. J. (1980). Direct inhibition of testicular function by gonadotropin-releasing hormone: Mediation by specific gonadotropin-releasing hormone receptors in interstitial cells. *Proc. Natl. Acad. Sci. USA,* **77,** 4459

Clayton, R. N. and Catt, K. J. (1981). Gonadotropin-releasing hormone receptors: characterization, physiological regulation, and relationship to reproductive function. *Endocr. Rev.*, **2,** 186

Clayton, R. N. and Huhtaniemi, I. T. (1982). Absence of gonadotropin-releasing hormone receptors in human gonadal tissue. *Nature (Lond.)*, **299,** 56

Coy, D. H., Coy, E. J., Vilchez-Martinez, J. A., de la Cruz, A., Arimura, A. and Schally, A. V. (1976*a*). Suppression of gonadotropin release and ovulation in animals by inhibitory analogs of luteinizing hormone-releasing hormone. In Labrie, F., Meites, J. and Pelletier, G. (eds.) *Hypothalamus and Endocrine Functions*, pp. 339–354. (New York: Plenum)

Coy, D. H., Vilchez-Martinez, J. A., Coy, E. J. and Schally, A. V. (1976*b*). Analogs of luteinizing hormone-releasing hormone with increased biological activity produced by D-amino acid substitutions in position 6. *J. Med. Chem.*, **19,** 423

Coy, D. H., Vilchez-Martinez, J. A. and Schally, A. V. (1977). Structure–function states of LRF. In Loffet, A. (ed.) *Peptides 1976*, pp. 463–469. (Brussels: Editions de L'Université de Bruxelles)

Coy, D. H., Mezo, I., Pedroza, E., Nekola, M. V., Vilchez, J., Piyachaturawat, P., Schally, A. V., Seprodi, J. and Teplan, I. (1979). LH-RH antagonists with potent antiovulatory activity. In Gross, E. and Meienhofer, J. (eds.) *Peptides: Structure and Biological Function. Proceedings of the Sixth American Peptide Symposium*, pp. 775–779. (Rockford, IL: Pierce Chemical Co.)

Coy, D. H., Horvath, A., Nekola, M. V., Coy, E. J., Erchegyi, J. and Schally, A. V. (1982). Peptide antagonists of LH-RH: large increases in antiovulatory activities produced by basic D-amino acids in the six position. *Endocrinology,* **110,** 1445

de la Cruz, A., Coy, D. H., Vilchez-Martinez, J., Arimura, A. and Schally, A. V. (1976). Blockade of ovulation in rats by inhibitory analogs of luteinizing hormone-releasing hormone. *Science,* **191,** 195

Erchegyi, J., Coy, D. H., Nekola, M. V., Pedroza, E., Coy, E. J., Mezo, I. and Schally, A. V.

(1981*a*). LH-RH antagonists: further analogs with ring-substituted aromatic residues. *Peptides,* **2,** 251

Erchegyi, J., Coy, D. H., Nekola, M. V., Schally, A. V., Mezo, I. and Teplan, I. (1981*b*). Luteinizing hormone-releasing hormone analogs with increased antiovulatory activity. *Biochem. Biophys. Res. Commun.,* **100,** 915

Fraser, H. M., Laird, N. C. and Blakely, D. M. (1980). Decreased pituitary responsiveness and inhibition of the luteinizing hormone surge and ovulation in the stumptailed monkey (*Macaca arctoides*) by chronic treatment with an agonist of luteinizing hormone-releasing hormone. *Endocrinology,* **106,** 452

Heber, D. and Swerdloff, R. S. (1980). Male contraception: synergism of gonadotropin-releasing hormone analog and testosterone in suppressing gonadotropin. *Science,* **209,** 936

Heber, D., Dodson, R. and Swerdloff, R. S. (1982). Pituitary receptor site blockade by a gonadotropin-releasing hormone antagonist in vivo: mechanism of action. *Science,* **216,** 420

Hsueh, A. J. W. and Jones, P. B. C. (1981). Extrapituitary actions of gonadotropin-releasing hormone. *Endocr. Rev.,* **2,** 437

Monahan, M. W., Amoss, M. S., Anderson, H. A. and Vale, W. (1973). Synthetic analogs of the hypothalamic luteinizing hormone releasing factor with increased agonist or antagonist properties. *Biochemistry,* **12,** 4616

Nekola, M. V., Ge, L.-J., Horvath, A., Altamirano, P., Coy, D. H. and Schally, A. V. (1982*a*). Investigation of an ovarian site of action in the blockade of ovulation produced by LH-RH antagonists. In Greenwald, G. and Terranova, P. F. (eds.) *Factors Regulating Ovarian Function,* pp. 251–255. (New York: Raven Press)

Nekola, M. V., Horvath, A., Ge, L.-J., Coy, D. H. and Schally, A. V. (1982*b*). Suppression of ovulation in the rat by an orally active antagonist of luteinizing hormone-releasing hormone. *Science,* **218,** 160

Patel, H. M. and Ryman, B. E. (1976). Oral administration of insulin by encapsulation within liposomes. *FEBS Lett.,* **62,** 60

Rabin, D., Linde, R., Doelle, G. and Alexander, N. (1981). Experience with a potent gonadotropin releasing hormone agonist in normal men: an approach to the development of a male contraceptive. In Zatuchni, G. I., Shelton, J. D. and Sciarra, J. J. (eds.) *LHRH Peptides as Female and Male Contraceptives,* pp. 296–306. (Philadelphia: Harper & Row)

Rees, R. W. A., Foell, T. J., Chai, S. and Grant, N. (1974). Synthesis and biological activities of analogs of the luteinizing hormone-releasing hormone (LH-RH) modified in position 2. *J. Med. Chem.,* **17,** 1016

Richards, J. S. and Bogovich, K. (1980). Development of gonadotropin receptors during follicular growth. In Mahesh, V. B., Muldoon, T. G., Sakena, B. B. and Sadler, W. A. (eds.) *Functional Correlates of Hormone Receptors in Reproduction,* pp. 223–244. (New York: Elsevier/North Holland)

Rivier, J. and Vale, W. (1978). [D-pGlu^{1},D-Phe^{2},D-Trp^{3,6}]-LRF. A potent luteinizing hormone releasing factor antagonist in vitro and inhibitor of ovulation in the rat. *Life Sci.,* **23,** 869.

Rivier, C., Rivier, J. and Vale, W. (1978). Chronic effects of [D-Trp^{6}-Pro^{9}-NEt] luteinizing hormone-releasing factor on reproductive processes in the female rat. *Endocrinology,* **103,** 2299

Rivier, C. and Vale, W. (1981). Temporal relationship between the abortifacient effects of GnRH antagonists and hormonal secretion. *Biol. Reprod.,* **24,** 1061

Rivier, C., Rivier, J. and Vale, W. (1981). Antireproductive effects of a potent GnRH antagonist in the female rat. *Endocrinology,* **108,** 1425

Saffran, M., Franco-Sainz, R., Kong, A., Papahadjopoulos, D. and Szoka, F. (1979). A model for the study of the oral administration of peptide hormones. *Can. J. Biochem.,* **57,** 548

Sandow, J. (1982). Gonadotropic and antigonadotropic actions of LH-RH analogues. In Müller, E. E. and MacLeod, R. M. (eds.) *Neuroendocrine Perspectives. Vol. 1.,* pp. 339–395. (Amsterdam: Elsevier Biomedical Press)

11
Biological activity of a highly potent LHRH antagonist

G. I. McRAE, B. H. VICKERY, J. J. NESTOR Jr., W. J. BREMNER and T. M. BADGER

The search for antagonistic analogs of LHRH which could form the basis of new methods of contraception (Schally and Kastin, 1971; Guillemin, 1972) met with early successes, although the potency of these analogs was low (Monahan *et al.*, 1972; Vale *et al.*, 1972; Guillemin *et al.*, 1973; Coy *et al.*, 1974; Rees *et al.*, 1974; Vilchez-Martinez *et al.*, 1975). For example, a dose level of 6 × 500 μg of [D-Phe^2,D-Ala^6]LHRH was required to inhibit ovulation in rats (Yardley *et al al.*, 1975). Developments in the antagonist field were therefore overshadowed when, starting in 1975, it was demonstrated that LHRH and its agonist analogs were capable of exerting 'paradoxical' antireproductive effects in doses of 0.5 μg per day or less (Oshima *et al.*, 1975).

In the meantime, continued synthetic manipulation of the LHRH molecule has slowly resulted in progressive increases in antagonistic potency. The most potent compounds at this time are: [N-Ac-$\Delta^{3,4}$-Pro^1,D-pF-Phe^2,D-Nal(2)^{3,6}]LHRH (Rivier *et al.*, 1984); [N-Ac-D-pCl-Phe^1,D-pCl-Phe^2,D-Trp^3,D-Arg^6,D-Ala^{10}]LHRH (Nekola and Coy, 1984); [N-Ac-Pro^1,D-p-F-Phe^2,D-Nal(2)^{3,6}]LHRH (RS-29226).

The last of these compounds, RS-29226, resulted from an extension of the studies on very hydrophobic, agonist analogs (Nestor *et al.*, 1984). Detailed studies of its biological activities form the focus of this chapter.

ANTIOVULATORY ACTIVITY

Initial evaluation of RS-29226 was made using an antiovulatory assay in rats. Adult female rats were acclimatized for 2 weeks while daily vaginal lavage was used to determine vaginal cytology. Only rats with a minimum of two consecutive 4-day cycles immediately preceding the test cycles were used for assay. The rats were treated by single subcutaneous injection at noon on the day of vaginal proestrus. On the following morning, the predicted day of estrus, the oviducts were examined for the presence of freshly ovulated eggs, still tightly enclosed in cumulus cells.

Table 11.1 Antiovulatory activity of [N-Ac-L-Pro^{1},D-pF-Phe^{2},D-Nal(2)^{3,6}]LHRH (RS-29226), [N-Ac-Δ^{3}-Pro^{1},D-pF-Phe^{2},D-Nal(2)^{3,6}]LHRH (Analog A) and [N-Ac-D-pCl-Phe^{1},D-pCl-Phe^{3},D-Trp^{3},D-Arg^{6},D-Ala^{10}]LHRH (Analog B) when injected subcutaneously at noon on proestrus in the female rat

	Ovulation rate			
	RS-29226		*Analog A*	*Analog B*
Dose	*In propylene glycol/ saline vehicle*	*In corn oil vehicle*	*In corn oil vehicle*	*In propylene glycol/ saline vehicle*
0.25 μg	—	—	—	90 %
0.5 μg	77 %	—	—	80
1.0 μg	86	100 %	100 %	50
2.0 μg	55	94	80	0
4.0 μg	22	50	20	0
8.0 μg	8	20	0	0
16.0 μg	0	—	—	—

Comparative data were obtained for RS-29226, [N-Ac-Δ^{3,4}-Pro^{1},D-pF-Phe^{2},D-Nal(2)^{3,6}]LHRH, and [N-Ac-D-pCl-Phe^{1},D-pCl-Phe^{2},D-Trp^{3},D-Arg^{6}, D-Ala^{10}]LHRH (Table 11.1). These data allow several conclusions: first, the substitution of positions 3 and 6 of the LHRH molecule by D-Nal(2) is very effective, yielding compounds with very high antagonist potency, as might be predicted from earlier work with agonistic analogs (Nestor *et al.*, 1982). Secondly, the readily available N-Ac-Pro modification can generate very potent analogs. Although it had been shown that N-Ac-Δ^{3}-Pro^{1} is a superior modification relative to [N-Ac-D-Pro^{1}] (Rivier *et al.*, 1981), this work demonstrates that N-Ac-Δ^{3,4}-Pro^{1} is not superior to N-Ac-L-Pro^{1}. Finally, the delivery vehicle may have a significant effect on the apparent potency. This may be due to a need for prolonged blood levels of antagonist to antagonize ovulation effectively. Previous studies with less hydrophobic analogs such as [N-Ac-D-Phe^{1},D-pCl-Phe^{2},D-Trp^{3,6}]LHRH had already demonstrated the importance of correct choice of vehicles (Coy *et al.*, 1979). This latter analog had an ED_{100} of 62 μg when delivered in propylene glycol/saline but an ED_{100} of 15 μg when corn oil was used as vehicle. On the other hand, a much more hydrophobic compound might partition so slowly from oil to plasma that a sufficient concentration in plasma for efficacy is not reached. The apparent biological potency would then be lower in oil than an aqueous based vehicle as shown for RS-29226 in the present studies. However, for instances in which maintained release is required for very long periods of time, oleaginous vehicles may still be preferable.

IN VITRO STUDIES

A perifusion pituitary cell culture system (Loughlin *et al.*, 1981) was standardized with a 20 ng/ml bolus of LHRH (Figure 11.1). Baseline levels of LH secretion were re-established within 30 min of challenge. A mixture of 22 mg/ml or less of RS-29226 had no effect on the response to a bolus challenge of 22 mg/ml

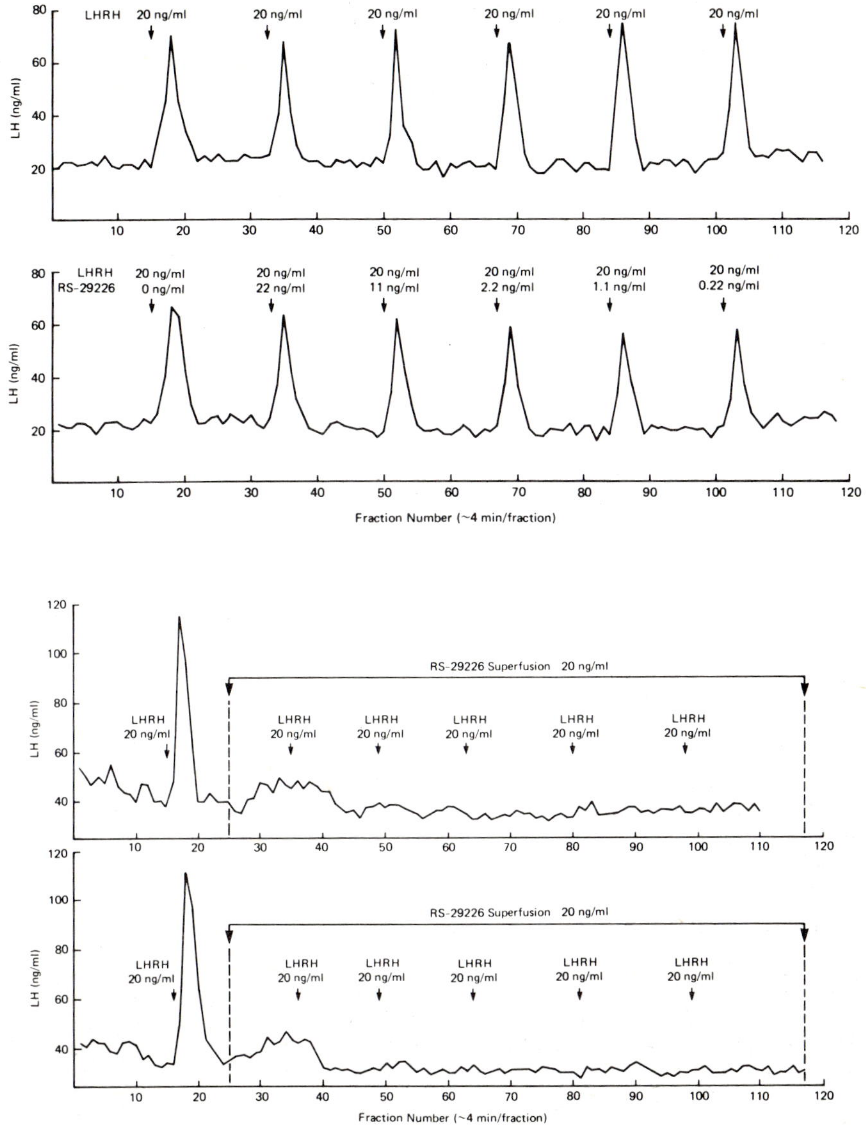

Figure 11.1 Top panel: LH secretion from perifusion pituitary cell culture systems challenged at hourly intervals with 20 ng/ml of LHRH alone or combined with concentrations of 0.22–22 ng/ml of RS-29226 ([N-Ac-L-Pro^1, D-pF-Phe^2, D-Nal(2)^{3,6}]LHRH). Bottom panel: LH secretion from perifusion pituitary cell culture systems challenged at hourly intervals with 20 ng/ml of LHRH and continuously superfused with 20 ng/ml of RS-29226.

LHRH. In separate experiments, however, a continuous superfusion of 20 ng/ml RS-29226 was given for 6 h with hourly bolus challenges of 20 ng LHRH beginning 1 h after the start of superfusion and continuing unil 1 h after stopping superfusion. Under these conditions, there was no detectable response to any challenge, while control cultures run concurrently showed the expected responses. These data indicate a slower rate of binding of RS-29226 than LHRH to the pituitary gonadotrope receptors. The prolonged biological activity of RS-29226 suggests either a slower dissociation rate or down regulation of the pituitary LHRH receptors to be possible. Although the latter hypothesis would be argued against by some recent studies (Clayton *et al.*, 1982), the dissociation kinetics of another highly potent antagonist [N-Ac-L-Ala^{1},D-pCl-Phe^{2},D-Trp^{3,6}]LHRH (Heber *et al.*, 1982) also exhibit a slow dissociation rate.

DURATION OF ACTION

Ovulation inhibition

Progressive shifting of the injection of RS-29226 to earlier time points, relative to noon on proestrus demonstrated a fivefold increase in compound requirement over the first 4 h, a 16-fold increase over 24 h, but little further change through 48 h. The lack of further increased dosage requirements suggests that these changes are not entirely due to simple factors such as biological half-life. The dramatically increased dose requirement over the first 4 h may be a reflection of tissue distribution. The flat dose response from 24 to 48 h suggests either that a whole body depot effect with later re-release into the circulation may occur or, alternatively, that pituitary receptor down regulation may be occurring, as suggested for this compound by the *in vitro* studies and for [N-Ac-Ala^{1},D-pCl-Phe^{2},D-Trp^{3,6}]LHRH previously (Heber *et al.*, 1982). Receptor number studies are required to substantiate this latter possibility.

Gonadotropin levels in castrate rats

Sixty day old male rats, castrated under ether anesthesia, were rested for 3 weeks and then the right atrium was cannulated. One day later the antagonist was injected subcutaneously as a solution in 50 : 50 propylene glycol : saline. RS-29226 was capable of suppressing LH levels for prolonged periods of time following single injection. A second study was extended to evaluate both LH and FSH levels in blood, and longer periods of follow-up were used. Increasing dose in this study influenced both the degree and the duration of suppression of circulating levels of the gonadotropins (Figure 11.2). At the highest dose level tested (500 μg/kg), LH levels were suppressed out through 72 h after injection. It is unlikely that these durations of effect are due to extended circulating levels of compound. The changes in FSH levels following RS-29226 are more ephemeral than those seen for LH. Changes in FSH upon stimulation with LHRH agonists also are more modest than those for LH and also tend to lag behind LH changes.

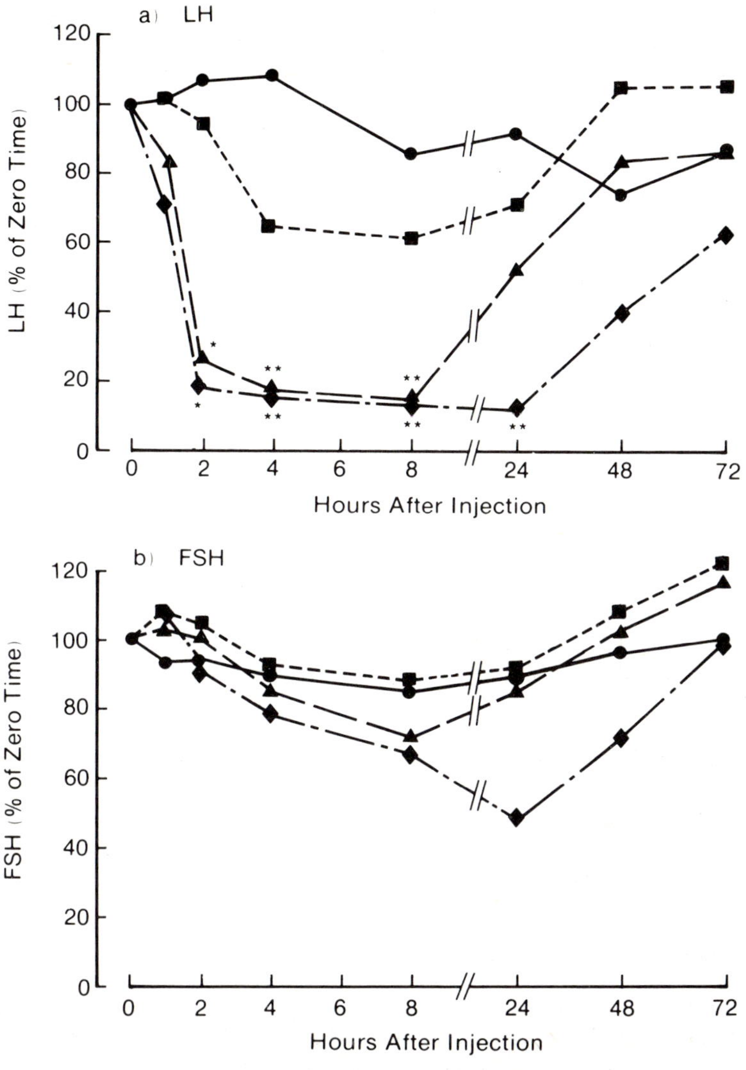

Figure 11.2 Effect of subcutaneous injection of RS-29226 as a solution in 1 : 1 propylene glycol : saline on circulating levels of LH and FSH in castrated male rats. (●——●) vehicle, $n = 5$; (■---■) 25 μg/kg, $n = 6$; (▲——▲) 100 μg/kg, $n = 4$; (◆----◆) 500 μg/kg, $n = 5$, * $p > 0.05$ and ** $p < 0.01$ when mean value for that group is compared to the mean value for the vehicle group at the same time by *t*-test.

ANTIREPRODUCTIVE EFFECTS IN FEMALES

Estrous cyclicity in rats

Daily subcutaneous administration of RS-29226 in corn oil to rats for 14 consecutive days caused a dose-related interference with estrous cyclicity.

The interference took the form of periods of continuous estrus in some animals but continuous diestrus in other animals. Regular cycling was abolished at 80 μg/rat per day. Similar studies were reported for [N-Ac-Δ^3-Pro^1,D-pCl-Phe^2,D-Trp^{3,6},N-MeLeu^7]LHRH for which 200 μg/rat per day, injected using corn oil as vehicle, were required to suppress normal cyclicity (Rivier *et al.*, 1981).

Pregnancy termination in rats

Administration of RS-29226 as a solution in corn oil to pregnant rats results in pregnancy termination. When administered subcutaneously on each of days 10–12 of pregnancy (day 1 = day of sperm detection) the lowest dose tested, 200 mg/rat per day, was totally effective. Pregnancy was also terminated in 90% of rats by this same dose administered once on day 10 only. For reference, [N-Ac-Δ^3-Pro^1,D-pCl-Phe^2,D-Trp^{3,6},N-MeLeu^7]LHRH terminated pregnancy in seven of eight rats when administered at a dose of 1 mg/rat per day on both of days 9 and 10 of pregnancy, and in eight of eight rats when the same dose was administered on both days 11 and 12 of pregnancy (Rivier *et al.*, 1981).

Placental effects

The presence and synthesis of an LHRH-like material (hCGnRH) was reported in human placental tissue (Siler-Khodr and Khodr, 1978, 1979; Khodr and Siler-Khodr, 1978, 1980). Stimulation of hCG and progesterone release from human placental tissue incubated *in vitro* with LHRH has led to the hypothesis that this hCGnRH regulates placental gonadotropin and progesterone (Siler-Khodr and Khodr, 1981, 1982).

We have examined the effect of RS-29226 upon gonadotropin and progesterone output *in vitro* from placental explants (Siler-Khodr *et al.*, 1983). A marked suppression of hCG, αhCG and progesterone levels in the medium was noted over the 8 days of culture of this mid-gestational (15 weeks) tissue when RS-29226 was present at 1 mg/ml. This inhibition was partially reversed by the addition of 10 mg/ml of LHRH, particularly over the first 1–2 days of culture. Although hCS release was also suppressed, the suppression occurred later and may be secondary to the other effects. The effects were presumably mediated through specific receptors (Currie *et al.*, 1981). This marked suppression of hCG and progesterone levels may have significance for the development of methods of pregnancy interruption.

ANTIREPRODUCTIVE EFFECTS IN MALES

Rats

The effects of RS-29226 on endocrine and reproductive parameters have been evaluated in male rats. Daily injection of RS-29226 as a solution in 50:50 propylene glycol : saline results in a precipitous fall in plasma testosterone and

LH levels at a dose of 1 mg/rat per day but has no effect at 0.1 mg/rat per day (Figure 11.3). Daily administration for as little as 14 days markedly suppressed reproductive organ weight (Table 11.2) and spermatogenesis (Figure 11.4). These findings are in keeping with previous reports of the effects of other antagonists to male rats (Rivier *et al.*, 1980, 1981). A study comparing the

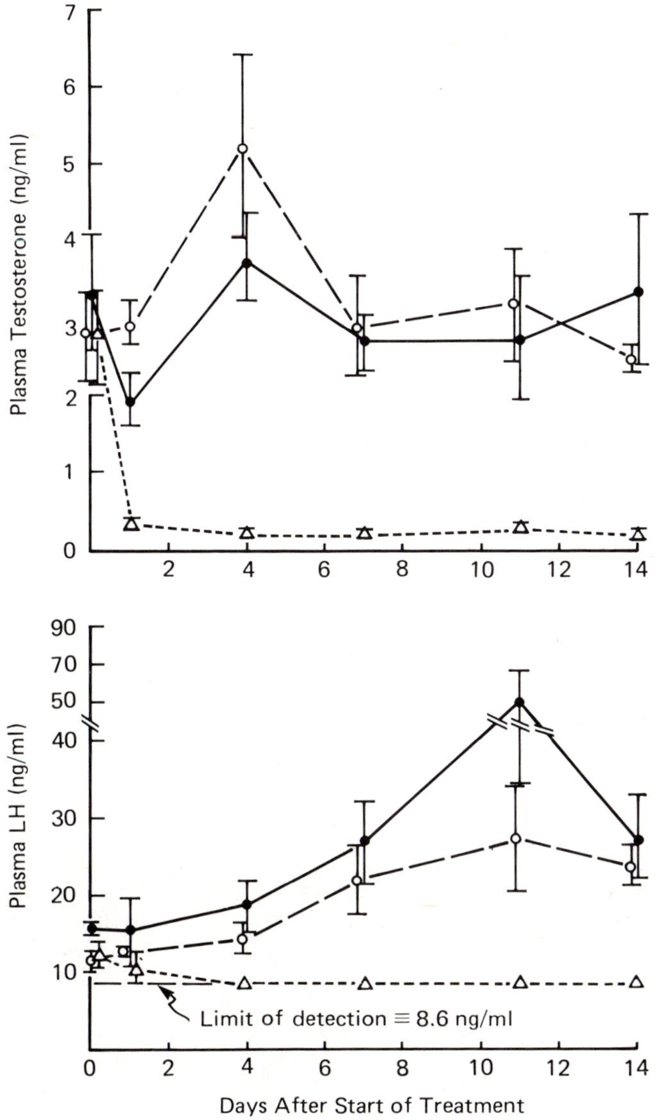

Figure 11.3 Plasma testosterone and LH in male rats treated with once-daily subcutaneous injections of RS-29226 for 14 days. (●——●) corn oil vehicle, (○– – –○) 0.1 mg/rat, (△– – –△) 1 mg/rat. $N = 6$ in all groups.

Table 11.2 Effect of 14 days of once-daily subcutaneous injections of [N-Ac-L-Pro[1],D-pF-Phe[2],D-Nal(2)[3,6]]LHRH as a solution in 50 : 50 propylene glycol : saline on reproductive organ weights in adult male rats

Dose per animal per day	n	*Testes weight* (g)	*Epididymides weight* (mg)	*Seminal vesicles weight* (mg)	*Ventral prostate weight* (mg)
Vehicle	6	3.1 ± 0.1	1113 ± 78	526 ± 36	375 ± 34
0.1 mg	6	3.2 ± 0.1	1021 ± 20	569 ± 39	358 ± 24
1.0 mg	6	1.6 ± 0.1[a]	414 ± 14[a]	252 ± 8[a]	43 ± 5[a]

[a] $p < 0.001$ versus controls by Student's *t*-test

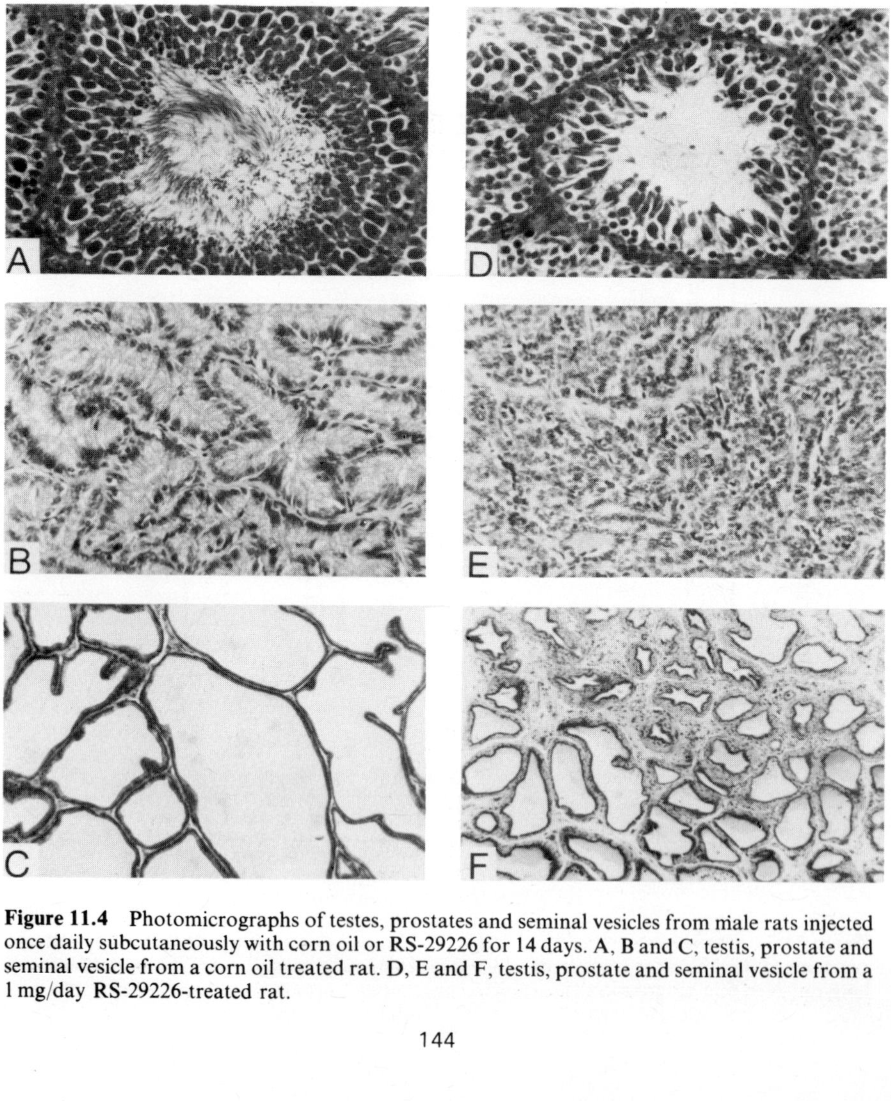

Figure 11.4 Photomicrographs of testes, prostates and seminal vesicles from male rats injected once daily subcutaneously with corn oil or RS-29226 for 14 days. A, B and C, testis, prostate and seminal vesicle from a corn oil treated rat. D, E and F, testis, prostate and seminal vesicle from a 1 mg/day RS-29226-treated rat.

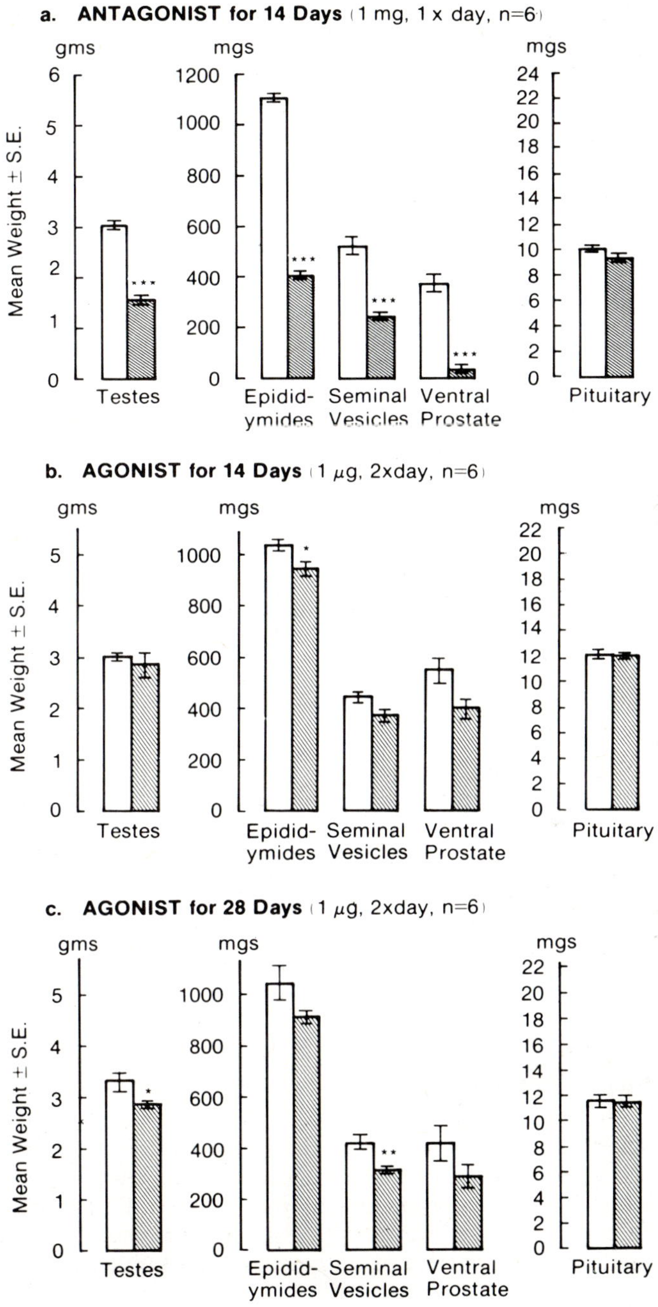

Figure 11.5 Comparative effects of LHRH antagonist, RS-29226, and LHRH agonist, [D-Nal(2)[6]]LHRH, on reproductive organ weights of mature male rats. *, **, and *** indicate $p < 0.05$, $p < 0.01$, and $p < 0.001$, respectively, by *t*-test. □ = vehicle; ▨ = LHRH analog.

ability of single injection of RS-29226 in different vehicles to lower testosterone levels for ≤ 24 h indicates that corn oil confers an apparent fivefold increase in potency on the compound versus the 50:50 propylene glycol : saline vehicle used. However, regardless of dose required, it is of interest to compare the degree of effect on testicular function to be achieved with the most potent agonists and this potent antagonist. Comparison shows that the degree of suppression of reproductive organ weight is markedly less with agonist than antagonist (Figure 11.5). An equivalent degree of suppression to that obtainable with RS-29226 has not been observed with an agonist, even when administered continuously at high dose levels from a pellet formulation (Vickery, 1982).

Dogs

RS-29226 has recently been evaluated for ability to suppress plasma testosterone and gonadotropin levels in male beagle dogs. Although equivocal responses were obtained with a dose of 10 mg/kg administered subcutaneously in corn oil, significant effects resulted with either 100 or 1000 mg/kg (Figure 11.6). The onset of suppression appears to be more rapid and the duration of suppression more prolonged at the higher dose. The persistence of significant suppression through 24 h following 1 mg/kg indicates that daily administration should abolish reproductive function.

Cynomolgus monkeys

Subcutaneous administration of 5 mg/kg of RS-29226 to male cynomolgus monkey suppressed circulating levels of testosterone for more than 24 h following injection (Figure 11.7). This suggests that daily administration should abolish male reproduction in the macaque. The result is of particular interest when compared to the effects of LHRH agonists in macaques. Male reproductive function in cynomolgus monkeys was not suppressed even by daily dosing with mg quantities of the most potent of agonists. In most species, the agonists exert their paradoxical antifertility effects at significantly lower doses than antagonists (Vickery and McRae, 1980).

POTENTIAL UTILITIES

LHRH antagonists may be useful in the range of utilities presently being explored using the paradoxical antireproductive and antisteroidal effects of LHRH agonists. These would include inhibition of ovulation and pregnancy termination in women, and contraception in men via inhibition of spermatogenesis, together with a variety of therapeutic possibilities deriving from an interference with reproductive endocrinology: endometriosis; breast, prostate and other reproductive tissue cancers; non-reproductive organ tumors and ectopic tumors, particularly those secreting chorionic gonadotropin. The basic animal studies exploring the contraceptive applications support this role.

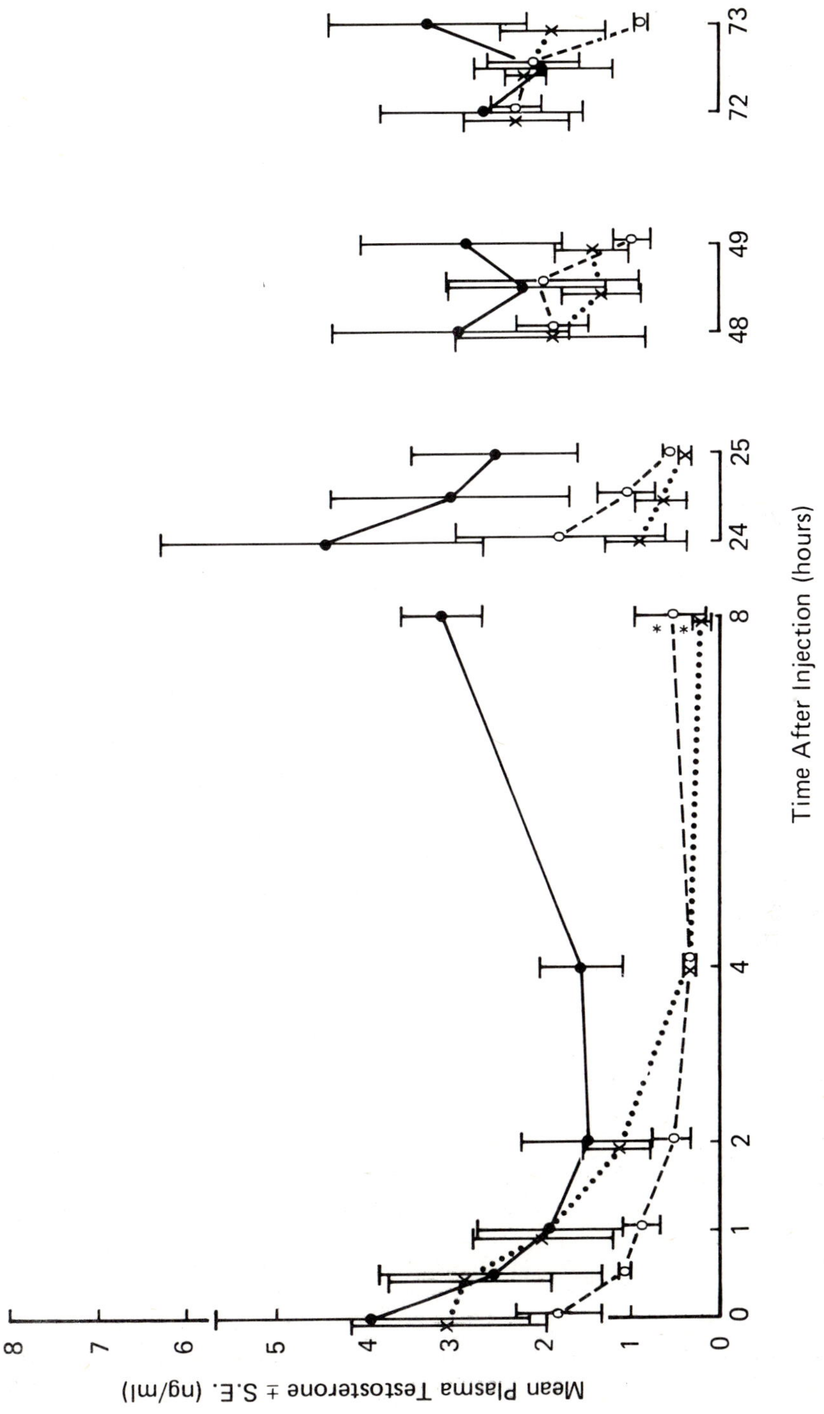

Figure 11.6 Plasma testosterone in male dogs following a single subcutaneous injection of vehicle or **RS-29226**. $N = 3$ for all groups; * $p < 0.05$ compared to vehicle group by *t*-test. (●——●) vehicle; (○– –○) 100 μg/kg; (x . . . . x) 1000 μg/kg

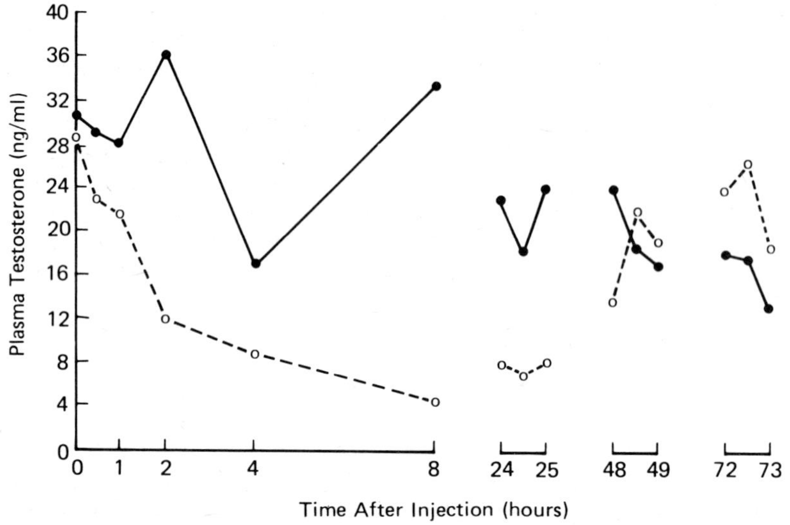

Figure 11.7 Plasma testosterone in two male cynomolgus monkeys following a single subcutaneous injection of vehicle or 5 mg/kg of RS-29226.

However, continuous administration of antagonists will result in gonadal hormone deficiency, a situation which does not seem to be always true with the agonists. Discontinuous administration or hormone replacement therapy will therefore be required for the contraceptive use. Although a single dose of 2–3 mg of [N-Ac-D-pCl-Phe^{1,2},D-Trp^{3},D-Phe^{6},D-Ala^{10}]LHRH administered on day 12 of an expected 28-day cycle in women was able to block ovulation in five of the eight subjects (Zárate *et al.*, 1981), the timing of treatment might be an insurmountable problem for the general population. A predictive test of impending ovulation (Tsibris *et al.*, 1982) might make such a discontinuous treatment feasible. The administration of LHRH antagonists for a short time during the early follicular phase with the object of inducing a subsequent defective or inadequate luteal phase (Sheehan *et al.*, 1982) might be a promising area.

The potential of RS-29226 for pregnancy termination offers promise. The limited studies in pregnant women with LHRH agonists have not been successful (Casper *et al.*, 1980; Tolis *et al.*, 1981). Although pregnancy is easily terminated in rats with LHRH antagonists, rodent assays have historically not been predictive of efficacy in primates. The direct placental effects of RS-29226 would encourage further work *in vivo*.

For LHRH antagonists to be useful as male contraceptives, testosterone supplementation will be required. Whether or not such supplementation will reverse the antispermatogenic effects of the antagonist is equivocal, based on published rat studies (Rivier *et al.*, 1979, 1980). The onset of pituitary and therefore gonadal suppression is faster and the degree of suppression is probably greater with antagonists than with LHRH agonists. The early stimulatory phase characteristic of agonists will not be associated with antagonists. This may be of particular importance in oncological therapy in minimizing the early stimulatory 'flare' seen during agonist therapy. Early studies with transplantable mammary tumors in immunosuppressed neonatal hamsters suggest that LHRH antagonists might be of use (Corbin, 1982). Direct actions on both gestational and non-gestational tumors should be pursued. There are possibly tumors which are directly responsive to gonadotropins (Meyskeus *et al.*, 1981) and these situations bear investigation. The rationale for the use of LHRH agonists to protect against the sterilizing effects of cancer chemotherapy (Glode *et al.*, 1981) is valid for LHRH antagonists.

CONCLUDING REMARKS

LHRH antagonist analogs, as typified by RS-29226, now have potencies one thousandfold greater than those of analogs first reported. The binding affinities of these most potent analogs are 30 times greater than LHRH itself and are similar to the highest reported for the best agonists. These compounds are available in sufficient quantity to permit evaluation in a variety of animal models and to begin to explore their clinical pharmacology in humans. Their major forte appears to be the rapidity and longevity of suppressive effects on pituitary and therefore gonadal function. Although very impressive increases in potency have been made, further increases may still be required to make the use of LHRH antagonists economically viable.

References

Casper, R. F., Sheehan, K. L. and Yen, S. S. C. (1980). Chorionic gonadotrophin prevents LRF-agonist-induced luteolysis in the human. *Contraception,* **21,** 471

Clayton, R. N., Channabasavaiah, K., Stewart, J. M. and Catt, K. J. (1982). Hypothalamic regulation of pituitary gonadotropin-releasing hormone receptors: Effects of hypothalamic lesions and a gonadotropin-releasing hormone antagonist. *Endocrinology,* **110,** 1108

Corbin, A. (1982). From contraception to cancer: A review of the therapeutic applications of LHRH analogues as antitumor agents. *Yale J. Biol. Med.,* **55,** 27

Coy, D. H., Coy, E. J., Schally, A. V., Vilchez-Martinez, J. A., Debeljuk, L., Carter, W. H. and Arimura, A. (1974). Stimulatory and inhibitory analogs of luteinizing hormone-releasing hormone. *Biochemistry,* **13,** 323

Coy, D. H., Mezo, I., Pedroza, E., Nekola, M. V., Vilchez-Martinez, J. A., Piyachaturawat, P., Schally, A. V., Seprodi, T., and Teplan, I. (1979). LH-RH antagonists with potent antiovulatory activity. In Gross, E. and Meienhofer, J. (eds.) *Peptides: Structure and Biological Function. Proceedings of 6th American Peptide Symposium,* p. 775. (Rockford, IL: Pierce Chemical Co.)

Currie, A. J., Fraser, H. M. and Sharpe, R. M. (1981). Human placental receptors for luteinizing hormone releasing hormone. *Biochem. Biophys. Res. Commun.,* **99,** 332

Glode, L. M., Robinson, J. and Gould, S. F. (1981). Protection from cyclophosphamide-induced testicular damage by an analogue of gonadotropin-releasing hormone. *Lancet,* **1,** 1132

Guillemin, R. (1972). Physiology and chemistry of the hypothalamic releasing factors for gonadotropins: a new approach to fertility control. *Contraception,* **5,** 1

Guillemin, R., Amoss, M., Blackwell, R., Burgus, R., Grant, G., Ling, N., Monahan, M., Rivier, J. and Vale, W. (1973). Polypeptide antagonists of the hypothalamic luteinizing hormone-releasing factors. *J. Reprod. Fertil.,* (Suppl.) **18,** 23

Heber, D., Dodson, R., Swerdloff, R. S., Channabasavaiah, K. and Stewart, J. M. (1982).

Pituitary receptor site blockade by a gonadotropin-releasing hormone antagonist in vivo: Mechanism of action. *Science,* **216,** 420

Khodr, G. S. and Siler-Khodr, T. M. (1978). Localization of luteinizing hormone releasing factor (LRF) in the human placenta. *Fertil. Steril.,* **29,** 523

Khodr, G. S. and Siler-Khodr, T. M. (1980). Placental LRF and its synthesis. *Science,* **207,** 315

Loughlin, J. S., Badger, T. M. and Crowley, W. F. Jr. (1981). Perifused pituitary cultures: A model for LHRH regulation of LH secretion. *Am. J. Physiol.,* **240,** E591

Meyskeus, F. L., Stouffer, R. S. and Sander, D. S. (1981). Luteinizing hormone modulates human melanoma tumor skin cell expression and binds to human melanoma cells. *Proc. 17th Ann. Mtg. Am. Soc. Clin. Oncol./Am. Assoc. Cancer Res.,* **21,** 152

Monahan, M. W., Rivier, J., Vale, W., Guillemin, R. and Burgus, R. (1972). (Gly 2) LRF and des-His 2-LRF. The synthesis, purification, and characterization of two LRF analogues antagonistic to LRF. *Biochem. Biophys. Res. Commun.,* **47,** 551

Nekola, M. and Coy, D. H. (1984). Physiology of LHRH antagonists in females. This volume, Chapter 10

Nestor, J. J. Jr., Ho, T. L., Simpson, R. A., Horner, B. L., Jones, G. H., McRae, G. I. and Vickery, B. H. (1982). The synthesis and biological activity of some very hydrophobic analogs of luteinizing hormone releasing hormone. *J. Med. Chem.,* **25,** 795

Nestor, J. J. Jr., Ho, T. L., Tahilramani, R., McRae, G. I. and Vickery, B. H. (1984). LHRH agonists and antagonists containing very hydrophobic amino acids. This volume, Chapter 3

Oshima, H., Nankin, H. R., Fan, D. F., Troen, P., Yanaihara, T., Niizato, N., Yoshida, K. I. and Ochiai K.-I. (1975). Delay in sexual maturation of rats caused by synthetic LH-releasing hormone: Enhancement of steroid Δ^4-5α-hydrogenase in testes. *Biol. Reprod.,* **12,** 491

Rees, R. W. A., Foell, T. J., Chai, S.-Y. and Grant, N. (1974). Synthesis and biological activities of analogs of the luteinizing hormone-releasing hormone (LH-RH) modified in position 2. *J. Med. Chem.,* **17,** 1016

Rivier, C., Rivier, J. and Vale, W. (1979). Chronic effects of [D-Trp^6,Pro^9-NEE] luteinizing hormone-releasing factor on reproductive processes in the male rat. *Endocrinology,* **105,** 1191

Rivier, C., Rivier, J. and Vale, W. (1980). Antireproductive effects of a potent gonadotropin-releasing hormone antagonist in the male rat. *Science,* **210,** 93

Rivier, C., Rivier, J. and Vale, W. (1981). Antireproductive effects of a potent GnRH antagonist in the female rat. *Endocrinology,* **108,** 1425

Rivier, J., Rivier, C., Perrin, M., Porter, J. and Vale, W. (1984). LHRH analogs as antiovulatory agents. This volume, Chapter 2

Schally, A. V. and Kastin, A. J. (1971). *Drug Ther.,* **1,** 29

Sheehan, K. L., Casper, R. F. and Yen, S. S. C. (1982). Luteal phase defects induced by an agonist of luteinizing hormone-releasing factor: a model for fertility control. *Science,* **215,** 170

Siler-Khodr, T. M. and Khodr, G. S. (1978). Luteinizing hormone releasing factor content of the human placenta. *Am. J. Obstet. Gynecol.,* **130,** 216

Siler-Khodr, T. M. and Khodr, G. S. (1979). Extrahypothalamic luteinizing hormone releasing factor (LRF): Release of immunoreactive LRF by the human placenta in vitro. *Fertil. Steril.,* **22,** 294

Siler-Khodr, T. M. and Khodr, G. S. (1981). Production and activity of placental releasing hormones. In Novy, M. J. and Reske, J. A. (eds.) *Fetal Endocrinology,* pp. 183–210. (New York: Academic Press)

Siler-Khodr, T. M. and Khodr, G. S. (1982). GnRH in the placenta. In McCann, S. (ed.) *Role of Peptides and Proteins in Control of Reproduction.* (New York: Elsevier/North Holland) (In press)

Siler-Khodr, T. M., Khodr, G. S., Vickery, B. H. and Nestor, J. J. Jr. (1983). Inhibition of hCG, αhCG and progesterone release from human placental tissue in vitro by a GnRH antagonist. *Life Sci.* (In press)

Tolis, G., Comaru-Schally, A. M., Mehta, A. E. and Schally, A. V. (1981). Failure to interrupt established pregnancy in humans by D-Trp^6 luteinizing hormone releasing hormone. *Fertil. Steril.,* **36,** 241

Tsibris, J. E. M., Thomason, J. L., Kunigk, A., Khan-Dawood, F. S., Kirschner, C. V. and Spellacy, W. N. (1982). Guaiacol peroxidase levels in human cervical mucus: A possible predictor of ovulation. *Contraception,* **25,** 59

Vale, W., Grant, G., Rivier, J., Monahan, M., Amoss, M., Blackwell, R., Burgus, R. and

Guillemin, R. (1972). Synthetic polypeptide antagonists of the hypothalamic luteinizing hormone-releasing factor. *Science,* **176,** 933

Vickery, B. H. (1982). Antigonadotropic, antisteroidogenic and antisteroidal activities of agonist analogs of luteinizing hormone releasing hormone as revealed by their antireproductive activities. In Agarwal, M. K. (ed.) *Hormone Antagonists,* pp. 623–660. (New York: de Gruyter)

Vickery, B. H., and McRae, G. I. (1980). Responses of the males of different laboratory species to continuous administration of an LHRH agonist. *J. Androl.,* **1,** 62

Vilchez-Martinez, J. A., Schally, A. V., Coy, D. H., Coy, E. J., Miller, C. M. III and Arimura, A. (1975). An in vivo assay for anti-LH-RH and anti-FSH-RH activities of inhibitory analogues of LH-RH. *Endocrinology,* **96,** 1130

Yardley, J. P., Foell, T. J., Beattie, C. W. and Grant, N. (1975). Antagonism of luteinizing hormone release and of ovulation by an analog of the luteinizing hormone-releasing hormone. *J. Med. Chem.,* **18,** 1244

Zárate, A., Canales, E. S., Schally, A. V., Coy, D. H. and Coumaru-Schally, A. M. (1981). The use of LHRH agonists and antagonists as antifertility agents in the human female. In Zatuchni, G. I., Shelton, J. D. and Sciarra, J. J. (eds.) *LHRH Peptides as Female and Male Contraceptives,* pp. 227–236. (Philadelphia: Harper and Row)

12
LHRH antagonists for male contraception

D. HEBER and R. S. SWERDLOFF

The potential of antagonistic analogs of LHRH as contraceptive agents was recognized shortly after the discovery and sequencing of LHRH (Schally *et al.*, 1971). LHRH agonists with prolonged duration of action compared to authentic LHRH were thought to be useful for the treatment of infertility due to LHRH deficiency. However, extensive studies in animals and humans with potent agonists revealed paradoxical inhibitory effects on male reproductive function (Pelletier *et al.*, 1978; Rivier *et al.*, 1980; Heber and Swerdloff, 1981; Linde *et al.*, 1981). While detailed and extensive clinical studies with potent LHRH agonists are well underway, preliminary human studies published to date have used much less potent antagonists (Gonzalez-Barcena *et al.*, 1977; Canales *et al.*, 1978). Since clinical studies using LHRH agonists are already initiated, why then propose studies of LHRH antagonists as potential male contraceptive agents? First, the efficacy of agonists in predictably suppressing spermatogenesis completely has not been demonstrated to date in man. Second, agonists have the potential disadvantage of a delay in the onset of their inhibitory effects caused by the initial stimulatory effects of agonist administration on gonadotropin and testosterone secretion (Sandow *et al.*, 1978; Happ *et al.*, 1978; Crowley *et al.*, 1980). Third, although the primary site of action of LHRH agonists in the human male is the pituitary gland (Heber *et al.*, 1983) irreversible effects of agonist treatment on testicular histology have been observed in rats (Vickery, 1981). While the focal necrosis observed in rat testes is not seen in any other species, histologic studies of rat testes following antagonist administration suggest a primary pituitary effect without direct toxic effects on the rat testis (Rivier *et al.*, 1980; Rivier *et al.*, 1981). Finally, while infertility has been demonstrated in rats following chronic antagonist administration (Rivier *et al.*, 1981), infertility has never been demonstrated in rats treated with LHRH agonist to date (C. Rivier, personal communications). Based on the above considerations LHRH antagonists are a promising new approach to male contraception.

RECEPTOR STUDIES

In order to define the mechanism of action of LHRH antagonists *in vivo* we administered two doses of a potent LHRH antagonist [N-Ac-Ala[1],D-pCl-

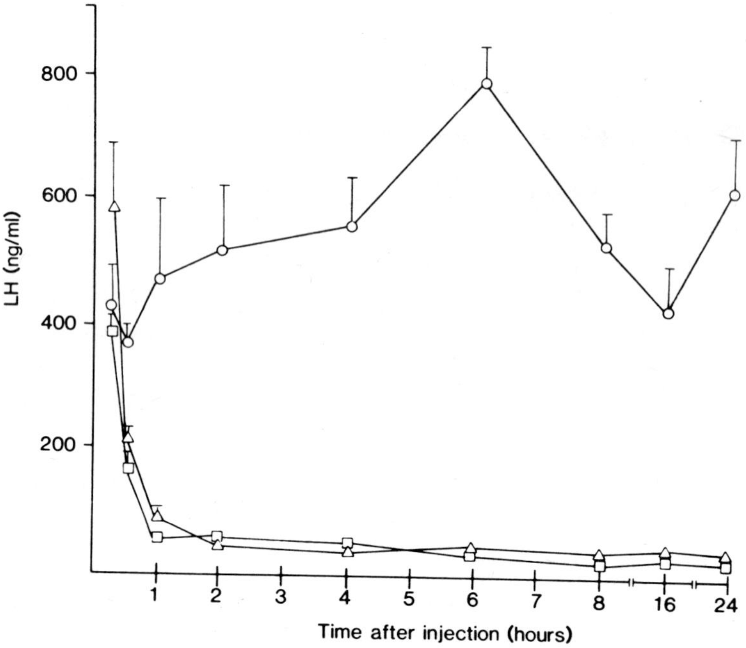
LH (ng/ml)
800
600
400
200
1
2
3
4
5
6
7
8
16
24
Time after injection (hours)

a

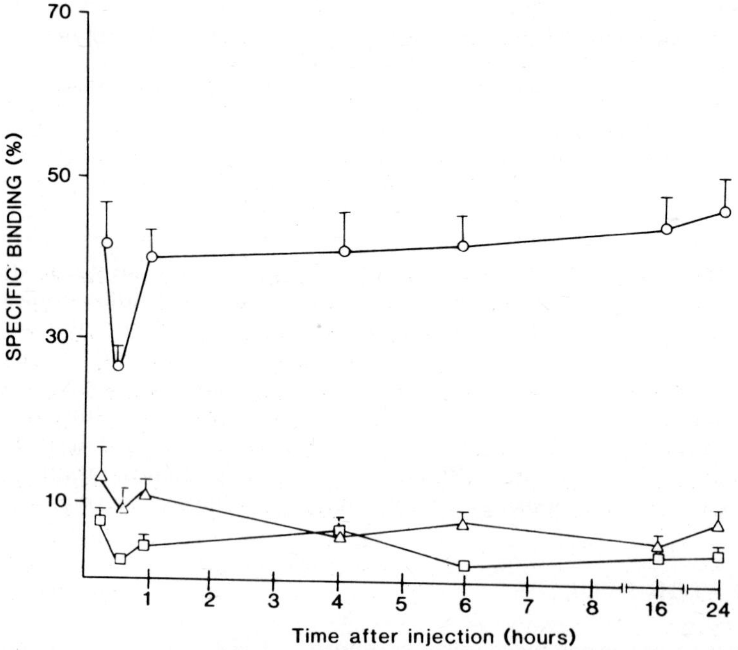
SPECIFIC BINDING (%)
70
50
30
10
1
2
3
4
5
6
7
8
16
24
Time after injection (hours)

b

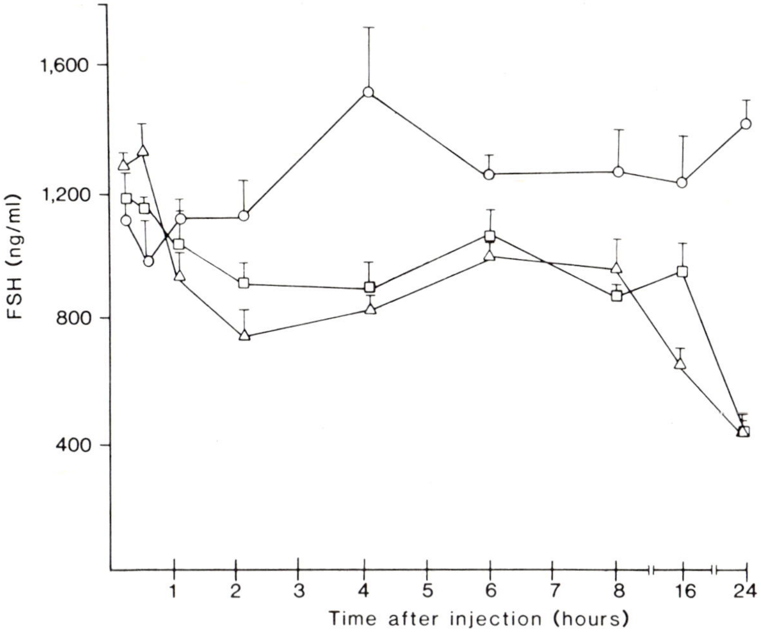

c

Figure 12.1 Effects of a single injection of vehicle alone (○), 100 μg of antagonist (Δ) or 1 mg of antagonist (□) on (**a**) serum LH, (**b**) specific binding of pituitary LHRH receptor and (**c**) serum FSH in castrated male rats. Groups of five rats from two treatment groups and the control group were killed at 15 min, 30 min, and 1, 2, 4, 6, 8, 16 and 24 h after antagonist injection. Pituitary receptor binding was measured by incubating the homogenates with 20 000 count/min of ^{125}I-labeled D-Leu^{6}des-Gly^{10} LHRH ethylamide (agonist) in assay buffer (0.01 mol/l tris-HCl buffer, pH 7.4, containing 1% recrystallized bovine serum albumin (Miles Pentex) with or without added 10^{-8} mol/l agonist at 4°C for 40 min. The bound and free hormone were separated by centrifugation at 15 000 *g*. Bars indicate ± standard error of mean.

Phe^2,D-Trp^{3,6}] LHRH (Antag A) to male rats castrated for seven days (Heber *et al.*, 1982). Either 100 μg or 1 mg of this antagonist was administered as a subcutaneous injection in corn oil. Groups of five animals in a control group and in two antagonist-treated groups were sacrificed at 15 min, 30 min and 1, 2, 4, 6, 8, 16 and 24 h after injection. Serum LH and FSH were determined by radioimmunoassay and pituitary LHRH receptor binding determined using an established pituitary LHRH radioreceptor assay. Pituitary LHRH receptor binding and serum LH levels fell within 1 h of antagonist administration and remained suppressed for over 24 h following injection. These changes (see Figure 12.1) were consistent with a rapid onset of receptor site blockade which mediated a rapid and prolonged inhibition of LH secretion. Serum FSH levels fell much more gradually over 24 h, consistent with the hypothesis that factors other than LHRH control FSH secretion in the rat.

Since receptor site blockade by the antagonist could mediate the observed effects on LH secretion, direct studies of the dissociation rate of antagonist from the pituitary LHRH receptor site were carried out using ^{125}I-labeled Antag-A and agonist ([D-Leu^6,Pro^9-NHEt] LHRH) ligands. Following a 40 min preincubation to allow analog association with the receptor to occur, a large excess (10 nmol/l) of unlabeled agonist or antagonist was added and the rate of exchange of labeled analogs off of the receptor site quantified (Figure 12.2). The antagonist dissociated at a rate fourfold slower than the LHRH agonist, indicating that persistent binding of antagonist at the pituitary receptor site was the likely mechanism for the prolonged duration of action of these agents.

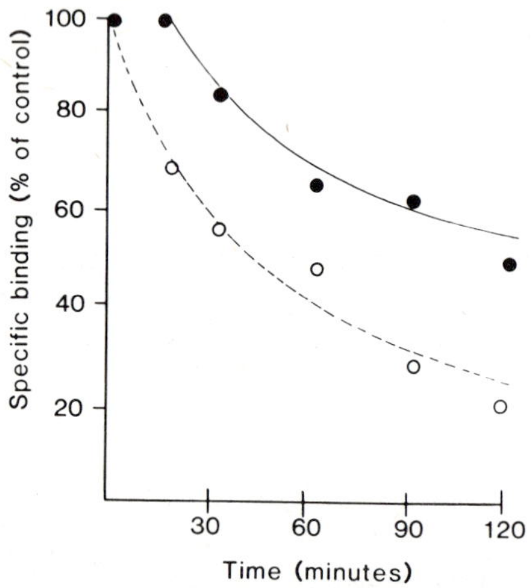

Figure 12.2 Specific pituitary LHRH receptor binding (see text) for radio-iodinated agonist (○) and antagonist (●) plotted against time in minutes after exposure to 10^{-8} mol/l concentrations of uniodinated agonist and antagonist, respectively.

Whether the slowed dissociation rate of LHRH antagonists is related to the lipophilic nature of these peptides, mediated by increased partitioning of the antagonist into the plasma membrane of the gonadotrope, is currently under study in our laboratories.

ANTAGONIST EFFECTS *IN VIVO*

In the male rat, chronic administration of 1 mg of the antagonist [Ac-Δ^3-Pro^1,D-pCl-Phe^2,D-Trp^{3,6},N-MeLeu^7]LHRH abolished mating behavior, gonadotropin secretion, testosterone secretion and spermatogenesis (Rivier *et al.*, 1980). An LHRH antagonist was shown to reverse the actions of LHRH on steroidogenesis in ovarian cell cultures (Hsueh and Ling, 1979). Since both gonadal and pituitary actions are possible for LHRH antagonists and agonists, we undertook studies assessing the actions and interactions of these compounds at the pituitary and gonadal levels in the male rat. Four groups of adult male rats were treated for 21 days with (1) vehicle alone (control), (2)

100 μg per day of [N-Ac-Ala^{1},D-pCl-Phe^{2},D-Trp^{3,6}]LHRH (antagonist-treated), (3) 200 ng per day of [D-Leu^{6},Pro^{9}-NHEt]LHRH (agonist-treated) or (4) both the agonist and antagonist in combination. The agonist and antagonist were administered in saline and corn oil, respectively. Antagonist treatment for 21 days resulted in a significant suppression of intratesticular sperm counts compared to controls (Table 12.1).

Table 12.1 Effects of analog treatment on spermatogenesis

Group	*Sperm count* ($\times 10^{6}$/*testis*)	*Testis weight* (g)
Control	239 ± 11	1.45 ± 0.04
Antagonist	158 ± 14	1.30 ± 0.05
Agonist	81 ± 11	1.05 ± 0.10
Antagonist/agonist	188 ± 11	1.35 ± 0.07

Agonist treatment resulted in more marked suppression of spermatogenesis at the dose employed than did antagonist. The combined treatment with agonist and antagonist was less effective in suppressing spermatogenesis than agonist alone. Serum LH, FSH, and testosterone following 21 days of treatment was determined in each group (Table 12.2).

Table 12.2 Effects of analog on gonadotropins and testosterone

Group	*Serum LH* (ng/ml RP-1)	*Serum FSH* (ng/ml RP-1)	*Serum T* (ng/dl)
Control	44 ± 10	383 ± 23	624 ± 110
Antagonist	16 ± 1[a]	<200	179 ± 33
Agonist	51 ± 1	536 ± 34	100 ± 9
Antag/Ag	16 ± 1[a]	284 ± 17	100 ± 18

[a] limit of detectability of LH is 15 mg/ml RP-1

While treatment with agonist results in elevated gonadotropins, both testosterone secretion and spermatogenesis are more markedly suppressed by agonist treatment than antagonist treatment. Combined agonist and antagonist treatment resulted in levels of FSH which were greater than those in the antagonist-treated group and levels of LH which were suppressed. Serum testosterone levels were as low as those in the agonist-treated group, yet spermatogenesis was less suppressed by combined treatment than by agonist alone. Thus, antagonist in combination with agonist counteracted agonist effects on spermatogenesis without altering serum testosterone levels. These data support previous observations from our laboratory (Heber and Swerdloff, 1981) and others (Hsueh and Ling, 1979) suggesting that LHRH agonists in the rat may act directly on gonadal spermatogenesis and steroidogenesis by mechanisms other than inhibition of gonadotropin secretion. Inhibition of testosterone secretion by LHRH agonist persisted in the combined treatment group despite inhibition of serum LH levels in analogy to observations in hypophysectomized male rats where agonist suppressed testosterone secretion in the absence of measurable serum gonadotropins (Hsueh and Ling, 1979).

INTERACTION OF TESTOSTERONE AND ANTAGONIST

The inhibitory effect of either LHRH agonist or antagonist treatment on testosterone secretion suggests the need for combined androgen and analog treatment to prevent the predictable occurrence of undermasculinization and impotence with effective analog therapy. This approach appears promising for agonists (Heber *et al.*, 1983; Bhasin *et al.*, 1983) and the preliminary studies described below in rats indicate that synergistic inhibition of spermatogenesis occurs when androgens and antagonist analogs are administered in combination.

In this study, two doses of testosterone were administered together with daily 100 μg subcutaneous injections of Antagonist-A for 30 days. A 20 mm Silastic testosterone capsule which we had previously demonstrated to suppress spermatogenesis synergistically in combination with injections of a LHRH agonist in the rat via enhanced gonadotropin inhibition was implanted in two groups of male rats both with and without LHRH antagonist treatment. A 200 mm Silastic implant reversed the effects of antagonist by replacing endogenous testosterone in the absence of gonadotropin secretion.

No histological abnormalities were noted in testis sections from the group receiving the 200 mm Silastic implants, while inhibition of spermatogenesis and of the germinal epithelium was noted in the group treated with antagonist and 20 mm Silastic testosterone implant. These data suggest that LHRH antagonist and testosterone in combination will synergistically suppress spermatogenesis in the human, while having the additional advantage of preventing symptoms associated with androgen deficiency which would inevitably result from effective inhibition of gonadotropin secretion in the male.

Table 12.3 Effects of antagonist, testosterone and the combination on spermatogenesis

Group (n = 10)	*Sperm count* (= 10^6/*testis*)	*Testis weight* (g)
Antagonist	235 ± 34	1.6 ± 0.2
20 mm T	129 ± 32	1.5 ± 0.2
200 mm T	196 ± 59	1.5 ± 0.2
Antag + 20 mm T	43 ± 28	0.6 ± 0.3
Antag + 200 mm T	229 ± 39	1.6 ± 0.1

CONCLUDING REMARKS

While detailed clinical studies with potent agonists are well underway, preliminary human studies published to date have used much less potent antagonists (Gonzalez-Barcena *et al.*, 1977; Canales *et al.*, 1980). Studies of LHRH antagonist actions in the human male with the current generation of more potent antagonists are now being planned. With the most potent antagonists now available, doses in the milligram per day range are anticipated for human studies. Such studies will need to define the dose–response characteristics of antagonists as well as their duration of action. Subsequent studies in the male will be directed at determining the effects of chronic LHRH antagonist treatment on spermatogenesis. It is likely, based on our studies in the rat, that the combination of antagonist with testosterone supplementation to prevent symptoms of underandrogenization will result in enhanced suppression of spermatogenesis. Such synergism of antagonist and testosterone may allow lower doses of LHRH antagonist to produce complete suppression of spermatogenesis.

The challenge of producing an effective male contraceptive is one of the greatest in clinical research. Continued clinical investigation of newly developed LHRH antagonists holds great promise for the development of agents for effective suppression of spermatogenesis via inhibition of gonadotropin secretion.

References

Bhasin, S., Heber, D., Peterson, M., Steiner, B. and Swerdloff, R. S. (1984). Hormonal effects of GnRH agonists in the human male. II. Testosterone enhances GnRH agonist-induced inhibition of gonadotropins. *Clin. Endocrinol.* (In press)

Canales, E. S., Montvelinsky, Zárate, A., Kastin, A. J., Coy, D. H. and Schally, A. V. (1978). Suppressive effect of an inhibitory LHRH analog on the gonadotropin response of LHRH in normal women. *Int. J. Fertil.*, **25,** 190

Crowley, W. F., Beitins, I. Z., Vale, W., Kliman, B., Rivier, J., Rivier, C. and McArthur, J. W. (1980). The biologic activity of a potent analogue of gonadotropin-releasing hormone in normal and hypogonadotropic men. *N. Engl. J. Med.*, **302,** 1052

Gonzalez-Barcena, D., Kastin, A. J., Coy, D. H. and Schally, A. V. (1977). Suppression of gonadotropin release in man by an inhibitory analogue of LHRH. *Lancet*, **2,** 997

Happ, J., Hartmann, U., Weber, T., Cordes, U. and Beyer, J. (1978). Gonadotropin and testosterone secretion in normal human males after stimulation with gonadotropin-releasing hormone (GnRH) or potent GnRH analogs using different modes of application. *Fertil. Steril.*, **30,** 666

Heber, D. and Swerdloff,R. S. (1981). Gonadotropin-releasing hormone analog and testosterone synergistically inhibit spermatogenesis. *Endocrinology*, **108,** 2019

Heber, D., Dodson, R., Swerdloff, R. S., Channabasavaiah, K. and Stewart, J. M. (1982). Pituitary receptor site blockade by a gonadotropin-releasing hormone antagonist in vivo: mechanism of action. *Science*, **216,** 420

Heber, D., Swerdloff, R. S., Steiner, B. and Rajfer, J. (1983). The pituitary gland: primary site of action of gonadotropin-releasing hormone agonists in the human male. *Clin. Res.*, **31,** 24A

Hsueh, A. J. W. and Ling, N. C. (1979). Effect of an antagonistic analog of gonadotropin-releasing hormone upon granulosa cell function. *Life Sci.*, **25,** 1223

Linde, R. B., Doelle, G. C., Alexander, N. and Rabin, D. (1981). Reversible inhibition of testicular steroidogenesis and spermatogenesis by a potent gonadotropin releasing hormone agonist in normal men: an approach to the development of a male contraceptive. *N. Engl. J. Med.*, **305,** 663

Pelletier, G., Cusan, L., Auclair, P., Kelly, A., Desey, L. and Labrie, F. (1978). Inhibition of spermatogenesis in the rat by treatment with $DAla^6desGlyNH_2{}^{10}$LHRH ethylamide. *Endocrinology*, **103,** 641

Rivier, C., Rivier, J. and Vale, W. (1980). Antireproductive effects of a potent gonadotropin-releasing hormone antagonist in the male rat. *Science,* **210,** 93

Rivier, C., Rivier, J. and Vale, W. (1981). Effect of a potent GnRH antagonist and testosterone propionate on mating behavior and fertility in the male rat. *Endocrinology,* **108,** 1988

Sandow, J., von Rechenberg, W., Konig, W., Hahn, M., Jerzabeck, G. and Fraser, H. (1978). Physiological studies with highly active analogues of LHRH. In Voelter, W. and Gupta, D., (eds.) *Proceedings of the 2nd European Colloquium on Hypothalamic Hormones,* Tubingen, Germany, pp. 307–26. (Weinkein: Verlag Cheime)

Schally, A. V., Coy, D. H. and Arimura, A. (1971). Isolation and properties of the FSH and LH releasing hormone. *Biochem. Biophys. Res. Commun.,* **43,** 393

Vickery, B. H. (1981). Physiology and antifertility effects of LHRH and agonist analogs in male animals. In Zatuchni, G. I., Shelton, J. D. and Sciarra, J. J. (eds.) *LHRH Peptides as Female and Male Contraceptives,* pp. 275–290. (Philadelphia: Harper & Row)

SECTION III
EXTRAHYPOPHYSIAL PARAMETERS

13
Direct antigonadal actions of LHRH

P. B. C. JONES and A. J. W. HSUEH

Since pituitary gonadotropins are essential for normal gonadal functions and since hypothalamic LHRH was believed to act solely on the pituitary gland, treatment with high doses of LHRH or its agonists had been predicted to be a potential means for enhancing fertility. However, early studies using LHRH as an ovulation-inducing agent in anovulatory women have been only partially successful. Similarly, the early use of LHRH and LHRH agonists in the therapy of hypogonadotropic hypogonadism in men resulted in only limited success, and actual decreases in testicular steroidogenesis were reported.

The paradoxical inhibitory actions of LHRH and agonists have been well-documented in animal models (reviewed in Hsueh and Jones, 1981). In female rats, the long term administration of pharmacological doses of LHRH or potent LHRH agonists inhibits ovarian steroidogenesis, ovulation, ovum transport, ovum implantation, pregnancy, uterine growth and ovarian-dependent mammary tumorigenesis. Similarly, in male rats, long term administration of high doses of LHRH or LHRH agonists has been shown to inhibit testicular steroidogenesis, spermatogenesis, and growth of male accessory sex organ and some prostate tumors.

At least three possible mechanisms can be proposed to explain the paradoxical, inhibitory actions of LHRH and its agonists (Figure 13.1): (1) chronic stimulation of the anterior pituitary by high doses of LHRH or its agonists may desensitize the gonadotrophs to hypothalamic LHRH, resulting in decreased circulating gonadotropins and subsequent atrophy of reproductive organs, (2) treatment with pharmacological doses of LHRH or its agonists may stimulate the release of high levels of LH which, in turn, results in LH-induced desensitization of gonadal cells to subsequent LH action and (3) LHRH and its agonists may exert an extrapituitary, direct inhibitory action upon gonadal cells.

A possible extrapituitary action of an LHRH agonist was suggested by the demonstration of an inhibitory effect of this peptide on the hCG-stimulated augmentation of ovarian and uterine weights in immature hypophysectomized rats (Rippel and Johnson, 1976). We have used an ovarian primary cell culture to provide conclusive evidence of the direct inhibitory effect of LHRH and its agonists on ovarian granulosa cell functions *in vitro*.

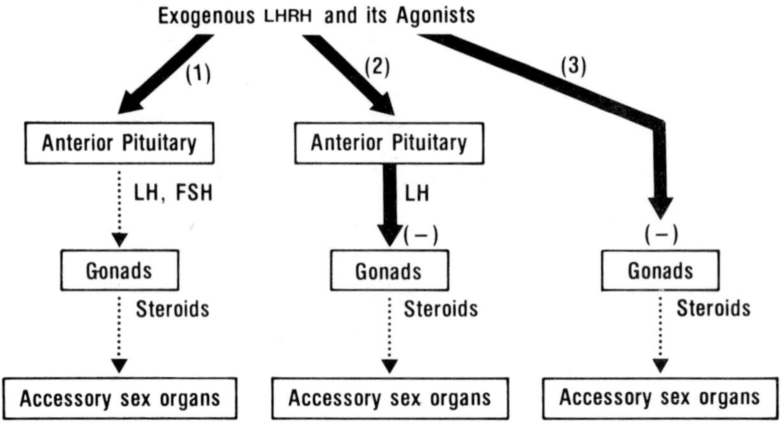

Figure 13.1 Three possible mechanisms involved in the paradoxical inhibition of gonadal functions by LHRH and its agonists. Dotted lines indicated decreased production of hormones. Heavy arrows indicate prolonged stimulation by pharmacological doses of hormones.

DIRECT MODULATION OF OVARIAN FUNCTIONS BY LHRH

Granulosa cells

Ovarian granulosa cells, obtained from preantral follicles of immature hypophysectomized rats, respond *in vitro* to follicle-stimulating hormone (FSH) with the production of estrogens and progestins. Concomitant treatment with LHRH or an LHRH agonist results in the inhibition of FSH-stimulated estrogen and progestin production (Hsueh and Erickson, 1979*b*; Hsueh and Ling, 1979; see Figure 13.2). LHRH inhibits FSH-stimulated estrogen and progestin production with ED_{50} values of 5×10^{-10} mol/l and 1.5×10^{-9} mol/l, respectively. Treatment with LHRH also inhibits the FSH-stimulated release of ^3H_2O from [1β–^{3}H] testosterone, indicating that LHRH inhibits gonadotropin-stimulated aromatase enzymes (Gore-Langton *et al.*, 1981).

The inhibition of FSH-stimulated steroidogenesis by LHRH can be blocked by concomitant treatment with an LHRH antagonist (Hsueh and Ling, 1979; Jones and Hsueh, 1981*b*). The counteractive effect of an LHRH antagonist on granulosa cell cultures treated with LHRH suggests that the actions of LHRH and its analogs are mediated through stereospecific recognition sites in the granulosa cells. Since the design of the LHRH analogs was based on their ability to modulate pituitary gonadotropin release, the stereospecificity of the ovarian recognition site may be similar to that of the pituitary LHRH receptors.

FSH stimulates LH and prolactin (PRL) receptor formation by cultured granulosa cells (reviewed in Hsueh *et al.*, 1983*a*). Concomitant treatment with LHRH or its agonists inhibits the FSH stimulation of LH and PRL receptor formation, and again the inhibitory effect of LHRH is blocked by an LHRH

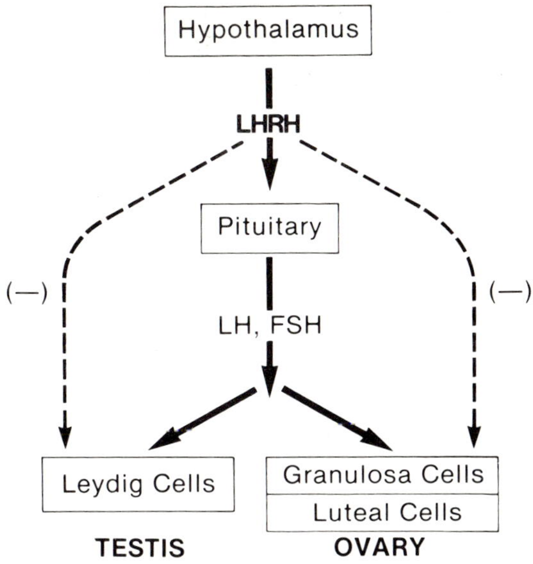

Figure 13.2 Diagrammatic representation of the direct inhibition of ovarian granulosa and luteal as well as testicular Leydig cell functions by LHRH.

antagonist (Hsueh and Ling, 1979; Hsueh *et al.*, 1980; Navickis *et al.*, 1982).

LHRH modulates various FSH-induced responses in granulosa cells from preantral follicles (Figure 13.3). In addition to the inhibitory effects of LHRH on FSH-stimulated steroidogenesis and receptor formation, LHRH inhibits FSH-stimulated cAMP formation (Clark *et al.*, 1980; Massicotte *et al.*, 1980). In contrast, LHRH enhances FSH-stimulated prostaglandin production (Clark *et al.*, 1980), and the FSH-stimulated increase in granulosa cell protein content (Jones and Hsueh, 1982*a*). LHRH has a biphasic effect on FSH-stimulated glycolysis – first enhancing, and then inhibiting, FSH action (Billig *et al.*, 1982). Furthermore, FSH induces a rise in the apparent cell membrane microviscosity in cultured granulosa cells and this action of FSH is inhibited by LHRH (Strulovici *et al.*, 1981).

The inhibitory effects of LHRH upon granulosa cells from preantral follicles are not limited to the interference with FSH actions. LHRH and its agonists inhibit the stimulation of steroidogenesis by cholera toxin, prostaglandin E_2 and cAMP analogs (Hsueh *et al.*, 1980; Jones and Hsueh, 1981*b*; Hillier *et al.*, 1981).

FSH treatment of cultured granulosa cells *in vitro* induces functional LH and PRL receptors and increases the responsiveness of granulosa cells to β_2-adrenergic agents (Hsueh *et al.*, 1983*a*). These FSH-treated granulosa cells acquire certain characteristics similar to those of luteal cells (Figure 13.4). Treatment of these granulosa-luteal cells with LH increases estrogen and progestin production (Wang *et al.*, 1981). In contrast, treatment with PRL or β_2-adrenergic agents stimulates progesterone production without affecting

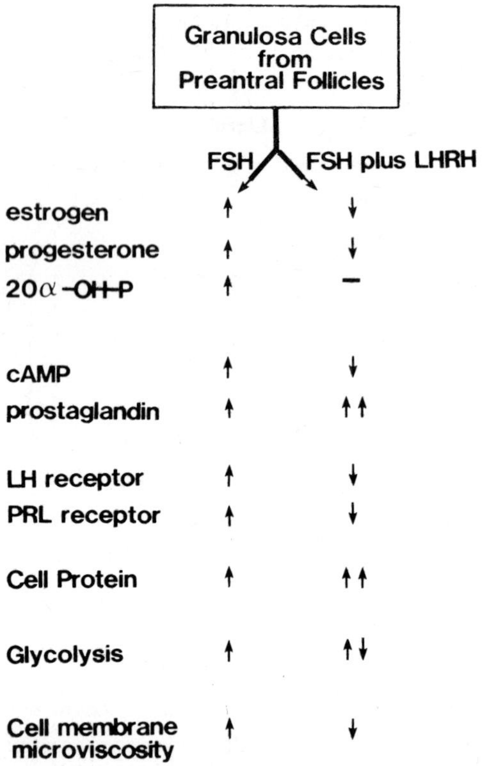

Figure 13.3 Direct regulation of diverse granulosa cell functions by LHRH and FSH *in vitro.*

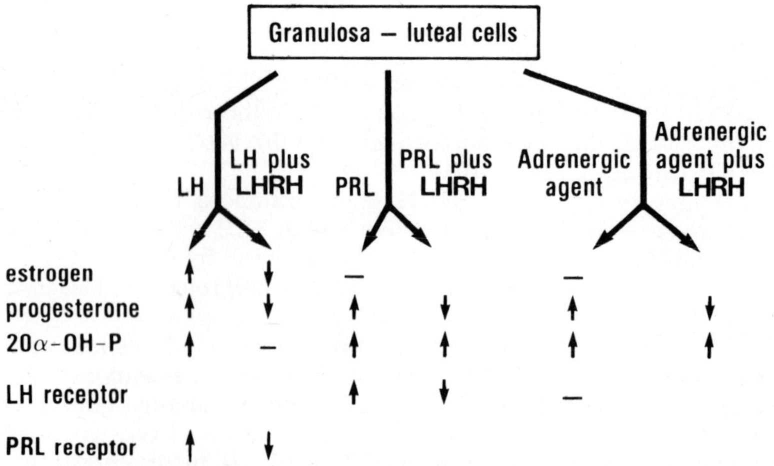

Figure 13.4 Direct regulation of ovarian steroidogenesis and gonadotropin receptor formation by LHRH in FSH-primed granulosa–luteal cells.

aromatase activity (Wang *et al.*, 1979; Adashi and Hsueh, 1981). Concomitant treatment with LHRH inhibits LH stimulation of estrogen production (Jones and Hsueh, 1981*b*). LHRH treatment also inhibits progesterone production stimulated by LH, PRL or β_2-adrenergic agents (Jones and Hsueh, 1981*b*; Jones *et al.*, 1982). Furthermore, PRL treatment increases LH receptor content, while LHRH treatment inhibits PRL action (Jones and Hsueh, 1981*b*). All of these inhibitory effects of LHRH are blocked by concomitant treatment with an LHRH antagonist.

The *in vitro* studies were extended to *in vivo* experiments using immature, hypophysectomized rats. Administration of high doses of LHRH or an LHRH agonist inhibits FSH-stimulated increases in ovarian weight, ovarian LH receptor content, and granulosa cell aromatase activity (Hsueh and Erickson, 1979*b*; Hsueh *et al.*, 1980). These inhibitory effects are blocked by *in vivo* treatment with an LHRH antagonist (Jones and Hsueh, 1981*b*). *In vivo* administration of LHRH or an LHRH agonist to hypophysectomized rats also inhibits hCG-stimulated ovarian growth (Rippel and Johnson, 1976; Mayer *et al.*, 1979). In hypophysectomized rats pretreated with pregnant mare's serum gonadotropin (PMSG) and hCG, LHRH agonist treatment decreases ovarian weight and ovarian LH/hCG receptor content (Arimura *et al.*, 1980). Ovarian LH and FSH receptors are also decreased, in a dose-dependent manner, by treatment of hypophysectomized rats with an LHRH agonist (Seguin *et al.*, 1981*b*).

Theca–interstitial cells

The direct inhibitory effect of LHRH on preovulatory follicles may not be restricted to ovarian granulosa cells. Whole cell dispersates of ovaries from immature rats respond to treatment with hCG, cholera toxin or 8-bromo-cAMP by the production of progesterone during a 3 h incubation period; preincubation of these cells with an LHRH agonist inhibits the action of the stimulatory agents (Reddy *et al.*, 1980). Since the stimulation of progesterone biosynthesis by granulosa cells (a cell type that is present in the whole ovarian dispersates) requires a latent period greater than 3 h, these data suggest a possible direct action of LHRH on ovarian theca or interstitial cells. LHRH also inhibits LH-stimulated androgen biosynthesis by whole ovarian dispersates during long term cultures; this inhibitory effect is blocked by an LHRH antagonist (Magoffin *et al.*, 1981). Thus, LHRH may act directly on ovarian interstitial and/or thecal cells.

Luteal cells

In vivo administration of LHRH or an LHRH agonist inhibits ovarian luteal functions in women, as well as in non-pregnant and pregnant animals (reviewed in Hsueh and Jones, 1981). The direct inhibition of luteal cell steroidogenesis by LHRH has been studied using short term incubations of rat luteal cells *in vitro*. Treatment with LHRH or an agonist inhibits luteal progesterone production stimulated by hCG, epinephrine (adrenaline) or LH

(Clayton *et al.*, 1979; Massicotte *et al.*, 1981; Harwood *et al.*, 1980*a*; Behrman *et al.*, 1980).

The extrapituitary inhibition of luteal functions by LHRH has also been demonstrated in hypophysectomized pregnant or pseudopregnant rats (Macdonald *et al.*, 1980; Harwood *et al.*, 1980*b*). The second half of pregnancy in rats is not dependent upon pituitary support, and hypophysectomy of female rats on day 11 or 12 of pregnancy does not result in abortion. This model was used to demonstrate that daily administration of LHRH or an agonist induces a dose-related increase in fetal resorption accompanied by decreased ovarian and adrenal weights, as well as depression of serum progesterone levels. The LHRH-induced inhibition of luteal progesterone production may be accompanied by decreased serum levels of rat placental lactogen (Bex and Corbin, 1981*b*). While these studies suggest that exogenous LHRH inhibits ovarian luteal functions *in vivo* by an extrapituitary mechanism, LHRH may also directly modulate placental functions as well (Vickery *et al.*, 1981).

The *in vivo* administration of LHRH or an LHRH agonist also antagonizes the action of exogenous luteotrophic hormones. Treatment with an LHRH agonist inhibits the luteotropic effects of PRL in hypophysectomized, nonpregnant rats (Jones and Hsueh, 1980; Macdonald *et al.*, 1980). In the rhesus monkey, hCG treatment increases serum progesterone levels and extends the cycle length, whereas administration of an LHRH agonist inhibits hCG action by shortening cycle length and decreasing serum progesterone (Vickery and McRae, 1980). The inhibition of hCG action by the LHRH agonist suggests a possible direct action of the LHRH agonist on luteal functions in primates.

MECHANISMS OF LHRH ACTION IN THE OVARY

LHRH inhibits hormone-stimulated ovarian steroidogenesis (estrogen and progesterone production) and gonadotropin (LH and PRL) receptor formation. These actions of LHRH are not the results of a general negative effect on cellular metabolism. Treatment of granulosa cells with LHRH alone enhances glycolysis (Billig *et al.*, 1982), increases cellular protein content (Jones and Hsueh, 1982*a*), stimulates progesterone production (Jones and Hsueh, 1982*a,b*) increases prostaglandin synthesis (Clark *et al.*, 1980), and increases phosphatidylinositol production (Davis *et al.*, 1982). LHRH, by itself, also stimulates oocyte maturation *in vitro* (Hillensjö and LeMaire, 1980) and induces ovulation in hypophysectomized rats (Ekholm *et al.*, 1981; Corbin and Bex, 1981).

Using radiolabeled LHRH agonists, specific high affinity ($K_D \sim 10^{-10}$ mol/l) binding sites have been demonstrated in granulosa (Jones *et al.*, 1980; Pieper *et al.*, 1981) and luteal cells (Clayton *et al.*, 1979; Harwood *et al.*, 1980*a,b*; Pieper *et al.*, 1981). LHRH receptors are widely distributed in luteal, thecal, and granulosa cells at all states of cellular differentation. Furthermore, LHRH binding sites have been characterized in granulosa cells using photoaffinity and fluorescence labeling methods (Hazum and Nimrod, 1982).

The rat granulosa cell culture system was used to examine the mechanism by which LHRH inhibits the FSH stimulation of progesterone production. LHRH-induced decreases in progesterone production may result from the inhibition of progesterone biosynthesis and/or the stimulation of the conversion of progesterone to its inactive metabolites.

FSH treatment *in vitro* markedly stimulates the activity of 3β-hydroxysteroid dehydrogenase (3β-HSD), which converts the precursor pregnenolone to progesterone (Jones and Hsueh, 1982*a*; Figure 13.5). FSH treatment also increases the activity of 20α-hydroxysteroid dehydrogenase (20α-HSD), which metabolizes progesterone to its inactive metabolite, 20α-hydroxypregn-4-en-3-one (20α-dihydroprogesterone). Concomitant treatment with LHRH partially inhibits the stimulatory effect of FSH on 3β-HSD activity, but further enhances the FSH stimulation of 20α-HSD activity – thereby both decreasing the conversion of pregnenolone to progesterone and increasing the breakdown of progesterone. The regulation of these two enzymes by LHRH is associated with changes in the maximal velocities of these enzymes with no effect on their substrate affinities. Furthermore, measurement of pregnenolone biosynthesis in granulosa cells treated with cyanoketone (an inhibitor of 3β-HSD activity) shows that FSH stimulates pregnenolone production and LHRH inhibits FSH action, suggesting that LHRH may affect additional steroidogenic enzymes (such as side chain cleavage enzymes) before pregnenolone production (Jones and Hsueh,

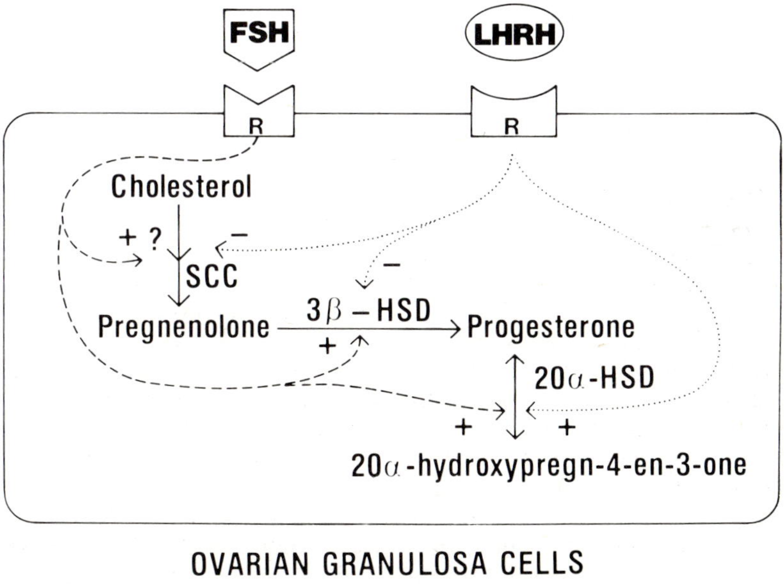

Figure 13.5 Mechanism of LHRH action in the granulosa cells: Modulation of steroidogenic enzymes by FSH and LHRH. SCC = side chain cleavage enzymes; 3β-HSD = 3β-hydroxysteroid dehydrogenase; 20α-HSD = 20α-hydroxysteroid dehydrogenase; 20α-hydroxypregn-4-en-3-one = 20α-dihydroprogesterone.

1982*b*). The major effects of LHRH are probably the decreased pregnenolone production coupled with the increased conversion of progesterone to 20α-dihydroprogesterone. Modulation of these steroidogenic enzymes by LHRH is blocked by concomitant treatment with LHRH antagonists. This suggests the involvement of stereospecific LHRH recognition sites in these processes.

In cultured granulosa cells, an inhibitory effect of LHRH on the FSH stimulation of cAMP production was suggested by short term (15 min) incubation of granulosa cells obtained from PMSG-treated rats (Clark *et al.*, 1980). Similarly, an LHRH agonist inhibits FSH-stimulated cAMP production in cultured porcine granulosa cells by 30–50 % (Massicotte *et al.*, 1980). Longer term (up to 2 days) studies of rat granulosa cells indicate that LHRH treatment inhibits FSH-stimulated cAMP production by approximately 80 %. This inhibitory effect of LHRH may be due to an inhibition of adenyl cyclase activity, as well as a stimulation of extracellular phosphodiesterase activity (Knecht and Catt, 1981). While the latter effect would result in decreased concentrations of cAMP in the culture medium, it is doubtful that a stimulation of extracellular phosphodiesterase activity would affect intracellular cAMP metabolism.

Cyclic AMP analogs stimulate progesterone production by cultured granulosa cells and this stimulatory effect is inhibited by LHRH or an agonist (Hillier *et al.*, 1981). The LHRH inhibition of 8-bromo-cAMP stimulated progesterone production is characterized by a decrease in progesterone and an increase in 20α-dihydroprogesterone production. In contrast, pregnenolone levels are not decreased (Jones and Hsueh, 1982*b*). This suggests that LHRH inhibits 8-bromo-cAMP action by stimulating 20α-HSD activity. LHRH, alone, stimulates 20α-HSD activity in granulosa cells (Jones and Hsueh, 1981*a*, *c*) and this effect appears to be mediated through a cAMP-independent pathway. Thus, at least one action of LHRH appears to involve site(s) independent of gonadotropin-stimulated cAMP production. The inhibition of FSH-stimulated progesterone production may involve two actions of LHRH: (1) an inhibition of FSH-stimulated adenyl cyclase, resulting in decreased pregnenolone production (LHRH does not inhibit pregnenolone production stimulated by a cAMP analog), and (2) a stimulation of 20α-HSD activity.

FSH-primed granulosa-luteal cells were used to examine the LHRH inhibition of progesterone production stimulated by PRL, a β_2-adrenergic agonist, or LH/hCG. Both PRL and the β_2-adrenergic agonist stimulate progesterone production by increasing pregnenolone production and 3β-HSD activity as well as by decreasing 20α-HSD activity (Jones *et al.*, 1982). The inhibitory effect of LHRH on PRL- or β_2-adrenergic agonist-stimulated progesterone production appears to result from a preferential increase in 20α-HSD activity (Figure 13.6). In contrast, hCG stimulates progesterone production in these cells by increasing pregnenolone production and 3β-HSD activity, and in this case LHRH inhibits hCG action through a preferential inhibition of pregnenolone production (Figure 13.7).

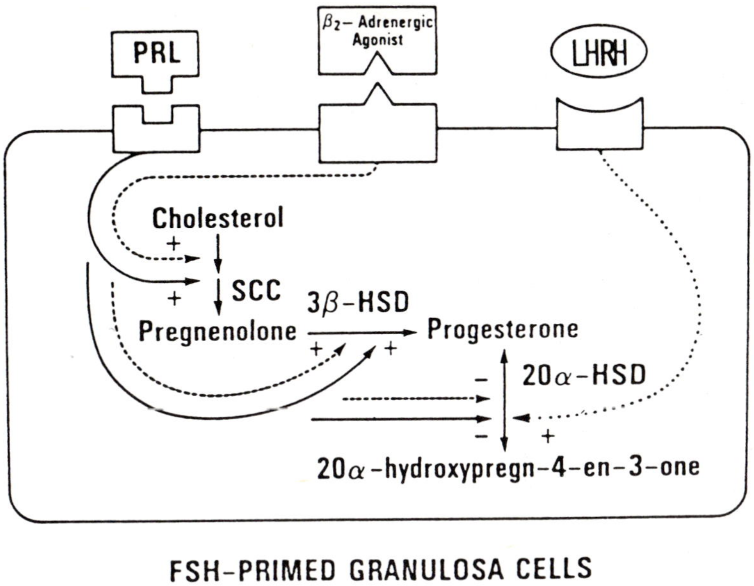

Figure 13.6 Regulation of steroidogenic enzymes by PRL and β_2-adrenergic agonist in FSH-primed granulosa cells: modulation by LHRH. For abbreviations, see Figure 13.5 legend.

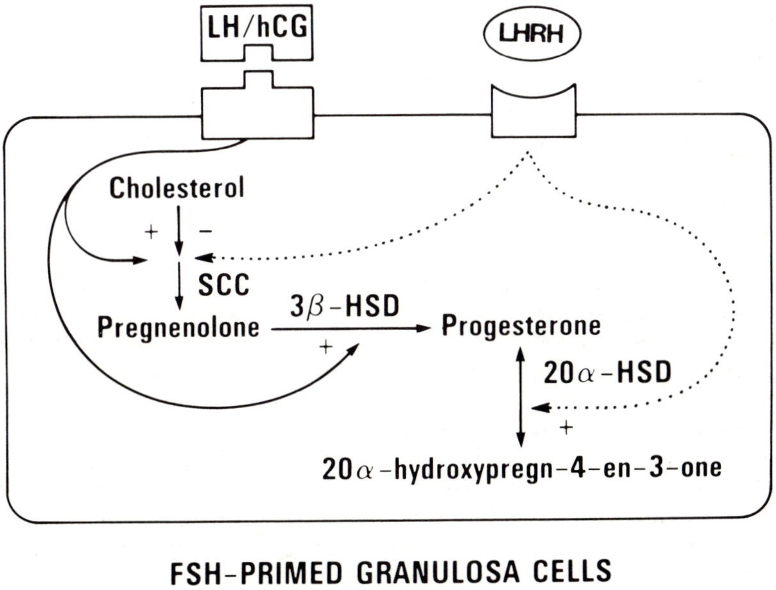

Figure 13.7 Regulation of steroidogenic enzymes by LH/hCG in FSH-primed granulosa cells: modulation by LHRH. For abbreviations, see Figure 13.5 legend.

DIRECT INHIBITORY EFFECTS OF LHRH ON TESTICULAR FUNCTIONS

Treatment with hCG substantially stimulates androgen production in cultured testicular cells obtained from hypophysectomized, immature or adult rats. Concomitant treatment with LHRH or an LHRH agonist results in a dose-dependent inhibition of androgen production (Hsueh *et al.*, 1981; Hsueh, 1982). Furthermore, the inhibitory effect of LHRH is blocked by concomitant treatment with a potent LHRH antagonist (Hsueh, 1982).

The adult testis culture system contains both Leydig and Sertoli cells, which are known to contain LH and FSH receptors, respectively. Since LHRH or its agonists inhibit testosterone production maintained by hCG (Hsueh, 1982) the most likely site of action of LHRH in these cultures is at the Leydig cells (Hunter *et al.*, 1982). Primary cultures of purified Sertoli cells have also been used to study LHRH action. Treatment with high doses of LHRH or an agonist does not interfere with aromatase activity or the synthesis of plasminogen activator stimulated by FSH, cholera toxin or a cAMP analog (Gore-Langton *et al.*, 1981). In contrast, treatment with an LHRH agonist inhibits the FSH stimulation of androgen binding protein secretion (Rich and Bardin, 1981).

An extrapituitary inhibitory effect of LHRH on testicular functions has been observed in hypophysectomized rats. Treatment with high doses of LHRH or an LHRH agonist for 5 days in immature, hypophysectomized male rats decreases the FSH maintenance of testis weight and Leydig cell androgen biosynthesis (Hsueh and Erickson, 1979*a*). Moreover, treatment with FSH or PRL and growth hormone in hypophysectomized immature or adult rats maintains testis weight, LH receptor content, and steroidogenic responsiveness, whereas concomitant treatment with LHRH or an agonist inhibits the action of the pituitary hormones (Bambino *et al.*, 1980). This decrease in testicular steroidogenesis is associated with a decrease in 17α-hydroxylase activity.

The *in vivo* administration of LHRH to hypophysectomized male rats decreases testicular LH (Hsueh and Erickson, 1979*a*; Clayton *et al.*, 1980; Labrie *et al.*, 1980; Séguin *et al.*, 1981*a*, *b*) and PRL (Clayton *et al.*, 1980; Séguin *et al.*, 1981*a*) receptor contents. Furthermore, treatment with LHRH agonists in hypophysectomized and adrenalectomized rats decreases testicular LH receptor content, ruling out the possible role of the adrenal gland in mediating the inhibitory action of LHRH (Clayton *et al.*, 1980).

The mechanism of action of LHRH on testicular Leydig cells has also been studied (Figure 13.8). Primary cultures of adult testicular cells were used to examine the mechanism of the LHRH inhibition of hCG-stimulated testosterone production. The inhibitory effect of LHRH on testicular androgen production appears to be the result of decreases in the activities of 17α-hydroxylase and 17–20 desmolase (Hsueh *et al.*, 1983*b*). This is not accompanied by decreases in hCG-stimulated cAMP production in LHRH-treated cells (unpublished data). Furthermore, LHRH inhibits testosterone production stimulated by a cAMP analog, suggesting that LHRH may act at steps distal to cAMP synthesis (Hsueh, 1982; Hsueh *et al.*, 1983*b*). These

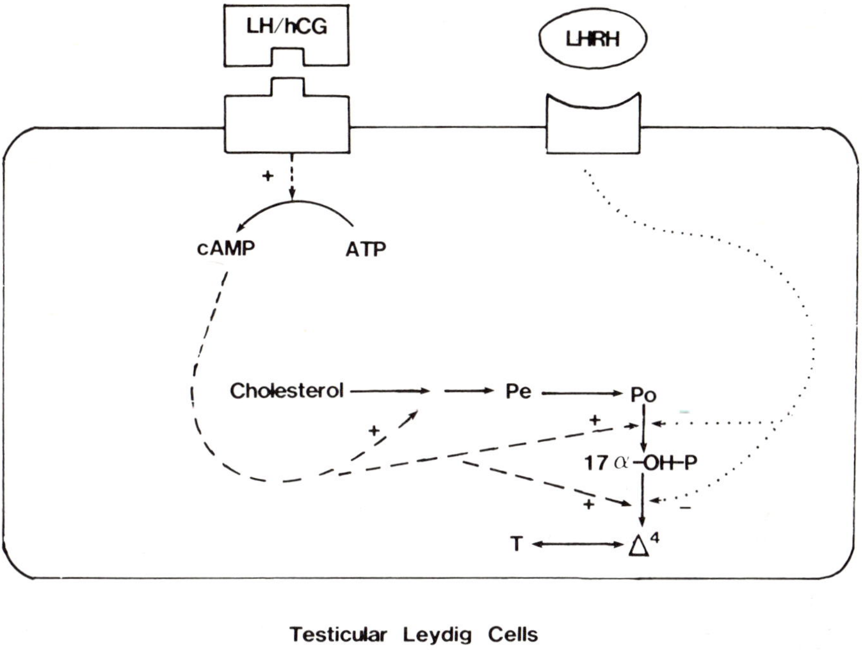

Figure 13.8 Regulation of testicular Leydig cell androgen biosynthesis by LH/hCG and LHRH. Pe = pregnenolone; Po = progesterone; 17α-OH-P = 17α-hydroxyprogesterone; Δ^4 = androstenedione; T = testosterone.

inhibitory effects of LHRH are believed to be mediated by the specific, high affinity ($K_D \sim 10^{-10}$ mol/l) LHRH binding sites which have been demonstrated in testicular Leydig, but not Sertoli, cells (Clayton *et al.*, 1980; Bourne *et al.*, 1980). In summary, LHRH and its agonists stimulate pituitary releases of LH and FSH which, in turn, enhance gonadal functions (Figure 13.2). In addition, administration of pharmacological doses of LHRH and its agonists exerts direct, extrapituitary actions by blocking estrogen and progesterone production in ovarian granulosa cells as well as by inhibiting testosterone production in testicular Leydig cells (Figure 13.2).

EXTRAPITUITARY ACTIONS OF LHRH: MULTIPLE TARGET ORGANS AND SPECIES VARIATION

Although the rat model has been used extensively to examine the direct effects of LHRH on gonadal functions, the direct gonadal action of LHRH is not limited to this species (Table 13.1). *In vitro* treatment with LHRH or its agonists modulates steroidogenesis in ovarian cells from woman (Lamberts *et al.*, 1982; Tureck *et al.*, 1982), rabbit (Koos *et al.*, 1982), pig (Massicotte *et al.*, 1980) and chicken (Hertelendy *et al.*, 1981). Additionally, LHRH treatment stimulates ovulation in perfused rabbit ovaries (Koos *et al.*, 1982). While there

Table 13.1 Direct *in vitro* effects of LHRH on gonadal functions: species specificity

	Animal species						
LHRH action	*Human*	*Rat*	*Mouse*	*Rabbit*	*Pig*	*Chicken*	*Frog*
Modulation of ovarian steroidogenesis	Yes	Yes	No	Yes	Yes	Yes	?
Stimulation of oocyte maturation/ovulation	?	Yes	?	Yes	?	?	?
Modulation of testicular steroidogenesis	?	Yes	No	?	?	?	Yes

are limited data on the species specificity of direct LHRH action on testicular steroidogenesis, LHRH treatment *in vitro* increases steroidogenesis in frog testes (Segal and Adejuwon, 1979). In contrast, the mouse appears to be resistant to the direct modulatory effects of LHRH in both females and males (Bex *et al.*, 1982; Hunter *et al.*, 1982; Sundaram and Wang, 1982).

In addition to their actions on the gonads, LHRH and its agonists also directly affect the functions of many other organs through extrapituitary actions (Table 13.2). LHRH treatment modulates the function of both female and male accessory sex organs, the placenta, fat cells and frog sympathetic

Table 13.2 Extrapituitary actions of LHRH and the presence of LHRH-like 'receptors'[a] outside the central nervous system

	LHRH effects	*LHRH 'receptors'*
(1) Ovary		
(a) Granulosa cells	Yes	Yes
(b) Luteal cells	Yes	Yes
(c) Theca and/or interstitial cells	Yes	Yes
(d) Oocytes	Yes	?
(2) Testis		
(a) Leydig cells	Yes	Yes
(b) Sertoli cells	Yes	No
(3) Male accessory sex organs	Yes	?
(4) Female accessory sex organs	Yes	?
(5) Placenta	Yes	Yes
(6) Sympathetic ganglia (frog)	Yes	Yes
(7) Adrenal	?	Yes
(8) Fat cells	Yes	?
(9) Kidney	Yes	?

[a] The use of the term 'receptor' here designates tissues in which [^{125}I]-LHRH agonist binding has been demonstrated or the observed direct actions of LHRH are blocked by LHRH antagonists

ganglia (reviewed in Hsueh and Jones, 1981). Additionally, LHRH exerts an antiandrogenic action in the mouse kidney (Lecomte *et al.*, 1982). Thus, the extrapituitary actions of LHRH are widespread.

LHRH AND OTHER REGULATORY PEPTIDES AS POTENTIAL GONADAL HORMONES

LHRH is different from most classical hormones in that the circulation of this neuropeptide is restricted to the brain portal vessel. While hypothalamic LHRH reaches sufficient concentrations in the brain portal circulation to interact effectively with pituitary LHRH receptors, the peripheral concentration of hypothalamic LHRH is believed to be lower than 10^{-11} mol/l. Thus, the hypothalamic neuropeptide is not present in the systemic circulation in sufficient concentration to interact with extrapituitary binding sites. While the extrapituitary actions of LHRH and its agonists on gonadal functions may represent an evolutionary vestigial phenomenon, recent evidence indicates that LHRH-like peptides are secreted by extrahypothalamic tissues.

The presence of LHRH-like peptides has been demonstrated in testicular, placental, mammary and pancreatic tissues (reviewed in Hsueh and Jones, 1981). LHRH-like peptides have also been found in rat testicular tissue (Sharpe and Fraser, 1980; Dutlow and Millar, 1981; Paull *et al.*, 1981) and placental tissues from women (Gibbons *et al.*, 1975; Khodr and Siler-Khodr, 1980; Lee *et al.*, 1981), rats (Gautron *et al.*, 1981) and rabbits (Nowak and Wiseman, 1982). Thus, LHRH or LHRH-like peptides may play an important paracrine role in the regulation of various extrapituitary organs.

The direct inhibitory actions of LHRH and its agonists on gonadal functions may explain, at least partially, the paradoxical inhibitory effect of these peptides on various male and female reproductive functions. Subsequent demonstration of LHRH receptors and LHRH-like peptides in the gonads further raises questions regarding a paracrine control role of this and other regulatory peptides in the gonads. Future studies on the intragonadal role of various regulatory peptides on gonadal development should afford important information regarding the maturation of ovarian follicles and testicular seminiferous tubules.

Acknowledgements

This work was supported by National Institutes of Health Research Grant HD-14084 and Program Project Grant HD-12303. A.J.W.H. is the recipient of Research Career Development Award HD-00375.

References

Adashi, E. Y. and Hsueh, A. J. W. (1981). Stimulation of β_2-adrenergic responsiveness by follicle-stimulating hormone in rat granulosa cells *in vitro*. *Endocrinology*, **108**, 2170

Arimura, A., Serafini, P., Talbot, S. and Schally, A. V. (1979). Reduction of testicular luteinizing hormone/human chorionic gonadotropin receptors by [D-Trp[6]]-luteinizing hormone releasing hormone in hypophysectomized rats. *Biochem. Biophys. Res. Commun.*, **90,** 687

Bambino, T. H., Schreiber, J. R. and Hsueh, A. J. W. (1980). Gonadotropin-releasing hormone and its agonist inhibit testicular luteinizing hormone receptor and steroidogenesis in immature and adult hypophysectomized rats. *Endocrinology*, **107,** 908

Behrman, H. R., Preston, S. L. and Hall, A. K. (1980). Cellular mechanism of the anti-gonadotropic action of luteinizing hormone-releasing hormone in the corpus luteum. *Endocrinology*, **107,** 656

Bex, F. J. and Corbin, A. (1981*b*). Luteinizing hormone-releasing hormone (LHRH) and LHRH agonist termination of pregnancy in hypophysectomized rats: extrapituitary site of action. *Endocrinology*, **108,** 273

Bex, F. J., Corbin, A. and France, E. (1982). Resistance of the mouse to the antifertility effects of LHRH agonists. *Life Sci.*, **30,** 1263

Billig, H., Magnusson, C., Ekholm, C. and Hillensjo, T. (1982). Biphasic effect of a GnRH agonist on glycolysis in cultured rat granulosa cells. *Biol. Reprod.*, **26**(Suppl.), 152A

Bourne, G. A., Regiani, S., Payne, A. H. and Marshall, J. C. (1980). Testicular GnRH receptors – characterization and localization on interstitial tissue. *J. Clin. Endocrinol. Metab.*, **51,** 407

Clark, M. R., Thibier, C., Marsh, J. M. and LeMaire, W. J. (1980). Stimulation of prostaglandin accumulation by luteinizing hormone-releasing hormone (LHRH) and LHRH analogs in rat granulosa cells in vitro. *Endocrinology*, **107,** 17

Clayton, R. N., Harwood, J. P. and Catt, K. J. (1979). Gonadotropin-releasing hormone analogue binds to luteal cells and inhibits progesterone production. *Nature* (*Lond.*), **282,** 90

Clayton, R. N., Katikeneni, M., Chan, V., Dufau, M. L. and Catt, K. J. (1980). Direct inhibition of testicular function by gonadotropin-releasing hormone: mediation by specific gonadotropin-releasing hormone receptors in interstitial cells. *Proc. Natl. Acad. Sci. USA*, **77,** 4459

Corbin, A. and Bex, F. J. (1981). Luteinizing hormone releasing hormone agonists induce ovulation in hypophysectomized proestrous rats: direct ovarian effect. *Life Sci.*, **29,** 185

Davis, J. S., Farese, R. V. and Clark, M. R. (1982). LH and GnRH acutely increase phosphatidylinositol levels in rat granulosa cells. *Biol. Reprod.*, **26** (Suppl.), 41A

Dutlow, C. M. and Millar, R. P. (1981). Rat testis immunoreactive LH-RH differs structurally from hypothalamic LH-RH. *Biochem. Biophys. Res. Commun.*, **101,** 486

Ekholm, C, Hillensjo, T. and Isaksson, O. (1981) Gonadotropin-releasing hormone agonists stimulate oocyte meiosis and ovulation in hypophysectomized rats. *Endocrinology*, **108,** 2022

Gautron, J. P., Pattou, E. and Kordon, C. (1981). Occurrence of higher molecular forms of LHRH in fractionated extracts from rat hypothalamus, cortex, and placenta. *Mol. Cell. Endocrinol.*, **24,** 1

Gibbons, J. M., Mitnick, M. and Chieffo, V. (1975). In vitro biosynthesis of TSH- and LH-releasing factors by the human placenta. *Am. J. Obstet. Gynecol.*, **121,** 127

Gore-Langton, R. E., Lacroix, M. and Dorrington, J. H. (1981). Differential effects of luteinizing hormone-releasing hormone on follicle-stimulating hormone-dependent responses in rat granulosa cells and Sertoli cells in vitro. *Endocrinology*, **108,** 812

Harwood, J. P., Clayton, R. N. and Catt, K. J. (1980*a*). Ovarian gonadotropin-releasing hormone receptors. I. Properties and inhibition of luteal cell function. *Endocrinology*, **107,** 407

Harwood, J. P., Clayton, R. N., Chen, T. T., Knox, G. and Catt, K. J. (1980*b*). Ovarian gonadotropin-releasing hormone receptors. II. Regulation and effects on ovarian development. *Endocrinology*, **107,** 414

Hazum, E. and Nimrod, A. (1982). Photoaffinity labeling and fluorescence distribution studies of gonadotropin-releasing hormone receptors in ovarian granulosa cells. *Proc. Natl. Acad. Sci. USA*, **79,** 1747

Hertelendy, R., Linter, F. and Takáts, A. (1981). Paradoxical effects of GnRH on LH-induced progesterone production in avian granulosa cells. *Biol. Reprod.*, **24** (Suppl.), 72A

Hillensjö, T. and LeMaire, W. J. (1980). Gonadotropin-releasing hormone agonists stimulate meiotic maturation of follicle-enclosed rat oocytes in vitro. *Nature* (*Lond.*), **287,** 145

Hillier, S. G., Reichert, L. E. and van Hall, E. V. (1981). Modulation of FSH-controlled steroidogenesis in rat granulosa cells: direct effects of LHRH and ICI-118630. *Mol. Cell. Endocrinol.*, **23,** 193

Hsueh, A. J. W. (1982). Direct effects of gonadotropin-releasing hormone on testicular Leydig cell functions. *Ann. NY Acad. Sci.*, **383,** 249

Hsueh, A. J. W. and Erickson, G. F. (1979*a*). Extra-pituitary inhibition of testicular function by luteinizing hormone releasing hormone. *Nature (Lond.)*, **281,** 66

Hsueh, A. J. W. and Erickson, G. F. (1979*b*). Extrapituitary action of gonadotropin releasing hormone: Direct inhibition of ovarian steroidogenesis. *Science*, **204,** 854

Hsueh, A. J. W. and Ling, N. C. (1979). Effect of an antagonistic analog of gonadotropin-releasing hormone upon ovarian granulosa cell function. *Life Sci.*, **25,** 1223

Hsueh, A. J. W., Wang, C. and Erickson, G. F. (1980). Direct inhibitory effect of gonadotropin-releasing hormone upon follicle-stimulating hormone induction of luteinizing hormone receptors and aromatase activity in rat granulosa cells. *Endocrinology*, **106,** 1697

Hsueh, A. J. W. and Jones, P. B. C. (1981). Extrapituitary actions of gonadotropin-releasing hormone. *Endocr. Rev.*, **2,** 437

Hsueh, A. J. W., Schreiber, J. R. and Erickson, G. F. (1981). Inhibitory effect of gonadotropin-releasing hormone upon cultured testicular cells. *Mol. Cell. Endocrinol.*, **21,** 43

Hsueh, A. J. W., Jones, P. B. C., Adashi, E. Y., Wang, C., Zhuang, L. Z. and Welsh, T. H. Jr. (1983*a*). Intraovarian mechanisms in the hormonal control of granulosa cell differentiation. *J. Reprod. Fertil.*, **69,** 325

Hsueh, A. J. W., Bambino, T. H., Zhuang, L. Z., Welsh, T. H. Jr. and Ling, N. C. (1983*b*). Mechanism of the direct action of gonadotropin-releasing hormone and its antagonist on androgen biosynthesis by cultured rat testicular cells. *Endocrinology*, **112,** 1653

Hunter, M. G., Sullivan, M. H. F., Dix, C. J., Aldred, L. F. and Cooke, B. A. (1982). Stimulation and inhibition by LHRH analogues of cultured rat Leydig cell function and lack of effect on mouse Leydig cells. *Mol. Cell. Endocrinol.*, **27,** 31

Jones, P. B. C. and Hsueh, A. J. W. (1980). Direct inhibitory effect of gonadotropin-releasing hormone upon luteal luteinizing hormone receptor and steroidogenesis in hypophysectomized rats. *Endocrinology*, **107,** 1930

Jones, P. B. C., Conn, P. M., Marian, J. and Hsueh, A. J. W. (1980). Binding of gonadotropin-releasing hormone agonist to rat ovarian granulosa cells. *Life Sci.*, **27,** 2125

Jones, P. B. C. and Hsueh, A. J. W. (1981*a*). Direct stimulation of ovarian progesterone metabolizing enzyme by gonadotropin-releasing hormone in cultured granulosa cells. *J. Biol. Chem.*, **256,** 1248

Jones, P. B. C. and Hsueh, A. J. W. (1981*b*). Direct effects of gonadotropin-releasing hormone and its antagonist upon ovarian functions stimulated by FSH, prolactin and LH. *Biol. Reprod.*, **24,** 747

Jones, P. B. C. and Hsueh, A. J. W. (1981*c*). Regulation of ovarian 20α-hydroxysteroid dehydrogenase by gonadotropin-releasing hormone and its antagonist in vitro and in vivo. *J. Steroid Biochem.*, **14,** 1169

Jones, P. B. C. and Hsueh, A. J. W. (1982*a*). Regulation of ovarian 3β-hydroxysteroid dehydrogenase by GnRH and follicle-stimulating hormone in cultured rat granulosa cells. *Endocrinology*, **110,** 1663

Jones, P. B. C. and Hsueh, A. J. W. (1982*b*). Pregnenolone biosynthesis by cultured rat granulosa cells: modulation by follicle-stimulating hormone and gonadotropin-releasing hormone. *Endocrinology*, **111,** 713

Jones, P. B. C., Fabics, C. and Hsueh, A. J. W. (1982). Mechanism of the regulation of progesterone biosynthesis by prolactin (PRL) and β_2-adrenergic agents in cultured rat granulosa cells: antagonistic effect of gonadotropin-releasing hormone (GnRH). *Biol. Reprod.*, **26** (Suppl.), 43A

Khodr, G. S and Siler-Khodr, T. M. (1980). Placental luteinizing hormone-releasing factor and its synthesis. *Science*, **207,** 315

Knecht, M. and Catt, K. J. (1981). Gonadotropin-releasing hormone: regulation of adenosine-3′:5′-cyclic monophosphate in ovarian granulosa cells. *Science*, **214,** 1346

Koos, R. D., Ahrén, K. E. B., Janson, P. O. and Lemaire, W. J. (1982). Effect of a GnRH agonist on the rabbit ovary perfused in vitro. *Endocrinology*, **110** (Suppl.), 178A

Labrie, F., Bélanger, A., Cusan, L., Séguin, C., Pelletier, G., Kelly, P. A., Reeves, J. J., Lefebvre, F.-A., Lemay, A., Gourdeau, Y. and Raynaud, J.-P. (1980). Antifertility effects of LHRH agonists in the male. *J. Androl.*, **1,** 209

Lamberts, S. W. J., Timmers, J. M., Oosterom, R., Verleun, T., Rommerts, F. G. and De Jong, F. H. (1982). Testosterone secretion by cultured arrhenoblastoma cells: suppression by a luteinizing hormone-releasing hormone agonist. *J. Clin. Endocrinol. Metab.*, **54,** 450

Lee, J.-N., Seppälä, M. and Chard, T. (1981). Characterization of placental luteinizing hormone-releasing factor-like material. *Acta Endocrinol.*, **96,** 394

Lecomte, P., Wang, N.-G., Sundaram, K., Rivier, J., Vale, W. and Bardin, C. W. (1982). The antiandrogenic action of gonadotropin-releasing hormone and its agonists on the mouse kidney. *Endocrinology,* **110,** 1

Macdonald, G. J., Greeley, L. K. and Beattie, C. W. (1980). Cessation of progesterone secretion by LH-RH in hypophysectomized pregnant and hypophysectomized, prolactin injected pseudopregnant rats. *Int. J. Fertil.*, **25,** 198

Magoffin, D. A., Reynolds, D. S. and Erickson, G. F. (1981). Direct inhibitory effect of GnRH on androgen secretion by ovarian interstitial cells. *Endocrinology,* **109,** 661

Massicotte, J., Veilleux, R., Lavoie, M. and Labrie, F. (1980). An LHRH agonist inhibits FSH-induced cyclic AMP accumulation and steroidogenesis in porcine granulosa cells in culture. *Biochem. Biophys. Res. Commun.*, **94,** 1362

Massicotte, J., Borgus, J.-P., Lachance, R. and Labrie, F. (1981). Inhibition of hCG-induced cyclic AMP accumulation and steroidogenesis in rat luteal cells by an LHRH agonist. *J. Steroid Biochem.*, **14,** 239

Mayer, M. R., Tarnovsky, G. K. and Reeves, J. J. (1979). Ovarian growth and uptake of iodinated D-Leu^6-des-Gly,NH_2^{10}-LHRH ethylamide in hCG treated rats. *Proc. Soc. Exp. Biol. Med.*, **161,** 216

Navickis, R. J., Jones, P. B. C. and Hsueh, A. J. W. (1982). Modulation of prolactin receptors in cultured rat granulosa cells by FSH, LH, and GnRH. *Mol. Cell. Endocrinol.*, **27,** 77

Nowak, R. and Wiseman, B. (1982). Secretion of a GnRH-like factor by the rabbit fetal placenta. *Biol. Reprod.*, **26** (Suppl.), 76A

Paull, W. K., Turkelson, C. M., Thomas, C. R. and Arimura, A. (1981). Immunohistochemical demonstration of a testicular substance related to luteinizing hormone-releasing hormone. *Science,* **213,** 1263

Pieper, D. R., Richards, J. S. and Marshall, J. C. (1981). Ovarian gonadotropin-releasing hormone (GnRH) receptors: characterization, distribution, and induction by GnRH. *Endocrinology,* **108,** 1148

Reddy, P. V., Azhar, S. and Mennon, K. M. J. (1980). Multiple inhibitory actions of luteinizing hormone-releasing hormone agonist on luteinizing hormone/human chorionic gonadotropin receptor-mediated ovarian responses. *Endocrinology,* **107,** 930

Rich, K. A. and Bardin, C. W. (1981). Direct inhibitory effect of a GnRH agonist on secretion of androgen binding protein (ABP) from Sertoli cells in primary culture. *Biol. Reprod.*, **24** (Suppl.), 133A

Rippel, R. H. and Johnson, E. S. (1976). Inhibition of hCG-induced ovarian and uterine weight augmentation in the immature rat by analogs of GnRH. *Proc. Soc. Exp. Biol. Med.*, **152,** 432

Segal, S. J. and Adejuwon, C. A. (1979). Direct effect of LHRH on testicular steroidogenesis in Rana pipiens. *Biol. Bull.*, **157,** 393

Séguin, C., Bélanger, A., Cusan, L., Pelletier, G., Reeves, J. J., Lefebvre, F.-A., Kelly, P. A. and Labrie, F. (1981*a*). Relative importance of the adenohypophyseal and gonadal sites of inhibitory action of LHRH agonists. *Biol. Reprod.*, **24,** 889

Séguin, C., Cusan, L., Bélanger, A., Kelly, P. A., Labrie, F. and Raynaud, J. P. (1981*b*). Additive inhibitory effects of treatment with an LHRH agonist and an antiandrogen on androgen-dependent tissues in the rat. *Mol. Cell. Endrocrinol.*, **21,** 37

Sharpe, R. M. and Fraser, H. M., (1980). HCG stimulation of testicular LHRH-like activity. *Nature* (*Lond.*), **287,** 642

Strulovici, B., Lindner, H. R., Shinitzky, M. and Zor, U. (1981). Elevation of apparent membrane viscosity in ovarian granulosa cells by follicle-stimulating hormone. *Biochim. Biophys. Acta,* **640,** 159

Sundaram, K. and Wang, N. (1982). Mice are insensitive to the antitesticular effects of LHRH agonists. *Endocrinology,* **110** (Suppl.), 90

Tureck, R.W., Mastroianni, L. Jr., Blasco, L. and Strauss, J. F. III (1982). Inhibition of human granulosa cell progesterone secretion by a gonadotropin-releasing hormone agonist. *J. Clin. Endocrinol. Metab.*, **54,** 1078

Vickery, B. H. and McRae, G. I. (1980). Antagonism by an LHRH agonist of the steroidogenic effects of exogenous human chorionic gonadotropin in the rhesus monkey. *Life Sci.*, **27,** 1409

Vickery, B. H., McRae, G. I. and Stevens, V. C. (1981). Suppression of luteal and placental function in pregnant baboons with agonist analogs of LHRH. *Fertil. Steril.*, **36,** 664

Wang, C., Hsueh, A. J. W. and Erickson, G. F. (1979). Induction of functional prolactin receptors by follicle-stimulating hormone in rat granulosa cells in vivo and in vitro. *J. Biol. Chem.*, **254,** 11330

Wang, C., Hsueh, A. J. W. and Erickson, G. F. (1981). LH stimulation of estrogen secretion in cultured granulosa cells. *Mol. Cell. Endocrinol.*, **24,** 17

14
Direct gonadal stimulation with LHRH

H. M. FRASER, R. M. SHARPE and R. M. POPKIN

The antifertility effects of LHRH and its agonists may result from three sites of action: (1) decreasing responsiveness of the anterior pituitary gonadotropes, (2) 'down regulation' of the gonads after abnormal gonadotropin stimulation and (3) direct action of LHRH on the testis and ovary. Investigation of chronic treatment with LHRH agonists showed the direct gonadal effects as inhibitory in nature (see Jones and Hsueh, 1984), a concept which fitted in well with the overall inhibitory actions of the treatment regimens. However, examination of short term actions of LHRH on the gonads revealed stimulatory effects. An understanding of these different actions of LHRH directly on the testis and ovary not only should help in evaluating their importance in the overall antifertility effects of LHRH, but also may reveal the physiological role of a putative LHRH-like factor which functions as an intragonadal regulator.

STIMULATORY EFFECTS OF LHRH ON THE OVARY

Oocyte maturation and ovulation

The most dramatic direct stimulatory effect of LHRH agonists on the ovary is the ability to cause ovulation in hypophysectomized rats by acting directly on preovulatory follicles. This was observed during experiments in which an agonist was tested for its effects on LH-induced ovulation in rats hypophysectomized at noon on the day of proestrus (Corbin and Bex, 1981; Ekholm *et al.*, 1981). The expected inhibitory effect of the agonist failed to occur. Instead, hypophysectomized rats receiving agonist alone ovulated (Figure 14.1). This also occurred when the agonist-treated rats were injected with antiserum to LH at the time of hypophysectomy, thus ensuring that ovulation was not mediated via agonist-induced LH release from residual pituitary tissue (Bex and Corbin, 1982). The specificity of the action of the agonist was demonstrated by the fact that it could be blocked by prior administration of an LHRH antagonist (Bex and Corbin, 1982).

LHRH can also act directly on the preovulatory follicle to stimulate meiosis.

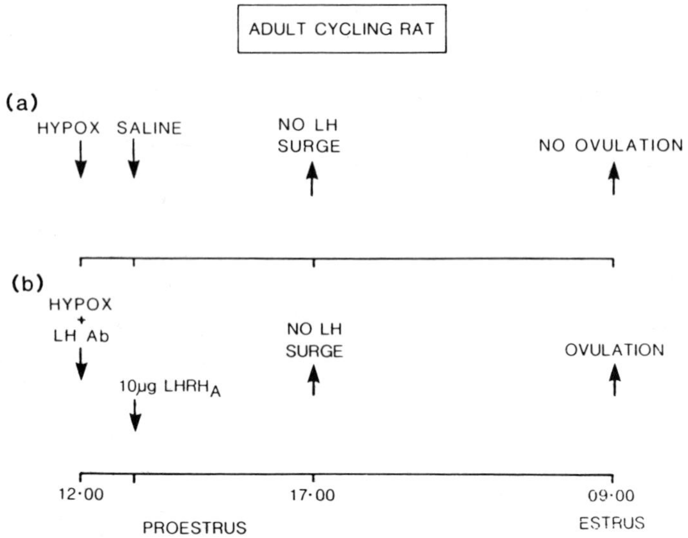

Figure 14.1 Diagram showing (a) absence of ovulation after hypophysectomy of rats in proestrus and (b) induction of ovulation by LHRH agonist in similar animals which have been both hypophysectomized and injected with LH antibody (Ab) to remove all sources of LH.

Oocyte maturation occurs as a result of the gonadotropin surge acting on granulosa cells within the preovulatory follicle, which, in turn, transmit a signal to the oocyte. It was expected that LHRH would inhibit the ability of LH to induce this process in follicle enclosed rat oocytes *in vitro*. Instead LHRH and its agonists added alone stimulated meiosis (Hillensjö and LeMaire, 1980). Other peptides were inactive, while the stimulatory effect was blocked by an LHRH antagonist (Ekholm *et al*., 1982*a*). The concept that LHRH might be mimicking the action of a substance generated by LH action on the follicle seems unlikely, however, since an antagonist failed to block LH-induced oocyte maturation (Ekholm *et al*., 1982*a*). It is not yet known whether LHRH acts directly on the oocyte to induce meiosis, or indirectly via other follicular compartments (Anderson and Hillensjö, 1982).

Effects on steroidogenesis

LHRH can exert a direct inhibitory action on the rat ovarian follicle. These effects have been shown, however, after prolonged (>24 h) exposure to LHRH, primarily on gonadotropin-stimulated events (Table 14.1). These studies have been performed using growing preantral follicles obtained from immature rats treated with diethylstilbestrol. In the preovulatory follicle LHRH has a stimulatory effect on steroidogenesis and, in contrast to its inhibitory influence, these stimulatory effects are observed on basal events during short term (<24 h) exposure (Table 14.2).

Table 14.1 Direct inhibitory actions of LHRH on rat ovarian follicles

Event *Gonadotropin induced*	*+LHRH*	*Site*	*Time* (days)
Estradiol ↑	Inhibits	Granulosa	2
Progesterone ↑	Inhibits	Granulosa	2
Androsterone ↑	Inhibits	Theca	4
cAMP ↑	Inhibits	Granulosa	2–4
LH receptor ↑	Inhibits	Granulosa	2
Cell differentiation	Inhibits	Granulosa	2
Ovarian weight gain	Inhibits		3–5
Phosphodiesterase ↓	Increases	Granulosa	1–2

Table 14.2 Direct stimulatory actions of LHRH on preovulatory rat follicle

Event	*Time*	*Site*
Binding	Immediate	Granulosa, theca, interstitial
cAMP *No effect*		
Androstenedione ↑	2–3 h	Theca?
Estradiol ↑	2–4 h	Granulosa
Progesterone ↑	4–6 h	Granulosa
PG ↑	3–6 h	Granulosa
Germinal vesicle breakdown	6–8 h	Oocyte
Oocyte meiosis	12 h	Oocyte
Serum progesterone ↑	6–8 h	
Ovulation	16–20 h	

Stimulation of progesterone release by LHRH and its agonists has been demonstrated using either isolated preovulatory follicles (Hillensjö *et al.*, 1982) or granulosa cells obtained from these follicles (Clark, 1982), derived from immature rats pretreated with pregnant mare's serum gonadotropin (PMSG). The presence of LHRH receptors on the granulosa cell and the stimulation of progesterone accumulation from isolated granulosa cells *in vitro* has established the granulosa cell as a site of action of LHRH. Using isolated follicles we have found that LHRH also causes a stimulation of androstenedione release. Since the theca is the main site of androstenedione production, LHRH may act on both cell types within the follicle.

When follicles isolated from immature rats (26–30 days old) primed 48 h earlier with 4 iu PMSG were incubated individually for periods up to 20 h, an LHRH agonist [D-Ser(tBu)^6,Pro^9-NHEt]LHRH, at 10^{-8} mol/l and native LHRH at 10^{-6} mol/l caused an increase in basal androstenedione, testosterone and progesterone release (Popkin *et al.*, 1983). This can be seen from the cumulative pattern of steroid release over a 20 h incubation period when medium is replaced every 2 h up to 8 h and again at 20 h (Figure 14.2).

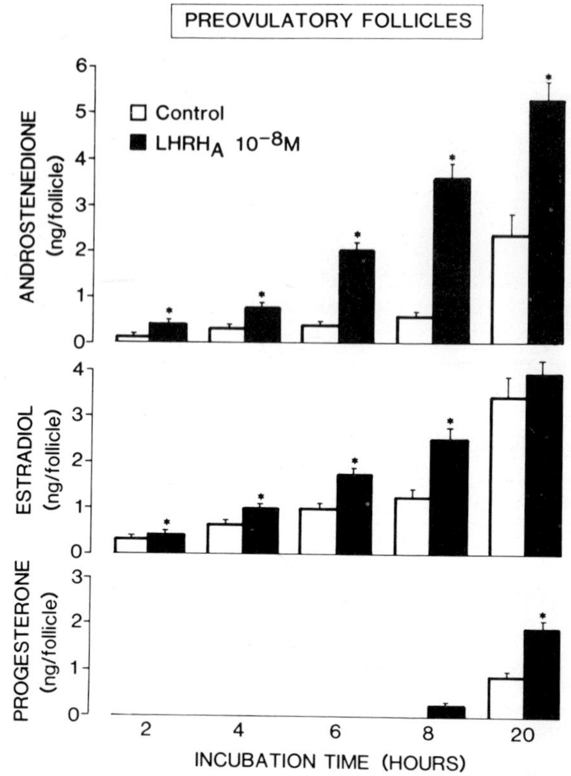

Figure 14.2 Time course of androstenedione, estradiol and progesterone release from isolated follicles obtained from PMSG primed immature rats and incubated with 10^{-8} mol/l [D-Ser(tBu)^6, Pro^9-NHEt]LHRH (■) or with medium alone (□). Medium was replaced after 2, 4, 6, 8 and 20 h. Data shown represent cumulative totals (mean ± SEM) of steroid production over the given time period (ten observations per group). *denotes $p < 0.05$ in comparison with respective control incubation. (From Popkin *et al.*, 1983*a*, by permission).

Androstenedione release was significantly increased in the presence of the LHRH agonist (2–5-fold over basal) during each 2 h period up to 8 h. The release between 8 and 20 h was not significantly greater than control but the cumulative total shows a significant increase. Progesterone release was stimulated by the LHRH agonist after 8 h. Estradiol levels were significantly stimulated by 10^{-8} mol/l LHRH agonist during each 2 h period; however, no further increase occurred between 8 and 20 h and the cumulative total after 20 h showed no significant stimulation of basal estradiol.

The stimulatory effect of the LHRH agonist on androstenedione and progesterone release was dose dependent (Figure 14.3). The lowest dose of the LHRH agonist found to elicit significant stimulation of both androstenedione and progesterone was 5×10^{-10} mol/l. LHRH also stimulated androstenedione and progesterone release at concentrations greater than 10^{-9} mol/l.

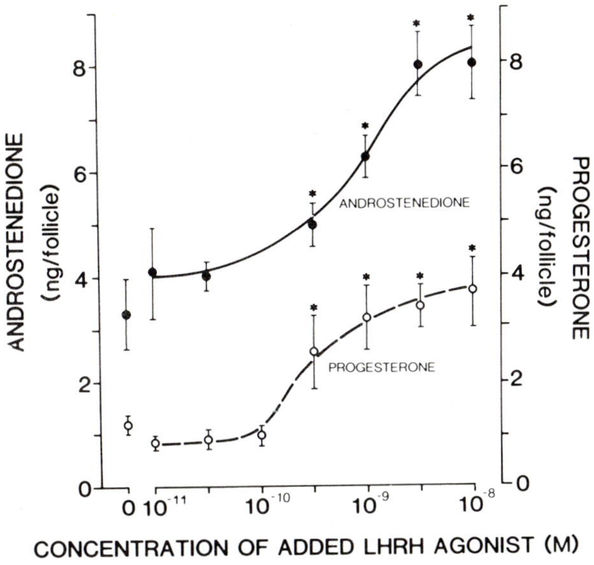

Figure 14.3 Dose dependent stimulation of androstenedione and progesterone release from follicles incubated with various concentrations of [D-Ser(tBu)^6,Pro^9-NHEt]LHRH for 18 h. Data shown are mean $\pm$ SEM with ten determinations in each group. * denotes $p < 0.05$ in comparison with basal steroid release. (From Popkin *et al.*, 1983, by permission).

The exact nature of the mechanism by which LHRH induces release of androstenedione from isolated follicles remains to be resolved. An entirely thecal action, mediated through LHRH receptors on theca/interstitial cells is the most likely explanation. However, while receptors for LHRH on granulosa and luteal cells are established, evidence for thecal cell binding is as yet indirect. For example, LHRH bound specifically to residual ovarian tissue left after removal of the majority of granulosa cells from ovaries from immature, estrogen treated, hypophysectomized rats (Pieper *et al.*, 1981). Autoradiography has shown the presence of LHRH grains to be distributed over most cell types within the rat ovary (Séguin *et al.*, 1982; R. M. Popkin *et al.*, 1983*b*).

Increased androgen release could be caused by an inhibition of granulosa cell aromatization resulting in accumulation of precursor. However, this seems unlikely as in no experiment have we shown any inhibitory effects of LHRH on estradiol release. Indeed, using isolated granulosa cells we find LHRH does not inhibit the conversion of testosterone to estradiol. Thus, the increase in progesterone is a direct stimulation at the level of the granulosa cells while the increased release of androstenedione is likely to be due to a stimulation of thecal androgen production.

The maximal stimulation of steroid release achieved with LHRH agonists is small and occurs over a different time course to that of LH or hCG on granulosa cells or isolated follicles (Clark, 1982; Hillensjö *et al.*, 1982; Popkin *et al.*, 1983*a*). Experiments in which follicles are exposed to both LHRH and LH indicate that LHRH cannot modify gonadotropin stimulated progesterone or androstenedione release (Clark, 1982; Hillensjö *et al.*, 1982; Popkin *et al.*, 1983).

While prior to ovulation LHRH mediates a series of stimulatory changes in steroid production and oocyte maturation, after ovulation an inhibitory influence on luteal function is evident. Both basal and hCG induced progesterone production by luteal tissue are inhibited in response to short term incubation with LHRH (Clayton *et al.*, 1979) although this effect is small and is overcome by high concentrations of gonadotropin.

Stimulatory effects on steroidogenesis *in vivo*

Little detailed information is available on direct stimulatory effects of LHRH on ovarian steroidogenesis *in vivo*. The obvious model in which to confirm the *in vitro* effects observed in preovulatory follicles is to administer LHRH agonist to rats hypophysectomized in proestrus. Rats which had been hypophysectomized on day 23 of age and treated consecutively with PMSG on day 27 and 2 days later with 1 μg [D-Ala^6,Pro^9-NHEt]LHRH produced only a small and insignificant increase in ovarian content of progesterone. Injection of hCG succeeded in raising progesterone concentrations in these animals (Clark, 1982). However, in similar experiments, using immature rats with preovulatory follicles but hypophysectomized only a few hours prior to administration of the agonist, a marked rise in plasma progesterone was observed (Ekholm *et al.*, 1981).

Mechanism of LHRH stimulation of steroidogenesis

The mechanism by which LHRH directly stimulates ovarian steroidogenesis has yet to be elucidated. Unlike LH, which stimulates a rapid increase in cAMP by the granulosa cell, LHRH agonists had no effect up to 2 h of incubation (Clark *et al.*, 1980). This observation was confirmed in studies on isolated follicles, although in this system a small rise in cAMP was observed after 4 h incubation (Hillensjö *et al.*, 1982).

In contrast, LHRH agonists can clearly stimulate PGE accumulation from granulosa cells *in vitro* (Clark *et al.*, 1980; Clark, 1982) and from isolated follicles (Hillensjö *et al.*, 1982) to a similar magnitude and on a similar time course to that found with LH (Figure 14.4). The effect of the agonist can be blocked by an LHRH antagonist *in vitro* and can be observed *in vivo* after agonist administration to hypophysectomized rats with preovulatory follicles, ovarian PGE content being elevated 6–8 h later (Clark, 1982; Ekholm *et al.*, 1982*b*). However, this rise in PGE does not appear to be of primary importance in agonist-induced stimulation of steroidogenesis or ovulation. Thus, the rise in PGE is blocked by treating the animals with the PG synthetase inhibitor indomethacin prior to agonist administration but the increased steroid release is unaffected. Although LHRH-induced oocyte meiosis is not inhibited when PG synthesis is prevented, the ability to cause ovulation is blocked, showing that LHRH-induced ovulation, like LH-induced ovulation, is dependent on increasing PG levels in the ovary (Ekholm *et al.*, 1981).

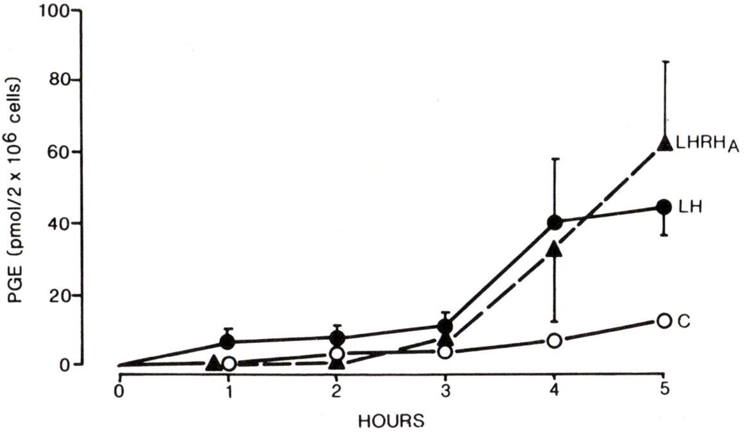

Figure 14.4 Time course of PGE accumulation in response to ovine LH and LHRH agonist. Granulosa cells were incubated in medium alone (○), with 1 μg/ml LH (●), or with 100 ng/ml LHRH agonist (▲) for the times indicated. Data shown here are mean ± SE of three experiments. The increases in PGE were first significant at 5 h for LH and LHRH agonist. (From Clark, 1982, with permission).

Physiological significance of stimulatory effects of LHRH

The fact that LHRH can influence these fundamental processes of ovarian function suggests that a naturally produced ovarian LHRH-like factor may have an important role in follicular development. Clearly, this hypothesis can only be proved once the putative substance is isolated and changes in its production measured in different stages of follicular maturation. An LHRH-like substance (gonadocrinin) isolated from follicular fluid has been described (Ying *et al.*, 1981), but the results have yet to be confirmed. However, the information on the stimulatory and inhibitory actions of LHRH on the ovary permits us to speculate on the role of such a substance (Figure 14.5). In the growing follicle, the gonadotropin-induced stimulation of growth and differentiation, steroidogenesis and LH receptor increase can all be inhibited by LHRH. This suggests that a locally produced LHRH-like factor may be involved in the induction of follicular atresia. However, in those follicles which develop to the preovulatory stage, production of the factor would result in the stimulatory effects which have been observed using LHRH, and be a positive influence in induction of ovulation. Once ovulation has taken place the action of 'ovarian LHRH' would switch again to inhibition.

STIMULATORY EFFECTS OF LHRH ON THE TESTIS

Within the testis the actions of LHRH are directed solely towards the Leydig cells (Bourne *et al.*, 1980; Sharpe and Fraser, 1980*a*), and until recently these effects were considered to be exclusively inhibitory. This belief stemmed from

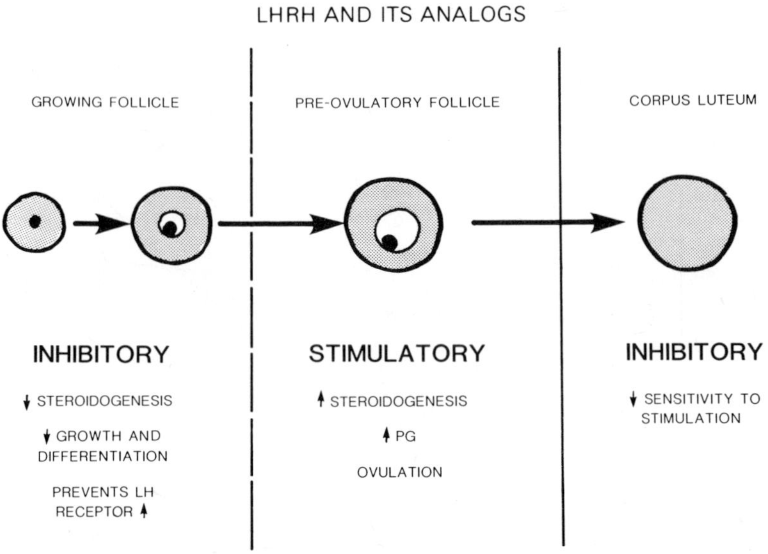

Figure 14.5 Diagram indicating possible physiological role of an ovarian LHRH-like factor, derived from studies on responses to LHRH and its agonists.

observations made in gonadotropin-primed hypophysectomized immature or adult rats which had been treated for 3–5 days with LHRH agonists. This treatment caused a reduction in LH-receptor numbers and in the capacity of the testis to secrete testosterone *in vitro* (Jones and Hsueh, 1983). Comparable inhibitory effects have also been demonstrated *in vitro*, but again these were only evident after continuous exposure of cultured testicular cells from hypophysectomized rats to LHRH agonist for 4–5 days (Hsueh *et al.*, 1981). However, it is now clear that the initial or short term effect of LHRH and its agonists on the Leydig cell is to stimulate steroidogenesis.

Stimulation of Leydig cell steroidogenesis *in vitro*

Incubation of collagenase-dispersed Leydig cells from adult rats for 4 h in the presence of increasing concentrations of native LHRH or an LHRH agonist, [D-Ser(tBu)^6,Pro^9-NHEt]LHRH, results in dose dependent stimulation of testosterone secretion. The concentrations of LHRH required to achieve a given level of stimulation were approximately 1000 times those of the LHRH agonist, a finding consistent with the different affinities of these two peptides for the Leydig cell LHRH-receptor (Sharpe and Fraser, 1980*a*). Stimulation of testosterone secretion by the same LHRH agonist has also been demonstrated in 4 h incubations of Leydig cells from immature (Sharpe and Cooper, 1982*a*) and pubertal (Sharpe, 1983) rats, as well as in short term (2–16 h) cultures of Percoll-purified rat Leydig cells (Hunter *et al.*, 1982).

The stimulatory effect of LHRH agonist on testosterone secretion *in vitro* is prevented by concomitant incubation with an LHRH antagonist [D-Phe^{2,6},Phe^3]LHRH (Figure 14.6) (Sharpe and Cooper, 1982*a*). Stimulation is

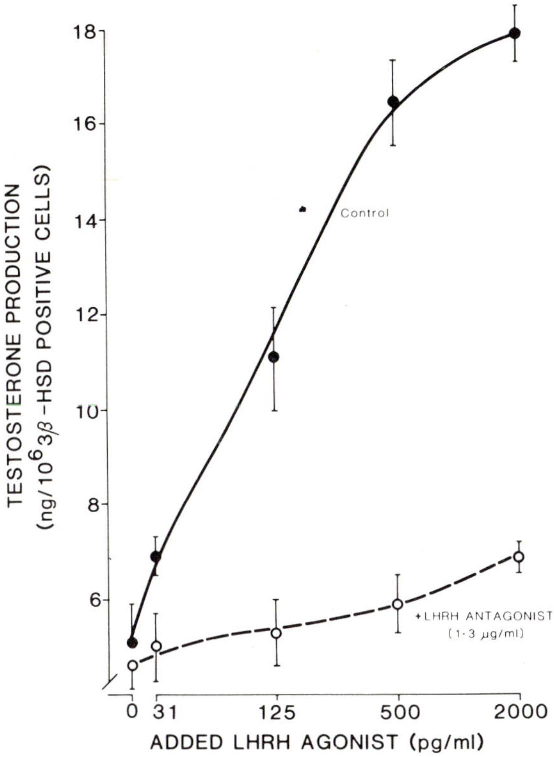

Figure 14.6 Reversal of the stimulatory effect of [D-Ser(tBu)^6,Pro^9-NHEt]LHRH on Leydig cell testosterone secretion *in vitro* by co-incubation in the presence of an LHRH antagonist [D-Phe^{2,6},Phe^3]LHRH. Each point is the mean ± SD of triplicate incubations.

dependent on the continuous presence of LHRH agonist in the incubation medium, as its removal leads to rapid dissociation of receptor-bound peptide and this results in termination of stimulation (Sharpe and Cooper, 1982*b*).

In addition to its stimulatory effect on basal testosterone secretion, the LHRH agonist can also enhance the testosterone response to LH, hCG and dibutyryl cyclic AMP (Hunter *et al*., 1982; Sharpe and Cooper, 1982*a*), even when these factors are present in maximally stimulating concentrations, although this positive interactive effect is not observed with every preparation of Leydig cells (Sharpe, unpublished data).

Stimulation of steroidogenesis in hypophysectomized rats

To test whether stimulatory effects of LHRH agonist comparable to those observed *in vitro* could be obtained *in vivo*, the effect of single or repeated daily injection of LHRH agonist into hypophysectomized rats was assessed. The rats used were 55 days of age (the time of maximum testosterone responsiveness) and had been hypophysectomized 3 days earlier – in this short interval there is no loss of testosterone responsiveness (Hauger *et al.*, 1977). At the end of the experiment, the completeness of hypophysectomy was checked both visually and by the measurement of serum LH levels, and any animals failing to meet the requisite criteria (Sharpe *et al.*, 1982*a*) were discarded.

Subcutaneous injection of hypophysectomized rats with 10 μg [D-Ser(tBu)^6,Pro^9-NHEt]LHRH resulted in a 10–15-fold increase in the serum levels of testosterone at $1\frac{1}{2}$–4 h after injection, although levels had returned to baseline (control) levels by 24 h (Figure 14.7). In control animals injected with the vehicle alone, the serum levels of testosterone remained low (0.2–0.5 ng/ml) throughout the 24 h period. In further experiments using hypophysectomized rats, a single injection of lower doses of the LHRH agonist (1 or 0.2 μg) caused comparable stimulation of testosterone secretion 2 h later (Table 14.3). However, daily injection of either of these two doses of LHRH agonist for 6 days resulted in total ablation of the testosterone response by the last day of treatment. This effect was not due to the length of time after hypophysectomy, as rats which had been treated for 5 days with the vehicle and then injected on the 6th day with LHRH agonist showed a 15-fold increase in the serum levels of testosterone (Table 14.3).

These results confirm the *in vitro* findings with isolated Leydig cells in showing that the initial effect of LHRH agonist on the Leydig cell *in vivo* is to stimulate steroidogenesis, to the extent that for 4 h at least the serum levels of testosterone are raised to within or above the normal range (1–8 ng/ml) for intact, untreated rats of this age and strain. However, this stimulatory effect is lost during repeated daily injection of LHRH agonist, and this may in part

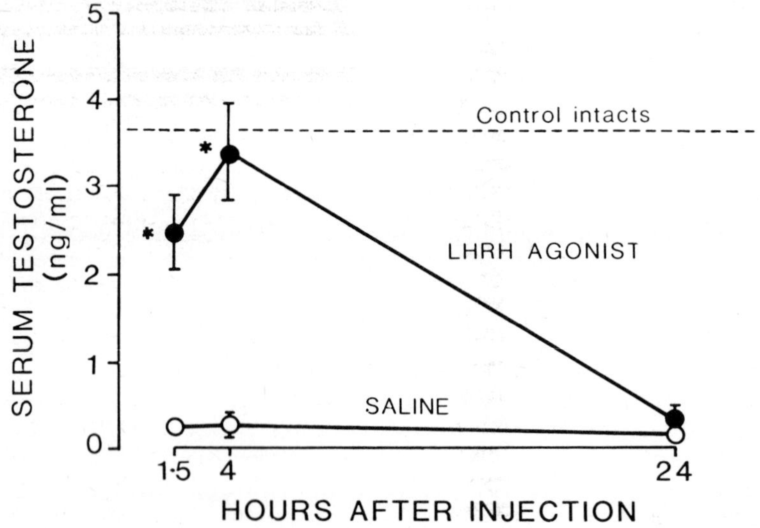

Figure 14.7 Serum levels of testosterone at intervals after subcutaneous injection of hypophysectomized 55-day-old male rats with either saline or 10 μg LHRH agonist. Blood samples were obtained serially from the tail vein of individual animals and are plotted as the mean ± SD for five rats per group. Asterisks indicate a significant ($p < 0.001$) difference between values for the two treatment groups. (From Sharpe *et al.*, 1982a; with permission.)

Table 14.3 Decline in testosterone responsiveness to [D-Ser(tBu)^6,Pro^9-NHEt]LHRH (LHRH-A) in hypophysectomized rats following repeated daily injection of the peptide

Injected material	*Duration of treatment* (days)	*Serum level of testosterone* (ng/ml)
Vehicle	1	0.4 ± 0.2
LHRH-A 1 μg	1	7.0 ± 1.9*
LHRH-A 0.2 μg	1	6.7 ± 2.1*
Vehicle	6	0.4 ± 0.1
LHRH-A 1 μg	6	0.3 ± 0.1
LHRH-A 0.2 μg	6	0.5 ± 0.1
Vehicle + LHRH-A 1 μg	5 + 1	5.9 ± 1.5*

Animals were injected daily as shown and a blood sample taken at 2 h after the 1st and 6th injections. Values are the mean ± SD for 3–5 animals per group and asterisks indicate a significant ($p < 0.001$) difference from the vehicle-injected (control) group

explain why inhibitory rather than stimulatory effects are observed during long term treatment of gonadotropin-primed hypophysectomized rats with LHRH and its agonists.

Stimulation of steroidogenesis in intact rats

The foregoing studies suggest that LHRH agonist may have stimulatory effects *in vivo* in intact rats, but there is a major obstacle to proving this. Because LHRH agonist will cause release of pituitary LH (and FSH) in intact rats, it becomes impossible to distinguish between direct effects of LHRH agonist on the Leydig cell and those mediated by LH release, particularly when either may result in the same effect, of increased testosterone secretion. We have found, however, that administration of LHRH agonist unilaterally into the right testis at a dose of 1 ng does not result in any significant LH release following its leakage or diffusion from the testis. Injection of the left testis with the injection vehicle alone acts as a control. In this way any testicular effects of the peptide resulting from LH release can be controlled for using the left testis. Other rats were injected intratesticularly bilaterally with the vehicle alone.

Because we were looking for a unilateral stimulatory effect of LHRH agonist on testicular testosterone secretion, we collected testicular interstitial fluid (IF) from left and right testes. At 1, 2 and 4 h after intratesticular injection of 1 ng LHRH agonist, the mean levels of testosterone in IF were increased compared with the left testis, as shown in Figure 14.8. However, because IF levels of testosterone vary considerably between animals, this increase is somewhat obscured. This obscurity can be reduced by assessing the difference in testosterone concentration between IF from left (control) and right (LHRH agonist-injected) testes from individual animals, a comparison that reveals no significant difference for control animals. In contrast, testosterone levels in IF

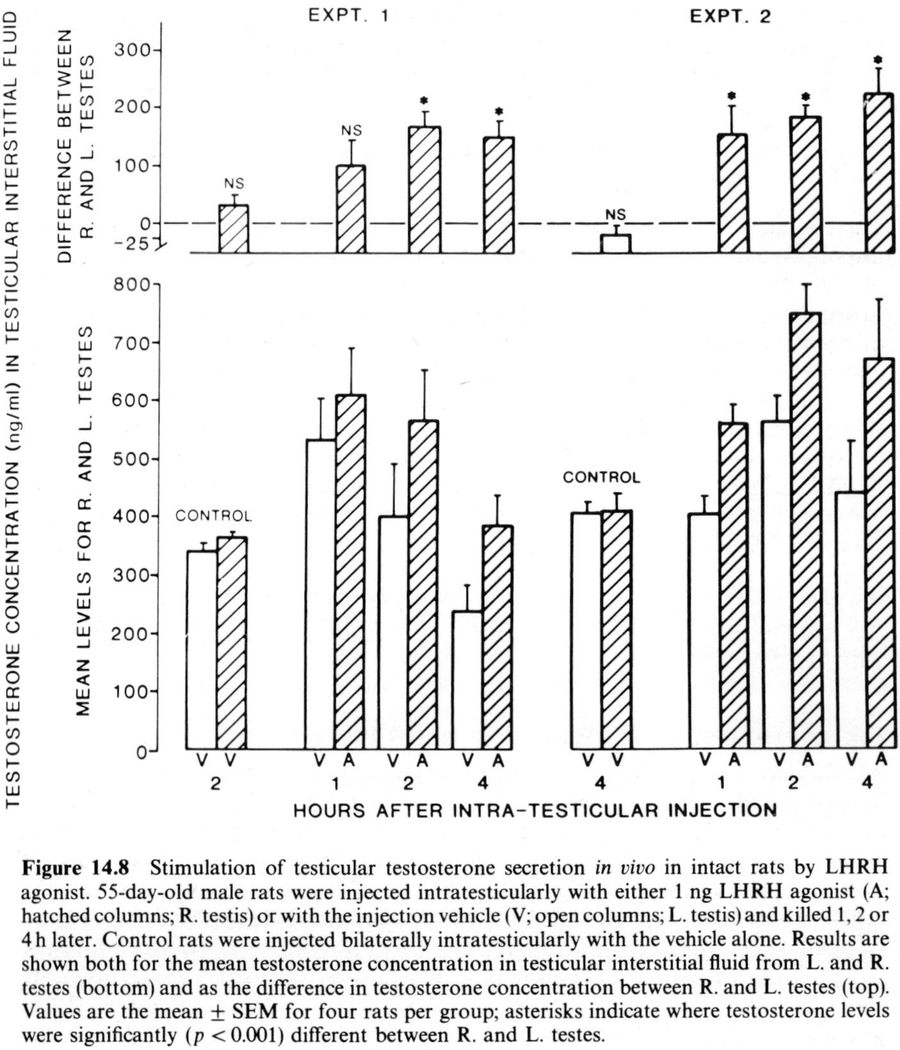

Figure 14.8 Stimulation of testicular testosterone secretion *in vivo* in intact rats by LHRH agonist. 55-day-old male rats were injected intratesticularly with either 1 ng LHRH agonist (A; hatched columns; R. testis) or with the injection vehicle (V; open columns; L. testis) and killed 1, 2 or 4 h later. Control rats were injected bilaterally intratesticularly with the vehicle alone. Results are shown both for the mean testosterone concentration in testicular interstitial fluid from L. and R. testes (bottom) and as the difference in testosterone concentration between R. and L. testes (top). Values are the mean ± SEM for four rats per group; asterisks indicate where testosterone levels were significantly ($p < 0.001$) different between R. and L. testes.

from testes injected with LHRH agonist were raised at all times in both experiments, and in only one instance did this increase fail to reach statistical significance. Testosterone levels in IF from the left (control) testis of animals injected contralaterally with LHRH agonist varied considerably between treatment groups, in some instances being raised compared with values for controls (i.e. injected bilaterally with vehicle) and in other instances lowered. These differences were not consistent between experiments, however, and could not be correlated with the serum levels of LH.

Thus, the initial effect of LHRH agonist on the Leydig cell *in vivo* is to stimulate testosterone secretion. This effect was remarkably consistent between animals, it lasted for at least 4 h and its magnitude appeared to be independent of the level of stimulation by endogenous LH, the levels of which varied considerably between animals in these experiments.

Physiological significance of the stimulatory effects of LHRH on the Leydig cell

The effects of LHRH agonist are directed towards the most fundamentally important aspect of testicular function, namely testosterone secretion. Because of the absolute dependence of spermatogenesis on testosterone from the Leydig cell, it would be logical for the seminiferous tubules to have some means of ensuring that the Leydig cells produce sufficient testosterone, and there is considerable indirect evidence to this effect (Sharpe, 1982). As the effects of testosterone on spermatogenesis are mediated via the Sertoli cells, it is logical that it should be the latter that communicate with the Leydig cells.

Thus, a 'testicular LHRH' could function as a communicator between the Sertoli and Leydig cells as a means of maintaining intratesticular levels of testosterone at the optimum required for the Sertoli cell in its support of spermatogenesis. We have previously demonstrated that an 'LHRH-like' factor can be extracted from rat seminiferous tubules. Its source is most likely the Sertoli cell and it is secreted *in vivo* into the interstitial fluid that surrounds the Leydig cells (Sharpe and Fraser, 1980*b*; Fraser *et al.*, 1982; Sharpe *et al.*, 1981, 1982*b*).

CONCLUDING REMARKS

Several parallels may be drawn between the action of LHRH on the ovary and testis. In both, LHRH has a stimulatory effect on steroidogenesis similar in many respects to that of LH, but of smaller magnitude and with a lag phase of some 2 hours before the effects are observed. A basic difference between the gonadal actions in the male and in the female is that in the testis LHRH acts on one cell type – the Leydig cell – while in the ovary it may act on all cell types.

The studies described relate to the rat, and it is important, both for assessing the significance of a 'gonadal LHRH' and in the evaluation of the role of direct gonadal actions in the mechanism of the antifertility effects of LHRH in the human, that these direct actions can be established in other species. There are obvious technical problems in investigating these effects *in vivo* because of the requirement for removing the influence of pituitary gonadotropin release after LHRH administration.

While receptors for LHRH and direct gonadal actions have been readily demonstrated in rat ovarian tissue and in the Leydig cells, their demonstration in other species has been less forthcoming. There are reports of absence of LHRH receptors on luteal tissue from rhesus monkeys (Asch *et al.*, 1981) and the human (Clayton and Huhtaniemi, 1982). However, we have found LHRH binding sites, apparently of low affinity, on human luteal tissue (Popkin *et al.*, 1983*a*). The mouse does not appear to have testicular LHRH receptors, nor do the Leydig cells respond to LHRH (Hunter *et al.*, 1982).

It seems that most of the initial difficulties in coming to terms with direct stimulatory and inhibitory actions of LHRH on the gonads can now be reconciled. In general, the initial effects of LHRH are stimulatory, with inhibitory actions becoming apparent after long term exposure (>24 h) particularly on gonadotropin-stimulated events. It might be suggested that short term actions are more likely to reflect the physiological actions of 'gonadal LHRH'. On the other hand, the long term inhibitory effects would appear to be the most important during chronic agonist treatment.

Acknowledgement

We wish to thank Dr J. Sandow (Hoechst AG) for gifts of LHRH and analogs used in our studies.

References

Anderson, L. D. and Hillensjö, T. (1982). Lack of effect of a gonadotropin-releasing hormone agonist upon meiosis in isolated porcine oocytes. *Acta Physiol. Scand.*, **114**, 623

Asch, R. H., Sickle, M. V., Rettori, V., Balmaceda, J. P., Eddy, C. A., Coy, D. H. and Schally, A. V. (1981). Absence of LHRH binding sites in corpora lutea from rhesus monkeys (Macaca mulatta). *J. Clin. Endocrinol. Metab.*, **53**, 215

Bex, F. J. and Corbin, A. (1982). Cyclic response of hypophysectomized (hpx) rats to ovulation induced by LHRH agonist (Ag): mediation by prostaglandins (PG). *Endocrinology*, **112**, 520A

Bourne, G. A., Regiani, S., Payne, A. H. and Marshall, J. C. (1980). Testicular GnRH receptors – characterization and localization on interstitial tissue. *J. Clin. Endocrinol. Metab.*, **51**, 407

Clark, M. R. (1982). Stimulation of progesterone and prostaglandin E accumulation by luteinizing hormone-releasing hormone (LHRH) and LHRH analogs in rat granulosa cells. *Endocrinology*, **110**, 146

Clark, M. R., Thibier, C., Marsh, J. M. and LeMaire, W. J. (1980). Stimulation of prostaglandin accumulation by luteinizing hormone-releasing hormone (LHRH) and LHRH analogs in rat granulosa cells in vitro. *Endocrinology*, **107**, 17

Clayton, R. N., Harwood, J. P. and Catt, K. J. (1979). Gonadotropin-releasing hormone analogue binds to luteal cells and inhibits progesterone production. *Nature* (*Lond.*), **282**, 90

Clayton, R. N. and Huhtaniemi I. T. (1982). Absence of gonadotropin-releasing hormone receptors in human gonadal tissue. *Nature* (*Lond.*), **299**, 56

Corbin, A. and Bex, F. J. (1981) Luteinizing hormone releasing hormone agonists induce ovulation in hypophysectomized proestrous rats: direct ovarian effect. *Life Sci.*, **29**, 185

Ekholm, C., Hillensjö, T. and Isaksson, O. (1981). Gonadotropin releasing hormone agonists stimulate oocyte meiosis and ovulation in hypophysectomized rats. *Endocrinology*, **108**, 2022

Ekholm, C., Hillensjö, T., LeMaire, W. J., Magnusson, C. and Sheela Rani, C. S. (1982*a*). A gonadotrophin-releasing hormone (GnRH) antagonist inhibits GnRH but not LH-induced meiosis in follicle-enclosed rat oocytes in vitro. *Acta Endocrinol.*, **101**, 264

Ekholm, C., Clark, M. R., Magnusson, C., Isaksson, O. and LeMaire, W. J. (1982*b*). Ovulation induced by a gonadotropin releasing hormone analog in hypophysectomized rats involves prostaglandins. *Endocrinology*, **110**, 288

Fraser, H. M., Sharpe, R. M., Lincoln, G. A. and Harmer, A. J. (1982). LHRH antibodies: Their use in the study of hypothalamic LHRH and testicular LHRH-like material, and possible contraceptive applications. In Jeffcoate, S. L. and Sandler, M. (eds.) *Progress Towards a Male Contraceptive*, pp. 41–78. (Chichester: Wiley).

Hauger, R. L., Chen, Y-D. I., Kelch, R. P. and Payne, A. H. (1977). Pituitary regulation of Leydig cell function in the adult male rat. *J. Endocrinol.*, **74**, 57

Hillensjö, T. and LeMaire, W. J. (1980). Gonadotropin releasing hormone agonists stimulate meiotic maturation of follicle-enclosed rat oocytes in vitro. *Nature* (*Lond.*), **287**, 145

Hillensjö, T., LeMaire, W. J., Clark, M. R. and Ahren, K. (1982). Effect of gonadotropin-releasing hormone (GnRH) and GnRH agonists upon accumulation of progesterone, cAMP and prostaglandin in isolated preovulatory rat follicles. *Acta Endocrinol.*, **101,** 603

Hsueh, A. J. W., Schreiber, J. R. and Erickson, G. F. (1981). Inhibitory effect of gonadotropin releasing hormone upon cultured testicular cells. *Mol. Cell. Endocrinol.*, **21,** 43

Hunter, M. G., Sullivan, M. H. F., Dix, C. J., Aldred, L. F. and Cooke, B. A. (1982). Stimulation and inhibition by LHRH analogues of cultured rat Leydig cell function and lack of effect on mouse Leydig cells. *Mol. Cell. Endocrinol.*, **27,** 31

Jones, P. B. C. and Hsueh, A. J. W. (1984). Direct antigonadal actions of LHRH. This volume, Chapter 13

Popkin, R. M., Fraser, H. M. and Jonassen, J. (1983*a*). Stimulation of androstenedione and progesterone release by LHRH and LHRH agonist from isolated preovulatory follicles. *Mol. Cell. Endocrinol.*, **29,** 169

Popkin, R. M., Fraser, H. M. and Gosden, R. G. (1983*b*). Effects of LH-RH agonist or LH-RH immunoneutralization on pituitary and ovarian LH-RH receptors in female rats. *J. Reprod. Fert.*, **69,** 245

Popkin, R. M., Branley, T. A., Currie, A., Shaw, R. W., Baird, D. T. and Fraser, H. M. (1983*c*). Specific binding of luteinizing hormone releasing hormone to human luteal tissue. *Biochem. Biophys. Res. Commun.*, **114,** 750

Pieper, D. R., Richards, J. S. and Marshall, J. C. (1981). Ovarian gonadotropin-releasing hormone (GnRH) receptors: characterization, distribution, and induction by GnRH. *Endocrinology,* **108,** 1148

Séguin, C., Pelletier, G., Dube, D. and Labrie, F. (1982). Distribution of luteinizing hormone-releasing hormone receptors in the rat ovary. *Regulatory Peptides,* **4,** 183

Sharpe, R. M. (1982). The hormonal regulation of the Leydig cell. In Finn, C. A. (ed.) *Oxford Reviews in Reproductive Biology.* (Oxford: Oxford UP) **4,** 241–317

Sharpe, R. M. (1983). Regulation of the Leydig cell by LHRH. In D'Agata, R. and van der Molen, H. J. (eds.) *Recent Advances in Male Reproduction: Molecular Bases and Clinical Implications.* (New York: Raven Press) Serono Symp. No 7, pp. 197–204

Sharpe, R. M. and Fraser, H. M. (1980*a*). Leydig cell receptors for luteinizing hormone-releasing hormone and its agonists and their modulation by administration or deprivation of the releasing hormone. *Biochem. Biophys. Res. Commun.*, **95,** 256

Sharpe, R. M. and Fraser, H. M. (1980*b*). HCG stimulation of testicular LHRH-like activity. *Nature (Lond.),* **287,** 642

Sharpe, R. M., Fraser, H. M., Cooper, I. and Rommerts, F. F. G. (1981). Sertoli–Leydig cell communication via an LHRH-like factor. *Nature (Lond.),* **290,** 785

Sharpe, R. M. and Cooper, I. (1982*a*). Stimulatory effect of LHRH and its agonists on Leydig cell steroidogenesis in vitro. *Mol. Cell. Endocrinol.*, **26,** 141

Sharpe, R. M. and Cooper, I. (1982*b*). The mode of action of LHRH agonists on the rat Leydig cell. *Mol. Cell. Endocrinol.*, **27,** 199

Sharpe, R. M., Doogan, D. G. and Cooper, I. (1982*a*). Stimulation of Leydig cell testosterone secretion in vitro and in vivo in hypophysectomized rats by an agonist of luteinizing hormone releasing hormone. *Biochem. Biophys. Res. Commun.*, **106,** 1210

Sharpe, R. M., Fraser, H. M., Cooper, I. and Rommerts, F. F. G. (1982*b*). The secretion, measurement and function of a testicular LHRH-like factor. *Ann. NY Acad. Sci.*, **383,** 272

Ying, S. Y., Ling, N., Bohlen, P. and Guillemin, R. (1981). Gonadocrinins: Peptides in ovarian follicular fluid stimulating the secretion of pituitary gonadotrophins. *Endocrinology,* **108,** 1206

15
Antisteroidal actions of LHRH agonists

K. SUNDARAM and C. W. BARDIN

The physiological role of LHRH is to regulate the secretion of LH and FSH by the pituitary and thereby control gonadal function and reproduction. It has been discovered that LHRH and its analogs can exert effects on a variety of tissues to reduce fertility (Schally, 1978). Among the effects of LHRH and its agonists are: (1) desensitization of the pituitary leading to impaired gonadotropin secretion (Rivier and Vale, 1979; Sandow *et al.*, 1980; Bergquist *et al.*, 1979; Sundaram *et al.*, 1982), (2) inhibition of steroidogenesis by testes and ovaries of rats (Hsueh and Erickson, 1979; Clayton *et al.*, 1979; Cao *et al.*, 1982) and (3) antagonism of the action of sex steroids on the reproductive tract (Pedroza *et al.*, 1980; Liu and Li, 1980; Sundaram *et al.*, 1981). The first two topics are reviewed extensively elsewhere in this volume. In this chapter we will review results which demonstrate the antisteroidal actions of LHRH and its agonists and discuss their clinical implications.

ANTIESTROGENIC ACTIONS

The antiestrogenic effects of LHRH agonists were first described by Pedroza *et al.* (1980), who found that [D-Trp^6]LHRH inhibited the action of estradiol on the uterus in rats. Immature hypophysectomized–ovariectomized rats were treated with 1 μg of estradiol and 1 μg of the agonist for 5 days. The agonist inhibited the estradiol-induced increase in uterine weight and in uterine estradiol receptors. The effect of LHRH agonists on the decidual response of pseudopregnant ovariectomized rats receiving optimal amounts of estradiol and progesterone has been reported (Liu and Li, 1980). The agonist treatment caused a 50 % decrease in the number of rats showing decidual response and a 30 % decrease in the uterine weights of rats that had a decidual response. An earlier report that administration of LHRH into one uterine horn of 5-day pregnant rats caused inhibition of pregnancy in the ipsilateral but not in the contralateral horn is consistent with a local effect of LHRH (Jones, 1979). These latter observations raise the possibility that LHRH agonists also interfere with the biological effects of progesterone.

The antiestrogenic effects of LHRH agonists have been confirmed and extended (Sundaram *et al.*, 1981). Immature ovariectomized rats were given estradiol (0.01 or 0.1 μg) with or without either LHRH (1 mg) or [D-His(B_3l)^6, Pro^9-NHEt]LHRH (LHRH-A) (10 μg) for 5 days. The results show that the uterotrophic action of estradiol was attenuated by LHRH as well as its agonist (Figure 15.1). At the end of the experiment the morphology of the cells in the vaginal lavage was examined. Only leukocytes were present in ovariectomized untreated animals. All eight animals that received estradiol (0.01 μg) had cornified epithelial cells in their vaginal smears. By contrast, in animals that received LHRH-A or LHRH with estradiol, only two of eight and three of eight, respectively, had cornified cells. There were no differences among the groups receiving the larger dose (0.1 μg) of estradiol, all of which showed the presence of cornified epithelial cells in their vaginal smears. A direct effect of LHRH agonists on the vagina was also proposed when it was found that chronic treatment of immature rats with 1 μg of [D-Trp^6]LHRH delayed vaginal opening without altering serum estradiol levels (Vilchez-Martinez *et al.*, 1979). The antiestrogenic experiments of LHRH agonists reported here were prompted by the studies of Bergquist and his colleagues. These investigators noted that, of the women treated for long periods of time with LHRH agonists, some developed amenorrhea-associated anovulation. When these women were injected with a progestin, withdrawal bleeding did not occur, even though estradiol levels present in serum were

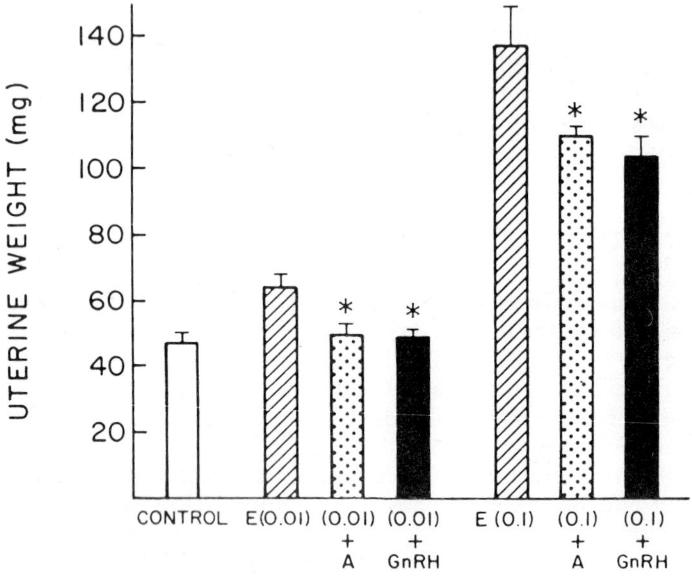

Figure 15.1 Effect of LHRH-A (A; 10 μg/day) and synthetic LHRH (1 mg/day) on uterine weight in ovariectomized estradiol-treated rats. Immature rats were ovariectomized and treated 1 week later with 0.01 or 0.1 μg of estradiol with or without one of the peptides for 5 days and killed on day 6. Values represent mean $\pm$ SE of eight rats. * = $p < 0.05$. (Reproduced, with permission, from Sundaram *et al.* (1981). Copyright 1981, Pergamon Press, Ltd.)

similar to those observed in the early follicular phase. These observations suggested that the activity of the estradiol on the endometrium had been blocked by some unknown mechanism. Also, subsequent examination of endometrial biopsies from women treated for long periods of time with LHRH agonists failed to demonstrate endometrial hyperplasia in spite of a high estrogen/progesterone ratio in blood (Bergquist *et al.*, 1981). There is no general agreement about this latter finding, however (Schmidt-Gollwitzer *et al.*, 1981).

ANTIANDROGENIC ACTIONS

Effect on ventral prostate and seminal vesicles in rats

The effect of administration of (LHRH-A) and [D-Trp[6],Pro[9]-NHEt]LHRH (LHRH-B) on testosterone propionate (TP) induced increase in the weights of ventral prostate and seminal vesicles is shown in Figure 15.2. Immature castrated male rats were given TP with or without one of the

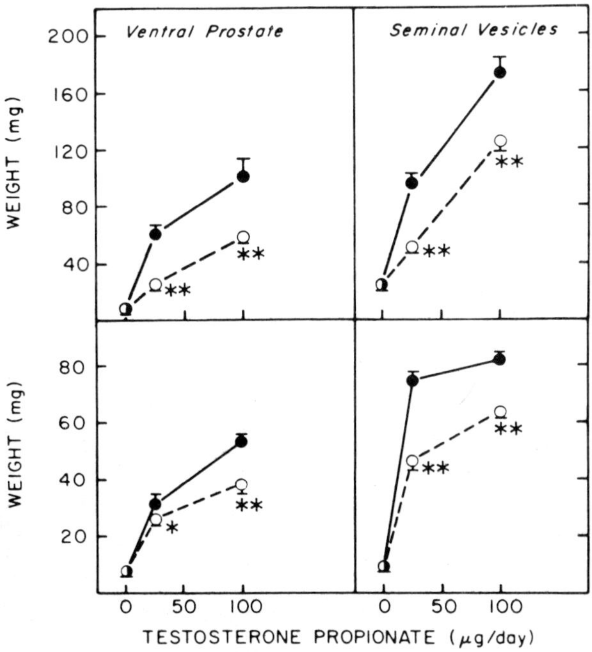

Figure 15.2 Effect of LHRH-A (upper panel) and LHRH-B (lower panel) on the weights of ventral prostate and seminal vesicles in androgen-treated rats. Immature male rats were castrated and treated with testosterone propionate (●) or testosterone propionate and the agonist (○) for 5 days. Each point represents the mean ± SE of eight animals. * = $p < 0.05$; ** = $p < 0.01$. (Reproduced, with permission, from Sundaram *et al.* (1981). Copyright, 1981, Pergamon Press, Ltd.)

agonists (10 μg/day) for 5 days and killed on day 6. Administration of TP caused a pronounced increase in the weights of ventral prostate and seminal vesicles. In animals receiving LHRH-A (upper panel) or LHRH-B (lower panel) along with TP, the ventral prostate and seminal vesicle weights were significantly lower. To exclude the possibility that this antiandrogenic action of LHRH analogs was mediated via the pituitary, similar experiments were performed in hypophysectomized castrated rats. LHRH-A inhibited the androgenic action of TP in hypophysectomized castrated rats also (Figure 15.3). That the antiandrogenic action may occur in the dog also was suggested by the finding that testosterone replacement therapy could not adequately restore prostate size and secretory function in dogs whose testicular function was suppressed by chronic treatment with an LHRH agonist (Vickery, 1981).

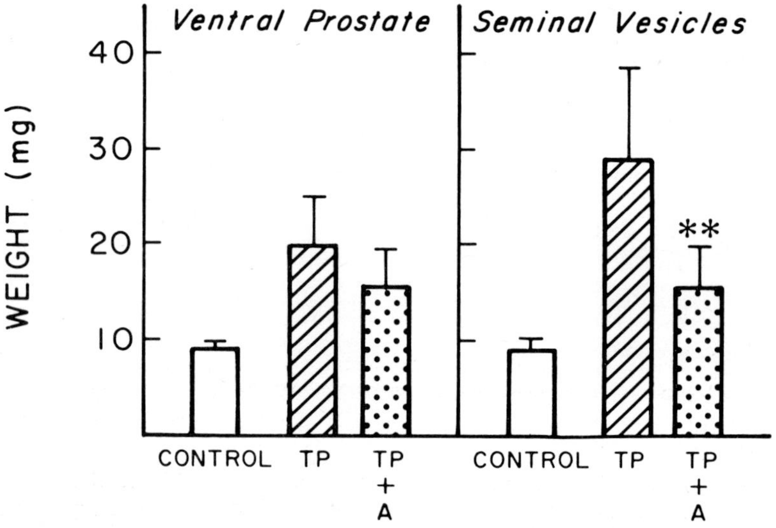

Figure 15.3 Inhibition of testosterone propionate (TP) induced increase in ventral prostate and seminal vesicle weights by LHRH-A (A) in hypophysectomized-castrated rats. Rats, hypophysectomized at 22 days of age, were castrated 1 week later. One week following castration, the animals received 100 μg of TP with or without 10 μg of agonist for 5 days. Mean ± SE of eight animals. ** = $p < 0.01$.

Effects on kidney β-glucuronidase in mice

The ability of agonistic peptides to modify the androgen-induced increase in β-glucuronidase activity in mouse kidneys was examined. Castrated male mice were given TP with or without LHRH-A or LHRH for 7 days and killed on day 8. The results showed that the androgen-induced increase in renal glucuronidase was inhibited by LHRH-A as well as LHRH (Figure 15.4). In another experiment, increasing doses of TP were given along with a fixed dose

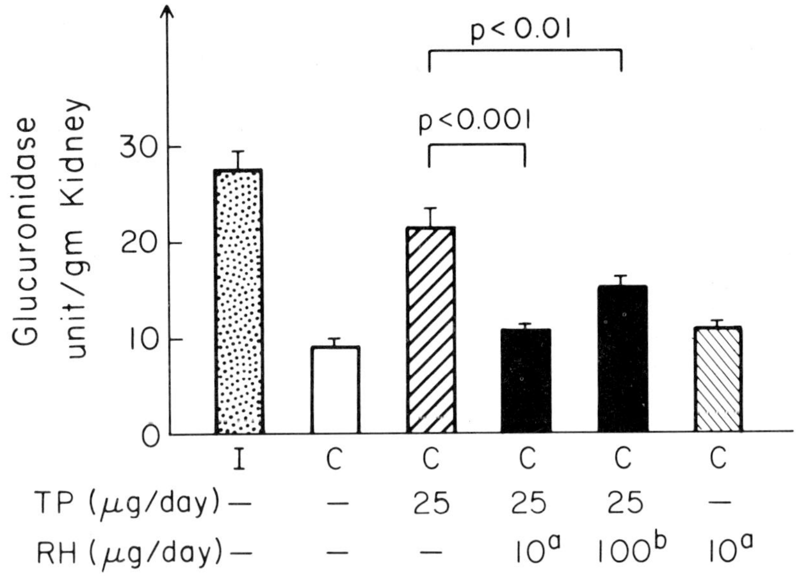

Figure 15.4 The antiandrogenic effect of (a) LHRH-A or (b) LHRH on mouse kidney β-glucuronidase. Adult male mice (ten per group) were castrated and given a daily injection of TP and twice daily injections of LHRH or its analog for 7 days. Mean (±SE) glucuronidase activities are also shown for intact (I) and castrated (C) untreated mice. (Reproduced, with permission, from Lecomte *et al.* (1982). Copyright, 1982, The Endocrine Society.)

(10 μg) of LHRH-A to castrated mice. LHRH-A caused a shift to the right of the dose response curve of kidney glucuronidase to TP (Figure 15.5). In addition, the magnitude of the antiandrogen action was related to the dose of the agonist.

It is of note, however, that this agonist did not block the action of testosterone on the seminal vesicle of the mouse. Furthermore, an anti-androgenic effect of the LHRH agonist could not be demonstrated on the kidneys of female mice that are as sensitive to androgens as those of males. These observations indicate that the antisteroidal effects of LHRH agonists are highly dependent on the sex of the test animal species and different organs within a given species. In this connection it should be noted that a pronounced difference between rats and mice in their sensitivity to the antitesticular effects of LHRH agonists exists (Wang *et al.*, 1983). Notwithstanding the results presented here, an antisteroidal effect of LHRH agonists could not be confirmed in rats (Furr and Nicholson, 1982).

CONCLUDING REMARKS

It is well recognized that LHRH and its agonists have effects on the pituitary and the gonads. A less well known property of these peptides is their ability to

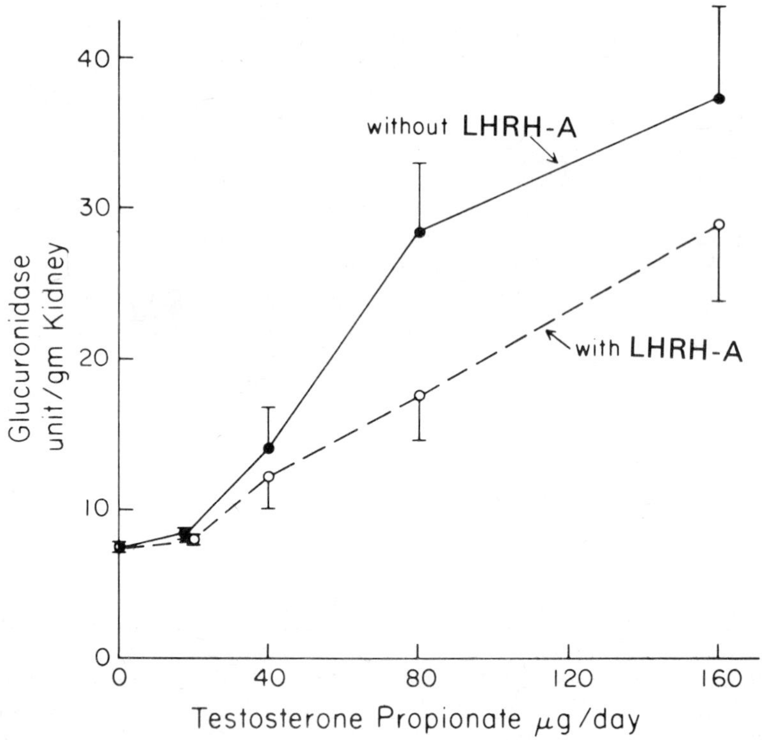

Figure 15.5 The antiandrogenic effect of LHRH-A on the stimulation of β-glucuronidase with increasing doses of TP in castrated male mice. Eight animals in each group were injected once daily with TP and twice daily with LHRH-A (10 μg/day) for 5 days. Means and SE are shown. (Reproduced, with permission, from Lecomte *et al.* (1982). Copyright, 1982, The Endocrine Society.)

inhibit the action of sex steroids on their target tissues. The evidence reviewed here shows that LHRH and its agonists can inhibit the biological activity of estradiol and testosterone.

LHRH agonists have been reported to cause regression of mammary tumors and prostate tumors in rats (DeSombre et al., 1976; Redding and Schally, 1981). Both these tumors are sex steroid dependent and regress after gonadectomy. Since chronic treatment with LHRH agonists leads to gonadal atrophy and decreased sex steroid production, the antitumor activity is believed to be mainly due to the effects of the agonist on the gonads. However, it is also possible that the antisteroidal actions of the LHRH agonists play a role in their antitumor activity.

The mechanism of the antisteroidal actions of LHRH agonists is not known. The uterine estradiol receptor concentration was increased with low doses and decreased with high doses of [D-Trp^6]LHRH (Pedroza *et al.*, 1980). On the other hand, the antiandrogenic action of LHRH-A on mouse kidney was not associated with changes in their androgen receptor content (Lecomte *et al.*, 1982). Also, in *in vitro* tests, LHRH agonists did not compete for binding sites on androgen receptors prepared from the mouse kidney. Most steroidal and non-steroidal compounds having antiandrogenic activity are believed to exert their effects by competing for receptor binding sites found in the cytoplasm and nucleus (Bardin *et al.*, 1973; Katzenellenbogen, 1980). In contrast, like other protein and peptide hormones, LHRH and its analogs bind to membrane receptors on their target tissues (Marshall and Odell, 1975; Perrin *et al.*, 1980; Reeves *et al.*, 1980; Clayton and Catt, 1981). So far, membrane receptors for LHRH have been demonstrated in pituitaries and gonads but not in the reproductive tract or sex accessory glands. An explanation for the mechanism of anti-sex-steroidal actions of LHRH agonists requires further experimentation. Whatever the mechanism of action chronic treatment with potent LHRH agonists may exert significant antisteroidal effects to enhance or modify their antifertility effects.

Acknowledgements

This work was supported by NIH Grant HD-13541, and undertaken as part of the contraceptive development program sponsored and coordinated by the International Committee for Contraception Research of the Population Council, Inc., New York, NY. The financial support provided by the International Development Research Centre of Canada, The U.S. Agency for International Development (Grant AID/pha 1116), the Ford Foundation, the Rockefeller Foundation and the Geo. J. Hecht Fund is gratefully acknowledged. The content does not necessarily reflect the policy of any of the funding sources.

References

Bardin, C. W., Bullock, L. P., Sherins, R. J., Mowszowicz, I. and Blackburn, W. R. (1973). Androgen metabolism and mechanism of action in male pseudohermaprhoditism. A study of testicular feminization. *Rec. Prog. Horm. Res.*, **29**, 65

Bergquist, C., Nillius, S. J., Bergh, T., Skarin, B. and Wide, L. (1979). Inhibitory effects of gonadotropin secretion and gonadal function in men during chronic treatment with a potent stimulatory luteinizing hormone-releasing hormone analogue. *Acta Endrocrinol.*, **91**, 601

Bergquist, C., Nillius, S. J., Wide, L. and Lingren, A. (1981). Endometrial patterns in women on chronic luteinizing hormone-releasing hormone agonist treatment for contraception. *Fertil. Steril.*, **36**, 339

Cao, Y.-Q., Sundaram, K., Bardin, C. W., Rivier, J. and Vale, W. (1982). Direct inhibition of testicular steroidogenesis and gonadotrophin receptor levels by [(imBzl)-D-His^6,Pro^9-NEt]GnRH and [D-Trp^6,Pro^9-NEt]GnRH, potent agonists of GnRH. *Int. J. Androl.*, **5**, 158

Clayton, R. N., Harwood, J. P. and Catt, K. J. (1979). Gonadotropin-releasing hormone analogue binds to luteal cells and inhibits progesterone production. *Nature* (*Lond.*), **282**, 90

Clayton, R. N. and Catt, K. J. (1981). Gonadotropin releasing hormone receptors: Characterization, physiological regulation and relationship to reproductive function. *Endocr. Rev.*, **2**, 186

DeSombre, E. R., Johnson, E. S. and White, W. F. (1976). Regression of rat mammary tumors effected by a gonadoliberin analog. *Cancer Res.*, **36**, 3830

Furr, B. J. A. and Nicholson, R. I. (1982). Use of analogues of luteinizing hormone-releasing hormone for the treatment of cancer. *J. Reprod. Fertil.*, **64**, 529

Hsueh, A. J. W. and Erickson, G. F. (1979). Extrapituitary inhibition of testicular function by luteinizing hormone-releasing hormone. *Nature* (*Lond.*), **281,** 66

Jones, R. C. (1979). Local antifertility effect of luteinizing hormone-releasing hormone (LRH). *Contraception,* **20,** 569

Katzenellenbogen, B. S. (1980). Dynamics of steroid hormone receptor action. *Ann. Rev. Physiol.,* **42,** 17

Lecomte, P., Wang, N.-G., Sundaram, K., Rivier, J., Vale, W. and Bardin, C. W. (1982). The antiandrogenic action of gonadotropin-releasing hormone and its agonists on the mouse kidney. *Endocrinology,* **110,** 1

Liu, Y. and Li, S. (1980). Studies on the mechanism of inhibitory action of a LHRH analogue on decidual formation. II. Experiments in pseudopregnant rats. *Acta Zool. Sinica,* **26,** 1

Marshall, J. C. and Odell, W. D. (1975). Preparation of biologically active [^{125}I] LHRH suitable for membrane binding studies. *Proc. Soc. Exp. Biol. Med.,* **149,** 351

Pedroza, E., Vilchez-Martinez, J. A., Coy, D. H., Arimura, A. and Schally, A. V. (1980). Reduction of LH-RH pituitary and estradiol uterine binding sites by a superactive analog of luteinizing hormone-releasing hormone. *Biochem. Biophys. Res. Commun.,* **95,** 1056

Perrin, M. H., Vaughan, J. M., Rivier, J. E. and Vale, W. W. (1980). High affinity GnRH binding to testicular membrane homogenates. *Life Sci.,* **26,** 2251

Redding, T. W. and Schally, A. V. (1981). Inhibition of prostate tumor growth in two rat models by chronic administration of D-Trp^6 analogue of luteinizing hormone-releasing hormone. *Proc. Natl. Acad. Sci. USA,* **78,** 6509

Reeves, J. J., Séguin, C., Lefebvre, F. A., Kelly, P. A. and Labrie, F. (1980). Similar luteinizing hormone-releasing hormone binding sites in rat anterior pituitary and ovary. *Proc. Natl. Acad. Sci. USA,* **77,** 5567

Rivier, C. and Vale, W. (1979). Hormonal secretion in male rats chronically treated with [D-Trp^6,Pro^9-NEt]-LRF. *Life Sci.,* **25,** 1065

Sandow, J., von Rechenberg, W., Jerzabek, G., Engelbart, K., Kuhl, H. and Fraser, H. (1980). Hypothalamic–pituitary–testicular function in rats after supraphysiological doses of a highly active LRH analogue (buserelin). *Acta Endocrinol.,* **94,** 489

Schally, A. V. (1978). Aspects of hypothalamic regulation of the pituitary gland. *Science,* **202,** 18

Schmidt-Gollwitzer, M., Hardt, W., Schmidt-Gollwitzer, K. and von der Ohe, M. (1981). The contraceptive use of buserelin, a potent LHRH agonist: Clinical and hormonal findings. In Zatuchni, G. I., Shelton, J. D. and Sciarra, J. J. (eds.) *LHRH Peptides as Female and Male Contraceptives.* (Philadelphia: Harper & Row).

Sundaram, K., Cao, Y.-Q., Wang, N.-G., Bardin, C. W., Rivier, J. and Vale, W. (1981). Inhibition of the action of sex steroids by gonadotropin-releasing hormone (GnRH) agonists: A new biological effect. *Life Sci.,* **28,** 83

Sundaram, K., Connell, K. G., Bardin, C. W., Samojlik, E. and Schally, A. V. (1982). Inhibition of pituitary-testicular function with [D-Trp^6] luteinizing hormone-releasing hormone in rhesus monkeys. *Endocrinology,* **110,** 1308

Vickery, B. H. (1981). Physiology and antifertility effects of LHRH and agonistic analogs in male animals. In Zatuchni, G. I., Shelton, J. D. and Sciarra, J. J. (eds.) *LHRH Peptides as Female and Male Contraceptives.* (Philadelphia: Harper & Row)

Vilchez-Martinez, J. A., Pedroza, E., Arimura, A. and Schally, A. V. (1979). Paradoxical effects of D-Trp^6-luteinizing hormone-releasing hormone on the hypothalamic–pituitary–gonadal axis in immature female rats. *Fertil. Steril.,* **31,** 677

Wang, N.-G., Sundaram, K., Pavlou, S., Rivier, J., Vale, W. and Bardin, C. W. (1983). Mice are insensitive to the antitesticular effects of LHRH agonists. *Endocrinology,* **112,** 331

SECTION IV
CONTRACEPTION IN WOMEN

16
LHRH agonists for female contraception

S. J. NILLIUS and C. BERGQUIST

The availability of synthetic LHRH made it possible to evaluate several approaches to contraception: disruption of the normal menstrual cycle by administration of LHRH in the early follicular phase; pinpointing of ovulation for the 'rhythm method' by administration of LHRH on a specific day of the cycle; an immunological approach by using an antiserum to LHRH and use of inhibitory analogs of LHRH (Schally *et al.*, 1972). However, none of these possible new leads to contraception has yet proven to be useful for control of human fertility.

Inhibition of ovulation can paradoxically be achieved by daily intranasal administration of an LHRH agonist and is the basis of a new approach to contraception (Bergquist *et al.*, 1979*a*). Another potential for contraception is induction of luteolysis by LHRH agonists (Lemay *et al.*, 1979; Casper and Yen, 1979) but this approach remains to be proven in women.

OVULATION INHIBITION BY CONTINUOUS TREATMENT

The first paradoxical inhibition of reproductive functions in women by administration of an LHRH agonist was achieved in 1978 with daily injections of 5 μg of [D-Ser(tBu)^6,Pro^9-NHEt]LHRH (Nillius *et al.*, 1978). Longer term studies used daily intranasal spray administration of the LHRH agonist which was practical and highly acceptable (Bergquist *et al.*, 1979*a*, 1982*a*; Schmidt-Gollwitzer *et al.*, 1981).

Contraceptive effectiveness

Seventy-one regularly menstruating women have used the nasal spray for contraception during 3–21 months (Table 16.1). Inhibition of ovulation occurred during 561 of the 564 treatment months. The failures were probably due to insufficient dosage because of problems with the first, technically deficient, spray applicator. No pregnancies have occurred.

Table 16.1 A summary of results from 71 female volunteers treated with single daily doses of 200–600 μg of the LHRH agonist for 3–21 months

Intranasal dose (μg)	*Subjects* (n)	*Treatment cycles* (months)	*Anovulatory treatment cycles* (months)
200	10	149	149
400	37	290	288
600	24	125	124
Total	71	564	561

Effects on menstrual bleeding patterns

The bleeding pattern during treatment varied from fairly regular bleeding intervals to amenorrhea (Bergquist *et al.*, 1982*a*) (Figure 16.1). The total bleeding index, i.e. the number of bleeding episodes per month, was 0.44. Short periods of spotting were reported during the first treatment months in three women. Prolonged and heavy bleedings did not occur. Representative hormone and bleeding patterns are shown in Figure 16.2. The estradiol levels in serum decreased during the course of the prolonged LHRH agonist treatment (Figure 16.3). However, no symptoms of estrogen deficiency, such as hot flushes or vaginal discomfort, were reported.

Serum progesterone levels were slightly raised, particularly during the first

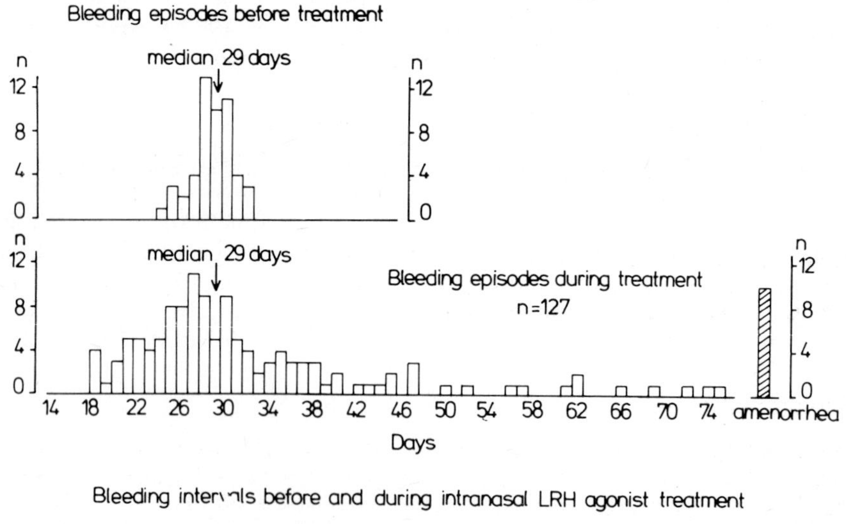

Figure 16.1 Bleeding intervals before and during 3–12 months of intranasal LHRH agonist treatment of regularly menstruating women. n = number of bleeding episodes. (From Bergquist *et al.* (1982*a*), reproduced by permission of the publisher, The American Fertility Society, Birmingham, AL.)

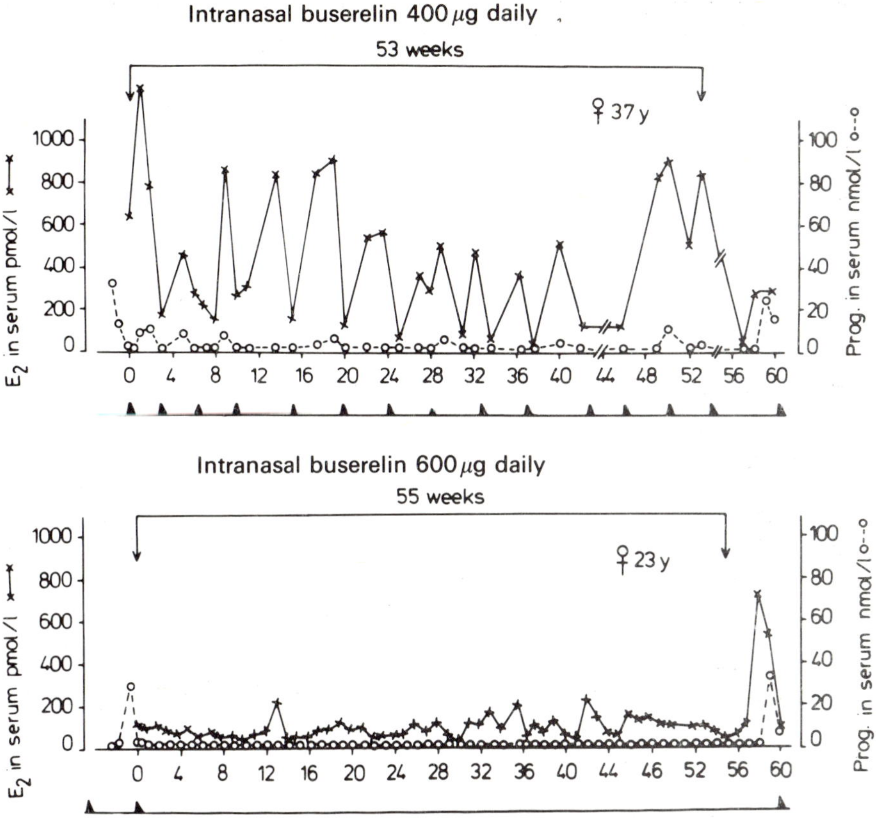

Figure 16.2 Hormone and bleeding patterns during prolonged intranasal LHRH agonist therapy. One woman had fairly regular uterine bleeding during 53 weeks of treatment (top), while the other woman had amenorrhea throughout 55 weeks of treatment (below). After cessation of treatment rapid return of normal ovulation. (From Bergquist *et al.* (1982*a*), reproduced by permission of the publisher, The American Fertility Society, Birmingham, AL.)

three months of treatment, interpreted as reactivation of corpus luteum at initiation of treatment, a defect in luteal function or luteinization of the follicle(s) (Bergquist *et al.*, 1982*b*) (Table 16.2).

Endometrial patterns

The predominant histologic picture from 50 biopsy specimens was inactive or weak proliferative glands with slightly atrophic stroma (Bergquist *et al.*, 1981). No signs of hyperplastic changes were observed. Early signs of hyperplasia of the endometrium have been noted by other investigators (Schmidt-Gollwitzer *et al.*, 1981). However, the findings decreased as treatment progressed. Nevertheless, further endometrial biopsies have to be performed in women on continuous LHRH agonist treatment to exclude hyperplastic changes.

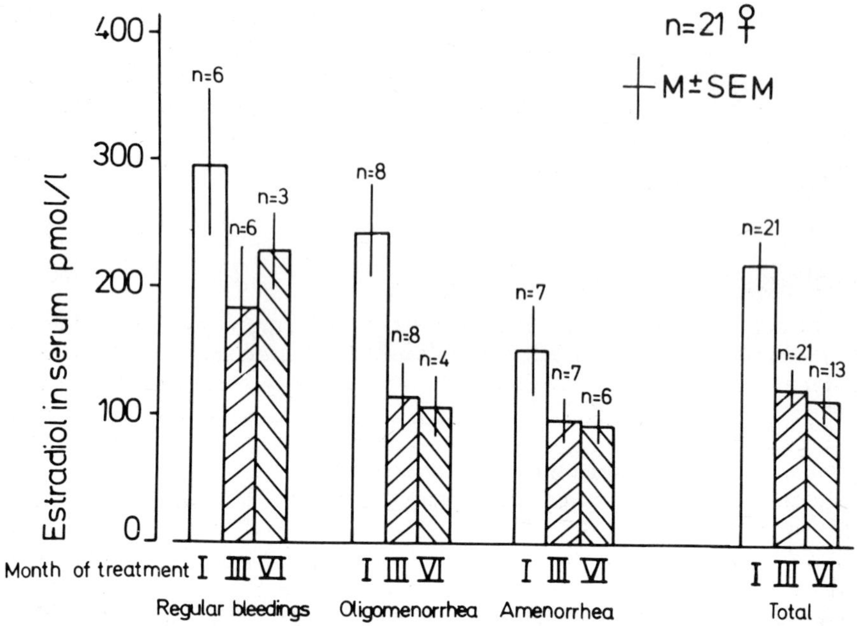

Figure 16.3 Mean serum estradiol levels and associated menstrual bleeding pattern during the 1st, 3rd and 6th month of prolonged intranasal LHRH agonist treatment. (From Bergquist *et al.* (1982*a*), reproduced by permission of the publisher, The American Fertility Society, Birmingham, AL.)

Table 16.2 Treatment months with raised progesterone levels during chronic intranasal LHRH agonist administration

Bleeding pattern during first 3 *months of treatment*	*Treatment months* (n)	*Reactivation of corpus luteum at initiation of treatment: Progesterone* > 5 nmol/l		*Luteinization of follicles: Progesterone* 5–9 nmol/l		*Defect luteal phase: Progesterone* 10–19 nmol/l		*Presumptive ovulation: Progesterone* > 20 nmol/l	
LHRH agonist dose (μg)		400	600	400	600	400	600	400	600
Cyclical uterine bleeding	51	0	2	3	3	3	1	1	0
Oligomenorrhea	69	2	2	3	4	2	1	1	1
Amenorrhea	30	0	0	0	0	0	0	0	0
Total	150	2	4	6	7	5	2	2	1

Resumption of ovulation

After cessation of prolonged LHRH agonist treatment, normal reproductive function was rapidly restored. The first ovulatory menstrual bleeding appeared after 33 days, on average, in 51 volunteers treated continuously for 3–12 months (Bergquist *et al.*, 1982*a*). Women with amenorrhea during treatment had their first ovulatory menstrual bleeding somewhat later (median 47 days) than the women who had uterine bleedings during treatment (median 33 days). Five volunteers who subsequently wanted to become pregnant had no difficulty in conceiving. Thus, there seems to be no question about the reversibility of this new contraceptive method.

Mechanisms of action

The mechanism by which LHRH agonists exert their paradoxical inhibitory effects on reproductive function is not known. Several possible mechanisms of action have been proposed: desensitization of the pituitary gonadotropes, down regulation of gonadal gonadotropin receptors and reduction of steroidogenic response of the ovary, and direct inhibitory actions of LHRH agonists on the reproductive organs.

Desensitization of the pituitary processes responsible for gonadotropin secretion is believed to be the main action of chronic LHRH agonist treatment. Repeated administration of [D-Ser(tBu)^6,Pro^9-NHEt]LHRH to either normally ovulating or postmenopausal women reduced the pituitary's ability to release gonadotropins (Bergquist *et al.*, 1979*b*,*c*; Dericks-Tan *et al.*, 1977). Furthermore, failure of positive feedback of estradiol has been demonstrated in chronic LHRH agonist treated women (Bergquist *et al.*, 1982*c*). The normal pulsatile LHRH and LH release from the hypothalamus and pituitary, respectively, may be abolished by the continuous administration of LHRH or by daily administration of potent, long acting LHRH agonists.

Extrapituitary effects of LHRH and its agonists have been clearly demonstrated in experimental animals (Hsueh and Jones, 1981). Such actions may partially explain the paradoxical inhibitory effects on reproductive functions in women. However, women respond to exogenous human gonadotropins with a similar estrogen increase both during and after chronic LHRH agonist treatment (Figure 16.4). Treatment with high doses of LHRH or its agonist did not alter the steroidogenic effect of FSH on cultured human granulosa cells (Casper *et al.*, 1982). Receptors for LHRH have so far not been detected in human gonads (Clayton and Huhtaniemi, 1982). Thus, LHRH agonists probably do not directly inhibit the human ovary.

LUTEOLYTIC APPROACHES TO CONTRACEPTION IN WOMEN

Early follicular phase administration

[D-Ser(tBu)^6,Pro^9-NHEt]LHRH was administered subcutaneously at a dose of 5–25 μg for 1–5 consecutive days in the early follicular phase (Skarin *et al.*, 1982*a*). The luteal phase during LHRH agonist treatment did not differ in length or progesterone concentrations from those of the control cycles although the highest doses resulted in a prolongation of the follicular phase

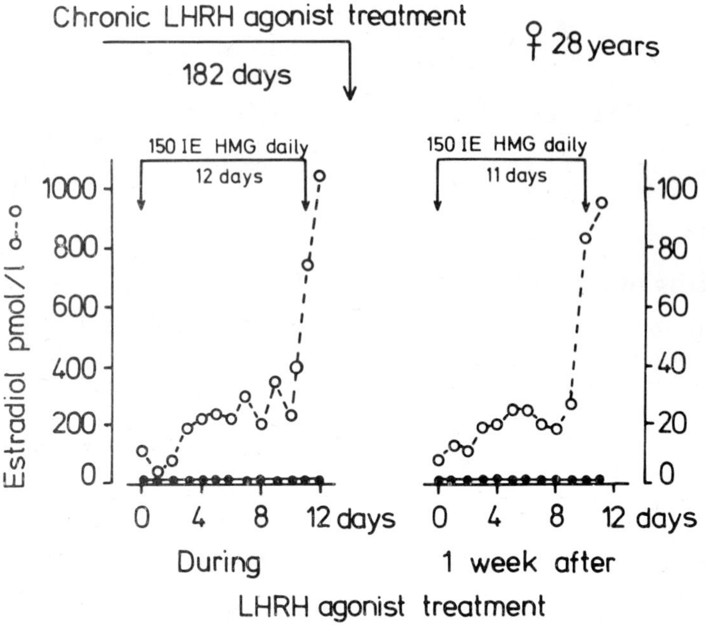

Figure 16.4 Estradiol response to HMG during and after chronic LHRH agonist treatment in a woman with amenorrhea during treatment.

(Figure 16.5). There was a positive correlation between the length of the follicular phase and the duration of the LHRH agonist administration. This is in contrast with another study in which subcutaneous administration of 50 μg of [D-Trp^6,Pro^9-NHEt]LHRH daily for the first 3 days after the onset of menstruation led to a shortened luteal phase with suboptimal levels of estradiol and progesterone (Sheehan *et al.*, 1982*a*).

Midluteal phase administration

Administration of an LHRH agonist on each of 2 consecutive days during the midluteal phase of the menstrual cycle has resulted in short luteal phase with premature decline of the progesterone level in serum and earlier onset of menstruation (Figure 16.6). A drawback to the use of this approach is the fact that the timing of the LHRH agonist administration is critical for its effectiveness. Successful luteolysis was achieved when [D-Trp^6,Pro^9-NHEt]LHRH was administered between 5 and 8 days after the LH peak (Sheehan *et al.*, 1982*b*). However, when the LHRH agonist treatment began within 5 days of the LH peak, induction of luteolysis failed to occur. The critical time or 'window' is narrow. The luteolytic action of an LHRH agonist is most effective when given 6–9 days after the LH surge as compared with days 1–5.

In further studies, hCG was administered daily for 10 days concomitantly with the postovulatory treatment with [D-Ser(tBu)^6,Pro^9-

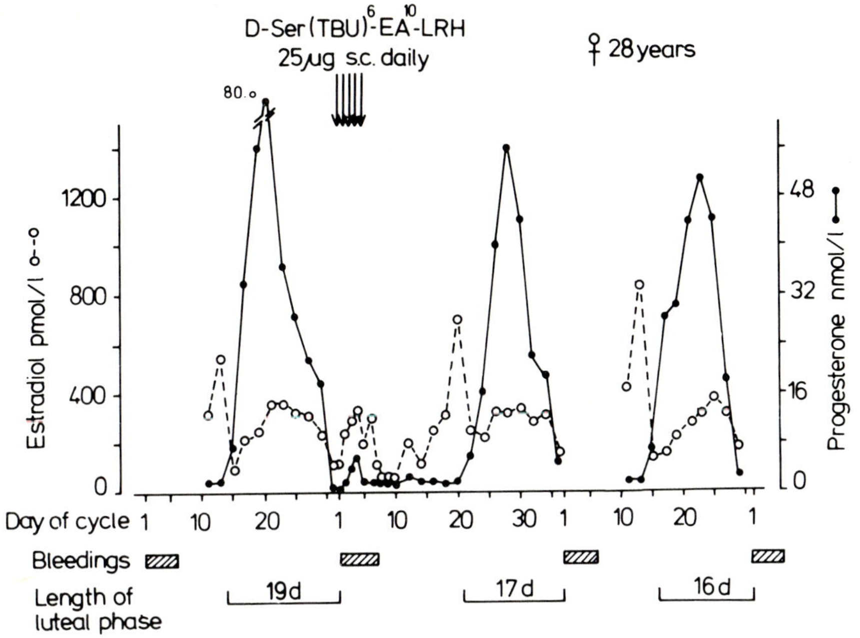

Figure 16.5 Plasma levels of estradiol and progesterone before, during and after administration of 25 µg LHRH agonist s.c. daily for 5 consecutive days during the early follicular phase of the menstrual cycle. The follicular phase length was 20 days during the treatment cycle compared with 13 days during the two control cycles. The luteal phase length was 16 days during the treatment cycle compared with 18 and 17 days during the control cycles. (From Skarin *et al.*, 1982*a*, with permission.)

NHEt]LHRH (Bergquist *et al.*, 1980). Raised progesterone levels in serum and a prolonged luteal phase were observed, i.e. the luteolytic effect of the LHRH agonist was completely prevented by the presence of hCG (Figure 16.6). Similar findings were made with [D-Trp^6,Pro^9-NHEt]LHRH (Casper *et al.*, 1980). Thus, the utility of LHRH agonists as postovulatory luteolytic agents is doubtful.

Administration during early pregnancy

Repeated doses of [D-Ser(tBu)^6,Pro^9-NHEt]LHRH (50–125 µg) were administered i.v. for 4 days to volunteers requesting legal abortion (Skarin *et al.*, 1982*b*). The LHRH agonist treatment did not induce any obvious changes in the estradiol or progesterone levels in serum in comparison with the serum levels observed during normal early human pregnancy (Figure 16.7). The hCG levels in serum continued to rise during and following the treatment and the pregnancies were terminated by suction curettage. The histopathological investigation of the uterine contents revealed normal pregnancy tissue. Similar

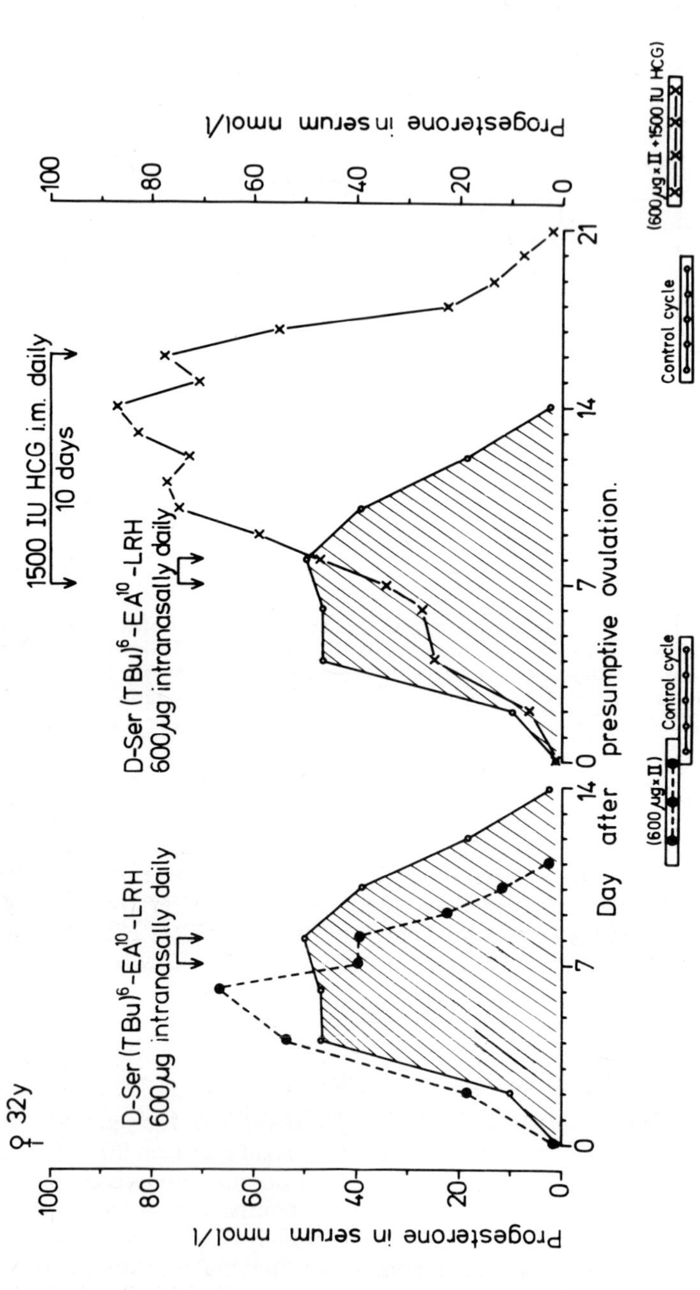

Figure 16.6 Serum progesterone levels and length of the luteal phases during one control cycle and two treatment cycles with the LHRH agonist only (left) and the LHRH agonist plus hCG (right). (Data from Bergquist *et al.*, 1980.)

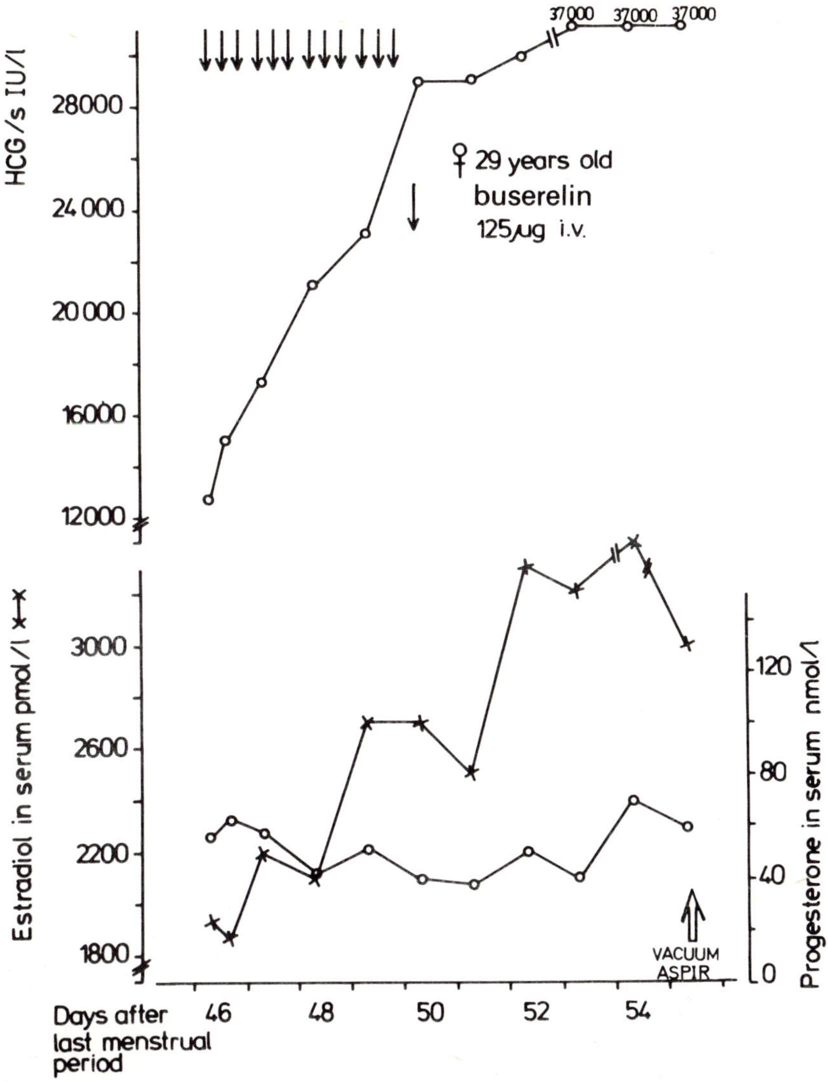

Figure 16.7 Serum levels of hCG, estradiol and progesterone before, during and after repeated intravenous injections (arrow) of [D-Ser(tBu)[6],Pro[9]-NHEt]LHRH (125 µg t.i.d. for 4 days) in a volunteer in early pregnancy 46 days after the last menstrual period. (From Skarin *et al.*, 1982*b*, with permission.)

results have been reported for [D-Trp[6]]LHRH and [D-Trp[6],Pro[9]-NHEt]LHRH (Casper *et al.*, 1980; Tolis *et al.*, 1981). Thus, the endogenous hCG secreted during early pregnancy prevented the luteolytic effects which are caused by LHRH agonists in the non-pregnant luteal phase.

CONCLUDING REMARKS

Long term clinical trials have demonstrated that continuous intranasal LHRH agonist treatment for inhibition of ovulation can provide safe, effective and reversible contraception in women. No serious side-effects have been observed. The only untoward effects are slight bleeding irregularities caused by the induced anovulation. Further clinical trials of this new lead to fertility control are clearly warranted. This approach to peptide contraception should provide a good safe complement to existing methods of steroid contraception. The contraceptive effectiveness of the luteolytic approach to peptide contraception, whether by early follicular phase or midluteal phase administration, remains to be proven in the human. Abortifacient effects of superactive LHRH agonists have not been observed during early human pregnancy. To date, ovulation inhibition by continuous LHRH superagonist treatment seems to be the most promising lead to peptide contraception.

Acknowledgements

The authors wish to express their sincere gratitude to Hoechst AG, FRG, for generous supply of the LHRH agonist, to Associate Professor L. Wide at the Department of Clinical Chemistry, University Hospital, Uppsala for the hormone determinations and to Mrs Birgitta Bohman for skillful technical assistance. This study was supported by the Swedish Medical Research Council (Grant No 13X-3145) and the International Committee for Contraception Research of the Population Council.

References

Bergquist, C., Nillius, S. J. and Wide, L. (1979*a*). Intranasal gonadotropin-releasing hormone agonist as a contraceptive agent. *Lancet,* **2,** 215

Bergquist, C., Nillius, S. J. and Wide, L. (1979*b*). Inhibition of ovulation in women by intranasal treatment with a luteinizing hormone-releasing hormone agonist. *Contraception,* **19,** 497

Bergquist, C., Nillius, S. J. and Wide, L. (1979*c*). Reduced gonadotropin secretion in postmenopausal women during treatment with a stimulatory LRH analogue. *J. Clin. Endocrinol. Metab.,* **49,** 472

Bergquist, C., Nillius, S. J. and Wide, L. (1980). Luteolysis induced by a luteinizing hormone-releasing hormone agonist is prevented by human chorionic gonadotropin. *Contraception,* **22,** 341

Bergquist, C., Nillius, S. J., Wide, L. and Lindgren, A. (1981). Endometrial patterns in women on chronic LRH agonist treatment for inhibition of ovulation. *Fertil. Steril.,* **36,** 339

Bergquist, C., Nillius, S. J. and Wide, L. (1982*a*). Long-term intranasal luteinizing hormone-releasing hormone agonist treatment for contraception in women. *Fertil. Steril.,* **38,** 190

Bergquist, C., Nillius, S. J. and Wide, L. (1982*b*). Intranasal LHRH agonist treatment for inhibition of ovulation in women: Clinical aspects. *Clin. Endocrinol.,* **17,** 91

Bergquist, C., Nillius, S. J. and Wide, L. (1982*c*). Failure of positive feedback of oestradiol during chronic intranasal luteinizing hormone-releasing hormone agonist treatment. *Clin. Endocrinol.,* **16,** 147

Casper, R. F. and Yen, S. S. C. (1979). Induction of luteolysis in the human with a long-acting analog of luteinizing hormone-releasing factor. *Science,* **205,** 408

Casper, R. F., Sheehan, K. L. and Yen, S. S. C. (1980). Chorionic gonadotropin prevents LRH-agonist-induced luteolysis in the human. *Contraception,* **21,** 471

Casper, R. F., Eriksson, G. F., Rebar, R. W. and Yen, S. S. C. (1982). The effect of luteinizing hormone-releasing factor and its agonist on cultured human granulosa cells. *Fertil. Steril.*, **37,** 406

Clayton, R. N. and Huhtaniemi, I. T. (1982). Absence of gonadotropin-releasing hormone receptors in human gonadal tissue. *Nature (Lond.)*, **299,** 56

Dericks-Tan, J. S. E., Hammer, E. and Taubert, H.-D. (1977). The effect of D-Ser(TBU)6-LH-RH-EA10 upon gonadotropin release in normally cyclic women. *J. Clin. Endocrinol. Metab.*, **45,** 597

Hsueh, A. J. W. and Jones, P. B. C. (1981). Extrapituitary actions of gonadotropin-releasing hormone. *Endocr. Rev.*, **2,** 437

Lemay, A., Labrie, F., Bélanger, A. and Raynaud, J.-P. (1979). Luteolytic effect of intranasal administration of (D-Ser(TBU)^6,DES-GLY-$NH_2{}^{10}$)-luteinizing hormone-releasing hormone ethylamide in normal women. *Fertil. Steril.*, **32,** 646

Nillius, S. J., Bergquist, C. and Wide, L. (1978). Inhibition of ovulation in women by chronic treatment with a stimulatory LRH analogue – a new approach to birth control? *Contraception*, **17,** 537

Schally, A. V., Kastin, A. J. and Arimura, A. (1972). The hypothalamus and reproduction. *Am. J. Obstet. Gynecol.*, **114,** 423

Schmidt-Gollwitzer, M., Hardt, W., Schmidt-Gollwitzer, K. and Nevinny-Stickel, J. (1981). Influence of the LH-RH analogue buserelin on cyclic ovarian function and on endometrium. A new approach to fertility control? *Contraception*, **23,** 187

Sheehan, K. L., Casper, R. F. and Yen, S. S. C. (1982*a*). Luteal phase defects induced by an agonist of luteinizing hormone-releasing factor: A model for fertility control. *Science*, **215,** 170

Sheehan, K. L., Casper, R. F. and Yen, S. S. C. (1982*b*). Induction of luteolysis by luteinizing hormone-releasing factor (LRF) agonist: sensitivity, reproducibility, and reversibility. *Fertil. Steril.*, **37,** 209

Skarin, G., Nillius, S. J. and Wide, L. (1982*a*). Early follicular phase luteinizing hormone-releasing hormone agonist administration – effects on follicular maturation and corpus luteum function in women. *Contraception*, **25,** 31

Skarin, G., Nillius, S. J. and Wide, L. (1982*b*). Failure to induce early abortion by huge doses of a superactive LRH agonist in women. *Contraception*, **26,** 457

Tolis, G., Comaru-Schally, A. M., Mehta, A. E. and Schally, A. V. (1981). Failure to interrupt established pregnancy in human by D-tryptophan-6-luteinizing hormone-releasing hormone. *Fertil. Steril.*, **36,** 241

17
Postcoital contraception with intranasal buserelin

A. LEMAY, N. FAURE, F. LABRIE and A. T. A. FAZEKAS

Pharmacological or repetitive doses of LHRH agonists lead to well-documented paradoxical antifertility effects. In female animals of several species, various treatments cause inhibition of ovulation, luteolysis and termination of pregnancy (Corbin and Bex, 1981; Balmaceda and Asch, 1981; Vickery, 1981; Puri and Csapo, 1981). In normal women treatment with LHRH agonists can induce luteolysis (Lemay *et al.*, 1978, 1979*a*,*b*, 1982; Casper and Yen, 1979; Sheehan *et al.*, 1982) and inhibit ovulation (Nillius *et al.*, 1978; Bauman *et al.*, 1980; Schmidt-Gollwitzer *et al.*, 1981).

Initial studies demonstrated induction of luteolysis by subcutaneous (s.c.) LHRH or intranasal (i.n.) [D-Ser(tBu)^6,Pro^9-NHEt]LHRH (buserelin) administration at midluteal phase in normal women (Lemay *et al.*, 1978, 1979*a*,*b*). This article summarizes the results of our three recent protocols conducted in 88 normal 20–40 year old women protected from pregnancy. We have now studied the effect of buserelin administered intranasally at different doses and days during the luteal phase. In addition, the LHRH agonist treatment has been administered at varying times before and during injections of hCG mimicking the beginning of a pregnancy.

DOSE-EFFECT OF INTRANASAL LHRH AGONIST AT MIDLUTEAL PHASE

A luteolytic effect was obtained when five 250 μg doses of native LHRH were injected s.c. every 4 hours (Lemay *et al.*, 1978). The treatment was more effective when the peptide was administered at midluteal phase (Lemay *et al.*, 1979*a*). Induction of luteolysis in women was demonstrated following a s.c. injection of 50 μg of a long acting LHRH analog on each of 2 successive days during midluteal phase (Casper and Yen, 1979). A window of maximal effectiveness for luteolysis on days 5–8 after ovulation has been reported (Sheehan *et al.*, 1982). In order to evaluate the efficacy of i.n. buserelin, we first studied the effects of increasing doses of the LHRH agonist during the midluteal phase.

Acute effects on serum gonadotropins and steroids

The serum LH and FSH responses to increasing doses (50–1500 μg) of buserelin administered i.n. 6–12 days after the midcycle LH peak can be expressed as areas under the 24 h serum response curves (Figure 17.1). Half-maximal response for both gonadotropins is obtained at a dose slightly above 100 μg i.n. Peak response is observed at 4 h for LH (10–15-fold) and at 6 h for FSH (4–5-fold) and is maximal at 200 μg. At the two highest doses (1000 and 1500 μg), the stimulation of gonadotropins is more prolonged, LH levels being elevated at 14 h after dosing. FSH levels are twice control values at the same time. Gonadotropin levels return to pretreatment control levels by 24 h.

Following the gonadotropin elevations, there was a transient elevation of serum estradiol and progesterone (Lemay *et al.*, 1982). The increase in progesterone levels was similar at all doses (200–250 %) and was maximal 8 h after the LHRH agonist treatment. The effect on estradiol levels was dose

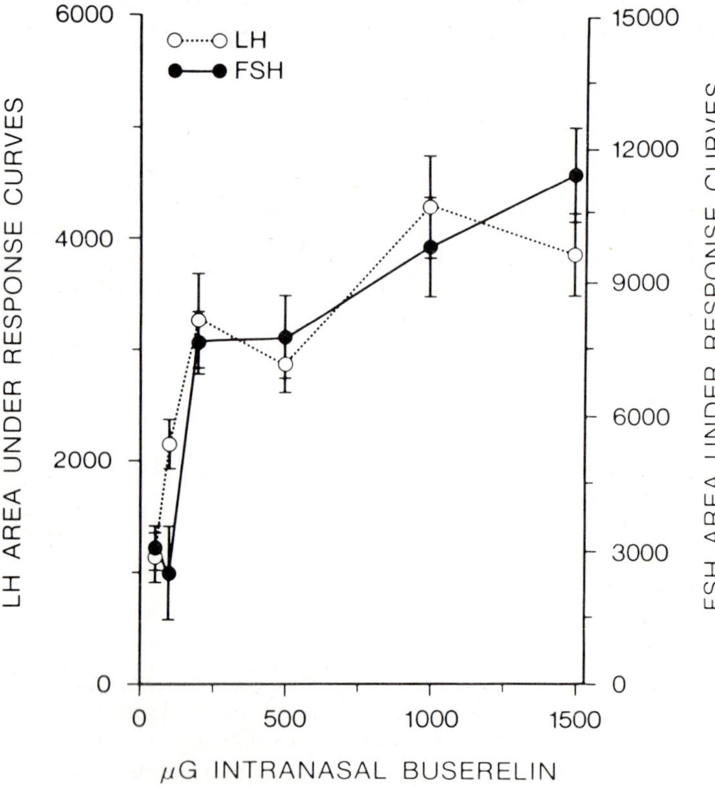

Figure 17.1 Effect of single increasing doses (50, 100, 200, 500, 1000 and 1500 μg) of intranasal buserelin on the 24 h serum LH and FSH areas under response curves. Blood samples were taken at $-\frac{1}{2}$, $-\frac{1}{4}$, 1, 2, 4, 6, 8, 11, 14 and 24 h relative to the time of LHRH agonist administration. The values are expressed as the mean ± the standard error of the mean of the cumulated 24 h serum LH and FSH levels in individual women.

related. At 24 h both steroids had returned to pretreatment control values in all groups.

Effects on corpus luteum function and luteal phase duration

Following these acute pituitary and corpus luteum responses, we measured serum estradiol and progesterone daily. The changes in the length of the luteal phase and the inhibition of daily serum progesterone and estradiol concentrations are related to increasing doses of i.n. buserelin (Figure 17.2). At doses of 50–200 μg of buserelin, there are no significant changes in the levels of serum sex steroids or in the length of the luteal phase. Decreased steroid levels are observed at the 500 μg dose and there is a corresponding shortening of the luteal phase in 56 % of treated cycles. At doses higher than 500 μg, the luteal phase is shortened in all the treated cycles. At the dose of 1000 μg, the shortening of the luteal phase averages 2.5 days and serum progesterone and estradiol levels are inhibited by 52 % and 54 % respectively.

Thus the corpus luteum is sensitive to single, high doses of buserelin i.n.

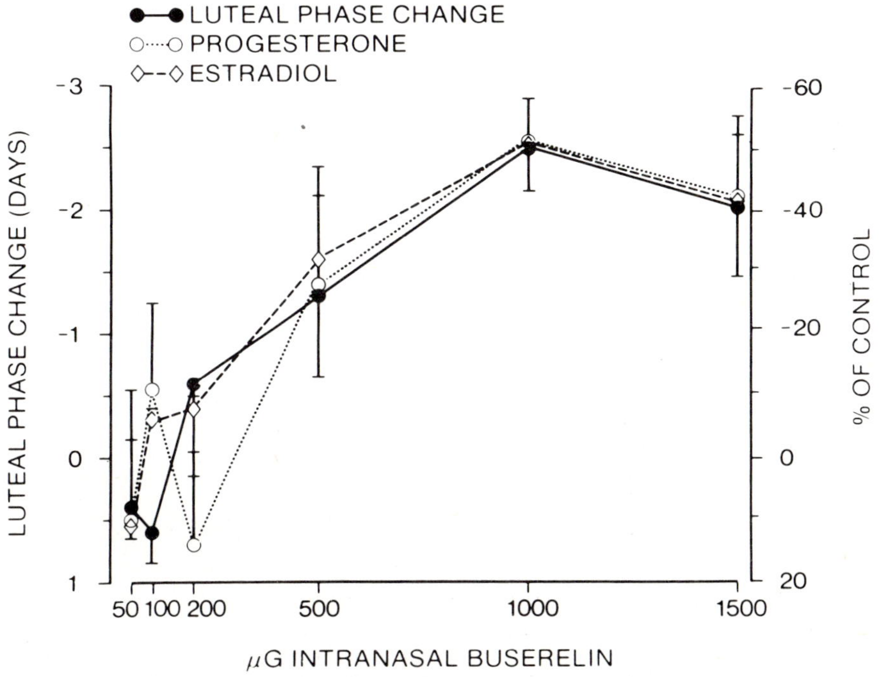

Figure 17.2 Effect of single intranasal insufflation of increasing doses (50, 100, 200, 500, 1000 and 1500 μg) of intranasal buserelin on luteal phase length and on serum progesterone and estradiol concentrations. The results are expressed as the mean ± the standard error of the mean of individual values as compared with pretreatment control cycles. The percentages of changes in progesterone and estradiol values have been calculated from the areas under the hormone curves in individual cases starting from the day of LHRH agonist treatment.

Although maximal amplitude of the response is observed at low doses, luteolysis results only after administration of a high dose which elicits more prolonged gonadotropin and estradiol responses.

TIME-EFFECT OF INTRANASAL LHRH AGONIST AFTER LH SURGE

Maximal sensitivity for the induction of luteolysis occurs when LHRH agonists are administered at midluteal phase (Lemay *et al.*, 1979*a*). The pituitary LH and FSH responses to LHRH or LHRH agonist treatment vary during the different phases of the menstrual cycle (Nillius and Wide, 1972; Yen *et al.*, 1972; Dericks-Tan *et al.*, 1977). Studies were performed on the pituitary and corpus luteum responses to i.n. LHRH agonist treatment at varying times during the luteal phase.

Since maximal increase of gonadotropins was observed at a 200 μg dose, and since luteolysis appeared to be related to prolonged hormonal stimulation, we administered two successive 300 μg doses at a 10 h time interval. This regimen was used on one of days 1–10 after the midcycle LH surge.

Acute effects on serum gonadotropins and steroids

After administration of the first dose, the stimulation of LH and FSH is of maximal amplitude on the first 2 days following the LH surge (Figure 17.3). On the following 2 days, the response decreases and remains stable on days 5–10. Ten hours after this initial dose, gonadotropins are still increased by 2–8-fold. Following the administration of the second dose on any day after the LH surge, the response is markedly blunted. The serum LH concentration is slightly increased 4 h after administration of the second dose whereas FSH levels remain stable. Fourteen hours after the second dose, both LH and FSH are slightly above pretreatment control levels.

On any day (1–10) after the LH surge, there is a progressive rise in serum estradiol levels following treatment (Figure 17.4, Panels D–F). A maximal stimulation (threefold) is obtained at 14 h (4 h after administration of the second dose) and the steroid hormone levels are still increased (twofold) at 24 h.

The acute effect on serum progesterone levels differs from the observed stimulation of serum estradiol levels. Basal progesterone blood levels are increasing between treatment days 1–4, but there is no stimulation following the LHRH agonist administration (Figure 17.4, Panels A and B). On treatment days 5–10 (Panel C), basal serum progesterone levels reach 20 ng/ml and are increased by 50 % 10 h after administration of the first dose of LHRH analog. However, at 14 h (4 h after the administration of the second dose), serum progesterone levels are decreasing and return to pretreatment levels at 24 h.

There is therefore a rapid refractoriness of the gonadotrope 10 h after i.n. administration of 300 μg of buserelin at any time during the luteal phase.

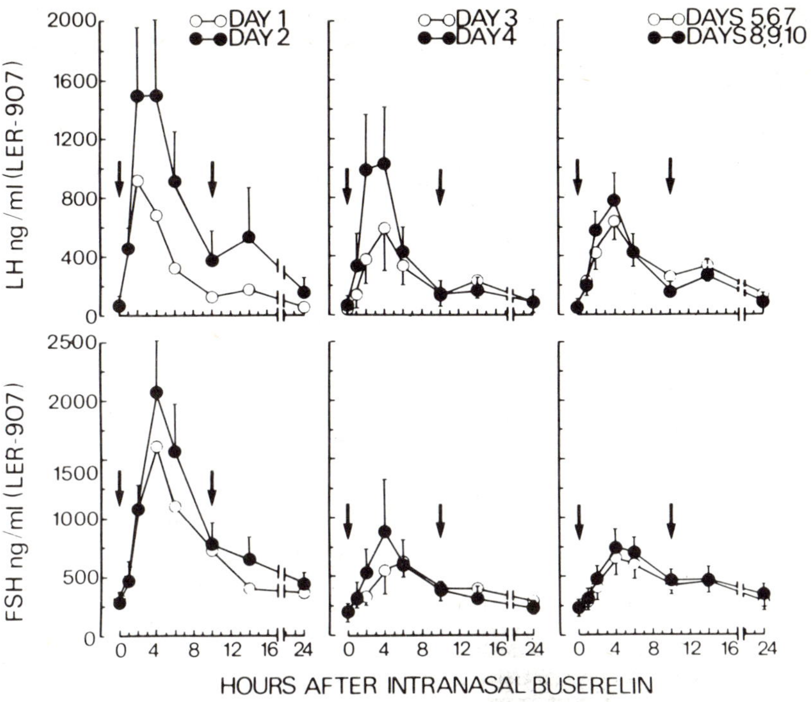

Figure 17.3 Effect of two successive doses of intranasal buserelin on acute serum LH and FSH responses at different days after the LH surge. 300 μg of the LHRH agonist were insufflated into the nose at 0 and 10 h on days 1–10 after the LH surge. Blood samples were obtained at times $-\frac{1}{2}$, 0, 1, 2, 4, 6 and 10 h relative to the first dose and at 4 and 14 h relative to the second dose.

Following the prolonged gonadotropin stimulation, there is a temporary rise in serum estradiol which is still twofold above control levels at 24 h. Progesterone levels are not stimulated during the first 4 days after the LH peak and increase in this steroid on days 5–10 is smaller and of shorter duration than estradiol, serum progesterone returning to normal control levels at 24 h.

Effects on corpus luteum function and luteal phase duration

The effect of the LHRH analog treatment on serum progesterone levels was analyzed for each day of the luteal phase (Figure 17.5). Control pre- and post-treatment curves are superimposable, demonstrating no effect of the treatment on the following control cycle (Panel A). When the treatment is administered early in the luteal phase (days 1–4 after the midcycle LH surge: Panels B and C), corpus luteum function is impaired and the serum progesterone levels are lower than in the pretreatment cycle. However, the length of the luteal phase is not modified.

When the treatment is given on day 5 (Panel D), there is a precocious fall of progesterone levels starting on day 8 but no significant changes in the length of

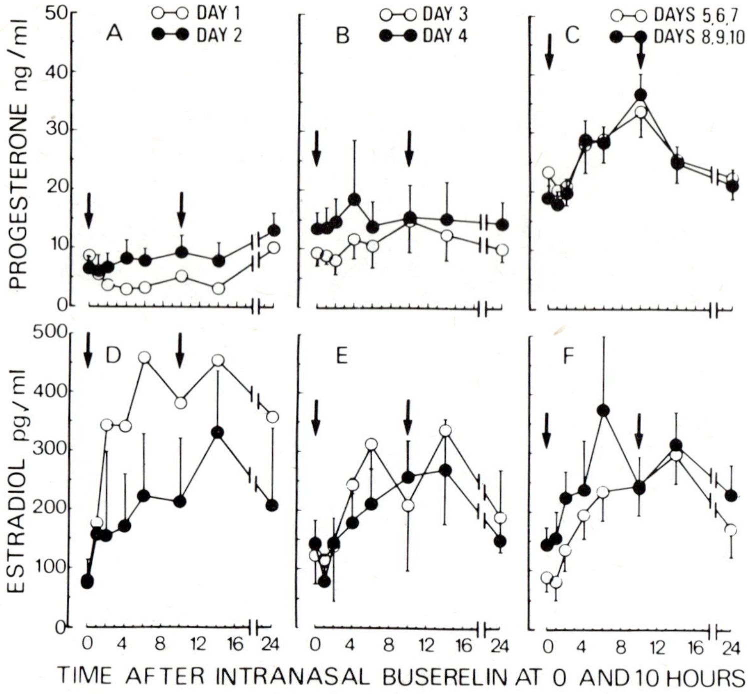

Figure 17.4 Effect of two successive doses (300 μg) of intranasal buserelin at different days after LH surge on acute serum estradiol and progesterone levels. Experimental conditions were as described for Figure 17.3.

the luteal phase. When treatment is on days 6–10, a luteolytic effect is evidenced by a more rapid drop in serum progesterone levels and shortening of the luteal phase (1–4 days) in all the treatment cycles (Panels D–F). When the treatment is administered late during the luteal phase, the fall in progesterone levels occurs sooner after the treatment.

The inhibition of serum progesterone is 30 % when treatment is applied on day 1 and decreases to 20 % in the following 3 days (Figure 17.6). There is no change in the duration of the luteal phase corresponding to this inhibitory effect. Maximal progesterone inhibition is observed following treatment on days 5–8 (42 ± 8 % on day 6) and is associated with a shortening of the luteal phase (3.1 ± 1.0 days on day 6). Although the fall of progesterone occurs sooner and is faster when the treatment is administered at a later time, the inhibition of progesterone levels and the shortening of the luteal phase appear to be diminished. This apparent decrease in the efficacy of treatment is probably related to the fact that the time of treatment is closer to the spontaneous regression of the corpus luteum.

Thus, when administered early in the luteal phase LHRH agonists impair the establishment of normal corpus luteum function, leading to luteal phase insufficiency without shortening of the luteal phase. On the other hand, when

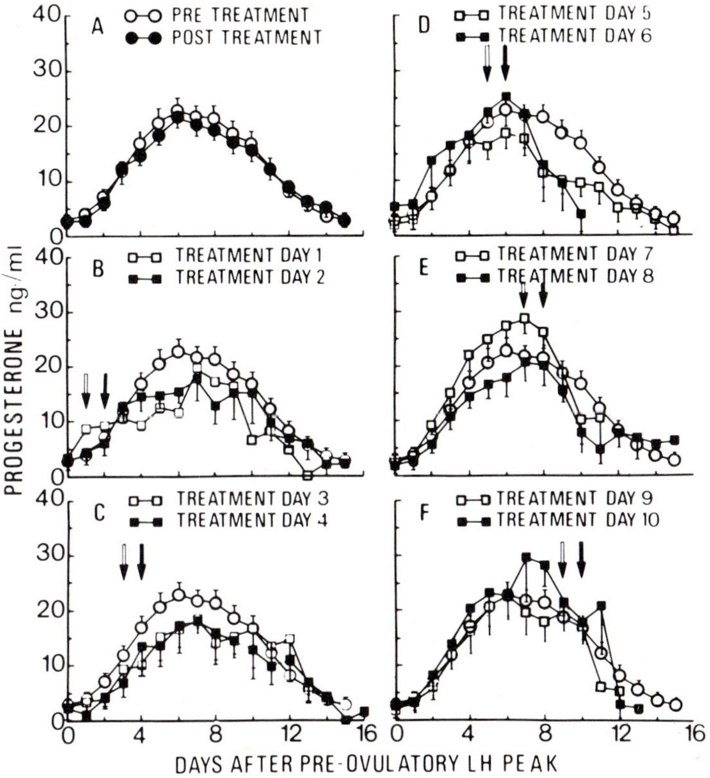

Figure 17.5 Daily serum progesterone levels after single day treatment using two successive doses (300 μg) of intranasal buserelin administered at varying times after the LH surge.

administered at midluteal phase, the LHRH agonist treatment induces luteolysis leading to precocious menses. These results are in agreement with other reports of inhibition of serum progesterone levels without shortening of the luteal phase after a 5 day treatment with [Pro^9-NHEt] LHRH starting early after ovulation (Koyama *et al.*, 1978). Marked inhibition of serum progesterone levels after daily administration of i.n. buserelin initiated immediately after presumptive ovulation has also been noted by Bergquist *et al.* (1980*a*).

INTRANASAL LHRH AGONIST BEFORE AND DURING hCG TREATMENT

For use of an intranasal LHRH agonist as a postcoital contraceptive, the obvious important question to be answered is the effectiveness of the treatment in the face of a possible onset of a pregnancy. Since hCG is secreted around the time of implantation and stimulates corpus luteum function,

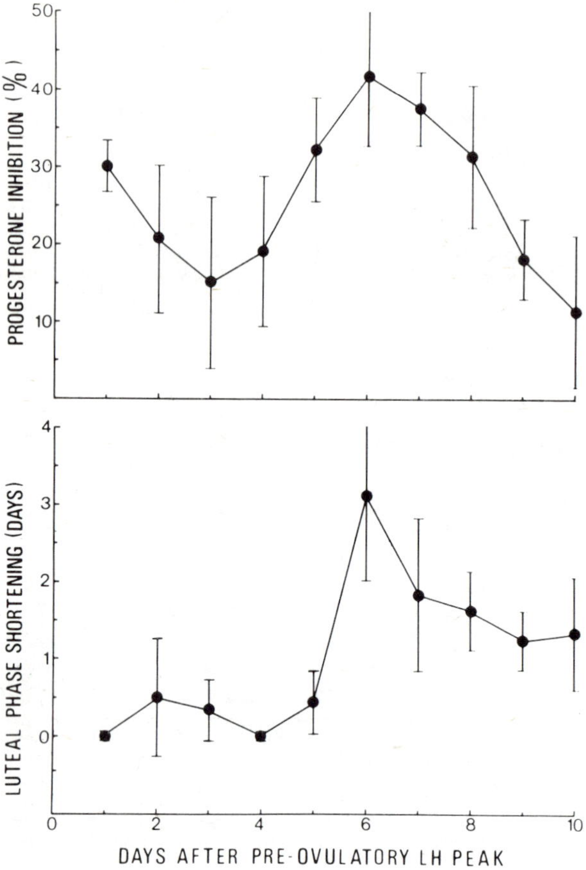

Figure 17.6 Mean inhibition of serum progesterone levels and shortening of the luteal phase after two successive doses (300 μg) of intranasal buserelin at varying times after LH surge. Progesterone levels were measured by calculating the surface areas under mean serum progesterone curves starting from the day of treatment.

LHRH agonist treatment should be able to prevent or intercept implantation. This problem can be addressed in non-pregnant women by administering hCG starting at midluteal phase and by studying the luteolytic efficacy of an optimal dose of LHRH agonist at various times during the luteal phase.

A protocol of intramuscular injection of increasing doses of purified hCG has been established. Starting on day 8–10 after LH peak, eight progressively increasing hCG doses (100–2000 IU) were administered every 12 h over 4 days. It has been established that this regimen increases β-hCG in a manner similar to the onset of pregnancy (Braunstein *et al.*, 1973).

LH, β-hCG and progesterone profiles of women were measured during consecutive cycles corresponding to control, hCG treatment, control, buserelin + hCG treatment and control cycles. In the hCG treatment cycle shown in Figure 17.7, β-hCG progressively increases to 60 mIU. The serum

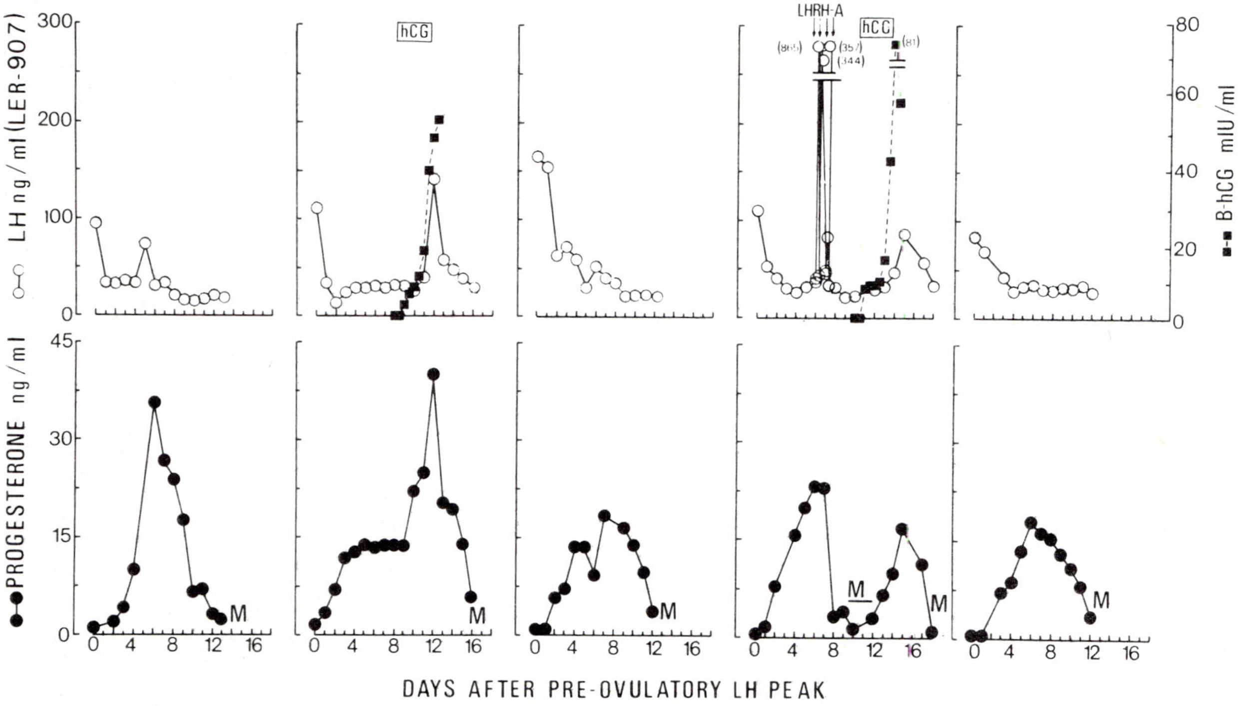

Figure 17.7 Daily serum LH and progesterone profiles in successive control and treatment cycles with hCG and intranasal buserelin in a woman. Increasing intramuscular doses of hCG (100–2000 iu) were injected twice daily for 4 days starting on day 8 of the 3rd and on day 10 of the 5th cycles. Two 300 μg doses of buserelin were insufflated into the nose every 12 h on days 5 and 6 of the 5th cycle. On the days of LHRH agonist treatment, LH was measured immediately before and 4 h after intranasal insufflation. β-hCG was measured on samples obtained twice daily before each injection and on the day following cessation of treatment.

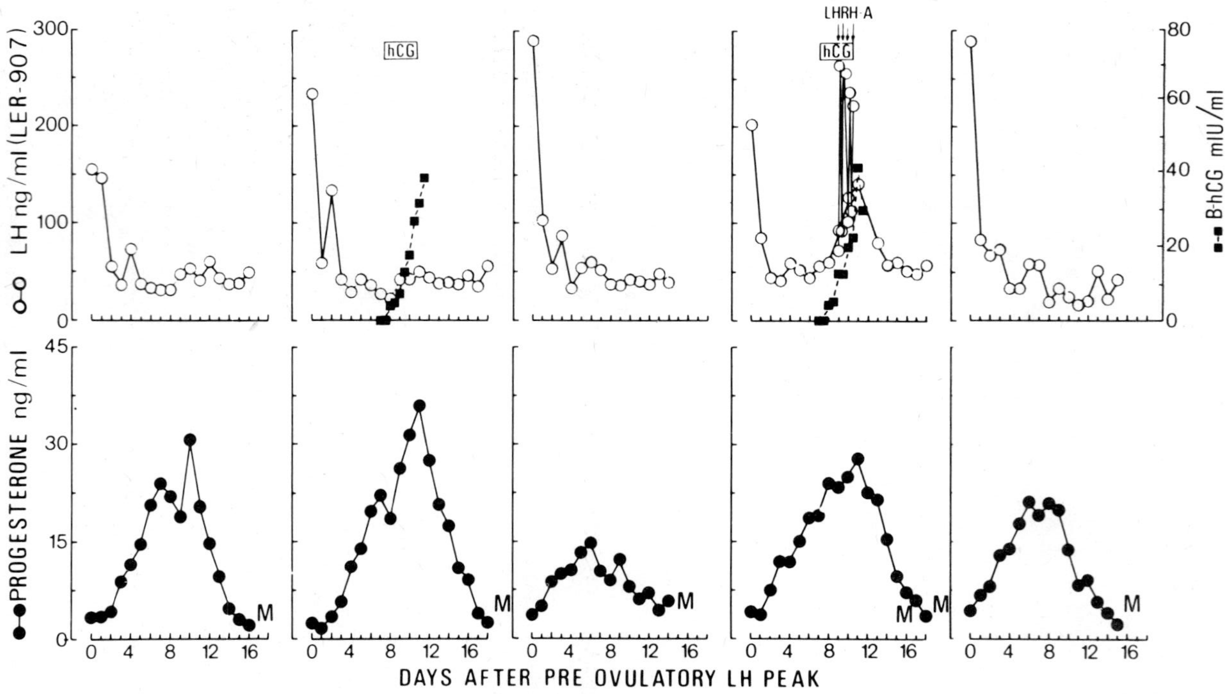

Figure 17.8 Daily serum LH, β-hCG and progesterone profiles in a woman in successive control and treatment cycles with hCG and intranasal buserelin. Experimental conditions were as described for Figure 17.7 except that hCG treatment was started on day 8 of the 3rd and 5th cycles. The LHRH agonist was administered on days 9 and 10 during hCG treatment of the 5th cycle.

progesterone levels increase progressively from 14 to 36 ng/ml during the hCG treatment and the luteal phase duration is slightly prolonged. The following control cycle is normal. On days 5 and 6 after the LH surge during the 4th cycle, 300 μg of buserelin is administered i.n. every 12 h. Serum progesterone remains at 15 ng/ml on day 7 but drops to 2.5 ng/ml on day 8. During the following 3 days, progesterone levels remain low and vaginal bleeding starts on day 10. At that time, hCG treatment is started. Bleeding continues for 3 days but stops when progesterone progressively increases to 15 ng/ml on day 15. A second vaginal bleeding occurs 2 days after cessation of hCG treatment.

In another woman, the LHRH agonist and hCG regimens were administered simultaneously (Figure 17.8). The hCG treatment was begun on day 8 whereas the buserelin was started on day 9 after the LH peak. Circulating levels of β-hCG increased to 40 mIU. There was no change in the serum progesterone levels nor in the duration of the luteal phase as compared to the control hCG cycle.

To evaluate the effect of LHRH agonist treatment, endometrial biopsies were performed before beginning hCG treatment. Although the number of biopsies are limited, endometrial dating revealed tissue which was clearly out of phase when the LHRH analog treatment was administered 4–5 days before hCG. Thus the preliminary results show luteolysis with vaginal bleeding or out of phase endometrial tissue when the LHRH agonist is administered a minimum of 4–5 days before the rise of hCG.

POSSIBLE MECHANISMS OF ACTION OF LHRH AGONISTS

Although the mechanism of action of LHRH or its analogs for the antifertility effects remains to be clarified, several possibilities based on animal and clinical observations can be considered.

Desensitization of ovarian gonadotropin receptors

In rats, the postcoital contraceptive effects of LHRH agonists are probably mediated in part by down regulation of LH and FSH gonadal receptors secondary to induced release of endogenous gonadotropins (Kledzik *et al.*, 1978*a,b*; Labrie *et al.*, 1979). Luteinization is associated with a biphasic increase in the number of receptors which may have a determining role in the regulation of follicular and corpus luteum development and function. The role of endogenous release of gonadotropins in the luteolytic action of LHRH agonist is also supported by the lack of luteolytic effect of LHRH superagonist in hypophysectomized versus intact rhesus monkeys (Asch *et al.*, 1981*a*; Balmaceda and Asch, 1981).

Refractoriness and down regulation of the gonadotropes

Another explanation for the inhibitory effects of LHRH agonists is the decreased gonadotropin responsiveness after pharmacological or repetitive doses of LHRH leading to hypogonadotropic hypogonadism (Sandow *et al.*, 1978; Rabin and McNeil, 1980). In the present studies, 10 h after i.n. administration of 300 μg of the agonist, the pituitary response was markedly blunted. The desensitized corpus luteum may secondarily lack support from the pituitary. The observation that the corpus luteum can be rescued by increasing doses of exogenous hCG is in keeping with this hypothesis.

Inappropriate increase in ovarian estradiol

There is an increase in serum estradiol levels following the gonadotropin stimulation in response to initial LHRH agonist treatment (Figure 17.4). The intraovarian increase in estradiol may interfere with the ovarian cycle. Exogenous estrogen can induce luteolysis in the monkey (Karsch *et al.*, 1973). In women, various synthetic estrogens given after ovulation inhibit serum progesterone levels (Johansson and Gemzell, 1971; Haspels *et al.*, 1977) and large doses of diethylstilbestrol can shorten the luteal phase (Gore *et al.*, 1973; Johansson, 1973). Estradiol directly inhibits LH- or FSH-stimulated synthesis of progesterone in ovarian cell cultures (Thanks and Channing, 1978; Williams *et al.*, 1979).

Direct inhibitory action of LHRH agonist at the ovarian level

LHRH analogs have a direct inhibitory effect at the gonad in hypophysectomized rats (Ying and Guillemin, 1979; Bex and Corbin, 1981). LHRH receptors have been identified in the rat ovary (Reeves *et al.*, 1980) and a direct inhibitory effect of LHRH and its agonists has been demonstrated on granulosa and luteal cells cultured *in vitro* (Clayton *et al.*, 1979; Massicotte *et al.*, 1980). In the male rat the main mechanism of action appears to be exerted through the pituitary, whereas in the female rat a direct action of LHRH at the gonadal level is more obvious (Séguin *et al.*, 1981, 1982; Hsueh and Jones, 1981). In the rhesus monkey, hypophysectomy prevents the induction of luteolysis by LHRH agonist treatment (Asch *et al.*, 1981*a*). LHRH binding sites appear to be absent from corpora lutea of this species (Asch *et al.*, 1981*b*). In human granulosa cell cultures, no inhibition of progesterone secretion by LHRH agonist was found by Casper *et al.* (1982) and Clayton and Huhtaniemi (1982), whereas Tureck *et al.* (1982) reported a dose dependent inhibition.

Decreased gonadotropin secretion and response to LHRH during hCG treatment and pregnancy

Luteolysis induced by LHRH agonist treatment in women is prevented by administration of exogenous hCG (Bergquist *et al.*, 1980*b*; Casper *et al.*, 1980). In these studies, fixed and relatively high doses of hCG were administered for 7 or 10 days starting at the same time as the 2 days of LHRH agonist administration. In the monkey, administration of increasing doses of hCG concomitantly with single or repetitive injections of an LHRH agonist could also prevent the luteolytic effect of the LHRH analog (Asch *et al.*, 1981*b*). High doses of LHRH agonists were unable to interfere with established pregnancies in women (Casper *et al.*, 1980; Tolis *et al.*, 1981).

A probable explanation for the lack of effect of LHRH agonist during pregnancy or during hCG treatment is the decreased pituitary responsivity in the presence of hCG. Basal FSH levels are decreased 2 weeks after artificial insemination successful in achieving a pregnancy, and at this early time there is already a marked blunting of the LH-FSH response to LHRH (Jeppson *et al.*, 1977). Intramuscular administration of 10 000 iu of hCG suppresses basal levels of LH in castrated women (Miyake *et al.*, 1977). At 6 weeks of pregnancy, gonadotropin responsiveness to LHRH is almost completely abolished (Jeppson *et al.*, 1977; Miyake *et al.*, 1977).

Direct inhibitory effects of LHRH agonists on the placenta

Continuous dosing using implants of LHRH agonist starting 4 days after ovulation could antagonize the effects of exogenous hCG both on luteal phase duration and on progesterone levels in the rhesus monkey and the baboon (Vickery and McRae, 1980; Vickery *et al.*, 1981). It is to be noted that these two primate species demonstrated continued acute responsitivity of both pituitary and corpus luteum. As mentioned earlier, the increased estrogens secretion by the corpus luteum may play a role in the luteolytic mechanism. In pregnant monkeys, a suppressive effect of LHRH agonist administration has been observed on endogenous chorionic gonadotropin secretion (Vickery *et al.*, 1981). The human placenta has been shown to synthesize and release LHRH (Khodr and Siler-Khodr, 1980) and LHRH has been reported to suppress progesterone production in organ culture of human placenta (Wilson and Jawad, 1980).

CONCLUDING REMARKS

Multiple doses or chronic administration of LHRH agonists after implantation are effective in intercepting and terminating pregnancy in small animals and infra-human primates. Even if administered early after implantation in the human, it appears that repetitive administration of large amounts of LHRH analogs would be required. Such a treatment does not appear to be practical and would probably interfere with the endocrine events of the following cycle. On the other hand, LHRH agonist treatment before implantation can inhibit corpus luteum function.

The corpus luteum is essential for implantation and maintenance of early pregnancy and luteal phase insufficiency is associated with infertility. Inhibition of the corpus luteum secondary to LHRH agonist treatment could be contraceptive. Luteolysis and vaginal bleeding occur 3–4 days after treatment at midluteal phase. Since serum hCG levels rise on day 10–11 after

LH surge and can rescue the corpus luteum, LHRH agonist treatment would be effective only if administered before day 8 after the midcycle LH surge. Administration of the treatment in the first 4 days after the LH surge would impair the establishment of a normal corpus luteum whereas treatment on days 5–8 would induce a precocious luteolysis. Under inadequate corpus luteum function and out-of-phase endometrium, implantation would not occur or defective hCG secretion would not be able to rescue the corpus luteum. Thus LHRH agonist treatment could be a postcoital contraceptive method that can be used in the first week after ovulation. In this case ovulation will be preserved and the following cycle would be normal.

It will be important to demonstrate the reproducibility and lack of side-effects of treatment in successive cycles in the same woman. The effect of an acute and optimal dose of LHRH agonist at varying times before ovulation needs further study. Preliminary results indicate that various effects can be obtained on ovulation and corpus luteum function during the treatment as well as the post-treatment cycle. Since the inhibitory action on the corpus luteum appears to be related mainly to the inappropriate release of gonadotropins, it is also possible that repetitive administration of smaller doses of the LHRH agonist would cause a more prolonged gonadotropin secretion leading to a more efficient inhibition.

Acknowledgements

These studies were supported through a contract of the National Institutes of Health (USA) and a grant from the Medical Research Council (Canada).

References

Asch, R. H., Eddy, C. A. and Schally, A. V. (1981*a*). Lack of luteolytic effect of D-Trp-6-LH-RH in hypophysectomized rhesus monkeys (Maccaca mulatta). *Biol. Reprod.*, **25,** 963

Asch, R. H., Sichle, M. V., Rettori, V., Balmaceda, J. P., Eddy, C. A., Coy, D. H. and Schally, A. V. (1981*b*). Absence of LH-RH binding sites in corpora lutea from rhesus monkeys (Maccaca mulatta). *J. Clin. Endocrinol. Metab.*, **53,** 215

Balmaceda, J. P. and Asch, R. H. (1981). The effects of LHRH agonistic analogs during the luteal phase of the rhesus monkey. In Zatuchni, G. I., Shelton, J. D. and Sciarra, J. J. (eds.) *LHRH Peptides as Female and Male Contraceptives*, pp. 86–100. (Philadelphia: Harper & Row)

Bauman, R., Kubil, H. Taubert, H. D. and Sandow, J. (1980). Ovulation inhibition by daily i.m. administration of a highly active LH-RH analog (D-Ser(TBU)6-LH-RH-(1–9)-nonapeptide-ethylamide. *Contraception,* **21,** 191

Bergquist, C., Nillius, S. J. and Wide, L. (1980*a*). Effects of a luteinizing hormone-releasing hormone agonist on luteal function in women. *Contraception,* **22,** 287

Bergquist, C., Nillius, S. J. and Wide, L. (1980*b*). Luteolysis induced by a luteinizing hormone-releasing hormone agonist is prevented by human chorionic gonadotropin. *Contraception,* **22,** 341

Bex, F. J. and Corbin, A. (1981). Luteinizing hormone-releasing hormone (LHRH) and LHRH agonist termination of pregnancy in hypophysectomized rats: extrapituitary site of action. *Endocrinology,* **108,** 273

Braunstein, G. D., Grodin, J. M., Vaitukaitis, J. and Ross, G. T. (1973). Secretory rates of human chorionic gonadotropin by normal trophoblast. *Am. J. Obstet. Gynecol.*, **115,** 447

Casper, R. F. and Yen, S. S. C. (1979). Induction of luteolysis in the human with a long-acting analog of luteinizing hormone-releasing factor. *Science,* **205,** 408

Casper, R. F., Sheehan, K., Erickson, G. and Yen, S. S. C. (1980). Neuropeptides and fertility control in the female. In Zatuchni, G. I., Labbok, M. H. and Sciarra, J. J. (eds.) *Research Frontiers in Fertility Regulation*, pp. 409–423. (Hagerstown: Harper & Row)

Casper, R. F., Erickson, G. F., Rebar, R. W. and Yen, S. S. C. (1982). The effect of luteinizing hormone-releasing factor and its agonist on cultured human granulosa cells. *Fertil. Steril.*, **37,** 406

Clayton, R. N., Harwood, J. P. and Catt, K. J. (1979). Gonadotropin-releasing hormone analogue binds to luteal cells and inhibits progesterone production. *Nature (Lond.)*, **282,** 90

Clayton, R. N. and Huhtaniemi, I. T. (1982) Absence of gonadotropin-releasing hormone receptors in human gonadal tissue. *Nature (Lond.)*, **299,** 56

Corbin, A. and Bex, F. J. (1981). Physiology and contraceptive effects of LHRH and agonistic analogs in female animals. In Zatuchni, G. I., Shelton, J. D. and Sciarra, J. J. (eds.) *LHRH Peptides as Female and Male Contraceptives*, pp. 68–84. (Philadelphia: Harper & Row)

Dericks-Tan, J. S. E., Hammer, E. and Taubert, H. D. (1977). The effect of D-Ser(TBU)^6-LH-RH-EA^{10} upon gonadotropin release in normally cycling women. *J. Clin. Endocrinol. Metab.*, **45,** 597

Gore, B. Z., Caldwell, B. V. and Speroff, L. (1973). Estrogen-induced human luteolysis. *J. Clin. Endocrinol. Metab.*, **36,** 615

Haspels, A. A., Linthorst, G. A. and Kicovic, P. M. (1977). Effect of post-ovulatory administration of a 'morning-after' injection on corpus luteum function and endometrium. *Contraception*, **15,** 105

Hsueh, A. J. W. and Jones, P. B. C. (1981). Extrapituitary actions of gonadotropin-releasing hormone. *Endocr. Rev.*, **2,** 437

Jeppson, S., Rannevik, G., Liedholm, P. and Thoull, J. I. (1977). Basal and LRH-stimulated secretion of FSH during early pregnancy. *Am. J. Obstet. Gynecol.*, **127,** 32

Johansson, E. D. B. (1973). Inhibition of the corpus luteum function of women taking large doses of diethylstilbestrol. *Contraception*, **8,** 27

Johansson, E. D. B. and Gemzell, C. (1971). Plasma levels of progesterone during the luteal phase in normal women treated with synthetic oestrogens. *Acta Endocrinol.*, **68,** 551

Karsch, F. J., Krey, L. C., Weick, R. F., Diershke, D. J. and Knobil, E. (1973). Functional luteolysis in the rhesus monkey: the role of estrogen. *Endocrinology*, **92,** 1148

Khodr, G. S. and Siler-Khodr, T. M. (1980). Placental luteinizing-hormone-releasing factor and its synthesis. *Science*, **207,** 315

Kledzik, G. S., Cusan, L., Auclair, C., Kelly, P. A. and Labrie, F. (1978*a*). Inhibitory effect of a luteinizing hormone (LH) releasing hormone agonist on rat ovarian LH and follicle stimulating hormone receptor levels during pregnancy. *Fertil. Steril.*, **29,** 560

Kledzik, G. S., Cusan, L., Auclair, C., Kelly, P. A. and Labrie, F. (1978*b*). Inhibition of ovarian luteinizing-hormone (LH) and follicle-stimulating hormone receptor levels by treatment with an LH-releasing hormone agonist during the estrous cycle in the rat. *Fertil. Steril.*, **30,** 348

Koyama, T., Ohkura, T., Kumasaka, T. and Saito, M. (1978). Effect of post-ovulatory treatment with a luteinizing hormone-releasing hormone analog on the plasma level of progesterone in women. *Fertil. Steril.*, **30,** 549

Labrie, F., Auclair, C., Lemay, A., Kledzik, G. S., Cusan, L., Kelly, P. A., Ferland, C., Séguin, C., Bélanger, A., Azadian-Boulanger, G. and Raynaud, J. P. (1979). Inhibition of ovarian receptor levels and function by treatment with LHRH or its agonists in the rat and possible luteolytic effects of LHRH in normal women. In Channing, C. P., Marsh, J. and Sadler, M. (eds.) *Ovarian Follicular and Corpus Luteum Function*, pp. 687–694. (New York: Plenum Press)

Lemay, A., Labrie, F., Azadian-Boulanger, G. and Raynaud, J. P. (1978). Action lutéolytique de la LHRH chez la femme. *C.R. Acad. Sci. [D] (Paris)*, **286,** 527

Lemay, A., Labrie, F., Ferland, L. and Raynaud, J. P. (1979*a*). Possible luteolytic effects of luteinizing hormone-releasing hormone in normal women. *Fertil. Steril.*, **31,** 29

Lemay, A., Labrie, F., Bélanger, A. and Raynaud, J. P. (1979*b*). Luteolytic effect of intranasal administration of [D-Ser(TBU)^6-des-Gly-NH_2^{10}] luteinizing hormone-releasing hormone ethylamide in normal women. *Fertil. Steril.*, **32,** 646

Lemay, A., Faure, N. and Labrie, F. (1982). Sensitivity of pituitary and corpus luteum responses to single intranasal administration of [D-Ser(TBU)^6-des-Gly-$NH_2{}^{10}$] luteinizing hormone-releasing hormone ethylamide (Buserelin) in normal women. *Fertil. Steril.*, **37,** 193

Massicotte, H., Veilleux, R., Lavoie, M. and Labrie, F. (1980). An LHRH agonist inhibits FSH-induced cyclic AMP accumulation and steroidogenesis in porcine granulosa cells in culture. *Biochem. Biophys. Res. Commun.*, **94,** 1362

Miyake, A., Tanizawa, O., Aono, T. and Kurachi, D. (1977). Pituitary responses in LH secretion to LHRH during pregnancy. *Obstet. Gynecol.*, **49,** 549

Nillius, S. J., Bergquist, C. and Wide, L. (1978). Inhibition of ovulation in women by chronic treatment with a stimulatory LRH analogue: a new approach to birth control? *Contraception,* **17,** 537

Nillius, S. J. and Wide, L. (1972). Variation in LH and FSH response to LH-releasing hormone during the menstrual cycle. *J. Obstet. Gynaecol. Br. Commonw.*, **79,** 865

Puri, C. P. and Csapo, A. I. (1981). Evaluation of antifertility effects of LHRH analogs in the guinea pig. In Zatuchni, G. I., Shelton, J. D. and Sciarra, J. J. (eds.) *LHRH Peptides as Female and Male Contraceptives,* pp. 126–133. (Philadelphia: Harper & Row)

Rabin, D. and McNeil, L. W. (1980). Pituitary and gonadal desensitization after continuous luteinizing hormone-releasing hormone infusion in normal females. *J. Clin. Endocrinol. Metab.*, **51,** 873

Reeves, J. J., Séguin, C., Lefebvre, F. A., Kelly, P. A. and Labrie, F. (1980). Similar luteinizing hormone-releasing hormone binding sites in rat anterior pituitary and ovary. *Proc. Natl. Acad. Sci. USA,* **77,** 5567

Sandow, J., von Rechenberg, W., Jerzabek, G. and Stoll, W. (1978). Pituitary gonadotropin inhibition by a highly active analog of luteinizing hormone-releasing hormone. *Fertil. Steril.*, **30,** 205

Schmidt-Gollwitzer, M., Hardt, W. and Schmidt-Gollwitzer, K. (1981). Influence of the LHRH analogue buserelin on cyclic ovarian function and on endometrium. A new approach to fertility control? *Contraception,* **23,** 187

Séguin, C., Bélanger, A., Cusan, L., Pelletier, G., Reeves, J. J., Lefebvre, F. A., Kelly, P. A. and Labrie, F. (1981). Relative importance of the adenohypophyseal and gonadal sites of inhibitory action of LHRH agonists. *Biol. Reprod.*, **24,** 889

Séguin, C., Bélanger, A., Labrie, F. and Hansel, W. (1982). Study of the direct action of luteinizing hormone-releasing hormone agonists at the testicular level in intact rats treated with an anti-luteinizing hormone serum. *Endocrinology,* **110,** 524

Sheehan, K. L., Casper, R. F. and Yen, S. S. C. (1982). Induction of luteolysis by luteinizing hormone-releasing factor (LRF) agonist: sensitivity, reproducibility and reversibility. *Fertil. Steril.*, **37,** 209

Thanks, K. H. and Channing, C. P. (1978). Effects of follicle-stimulating hormone and estradiol upon progesterone secretion by porcine granulosa cells in tissue culture. *Endocrinology,* **103,** 74

Tolis, G., Comaru-Schally, A. M., Mehta, A. E. and Schally, A. V. (1981). Failure to interrupt established pregnancy in humans by D-tryptophan-6-luteinizing hormone-releasing hormone. *Fertil. Steril.*, **36,** 241

Tureck, R. W., Mastroianni, L., Blasco, L. and Strauss, J. F. III (1982). Inhibition of human granulosa cell progesterone secretion by a gonadotropin-releasing hormone agonist. *J. Clin. Endocrinol. Metab.*, **54,** 1078

Vickery, B. H. (1981). Female contraceptive potential of 'super' agonists of LHRH as assessed in infrahuman primates. In Zatuchni, G. I., Shelton, J. D. and Sciarra, J. J. (eds.) *LHRH Peptides as Female and Male Contraceptives,* pp. 109–125. (Philadelphia: Harper & Row)

Vickery, B. H. and McRae, G. (1980). Antagonism by an LHRH agonist of the steroidogenic effects of exogenous human chorionic gonadotrophin in female rhesus. *Life Sci.*, **27,** 1409

Vickery, B. H., McRae, G. I. and Stevens, V. C. (1981). Suppression of luteal and placental function in pregnant baboons with agonist analogs of luteinizing hormone-releasing hormones. *Fertil. Steril.*, **36,** 664

Williams, M. T., Roth, M. S., Marsh, J. M. and Le Maire, W. J. (1979). Inhibition of human chorionic gonadotropin-induced progesterone synthesis by estradiol in isolated human luteal cells. *J. Clin. Endocrinol. Metab.*, **48,** 437

Wilson, E. A. and Jawad, M. J. (1980). Luteinizing hormone-releasing hormone suppression of human placental progesterone production. *Fertil. Steril.*, **33,** 91

Yen, S. S. C., Vandenberg, G., Rebar, R. and Ehara, Y. (1972). Variation of pituitary responsiveness to synthetic LRH during different phases of the menstrual cycle. *J. Clin. Endocrinol. Metab.*, **35,** 931

Ying, S. Y. and Guillemin, R. (1979). (D-Trp^6-Pro^9-NET)-luteinizing hormone-releasing factor inhibits follicular development in hypophysectomized rats. *Nature (Lond.),* **280,** 593

18
Antifertility by discontinuous treatment with buserelin in women

W. HARDT, T. GENZ and M. SCHMIDT-GOLLWITZER

PROBLEMS OF CONTINUOUS TREATMENT WITH LHRH ANALOGS

Paradoxical antifertility effects of LHRH agonists in various species have been described (Corbin and Bex, 1981). In women the continuous application of the LHRH agonist, buserelin, leads to inhibition of ovulation (Bergquist *et al.*, 1979; Hardt *et al.*, 1981). Progesterone secretion is dose-relatedly suppressed; estradiol production, however, shows a marked intra- and interindividual variance, even at contraceptive doses of buserelin. In the majority of women treated with such doses, this leads to irregular bleeding, in some cases going as far as amenorrhea. This results, on the one hand, in phases of endometrial stimulation of longer duration and, on the other hand, in phases of inadequate estradiol secretion accompanied by endometrial inactivity and estrogen deficiency symptoms. Because of these disadvantages a continuous long term treatment with LHRH analogs cannot be recommended for contraceptive purposes (Schmidt-Gollwitzer *et al.*, 1983).

PROBLEMS OF DISCONTINUOUS TREATMENT WITH LHRH ANALOGS

The continuous application of buserelin has now been compared with the results of discontinuous application, using 22 days of therapy with a 6-day break. Contraceptive efficacy was not noticeably influenced by the break in treatment. During this week a complete resensitization of the pituitary could be recognized. In most women this produces follicle maturation accompanied by cyclic estradiol secretion, but not, however, regular bleeding in the interval between treatments. For the above reasons, the 22-day buserelin therapy was combined with a short term gestagen treatment, to ensure a largely regular bleeding pattern.

DISCONTINUOUS TREATMENT WITH GESTAGEN-INDUCED BLEEDING

The recent study addresses the combination of discontinuous buserelin therapy with 3 days of gestagen treatment. The selected daily dose of 400 μg had proved adequately contraceptive in the other studies of continuous application (Schmidt-Gollwitzer *et al.*, 1981). Subjects received a daily dose of 400 μg buserelin over a period of 22 days starting on the day of menstruation. Between the 20th and 22nd days of treatment, 10 mg daily of norethisterone acetate were also administered. After a 6-day break the treatment was continued along the same lines.

Contraceptive effectiveness

The progesterone levels remained below 1 ng/ml in the majority of treated cycles. In some cycles a transient increase to no more than 3 ng/ml was noted, thus anovulation occurred in 95% of treated cycles. In five of the remaining six cycles a transient increase in the progesterone level up to values between 3 and 6 ng/ml was observed. A contraceptive effect was probable in these cases. A progesterone level consistent with normal corpus luteum function was observed in only 1 month of therapy (Figure 18.1). In this case however, treatment was started on the 7th, rather than the 1st, day of cycle. In the subsequent months of treatment this subject was anovulatory. No other means of contraception was used during the trials. No pregnancy occurred during the period of observation. Therefore the discontinuous intranasal treatment application of buserelin combined with a short period of gestagen administration is comparable with continuous treatment from the point of view of its contraceptive effectiveness.

Hormone profiles

The serum estradiol levels revealed two characteristic secretion patterns. In 17 women a regular increase in serum estradiol concentrations, in part attaining preovulatory levels, was observed at the beginning of therapy and after the 6-day break. A fall in estradiol levels occurred during the last week of treatment which, together with 3-day gestagen treatment, then led to the regular withdrawal bleeding. However, particularly in the first month and where treatment was started late (on the 6th or 7th instead of on the 1st day of cycle) hypersecretion of estradiol was noted (Figure 18.2). Occasionally a marked suppression of estrogen production followed the initial stimulation and in these cases hot flushes were noted. In these, ovarian function was completely inhibited.

Similarly to the estradiol secretion, a short-lived increase in release of gonadotropins was commonly observed in the first days of treatment cycles, LH notably more so than FSH. In the course of the 3 weeks of treatment the pituitary stimulation decreased markedly. Basal LH level remained in the normal range in contrast to the serum FSH level which dropped below the

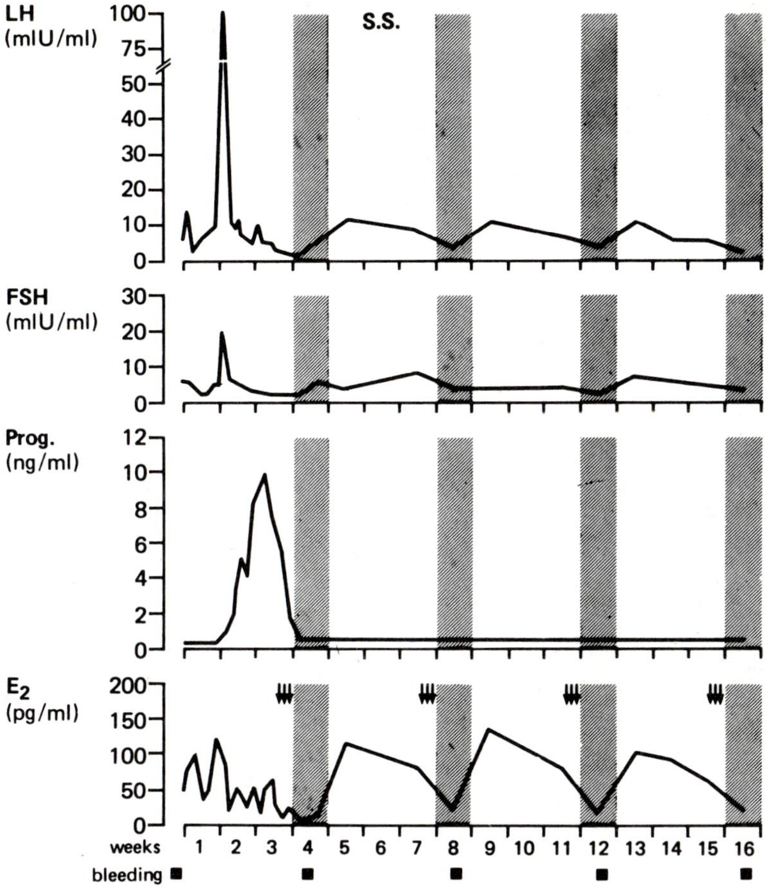

Figure 18.1 Hormone profile of volunteer S.S. undergoing discontinuous treatment with 400 μg buserelin and short term administration of gestagen (arrow corresponds to 10 mg norethisterone acetate). Marked progesterone increase in 1st month of treatment after late start of therapy (7th day of cycle).

normal range. This dissociation of gonadotropin secretion was particularly marked in women with strongly suppressed estradiol secretion. In the weeks without treatment, neither estradiol increase nor gonadotropin peaks nor the start of progesterone secretion was observed.

In conclusion, daily pituitary stimulation by long term effective LHRH analogs, such as buserelin, leads to a reduction and dissociation of gonadotropin release. The antifertility effect of buserelin, both continuously or discontinuously applied, involves the influence of unphysiological gonadotropin secretion on follicle maturation (Sheehan and Yen, 1981), thus leading to inhibition of ovulation or to corpus luteum insufficiency.

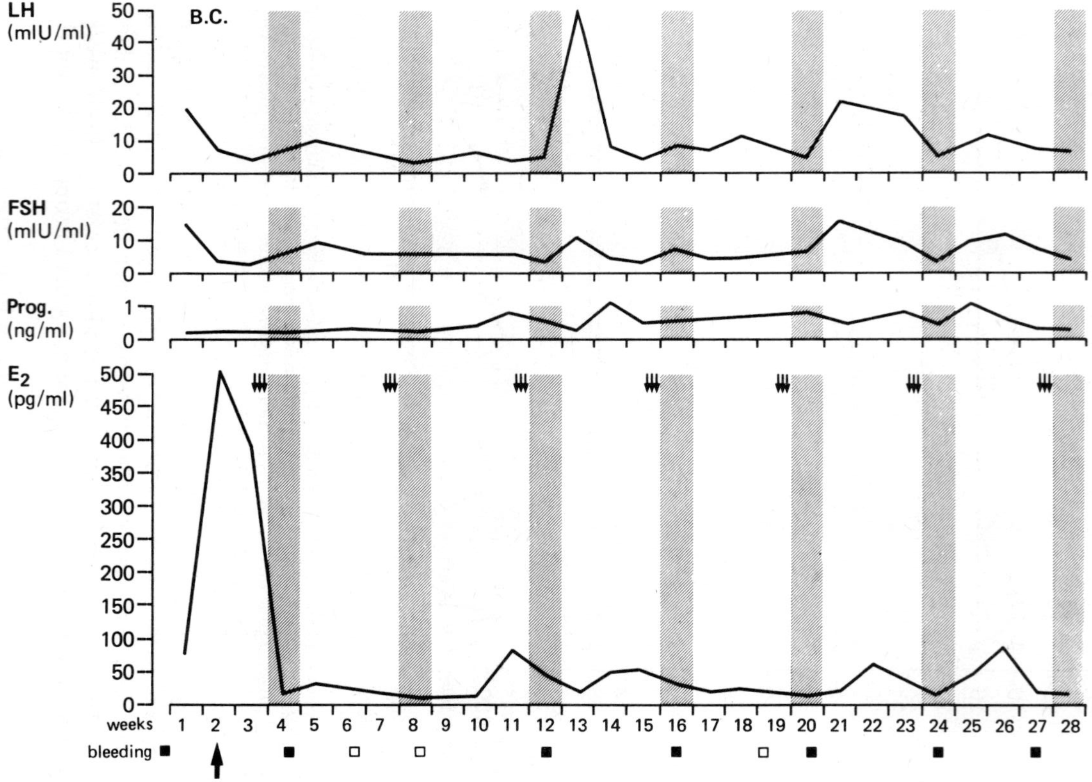

Figure 18.2 Maximal estradiol secretion after delayed start of treatment (6th day of cycle) in 1st month, marked suppression of estrogen synthesis in the course of subsequent months of therapy.

Influence on the target organ endometrium

The endometrial biopsies, carried out in the later days of treatment and prior to gestagen administration (18th–20th day, $n = 6$), revealed a histological picture consistent with a moderate level of proliferation (corresponding to the 9th–12th day of cycle), with no signs of the beginnings of hyperplasia. One biopsy revealed early secretory changes, consistent with the observed increase in endogenous progesterone up to 2 ng/ml. Biopsies carried out at the beginning of bleeding showed secretional transformation and the start of the breakdown of the endometrium ($n = 5$). The biopsies performed after bleeding invariably gave the histological picture of early proliferation corresponding to the first postmenstrual days of a normal cycle ($n = 8$).

Compared to continuous treatment with buserelin no pathological changes of the endometrium occurred. Unopposed estrogen effects on endometrium which may play a role in the development of endometrial cancer are prevented by the short term gestagen administration.

Acceptability

Regular, gestagen-induced bleeding occurred in 97% of the treated cycles, usually starting between the 2nd and 4th day of the break in treatment. The bleeding was less and of shorter duration than normal menstruation. In addition to the gestagen-induced withdrawal bleeding, a spotting, lasting 1 or 2 days, was reported in 25% of the cycles. In 17 of the volunteers only 11 occurrences of breakthrough bleeding were reported during 81 months of treatment. These women thus showed no appreciable detrimental effect on the pattern of bleeding (Figure 18.3). Four test persons reported 14 breakthrough bleedings combined with very weak or absent withdrawal bleeding in 20 therapy months. Regular, controlled bleeding is thus no longer apparent in these women (Figure 18.4).

In conclusion, in four fifths of the women treated, the 22-day therapy combined with short term gestagen treatment produced regular withdrawal bleeding, compared with one quarter during continuous treatment (Hardt *et al.*, 1981).

With the exception of slight irritation of the nasal mucous membranes and short-lived headaches at the beginning of treatment, no serious side-effects were reported. The strong suppression of estradiol secretion led to hot flushes in two volunteers, which diminished over the course of continued treatment. The intranasal spray application of buserelin was well tolerated. Women who had complained of side-effects with steroidal contraceptives reported no problems with buserelin.

CONCLUDING REMARKS

Compared to continuous treatment with buserelin, discontinuous administration with gestagen-induced bleeding is the preferable method of contraception with LHRH analogs. Because of the cyclic nature of the treatment, it

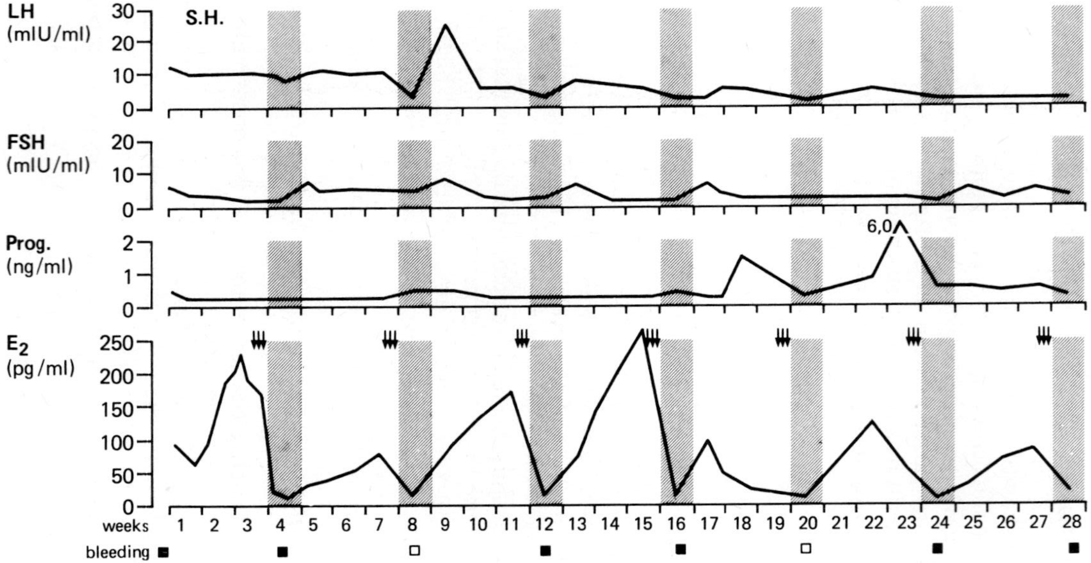

Figure 18.3 Hormone profile of volunteer S.H. Cyclic stimulation of estradiol production and regular pattern of bleeding of 7 months. ■ = bleeding of menstrual strength; □ = light bleeding.

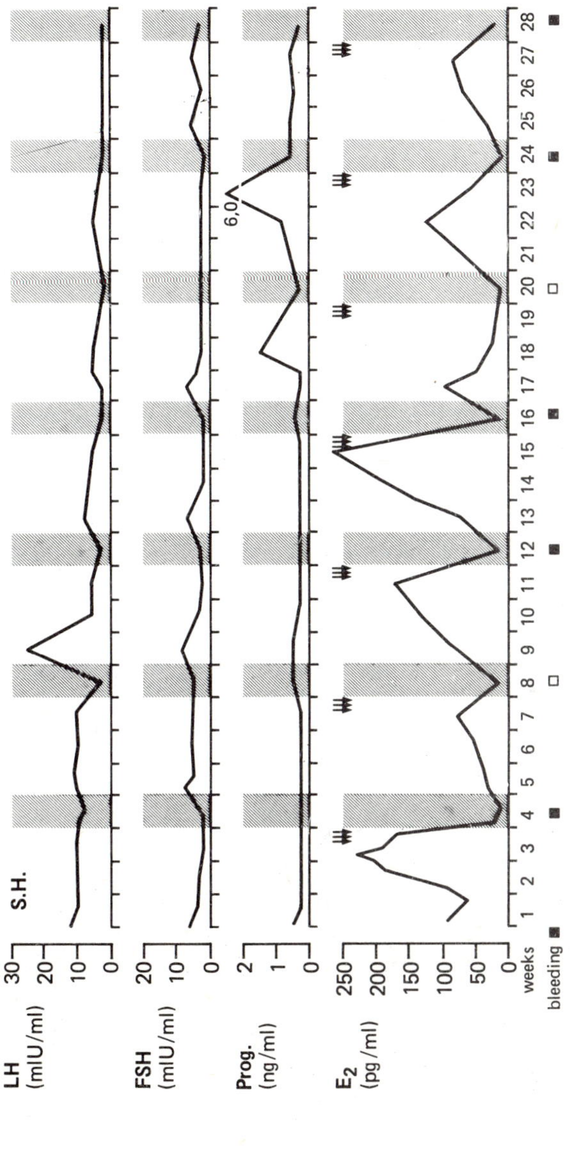

Figure 18.4 Hormone profile of volunteer K.P. Irregular pattern of bleeding. ■ = bleeding of menstrual strength; □ = light bleeding.

corresponds more closely to the physiological course of events regulating the sexual steroids and the changes these produce in the female reproductive organs. Phases of stronger and lengthier stimulation could thus be avoided, as clearly shown by the endometrial biopsies. The gestagen-induced withdrawal bleeding leads to the complete shedding of the endometrium, as shown by the biopsies performed during and after bleeding. At present we are investigating whether different dose schedules of gestagens could improve bleeding behavior.

Acknowledgement

Our thanks to Dr Marianne von der Ohe, Hoechst AG, Frankfurt, Germany, for kindly providing the buserelin.

References

Bergquist, C., Nillius, S. J. and Wide, L. (1979). Intranasal gonadotropin releasing hormone agonist as a contraceptive agent. *Lancet,* **2,** 215

Corbin, A. and Bex, F. J. (1981). Physiology and contraceptive effects of LHRH and agonistic analogues in female animals. In Zatuchni, G. I., Shelton, J. D. and Sciarra, J. J. (eds.) *LHRH Peptides as Female and Male Contraceptives,* pp. 68–84. (Philadelphia: Harper & Row)

Hardt, W., Schmidt-Gollwitzer, M. von der Ohe, M. and Nevinny-Stickel, J. (1981). Der Einfluß der Dauermedikation des LH-RH Analogons Buserelin auf die Zyklusregulation. *Geburtsh. Frauenheilk.,* **41,** 791

Schmidt-Gollwitzer, M., Hardt, W., Schmidt-Gollwitzer, K.. von der Ohe, M. and Nevinny-Stickel, J. (1981). Influence of the LH-RH analogue buserelin on cyclic ovarian function and on endometrium. *Contraception,* **23,** 187

Schmidt-Gollwitzer, M., Hardt, W. and Schmidt-Gollwitzer, K. (1983). Risks and benefits of LHRH agonists as antifertility agents. This volume, Chapter 19

Sheehan, C. and Yen, S. S. C. (1981). LHRH peptides as female and male contraceptives. In Zatuchni, G. I., Shelton, J. D. and Sciarra, J. J. (eds.) *LHRH Peptides as Female and Male Contraceptives,* pp. 237–242. (Philadelphia: Harper & Row)

19
Risks and benefits of LHRH agonists as antifertility agents

M. SCHMIDT-GOLLWITZER, W. HARDT and K. SCHMIDT-GOLLWITZER

ANTIGONADAL PROPERTIES OF LHRH AGONISTS

Deletion and substitution of certain amino acids of LHRH led to analogs with potent agonistic and antagonistic properties (Sandow, 1982). One of the most potent LHRH agonists, the nonapeptide [D-Ser(tBu^6),Pro^9-NHEt]LHRH (buserelin, HOE766) has been estimated to exceed the effectivity of LHRH in fertile women by a factor of 40 (Dericks-Tan *et al.*, 1977; Sandow *et al.*, 1981).

Although the LHRH agonists provide a new therapeutical approach to endocrine infertility, only limited success has been reported (Canales *et al.*, 1980; Katzorke *et al.*, 1980). In patients with hypogonadotropic amenorrhea, chronic administration of buserelin produced, after initial stimulation, a subsequent suppression of gonadal function (Figure 19.1) (Schmidt-Gollwitzer *et al.*, 1979). This paradoxical antifertility effect of buserelin led to the consideration of a possible contraceptive use as also suggested by studies of the antireproductive properties of LHRH analogs in animals (Fraser *et al.*, 1980; Sandow, 1982).

The possibility of using potent and long acting LHRH agonists such as buserelin via chronic subcutaneous or intranasal application for fertility control in women has now been well documented and may offer advantages compared to other hormonal contraceptive methods (Bergquist *et al.*, 1979*a*; Nillius *et al.*, 1978; Schmidt-Gollwitzer *et al.*, 1981). To establish the contraceptive feasibilities of this compound we have extended our recently published study and have investigated different dose regimens which are reported in this chapter.

DOSE-DEPENDENT CONTRACEPTIVE EFFECTIVENESS OF BUSERELIN

Daily intranasal administration of buserelin (100–1200 μg) was started normally on the first day of menstrual bleeding following the control cycle and was continued up to 12 months. Doses used were 100 μg of buserelin once or twice

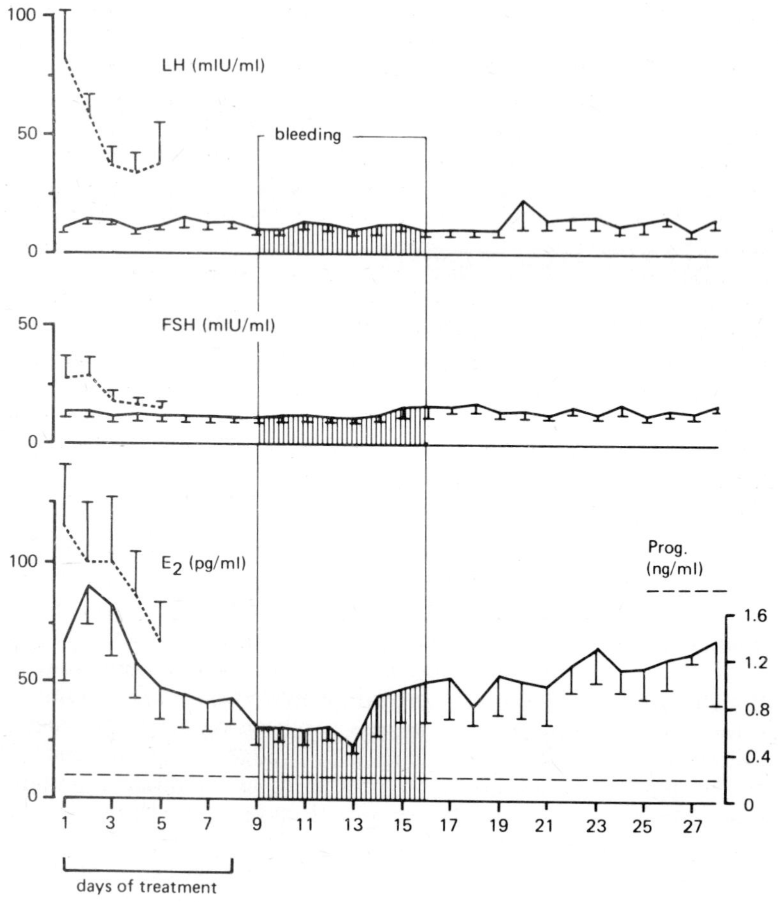

Figure 19.1 Serum values of gonadotropins (LH, FSH) estradiol (E2) and progesterone (Prog.) of ten patients with amenorrhea during and after the s.c. treatment with 87 μg/day buserelin (MD ± SD).

daily, 200 μg or 400 μg daily, 400 μg twice or thrice daily. All women receiving 100 μg daily used an additional means of contraception, since preliminary results indicated insufficient inhibition of ovulation. The compliance was monitored by clinical examinations and frequent blood samples for determination of FSH, LH, estradiol and progesterone by radioimmunoassay.

Altogether 451 treatment months with different doses of buserelin were recorded. Only the 65 women using more than 100 μg buserelin did not use an additional contraceptive method. Thus, only 377 treatment months can be considered in terms of contraceptive effectiveness. One pregnancy occurred. This volunteer reduced the daily dose from 200 μg to 100 μg buserelin on her own initiative. Ovulation occurred approximately 1 week after reduction of medication. Pregnancy was confirmed by detection of hCG. This woman had a miscarriage 7 weeks postconception.

In 329 out of 451 treatment months, progesterone levels were consistently below 1 ng/ml (Table 19.1). The incidence of anovulation was dose-related and decreased from 95% (800/1200 μg) to 87% (400 μg), to 67% (200 μg) and 46% (100 μg buserelin). Progesterone secretion did not exceed 3 ng/ml during 68 treatment cycles, indicating impaired corpus luteum function or luteinization only. In the other 54 treatment months, progesterone reflected minor suppression of corpus luteum steroidogenesis. In spite of these subnormal progesterone values no pregnancy occurred during 31 months of treatment in women using no further contraceptive method beside buserelin. In women treated with 100 μg buserelin and using an additional intrauterine device, subnormal and normal progesterone values (⩾6 ng/ml), and luteal phases of more than 10 days were observed (Figure 19.2).

Anovulation and severe corpus luteum insufficiency were found in 100%, 97.2%, 84.5% and 69% of the recorded treatment months in the decreasing dose groups (800/1200, 400, 200 and 100 μg buserelin). Concerning the contraceptive effectiveness of buserelin, daily doses of 400 μg and more lead to a sufficient inhibition of reproductive function in women, mainly as a result of inhibition of ovulation.

Table 19.1 Distribution of serum progesterone levels of 79 volunteers during the course of treatment with different doses of buserelin

Dose (μg/day)	*Progesterone* (ng/ml)				Months
	1	1–3	3–6	6	
100	34(46%)	17(23%)	14(19%)	9(12%)	74
200	121(67%)	33(18%)	22(12%)	5(3%)	181
400	136(87%)	16(10%)	4(3%)	0(0%)	156
800/1200	38(95%)	2(5%)	0(0%)	0(0%)	40

RISKS OF LONG TERM TREATMENT

The main problem concerning this new approach of fertility control seems to be finding the threshold doses which possess antifertility effectiveness combined with sufficient control of bleeding and low undesirable effects on target organs such as breast and endometrium. It is well known that unopposed estrogen stimulation may play a co-carcinogenic role in the development of endometrial cancer (Berenblum, 1974; Gusberg, 1947; Lipsett, 1977). On the other hand, prolonged periods of estrogen deficiency may provoke problems such as osteoporosis. This has to be extensively investigated before this pharmalogic advance can be used as a safe and effective contraceptive.

Bleeding control

Regardless of the dose regimen, 22 women developed amenorrhea with the onset of medication (Table 19.2, Figure 19.3). It is interesting to note that ten of

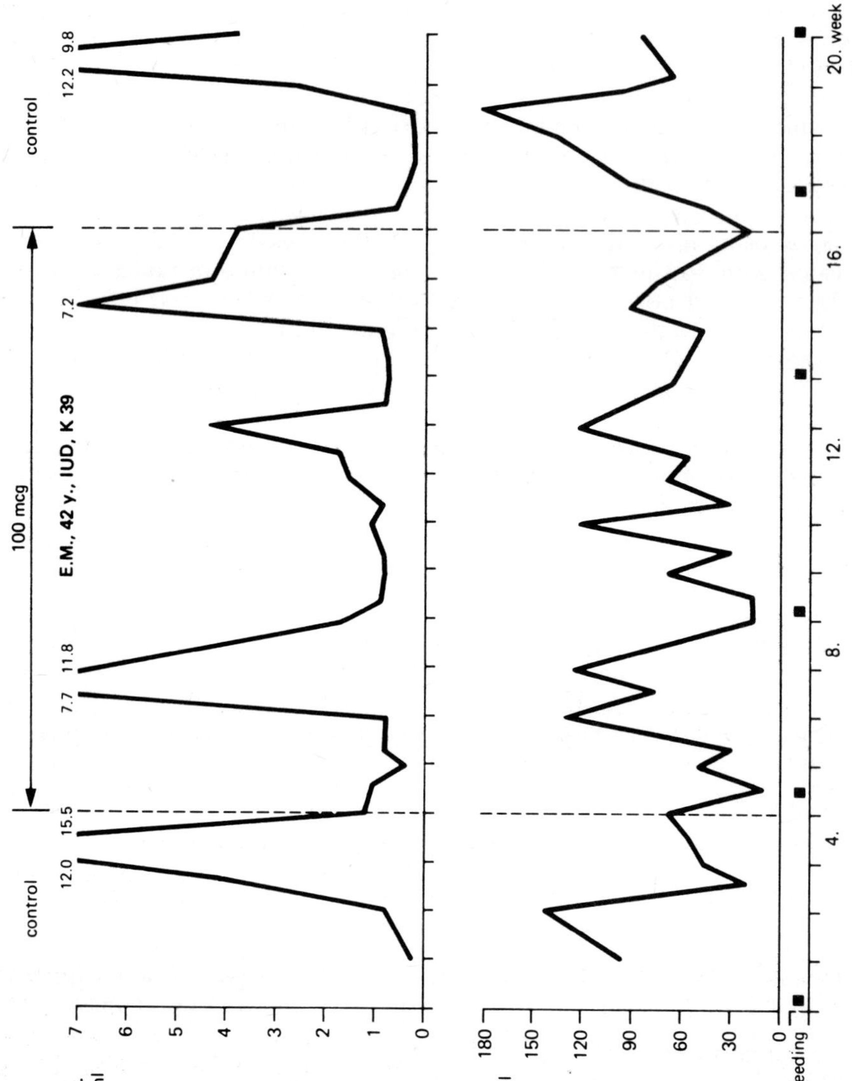

Figure 19.2 Serum values of estradiol (E2) and progesterone (Prog.) of the volunteer E.M. before, during and after the course of treatment with 100 μg/day buserelin.

Table 19.2 Distribution of bleeding pattern of 79 volunteers during the course of i.n. treatment with different doses of buserelin. Regular bleeding: intervals of 3–6 weeks; irregular bleeding: more than 6 weeks

Dose (μg)		*Bleeding pattern*		n
	None	*Regular*	*Irregular*	
100	1	4	9	14
200	11	3	14	28
400	7	14	7	28
800/1200	3	6	0	9

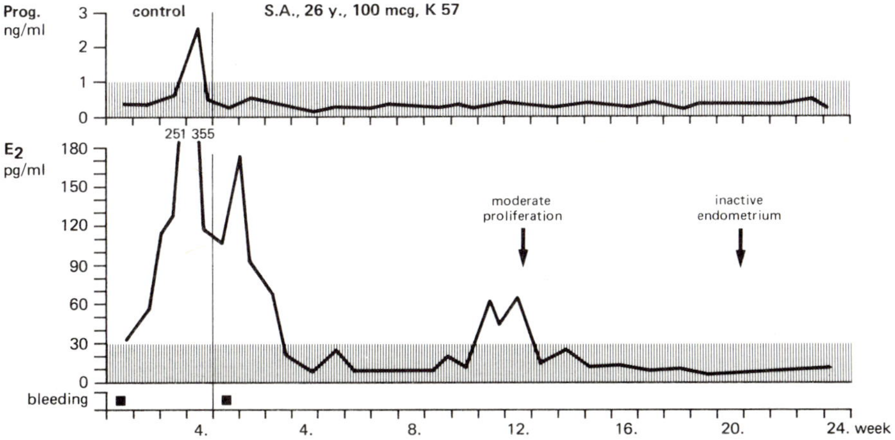

Figure 19.3 Serum values of estradiol (E2) and progesterone (Prog.) of the volunteer S.A. during the course of i.n. treatment with 100 μg/day buserelin. Shaded portions indicate the area of the hormone values of early follicular phase. Arrows indicate day of endometrial biopsy.

these volunteers had a pretreatment history of cyclic disturbance. Whereas the incidence of amenorrhea was equal in the higher dose regimens, it occurred significantly less frequently in the group using 100 μg. With 800 and 1200 μg, all 9 volunteers developed amenorrhea with estrogen deficiency symptoms (hot flushes) in the progress of treatment (Figure 19.4). Women receiving 400 μg had rather irregular bleeding intervals or developed amenorrhea during the second half of the observation period of 6 months (Figure 19.5). The occurrence of irregular bleeding intervals was significantly less frequent with the lower dose regimens.

Comparing bleeding events with preceding hormonal pattern revealed that estrogen-dependent breakthrough or withdrawal bleeding was the normal event with high doses and quite common at lower dose levels. Because of the higher incidence of residual cyclic progesterone activity, bleeding in the 100 and 200 μg group was mainly produced by progesterone withdrawal (Figure 19.6). This may minimize the risk of unopposed estrogen effects. However, the

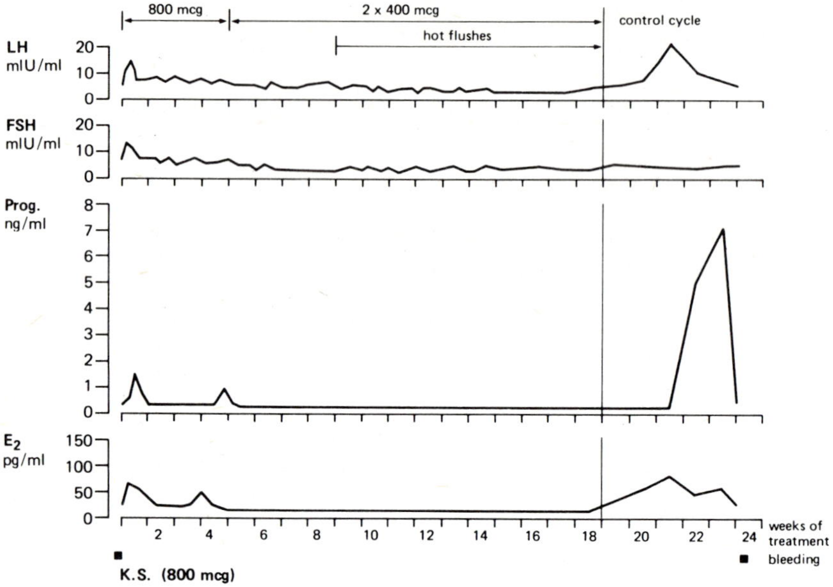

Figure 19.4 Serum values of gonadotropins (LH, FSH), estradiol (E2) and progesterone (Prog.) of the volunteer K.S. during and after the course of i.n. treatment with 800 μg/day buserelin.

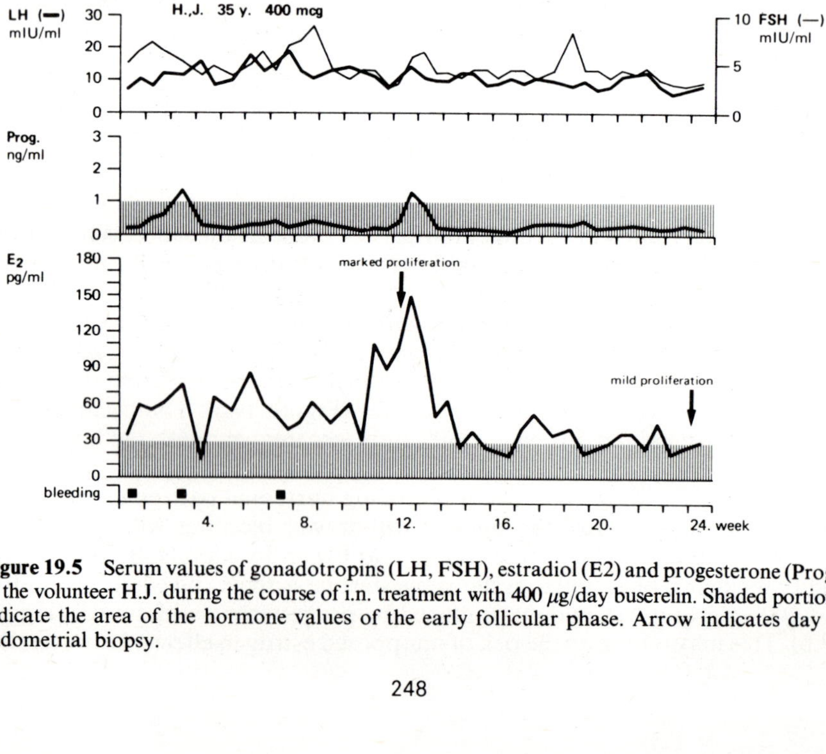

Figure 19.5 Serum values of gonadotropins (LH, FSH), estradiol (E2) and progesterone (Prog.) of the volunteer H.J. during the course of i.n. treatment with 400 μg/day buserelin. Shaded portions indicate the area of the hormone values of the early follicular phase. Arrow indicates day of endometrial biopsy.

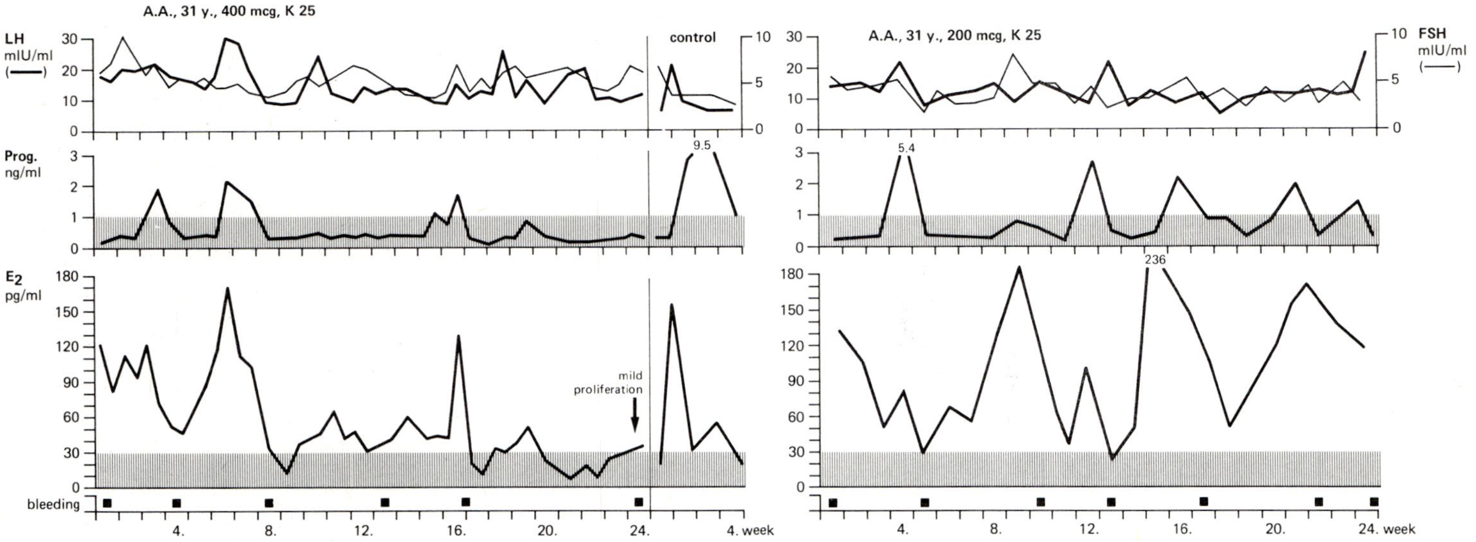

Figure 19.6 Serum values of gonadotropins (LH, FSH) estradiol (E2) and progesterone (Prog.) of the volunteer A.A. during the course of treatment with 400 and 200 μg buserelin per day. Shaded portions indicate the area of the hormone values of early follicular phase. Arrow indicates day of endometrial biopsy.

administration of 100 μg buserelin which leads to almost regular bleeding intervals is not sufficient to inhibit, in some cases, normal follicular maturation, ovulation and subsequently normal corpus luteum function. The critical contraceptive threshold dose seems to be between 200 and 400 μg buserelin. With these doses, however, the pattern of estradiol secretion cannot be predicted.

Unopposed estrogen secretion

In view of the reports of the Swedish group, unopposed estrogen secretion seems no problem in this contraceptive approach. Amenorrhea combined with reduced estrogen secretion was routinely noted. Endometrial biopsies showed mild proliferation in menstruating and inactive endometrium in amenorrheic women (Bergquist *et al.*, 1979*a,b*). However, our findings indicate that inhibition of follicular maturation, implied by consistently low estradiol secretion, could not be observed in all volunteers.

Only with doses of 800 and 1200 μg did the estradiol values decrease to postmenopausal levels in all volunteers with corresponding estrogen deficiency symptoms (Figure 19.4). Even with 400 μg the estradiol levels of three of 28 women were consistently suppressed (Figure 19.7). Generally, with doses up to 400 μg buserelin women showed serum estradiol concentrations within the normal and subnormal range. In the 400 μg group, women showed marked fluctuations of the estradiol values, at times reaching preovulatory levels (Figure 19.7). In some women estradiol secretion was not suppressed and marked fluctuation occurred throughout treatment. Prolonged estradiol secretion caused marked proliferation of the endometrium and was often not interrupted by withdrawal bleeding (Figure 19.7). At the lower doses, periods of prolonged and elevated estradiol secretion were infrequent because of the higher incidence of withdrawal bleedings.

Effects on the endometrium

The morphological findings ranged from inactive endometrium to marked proliferation as well as secretory transformation (Table 19.3). The morphological alterations could be readily correlated with the hormone profiles and bleeding intervals (Table 19.4). At the highest dose levels, all biopsies taken at the end of therapy showed atrophic changes. Full secretory transformation of the endometrium was only found in the 100 μg group, whereas at the higher doses early transformation with a shortened luteal phase or a picture similar to that found in corpus luteum insufficiency was found.

The highest incidence of marked proliferation was in the 400 μg group and could be readily correlated to the prolonged periods of anovulation with unsuppressed or slightly suppressed estradiol secretion (Figure 19.7). Similar results have been found in rhesus monkeys during long term treatment with LHRH agonists.

In conclusion, with doses of buserelin not leading consistently to estrogen deficiency the behavior of estradiol secretion, and thus the influence on target

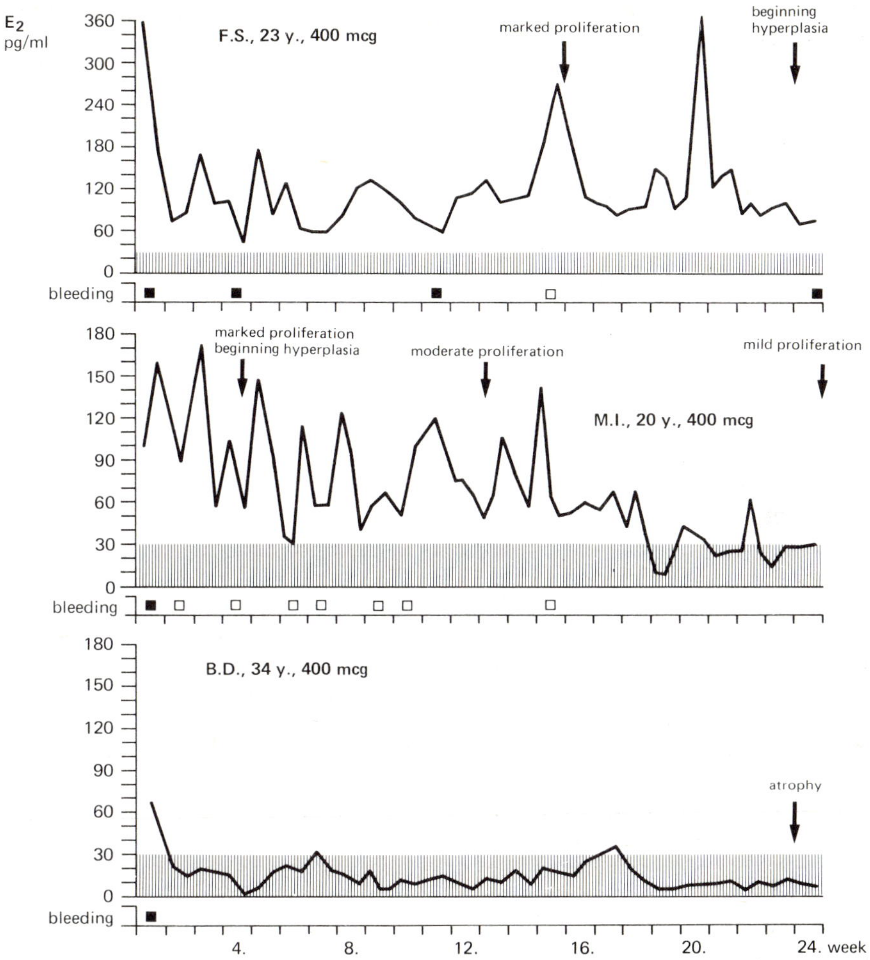

Figure 19.7 Typical pattern of estradiol (E2) secretion during the course of i.n. treatment with 400 μg buserelin in three volunteers. Shaded portions indicate the area of the hormone values of the early follicular phase. Arrows indicate the day of endometrial biopsies.

Table 19.3 Morphological findings of the endometrium of 64 volunteers during the course of i.n. treatment with different doses of buserelin

Dose (μg)		*Proliferation*			*Secretion*	n
	Inactive	*Mild*	*Moderate*	*Marked*		
100	1	5	2	6	3	17
200	15	18	15	6	7	61
400	4	4	9	12	2	31
800/1200	3	1	0	0	0	4

Table 19.4 Bleeding intervals of volunteers with marked proliferation of endometrium during the course of treatment with different doses of buserelin

Dose (μg)	n	*Days* (*M* ± *SD*) (*range*) *Last*	*Next*	*No*
100	6	22.5 (11–25)	10.5 (9–19)	4
200	6	20.5 (16–25)	13.5 (2–44)	1
400	12	33 (8–84)	8.5 (2–21)	4
800/1200	0	—	—	—

organs, cannot be predicted. In contrast to other groups (Bergquist *et al.*, 1982) we have stopped the chronic administration of LHRH agonists for general contraceptive use. The fact that these compounds do not cause general metabolic problems and that the intranasal administration was well tolerated by the volunteers encouraged us to investigate other treatment approaches. A promising way seems to be the combination of discontinuous treatment with buserelin in combination with gestagens (Hardt *et al.*, 1982).

BENEFITS OF LONG TERM TREATMENT

The disadvantage of high doses of LHRH agonists, such as complete suppression of estradiol production, for contraceptive purposes offers new ways in the treatment of sexual steroid dependent diseases. Whereas basal secretion of both gonadotropins remained nearly unaltered during the whole treatment course with the dose schedules up to 400 μg, with higher doses basal gonadotropin values were suppressed below the normal range. Intranasal administration of buserelin evokes a pronounced release of LH, FSH and estradiol during the first day of treatment. The stimulatory effect clearly decreased as treatment progressed (Figure 19.8). This was only a constant phenomenon in the higher dose regimen groups, and led to a suppression of estradiol values to postmenopausal levels in all volunteers (Figure 19.4). Therefore a higher dose regimen cannot be used for contraceptive purposes but could be used for reversible pharmacological castration (Hardt *et al.*, 1983).

Over a period of 1 year we have used this high dose regimen for pharmacological oophorectomy in 22 patients with endometriosis. The results clearly indicate that this therapeutical approach is superior, in comparison to the use of danazol for example.

CONCLUDING REMARKS

The main problem concerning long term treatment with LHRH agonists for contraceptive purposes is to find the threshold dose which possesses high antifertility effectiveness combined with normal menstrual-like bleeding and

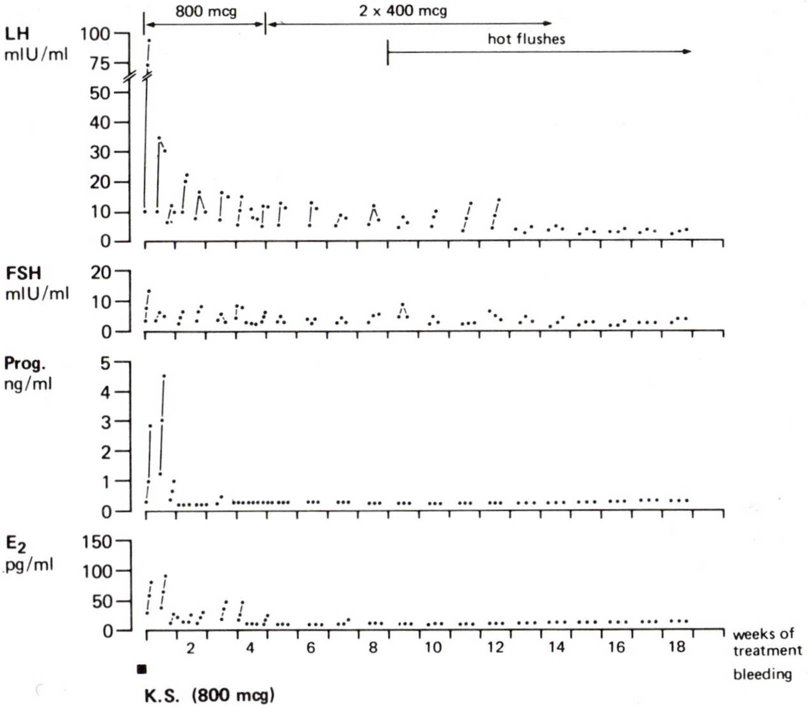

Figure 19.8 Serum values of gonadotropins (LH, FSH), estradiol (E2) and progesterone (Prog.) in a volunteer K.S. after stimulation with 800 μg/day buserelin (0, 4, 8 h) during different weeks of treatment (Basal values: Figure 19.4). Arrows: Day of endometrial biopsy.

low undesirable effects on target organs such as the endometrium. As far as the antifertility effect of buserelin is concerned, daily doses of 400 μg lead to sufficient inhibition of reproductive function in women, mainly as a result of inhibition of ovulation. However, with these doses the pattern of estradiol secretion and the influence on target organs cannot be predicted. As shown by the hormonal pattern and endometrial biopsies, periods of prolonged unopposed estrogen stimulation of the endometrium can occur, as well as phases of estrogen deficiency. Because of these disadvantages, continuous long term treatment with LHRH agonists cannot be recommended for general contraceptive use. Higher dose regimens lead consistently to suppression of estradiol secretion to postmenopausal values and offer a new possibility for treatment of hormone dependent diseases in women.

Acknowledgements

The authors would like to record their particular thanks to Hoechst AG, Frankfurt, FRG, who generously supplied buserelin, and to the nursing staff of the outpatient clinic of the Universitätsfrauenklinik Charlottenburg for their assistance in the care of our volunteers.

References

Berenblum, J. (1974). *Carcinogenesis as a Biological Problem.* (New York: Elsevier)

Bergquist, C., Nillius, S. J. and Wide, L. (1979*a*). Intranasal gonadotropin-releasing hormone agonist as a contraceptive agent. *Lancet,* **2,** 215

Bergquist, C., Nillius, S. J. and Wide, L. (1979*b*). Inhibition of ovulation in women by intranasal treatment with a luteinizing hormone-releasing hormone agonist. *Contraception,* **19,** 497

Bergquist, C., Nillius, S. J. and Wide, L. (1982). Peptide contraception in women. Xth World Congress of Gynecology and Obstetrics, San Francisco, Abstract 1148

Canales, E. S., Montvelinsky, H., Fonseca, E., Zárate, A., Coy, D. and Schally, A. V. (1980). The use of a potent stimulatory LHRH analog (D-Trp-6-LHRH) in the induction of ovulation. *Int. J. Fertil.,* **25,** 193

Dericks-Tan, J. S. E., Hammer, E. and Taubert, H.-D. (1977). The effect of D-Ser(TBU)6-LH-RH-EA10 upon gonadotropin release in normally cyclic women. *J. Clin. Endocrinol. Metab.,* **45,** 597

Fraser, H. M., Laird, N. C. and Blakeley, D. M. (1980). Decreased pituitary responsiveness and inhibition of the luteinizing hormone surge and ovulation in the stumptailed monkey (macaca arctoides) by chronic treatment with an agonist of luteinizing hormone-releasing hormone. *Endocrinology,* **106,** 452

Gusberg, S. B. (1947). Precursors of corpus carcinoma: estrogens and adenomatous hyperplasia. *Am. J. Obstet. Gynecol.,* **54,** 905

Hardt, W., Schmidt-Gollwitzer, K., Nevinny-Stickel, J. and Schmidt-Gollwitzer, M. (1982). Progress in the contraceptive use of the LH-RH agonist buserelin by intermittent medication with withdrawal bleeding induced by a progestational agent. *Geburtsh. Frauenheilk.,* **42,** 874

Hardt, W. and Schmidt-Gollwitzer, M. (1983). Sustained gonadal suppression in fertile women with the LH-RH-agonist Buserelin. A new therapeutical approach? *Clin. Endocrinol.* (Submitted for publication).

Katzorke, T. (1980). Clinical evaluation of the effects of a new long acting superactive luteinizing-releasing hormone (LH-RH) analog, D-Ser(TBU)6-des-Gly-Ethylamide-LH-RH, in fertile women. *Fertil. Steril.,* **33,** 35

Lipsett, M. B. (1977). Estrogen use and cancer risk. *J. Am. Med. Assoc.,* **237,** 1112

Nillius, S. J., Bergquist, C. and Wide, L. (1978). Inhibition of ovulation in women by chronic treatment with a stimulatory LRH analogue – a new approach to birth control? *Contraception,* **17,** 537

Sandow, J. (1982). Gonadotropic and antigonadotropic actions of LH-RH analogues. In Müller, E. E. and McLeod, R. M. (eds.) *Neureoendocrine Perspectives.* Vol. 1, pp. 339–395. (Amsterdam: Elsevier Biomedical)

Sandow, J., Clayton, R. N. and Kuhl, H. (1981). Pharmacology of LH-RH and its analogues. In Crosignani, P. and Rubin, B. L. (eds.) *Endocrinology of Human Infertility: New Aspects,* pp. 221–246. (London: Academic Press)

Schmidt-Gollwitzer, K., Hardt, W., Rebholz, G. and Schmidt-Gollwitzer, M. (1979). The effect of a new longacting LH-RH analogue (HOE 766) on gonadotrophin and steroid secretion in amenorrhoic women. *Acta Endocrinol.* (Suppl.), **225,** 357

Schmidt-Gollwitzer, M., Hardt, W., Schmidt-Gollwitzer, K. and Nevinny-Stickel, J. (1981). Influence of the LH-RH analogue buserelin on cyclic ovarian function and on endometrium. A new approach to fertility control? *Contraception,* **22,** 187

SECTION V
CONTRACEPTION IN MEN

20
Effects of nafarelin acetate in men

D. HEBER, R. S. SWERDLOFF and M. HENZL

Agonists and antagonists of LHRH would appear, by their nomenclature, to have opposite effects on the reproductive axis and thus different pharmacologic utilities. In fact, both classes of analogs, when administered chronically, are potent inhibitors of the pituitary–testicular axis. The antagonists were designed as such, while the agonists were intended to be used to treat hypogonadal patients with LHRH deficiency (Schally *et al.*, 1971).

These observations have led to clinical testing of LHRH agonists as hormonal treatments for precocious puberty (Comite *et al.*, 1981), for androgen sensitive neoplasms (i.e. prostatic carcinoma) (Faure *et al.*, 1982), and as male contraceptives (Rabin *et al.*, 1981). Their potent inhibitory action on Leydig cell function was a necessary and acceptable side-effect in the treatment of prostate cancer. However, decreased testosterone secretion, impotence and decreased libido would be highly undesirable side-effects of a male contraceptive. The combination of testosterone and LHRH analogs is doubly attractive since replacement testosterone treatment prevents the undesirable side-effects of impotence and diminished libido; and the combination should exert additive or synergistic effects on the suppression of spermatogenesis.

SYNERGISTIC INHIBITION OF GONADOTROPINS BY LHRH AGONIST AND TESTOSTERONE

Groups of adult male Wistar rats were castrated and treated with either vehicle, [D-Leu^6,Pro^9-NHEt]LHRH, testosterone or both LHRH agonist and testosterone for 7 days.

The animals were sacrificed after 7 days and serum LH and FSH measured (Table 20.1). Testosterone had additive or synergistic suppressive effects on gonadotropin secretion when administered concomitantly with maximally suppressive doses of analog (Heber and Swerdloff, 1980), suggesting that LHRH analogs and testosterone inhibit gonadotropin secretion by independent mechanisms.

Intact adult male rats were then treated with daily injections of vehicle (control), daily injections of LHRH analog alone, a subcutaneous tes-

Table 20.1 Effects of testosterone implants and/or [D-Leu[6],Pro[9]-NHEt]LHRH on serum gonadotropin levels in castrate male rats

	LH	*FSH*
1. Control	514 ± 42*	1251 ± 50
2. Testosterone implant	407 ± 50	1100 ± 66
3. Analog alone, 20 ng $(100\,g\,bw)^{-1}\,day^{-1}$	275 ± 82	1088 ± 53
4. Analog alone, 60 ng $(100\,g\,bw)^{-1}\,day^{-1}$	131 ± 15	692 ± 34
5. Analog alone, 200 ng $(100\,g\,bw)^{-1}\,day^{-1}$	134 ± 20	611 ± 35
6. Analog (20 ng) plus T	124 ± 30	975 ± 50
7. Analog (60 ng) plus T	77 ± 20	575 ± 30
8. Analog (200 ng) plus T	78 ± 18	384 ± 35

* Data are ng/ml; $x \pm$ SEM; $n = 10$ for all groups

tosterone implant, or analog and testosterone in combination (Heber and Swerdloff, 1981). After 20 days of treatment, intratesticular sperm counts and serum testosterone levels were significantly lowered by analog or analog plus testosterone (Figure 20.1), despite elevated serum levels of LH and FSH

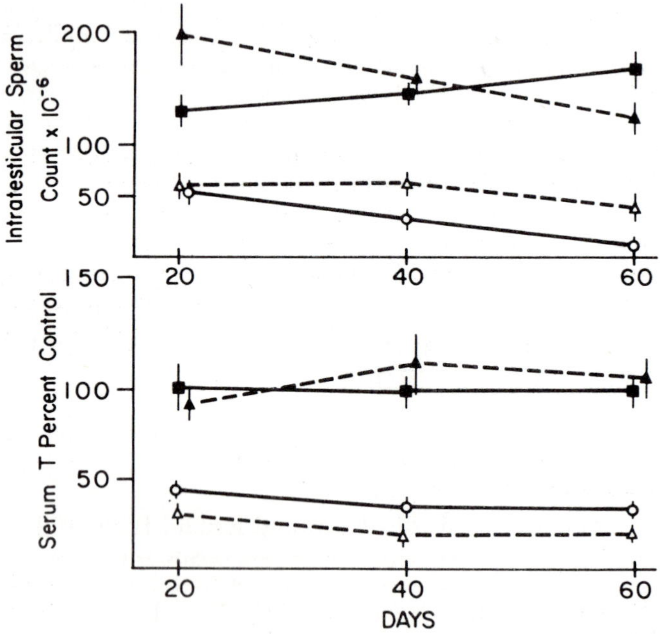

Figure 20.1 Intratesticular sperm counts (million per testis) and serum testosterone (T) (percentage of control) in vehicle-treated (■), testosterone-treated (▲), LHRH analog-treated (△) and LHRH analog plus testosterone-treated (○) adult male rats. Duration of treatment in days is shown on the abscissa. (From Heber and Swerdloff, 1981, with permission).

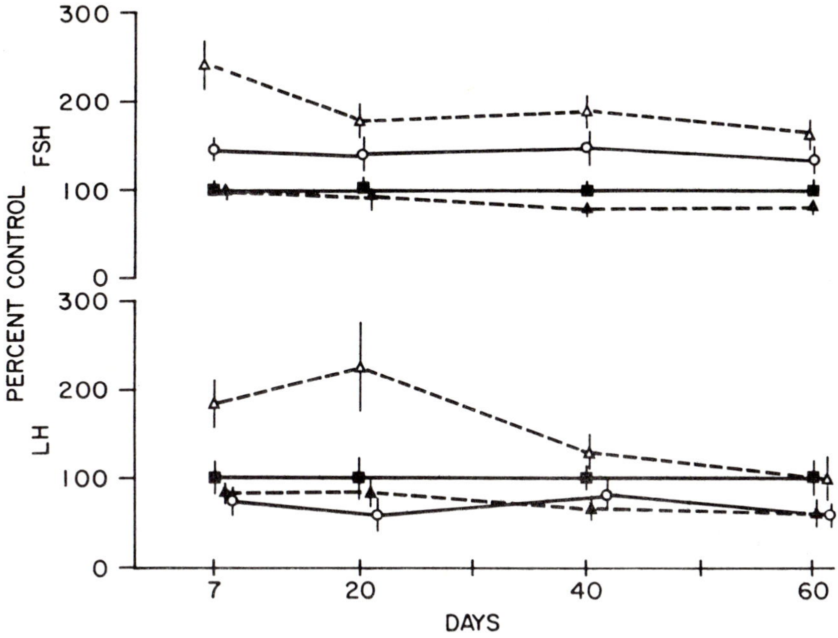

Figure 20.2 Serum FSH and LH as percentage of control values in vehicle-treated (■), testosterone-treated (▲), analog-treated (Δ), and LHRH analog plus testosterone-treated (○) adult male rats. Duration of treatment in days is shown on the abscissa. (From Heber and Swerdloff, 1981, with permission).

(Figure 20.2). At 40 and 60 days of treatment, analog treatment decreased sperm counts in the face of normal LH levels. The concomitant administration of analog and testosterone suppressed intratesticular sperm counts to a greater degree than either individual agent (Table 20.2).

Testosterone prevented the analog-induced increases in serum LH, but not FSH. At 40 and 60 days, the combined treatment regimen suppressed LH, but not FSH, to below control levels. Analog inhibition of testosterone secretion

Table 20.2 Intratesticular sperm counts (million/testis) after chronic treatment with [D-Leu^6,Pro^9-NHEt]LHRH testosterone implants or both

Group	*Day 40*	*Day 60*
Control	145 ± 7*	169 ± 13
Testosterone implanted	156 ± 15	122 ± 16
Analog at 200 ng	62 ± 10	44 ± 11
Analog plus testosterone	34 ± 7	9 ± 1.6

* Data are ng/ml; $x \pm$SEM; $n = 10$ for all groups

and spermatogenesis occurred when serum LH was normal at 40 and 60 days, suggesting that the major inhibitory effect of chronic LHRH analog treatment in the male rat is a direct inhibition of testis function. Concomitant analog and testosterone lowered both serum LH and FSH below that observed following analog treatment alone and further suppressed spermatogenesis. Testosterone appeared to enhance the analog effect in the intact male rat by lowering gonadotropin levels leading to further suppression of spermatogenesis.

In the castrate rat, synergistic inhibitory actions of testosterone and LHRH analog were demonstrated at a hypothalamic–pituitary level. In intact rats, the synergistic inhibition of spermatogenesis appeared to result from an inhibitory effect of testosterone on the secretion of gonadotropins combined with both direct gonadal and later pituitary inhibitory effects of LHRH agonists.

The mechanism by which LHRH agonists alone and in combination with testosterone influence available LHRH receptors was further studied. Studies in LHRH receptor number during the above treatment protocol in intact rats are described below (Heber *et al.*, 1982*a*).

Pituitary LHRH receptor binding was increased by analog treatment at 20 days and returned to control levels at 40 and 60 days treatment in parallel to the observed changes in serum LH (Table 20.3). Testosterone administration decreased pituitary LHRH receptor binding. Concomitant administration of LHRH analog and testosterone prevented the increase in pituitary LHRH receptors observed with analog administration alone. The changes in pituitary LHRH receptor binding correlated with changes in serum LH and the stimulatory effects of analog administration on LH were sensitive to inhibition by small doses of testosterone.

Table 20.3 Effects of LHRH analog and testosterone on LHRH receptor number (fmol/mg) in the intact male rat

Group	*20 Days*	*40 Days*	*60 Days*
Control	85 ± 20	119 ± 33	108 ± 21
Testosterone	42 ± 14	77 ± 14	92 ± 17
Analog	199 ± 57	121 ± 14	99 ± 32
Analog plus testosterone	83 ± 10	82 ± 4	132 ± 13

Subsequent studies support the findings that, in rat, both the testes and the pituitary are directly inhibited by chronic LHRH agonist treatment (Heber *et al.*, 1982*b*). The pituitary inhibition results from both decreased available receptor number and postreceptor blocking effect (Clayton, 1982).

STUDIES OF LHRH AGONIST IN MEN

Treatment of normal men for 17 weeks with 5 μg daily of [D-Ser(tBu)^6,Pro^9-NHEt]LHRH had little effect on spermatogenesis, while LH, FSH and testosterone levels fell significantly (Bergquist *et al.*, 1979). The administration of 50 μg of [D-Trp^6,Pro^9-NHEt]LHRH daily to normal men resulted in a marked fall in serum testosterone levels with a mean nadir of 60 ng/dl by the fourth week of treatment (Linde *et al.*, 1981). Gonadotropin levels were measured bimonthly and demonstrated incomplete inhibition, although a nadir value of 50% of mean pretreatment levels of LH was observed in the eight subjects tested. In these studies, agonist treatment was discontinued after 6 or 7 weeks in five of eight subjects because of impotence. Libido and potency returned 2 weeks after stopping agonist therapy. Only one of three subjects who completed 10 weeks of therapy was azoospermic. Recovery of spermatogenesis occurred within 10 weeks of cessation of therapy in all but the one azoospermic subject, who recovered after 14 weeks.

Studies in our laboratories defined the stimulatory and inhibitory effects of nafarelin acetate [D-Nal(2)^6]LHRH at two doses, 10 μg and 100 μg, in two groups of seven normal men treated for 10 days. Both doses of agonist initially increased LH, FSH and testosterone, with a return to pretreatment levels by day 10 (Figure 20.3). There was a dose-related inhibition of the integrated LH, FSH and testosterone responses to analog on day 10 vs day 1. Comparison of serum levels of LH and FSH following the first and tenth dose of 100 μg of analog reveals the pituitary down regulatory effects of the LHRH agonist (Figure 20.4). Stimulation of gonadotropins and testosterone in the human is transient following daily LHRH agonist treatment and is completed by 10 days, when down regulation to agonist stimulation is evident.

Human chorionic gonadotropin was injected during the control period and on the day after the last analog injection. Basal levels of serum testosterone were lowered by treatment with agonist, but increased after hCG in a parallel fashion to that seen during the pretreatment test. The predominant inhibitory effect of short term (10 day) LHRH agonist treatment in men is thus exerted on the pituitary gland.

STUDIES OF CONCOMITANT LHRH AGONIST AND TESTOSTERONE IN MEN

Men who had received daily agonist treatment previously were given the same dose (either 10 μg or 100 μg) together with a single injection of testosterone enanthate at the time of the first analog injection (Bhasin *et al.*, 1983). Combined low dose agonist (10 μg) and testosterone treatment exerted greater inhibitory effects on gonadotropin levels than did the 10 μg analog treatment alone.

Daily mean basal levels of LH and FSH were lowered to a greater degree by LHRH agonist plus testosterone enanthate than by analog alone (Figure 20.5). Serum FSH was more effectively suppressed than was LH by combined treatment. All FSH values were below the limits of detection of the assay on the 10th and 11th day of treatment. There was a marked inhibition of integrated FSH and LH responses to analog injection on day 10 as compared to day 1 in both the 10 and 100 μg groups (Figure 20.6). In the 10 μg group, there was no difference between the combined analog/testosterone or analog-treated group in integrated LH or FSH responses on day 1 or 10. In contrast, combined treatment with testosterone and 100 μg of analog led to enhanced inhibition of LH as well as FSH secretion on day 10 compared to 100 μg of analog alone. Thus concomitant treatment with testosterone enanthate and LHRH agonist leads to more effective suppression of gonadotropin secretion than does agonist alone.

The administration of 50 μg of [D-Trp,^{6}Pro^9-NHEt]LHRH subcutaneously every fourth day is not as effective as is daily administration in

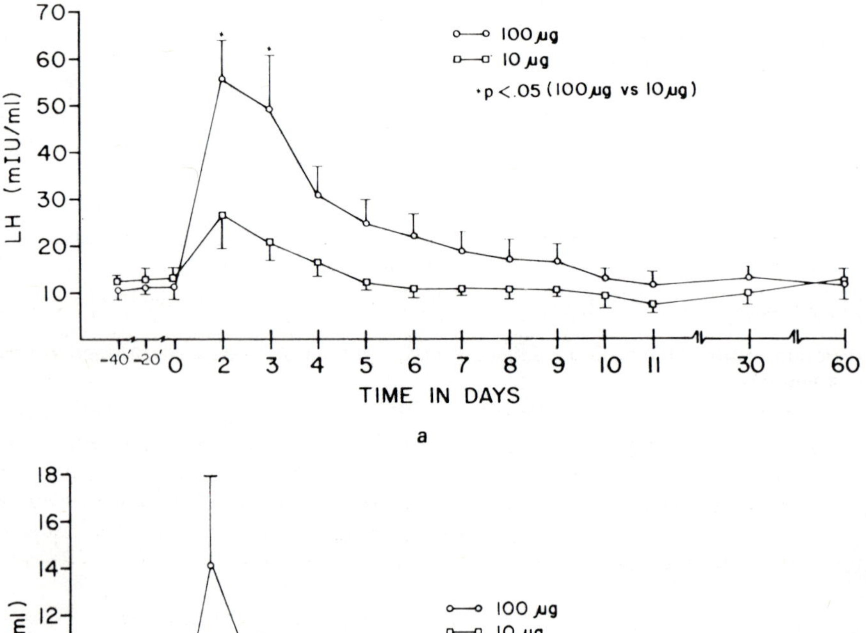

a

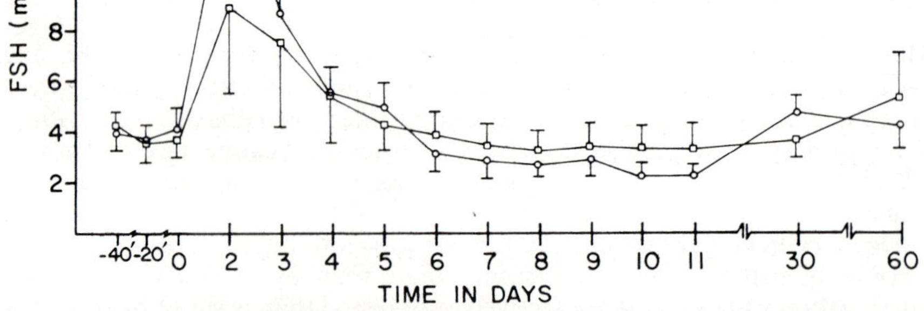

b

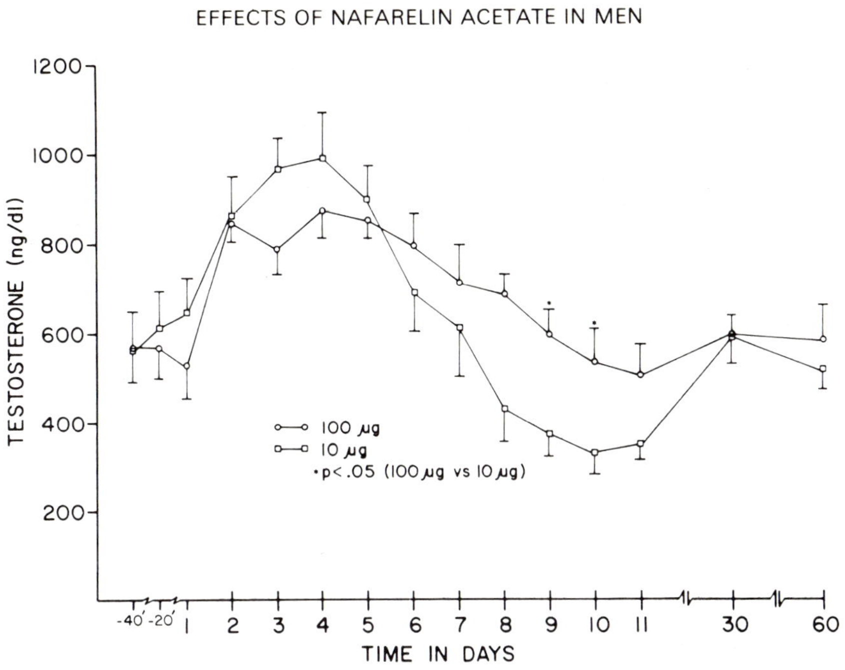

Figure 20.3a–c Serum LH, FSH and testosterone before treatment (−40, −20 and 0 min) during treatment (24 h after each daily intramuscular dose of [D-Nal(2)^6]LHRH – days 2–11) and after discontinuing LHRH analog treatment (days 30 and 60). (From Heber *et al.*, 1984, with permission).

suppressing spermatogenesis (Rabin *et al.*, 1981). Daily 50 µg subcutaneous injections of this agonist and bimonthly injections of 100 mg of testosterone enanthate resulted in a degree of oligospermia observed in six subjects which was similar to that reported following analog treatment alone. Azoospermia was not achieved during a 20-week treatment period in any subject (Rabin *et al.*, 1981).

[D-Trp^6,Pro^9-NHEt]LHRH and [D-Nal(2)^6]LHRH are approximately equipotent in their ability to stimulate LH release in an *in vitro* pituitary cell culture assay system (Heber and Swerdloff, unpublished observations). It is possible that the reported studies on [D-Trp^6,Pro^9-NHEt]LHRH have utilized too low a dose of both LHRH agonist and of testosterone. We presently have ongoing trials of 200 µg per day of [D-Nal(2)^6]LHRH together with a dose of testosterone enanthate that was previously demonstrated to suppress spermatogenesis to test this possibility (Swerdloff *et al.*, 1978).

THE SITE OF LHRH AGONIST ACTION IN MAN

In order to determine the site of LHRH agonist action in men our laboratories conducted studies of another LHRH agonist, [D-Leu^6,Pro^9-NHEt]LHRH, as

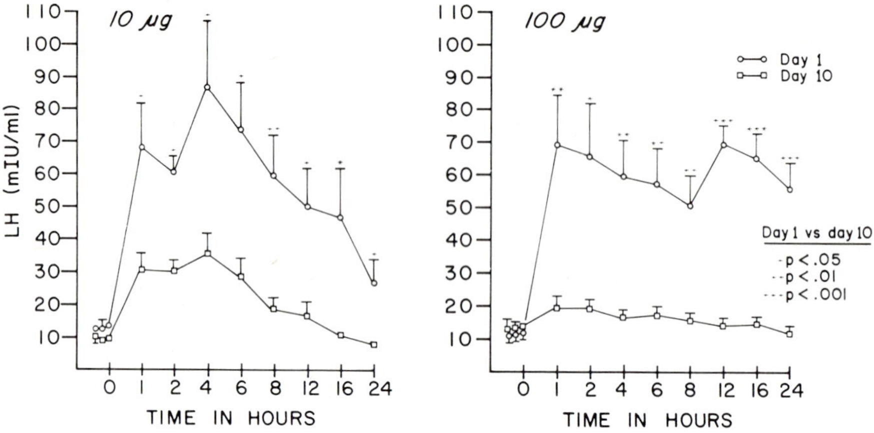

a

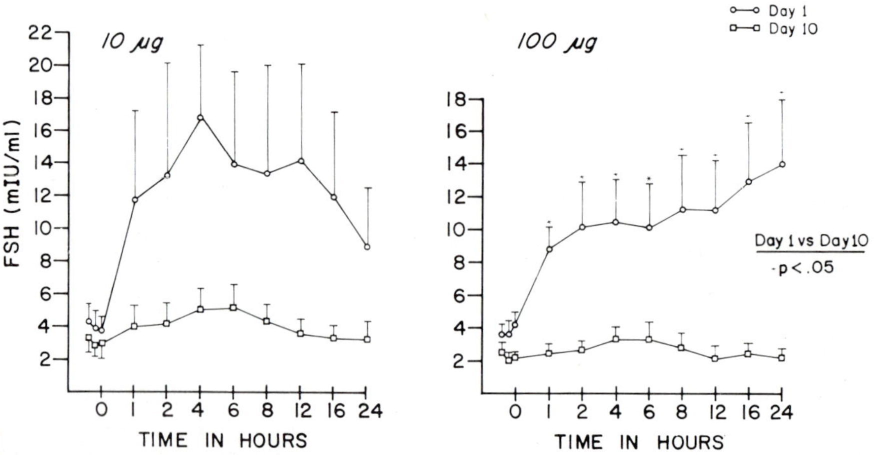

b

Figure 20.4a, b Serum LH and FSH during a 24 h period after the first dose (day 1) and the 10th dose (day 10) of 100 µg of [D-Nal(2)[6]]LHRH. (From Heber *et al.*, 1984, with permission).

part of the Tap-Abbott Cooperative Prostatic Cancer Study Group (Heber *et al.*, 1983). Men with metastatic prostate cancer were given daily subcutaneous injections of 1 mg of [D-Leu[6],Pro[9]-NHEt]LHRH, as part of this study. Both basal (preinjection) and peak increments of LH and FSH following agonist injection were significantly suppressed after day 56 of therapy (Figure 20.7). Suppression of basal and maximal gonadotropin secretion after agonist injection occurred in the face of markedly suppressed levels of serum testosterone. As low levels of testosterone would be expected to increase gonadotropin secretion by feedback mechanisms, this suggests that the

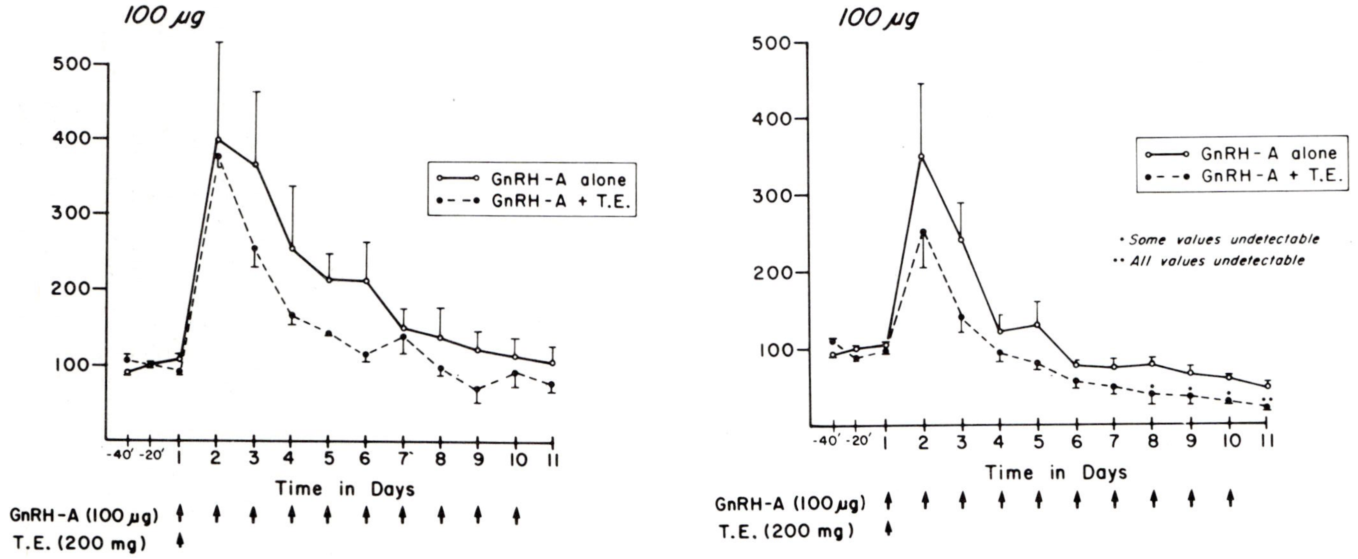

Figure 20.5 Serum LH and FSH measured 24 h after each daily dose of either 100 μg of [D-Nal(2)^6]LHRH (LHRH-A) (○—○) or 100 μg of LHRH-A given with a single 200 mg intramuscular injection of TE on day 1 (●—●). (From Bhasin *et al.*, 1983, with permission).

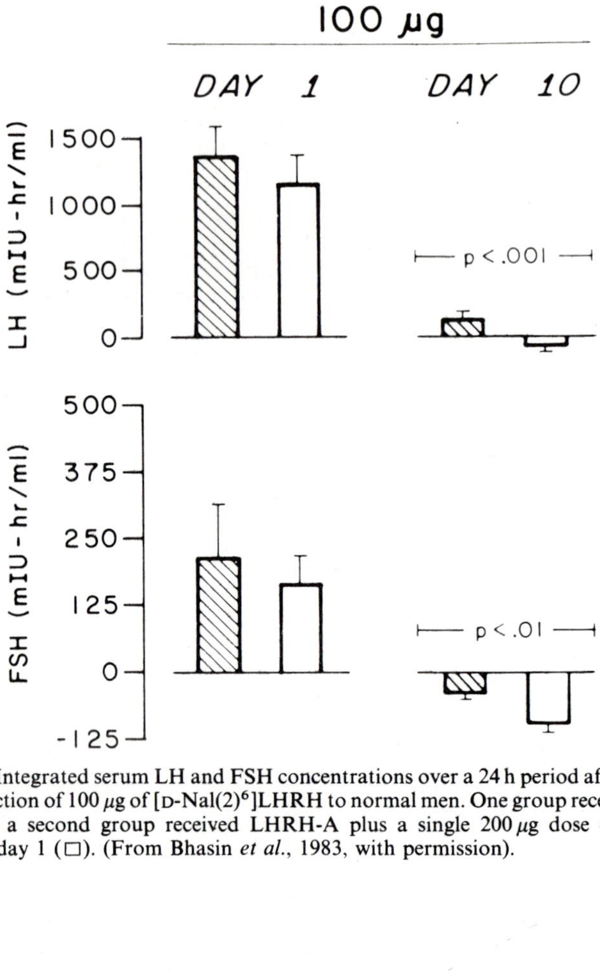

Figure 20.6 Integrated serum LH and FSH concentrations over a 24 h period after the first and 10th daily injection of 100 μg of [D-Nal(2)^6]LHRH to normal men. One group received LHRH-A alone (■) and a second group received LHRH-A plus a single 200 μg dose of testosterone enanthate on day 1 (□). (From Bhasin *et al.*, 1983, with permission).

pituitary gland is the primary site of action of LHRH agonist in the human male.

Despite the similarity of agonist effects on testosterone secretion and spermatogenesis in humans and rats, the mechanisms by which these agents affect the testes appear to be different in the two species. In man, LHRH agonists have an early stimulatory effect on LH and FSH secretion with pituitary down regulation evident by the 10th day of daily treatment. Longer duration of treatment suppresses circulating levels of LH, FSH and testosterone. In the rat, the stimulation of LH and FSH secretion by LHRH agonists persisted for a much longer period of time (20–60 days). In the rat, direct testicular effects of analog were the most likely cause of early suppression of testosterone and impaired sperm production while in man the pituitary gland is the primary site of agonist effects.

CONCLUDING REMARKS

The studies discussed in man and experimental animal models point to a primary effect of LHRH agonists at the pituitary which results in gonadotropin inhibition via pituitary desensitization. Our own studies point to the possibility that LHRH agonists and testosterone in combination may more effectively suppress spermatogenesis in man, since these two classes of agents independently and synergistically suppress gonadotropin secretion via effects on the hypothalamic–pituitary axis. Studies in man indicate that enhanced inhibition of gonadotropin secretion results from the combined use of testosterone and LHRH agonists for short periods. Clinical studies of combined androgen/agonist administration in the past have failed to demonstrate enhanced suppression of spermatogenesis. Studies currently underway in our laboratories using higher doses of agonist and testosterone as well as alternate routes and modes of administration will hopefully provide further information on the utility of this approach to male contraception.

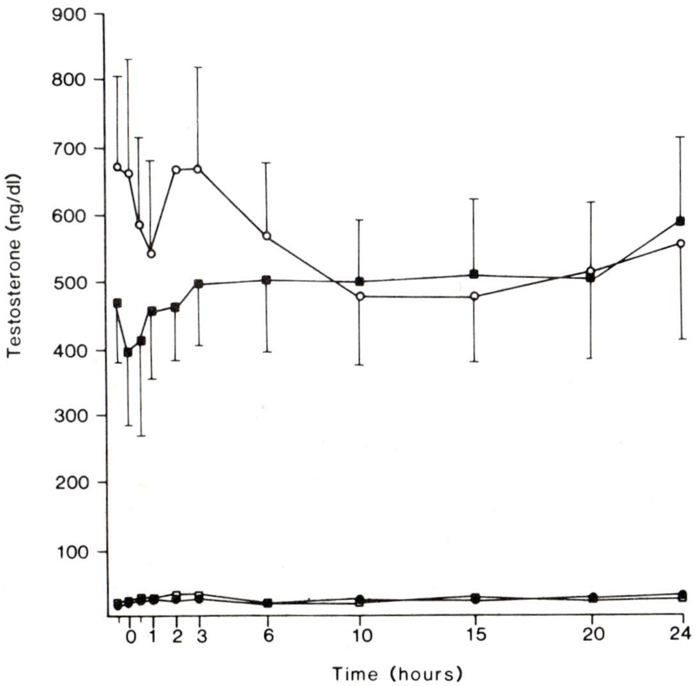

Figure 20.7a

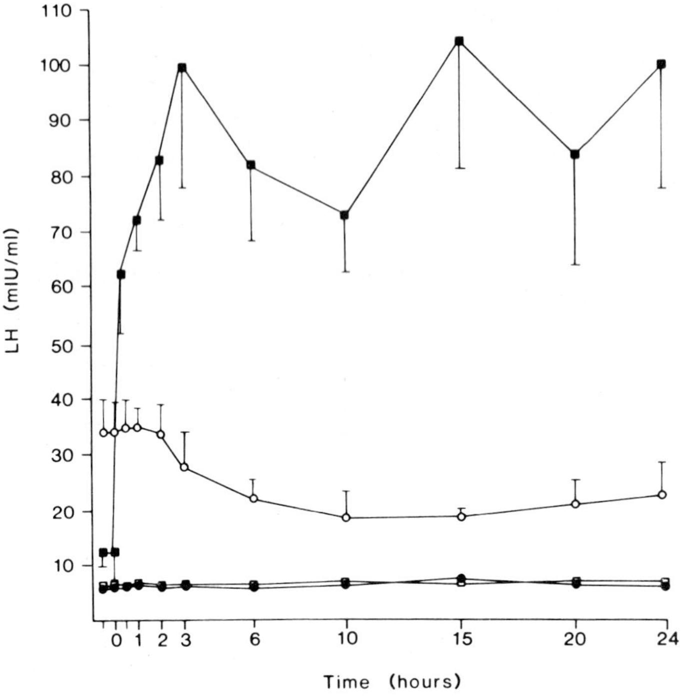

b

Figure 20.7a,b Testosterone (ng/dl) and serum LH (miu/ml) versus time in hours after injection of 1 mg of [D-Leu^6,Pro^9-NHEt]LHRH on days 1 (■), 5 (○), 56 (□), and 180 (●) of daily analog treatment. By 56 days of treatment, basal levels of LH and testosterone are suppressed with essentially no increment seen after GnRH administration.

References

Bergquist, C., Nillius, S. J., Bergh, T., Skarin, G. and Wide, L. (1979). Inhibitory effects on gonadotropin secretion and gonadal function in men during chronic treatment with a potent stimulatory LHRH analogue. *Acta Endocrinol.*, **91,** 601

Bhasin, S., Heber, D., Steiner, B. and Swerdloff, R. S. (1983). Enhanced inhibition of gonadotropin secretion in man by combined GnRH agonist and testosterone in the male. *Clin. Endocrinol.*, (In press)

Clayton, R. N. (1982). Gonadotropin releasing hormone modulation of its own pituitary receptors: evidence for biphasic regulation. *Endocrinology,* **11,** 152

Comite, F., Cutler, G. B., Rivier, J., Vale, W. W., Loriaux, D. L. and Crowley, W. F. (1981). Short-term treatment of idiopathic precocious puberty with a long-acting analogue of LHRH. *N. Engl. J. Med.,* **305,** 1546

Faure, H., Lemay, A., Bélanger, A. and Labrie, F. (1982). Inhibition of testicular steroidogenesis by chronic administration of a potent LHRH agonist, HOE 766, to patients with cancer of the prostate. *J. Androl.,* **3,** 43

Heber, D. and Swerdloff, R. S. (1980). Male contraception: synergism between superactive GnRH analog and testosterone in suppressing gonadotropin secretion. *Science,* **209,** 936

Heber, D. and Swerdloff, R. S. (1981). Gonadotropin-releasing hormone analog and testosterone synergistically inhibit spermatogenesis. *Endocrinology,* **108,** 2019

Heber, D., Dodson, R., Stoskopf, C., Peterson, M. and Swerdloff, R. S. (1982*a*). Pituitary desensitization and the regulation of pituitary GnRH receptors following chronic administration of superactive GnRH analog and testosterone. *Life Sci.,* **30,** 2301

Heber, D., Dodson, R., Nowak, F., Channabasavaiah, K., Stewart, J. M., and Swerdloff, R. S. (1982*b*). Actions and interactions of a potent GnRH agonist and antagonist in the male rat. *Clin. Res.,* **30,** 30A

Heber, D., Bhasin, S., Steiner, B. and Swerdloff, R. S. (1984). The stimulatory and inhibitory effects of a gonadotropin-releasing hormone agonist in man. *J. Clin. Endocrinol. Metab.* (In press)

Heber, D., Swerdloff, R. S., Steiner, B., Peterson, M. and Rajfer, J. (1983*b*). The pituitary gland: primary site of action of GnRH agonist in the human male. *J. Clin. Endocrinol. Metab.* (In press)

Linde, R. B., Doelle, G. C., Alexander, N., Kirchner, F., Vale, W., Rivier, J. and Rabin, D. (1981). Reversible inhibition of testicular steroidogenesis and spermatogenesis by a potent GnRH agonist in normal men: An approach toward the development of a male contraceptive. *N. Engl. J. Med.,* **305,** 663

Rabin, D., Linde, R., Doelle, G. and Alexander, N. (1981). Experience with a potent GnRH agonist in normal men: an approach to the development of a male contraceptive. In Zatuchni, G., Shelton, J. and Sciarra, J. (eds.) *LHRH Peptides as Female and Male Contraceptives,* pp. 296–306. (Philadelphia: Harper & Row)

Schally, A. V., Nair, R. M.G., Redding, J. W. and Arimura, A. (1971). Isolation of the luteinizing hormone and follicle stimulating hormone-releasing hormone from porcine hypothalami. *J. Biol. Chem.,* **246,** 7230

Swerdloff, R. S., McClure, R. D., Palacios, A., Campfield, L. A. and Brosman, S. A. (1978). Clinical evaluation of testosterone enanthate in the reversible suppression of spermatogenesis in the human male: efficacy, mechanism of action and adverse effect. In Patenelli, D. J. (ed.) *Proc. Hormonal Control of Male Fertility, 1977,* p. 41. (Washington: U.S. Department of Health, Education and Welfare, NIH)

21
Antifertility effects of an LHRH agonist in men

G. C. DOELLE, R. M. EVANS, A. N. ALEXANDER and D. RABIN

Research efforts toward development of a male contraceptive agent have proceeded in two general directions. Early studies dealt with agents having a direct effect on the seminiferous tubule. A number of compounds, notably the nitrofurans and diamines, were investigated, but all were found to have undesirable side-effects or a narrow and unacceptable therapeutic index. Recent efforts, primarily in the People's Republic of China, have utilized gossypol as an antifertility agent. Initial optimistic reports by the Chinese (National Coordinating Group on Male Antifertility Agents, 1978) have not yet been confirmed; current studies are designed to provide the answer to gossypol's contraceptive potential.

A second approach to male contraception has utilized hormonal intervention. Androgens singly (Steinberger and Smith, 1977) or in combination with progestins (Schearer, 1978) have been shown to induce oligospermia, though results have been inconsistent (Paulsen *et al.*, 1978). The development of potent agonistic analogs of gonadotropin-releasing hormone (LHRH) was followed by the demonstration of paradoxical antigonadal effects of these agents in laboratory animals. We have administered the LHRH agonist [D-Trp^6,Pro^9-NHEt]LHRH chronically to normal adult males, attempting to utilize the antigonadal properties of this agent toward the development of reversible male contraception.

LHRH AGONISTS IN EXPERIMENTAL ANIMALS AND MAN

The LHRH analog [D-Trp^6,Pro^9-NHEt]LHRH (LHRH-A) has a potency 144 times that of native LHRH in eliciting release of LH from pituitary cells *in vitro* (Vale *et al.*, 1977). When this LHRH analog was administered chronically to animals, however, the expected response did not occur; there was, in fact, an attenuation of gonadal activity (Rivier and Vale, 1979; Rivier *et al.*, 1980). This unexpected response in which an agonist behaved as an antagonist *in vivo* suggested that LHRH-A might have potential application in the human. Indeed, long term treatment with the LHRH agonist [D-Ser(tBu)^6,Pro^9-NHEt]LHRH resulted in a reduction of serum gonadotropin and testosterone concentrations in adult men (Bergquist *et al.*, 1979; Wiegelman *et al.*, 1977); treatment of men with [D-Trp^6]LHRH for 3–6 months led to a fall in plasma testosterone and dihydrotestosterone concentrations to castrate levels, with an associated decrease in beard growth, acne and erectile potency (Tolis *et al.*, 1981).

Several mechanisms have been identified which might explain the paradoxical effects of LHRH agonists. They (1) result in reduced pituitary responsiveness leading to impaired gonadotropin release, (2) lead to the loss of testicular LH and prolactin receptors and reduced steroidogenic activity and (3) inhibit peripheral androgen action.

Impaired gonadotropin responsiveness has been observed with chronic LHRH agonist administration both *in vitro* (Rivier and Vale, 1979) and *in vivo* (Sandow *et al.*, 1978). Decreased plasma and pituitary LH and FSH concentrations suggest decreased gonadotropin synthesis as well as reduced gonadotropin secretion. In the adult male, a significantly decreased LH response is seen after 1 week of daily administration of an LHRH agonist (Smith *et al.*, 1979), although the pituitary responds briskly to the initial administration of the agonist. Thus, while initial administration of LHRH agonists results in stimulation of pituitary gonadotropin release, chronic administration is followed by blunting of the gonadotrope response to further stimulation.

LHRH and its agonistic analogs also have effects at the level of the gonad. Adult male rats treated with the LHRH agonist [D-Leu^6,Pro^9-NHEt]LHRH demonstrate a marked decline in LH receptor number in testicular tissue (Auclair *et al.*, 1977), after both acute and chronic administration. That the decrease in LH receptor number is at least in part mediated by the acute release of endogenous LH is suggested by a similar decline in receptor number following administration of hCG or LH (Auclair *et al.*, 1977; Hsueh *et al.*, 1976, 1977). While tempting to attribute the antigonadal effects of LHRH agonists to acute release of endogenous LH, it has none the less been shown that direct gonadal effects of LHRH and its agonistic analogs do occur in the rat (Rippel and Johnson, 1976; Hsueh and Erickson, 1979*a*,*b*). The presence of specific LHRH receptors in testicular interstitial tissue (Clayton *et al.*, 1980) provides further evidence of direct gonadal activity of these compounds.

In addition to pituitary and gonadal sites of action, LHRH agonists may be capable of peripheral antisteroidal activity. The LHRH agonist [D-His(Bzl)^6, Pro^9-NHEt]LHRH is capable of inhibiting the testosterone-induced increase in weight of ventral prostate and seminal vesicles in castrate and castrate-hypophysectomized rats (Sundaram *et al.*, 1981). Furthermore, this LHRH agonist does not interact with the androgen receptor (Lecomte *et al.*, 1982), suggesting that the antisteroidal properties are mediated via another, possibly postreceptor mechanism.

ADMINISTRATION OF LHRH-A TO MEN

Over the range of 10–100 μg, a linear dose–response relationship exists between a single injection of LHRH-A and the rise in serum gonadotropin concentration (Crowley *et al.*, 1980). The gonadotropin response is sustained through 48 h at the 50 and 100 μg dose levels. Despite the augmentation of LH and FSH release with acute administration, continuous administration of LHRH agonists inhibits pituitary–gonadal function. The antigonadal activity of these compounds led us to examine their contraceptive potential in men.

Daily administration of LHRH-A

Eight healthy male subjects, age 28–42 years, were asked to defer planned vasectomy (Linde *et al.*, 1981). Semen analysis and blood hormone profiles were obtained at 2-week intervals for a 10-week control period. Thereafter, subjects received daily subcutaneous injections of 50 μg LHRH-A. The period of drug administration was scheduled to last 10 weeks, followed by a post-treatment period designed to observe full recovery in each subject.

Individual sperm density results varied widely during the control period, and individual mean sperm density during this period ranged from 20 to 195×10^6/ml (Figure 21.1). Six of the eight subjects demonstrated a fall in sperm density to values of 6×10^6/ml or less between the 7th and 18th week after the beginning of treatment. In the other two subjects, sperm density fell 70 and 86% below mean control values. In the three subjects who completed 10 weeks of LHRH-A treatment (*see below*), sperm densities of 4.6×10^6/ml (Subject F), 1.4×10^6/ml (Subject H), and O (Subject C) were observed. Sperm density returned to within control range during the post-treatment period in each subject.

Basal concentrations of serum gonadotropins and gonadal steroids were normal in all subjects (Table 21.1). With treatment, each subject demonstrated a rapid decline in serum testosterone; subnormal levels (i.e. less than 2.0 ng/ml) were achieved in five subjects within 2 weeks of instituting treatment, and levels of 1.3 ng/ml or less were noted in all subjects by the 4th treatment week. The fall in testosterone concentration was associated with diminished libido in all subjects; impotence developed in five of the eight subjects between the 6th and 7th treatment weeks, necessitating premature discontinuation of LHRH-A. Testosterone concentration and sexual function returned to pretreatment levels by the 4th post-treatment week.

A similar treatment period decline was also noted for serum 17β-estradiol, 17α-hydroxyprogesterone and progesterone. While the decline in all gonadal steroids was significant, the decline in progesterone concentration was of lesser magnitude than that of the other steroids, consistent with partial inhibition of 17α-hydroxylase (Labrie *et al.*, 1980).

Despite the pronounced fall in testosterone concentration noted during the period of LHRH-A administration, serum gonadotropin concentrations were unchanged during treatment (Table 21.1), an observation consistent with the phenomenon of pituitary 'desensitization'. Mean gonadotropin concentrations remained within the range of basal values after discontinuation of LHRH-A.

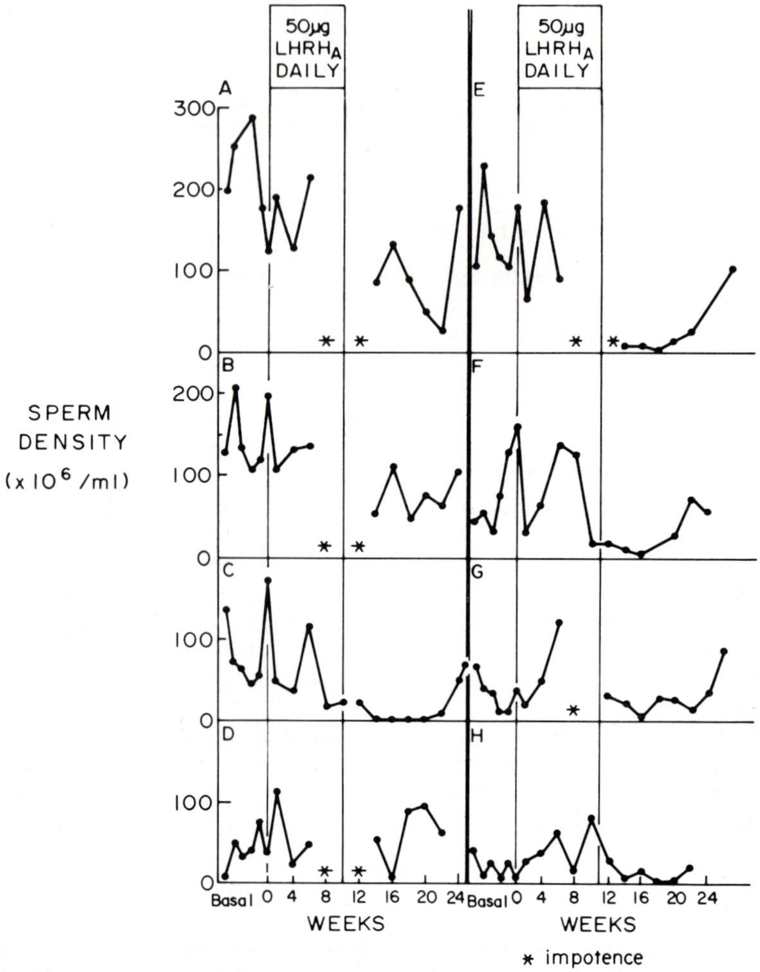

Figure 21.1 Individual sperm density results for subjects receiving LHRH-A daily. Results shown are for basal, treatment and post-treatment periods. (*) indicates inability to obtain semen sample due to impotence (see text).

Every fourth day administration of LHRH-A

In the male rat, intermittent administration of LHRH-A also exerted antigonadal properties (Rivier and Vale, 1979). We, therefore, utilized intermittent administration of LHRH-A in a second group of adult men (Doelle *et al.*, 1982). Seven subjects self-administered 50 µg LHRH-A by subcutaneous injection every 4th day, following a 10-week control period. Semen analysis and hormone profiles were obtained as outlined previously. Individual mean sperm density during the control period varied between 69

Table 21.1 Hormone profile for subjects receiving LHRH-A daily

Hormone	*Basal*	*Treatment* *Week 4*	*Treatment* *Week 8*	*Post-treatment* *Week 10*
Testosterone (ng/ml)	4.71 ±0.22	0.70 ±0.13[a]	0.73 ±0.21[a]	4.17 ±0.41
Progesterone (ng/ml)	0.71 ±0.03	0.65 ±0.07	0.59 ±0.07	0.59 ±0.06
17-OH Progesterone (ng/ml)	1.12 ±0.06	0.26 ±0.06[a]	0.34 ±0.14[a]	1.18 ±0.21
Estradiol (pg/ml)	29.7 ±1.33	10.0 ±1.9[a]	16.7 ±6.7	21.9 ±2.1
LH (mIU/l)	10.9 ±0.7	7.4 ±1.3	7.9 ±1.1	13.5 ±2.2
FSH (mIU/ml)	4.7 ±0.3	5.5 ±1.6	4.1 ±0.8	4.6 ±0.6

Basal values are the means of six samples from each subject. All values are means ± SEM.
[a] $p < 0.005$ compared to basal mean result

and 137 × 10^6/ml. Only inconsistent and statistically insignificant declines in sperm density were observed; sperm density fell consistently below 20 × 10^6/ml in only one subject. No side-effects were observed and libido and potency were maintained. This regimen did not consistently suppress the pituitary–gonadal axis. During treatment, elevated LH and testosterone concentrations were observed on eight and seven occasions, respectively, corresponding to samples obtained 24 and 48 h after LHRH-A injection. Depressed serum testosterone concentrations were observed on ten occasions in six subjects, and all but one corresponded to samples obtained 72–96 h after the previous LHRH-A injection. These results suggest retention of the pituitary and gonadal responses to LHRH-A administered every 4th day, and concur with earlier observations noting an LH response and increase in testicular size in men with hypogonadotropic hypogonadism treated with LHRH-A every other day (Crowley *et al.*, 1979); in these subjects, responses were extinguished when treatment was increased to daily frequency.

Administration of LHRH-A and testosterone

While administration of LHRH-A every 4th day yielded disappointing results, we were encouraged by the suppressive effect of daily LHRH-A administration on sperm density. The latter protocol was accompanied by marked suppression of testosterone concentration and an associated diminution of libido and potency. In an attempt to maintain sexual function while preserving LHRH-A's suppressive effect on spermatogenesis, we have administered identical dosages of LHRH-A in combination with testosterone enanthate. As a single agent, testosterone enanthate can produce oligospermia or azoospermia if administered at a dosage and frequency sufficient to inhibit gonadotropin secretion (Steinberger and Smith, 1977). Combined administration of an LHRH agonist with doses of testosterone which alone lower sperm count is synergistic in suppressing serum gonadotropin levels and spermatogenesis in the rat (Heber and Swerdloff, 1980, 1981). We chose a dose of testosterone enanthate which we thought would be insufficient to inhibit spermatogenesis if given as a single agent, yet which might prevent changes in sexual function during treatment with LHRH-A.

Accordingly, a third group of subjects was examined by semen analysis and hormone profile at 2-week intervals during a control period, 20-week treatment period, and post-treatment period. Six subjects received daily injections of 50 μg LHRH-A in combination with testosterone enanthate, 100 mg intramuscularly, every 2 weeks. Three subjects served as control and received testosterone enanthate alone on an identical schedule. (Doelle *et al.*, 1983)

Gonadotropin and gonadal steroid results were normal in all subjects during the control period (Table 21.2). A decline in plasma testosterone was evident by the 4th treatment week in subjects receiving LHRH-A and testosterone enanthate and suppressed testosterone concentrations were maintained throughout the treatment period. Mean testosterone concentrations at week 10 and week 20 of treatment were 1.2 ng/ml and 1.8 ng/ml, respectively. These samples were obtained just prior to the next testosterone injection. These nadir values were, none the less, higher than random testosterone concentration measured in subjects treated with LHRH-A alone. Libido and potency were maintained in subjects receiving combination treatment. No change in sexual function was reported by subjects or sexual partners, and no subject demonstrated any change in frequency of ejaculation during or following the period of drug administration. All subjects were able to complete the full 20-week treatment period.

Sperm density for subjects receiving LHRH-A and testosterone enanthate varied widely throughout the control period (Figure 21.2). Treatment response was variable, however; a consistent decline in sperm density occurred in all subjects, with nadir values achieved on the final week of treatment or 2 weeks later. Because of individual variability in the time course of treatment response, we compared mean sperm density of the control period with that of the latter 6 weeks of treatment and first 4 weeks of recovery, both 10-week intervals comprising an identical number of semen analyses from each subject. Mean control sperm density was 77×10^6/ml, with a range from 32 to 133×10^6/ml. Mean sperm density during the 10-week period at the termination of treatment ($25 \pm 3.1 \times 10^6$/ml, range $3\text{–}39 \times 10^6$/ml) was significantly less than the mean pretreatment value.

No consistent change in sperm density was observed in the three subjects receiving only testosterone enanthate. Mean control sperm density in this

Table 21.2 Hormone profile for subjects receiving LHRH-A and testosterone enanthate

		Treatment		Post-treatment
Hormone	*Basal*	*Week 10*	*Week 20*	*Week 10*
Testosterone (ng/ml)	3.76 ± 0.24	1.20 ± 0.34^a	1.77 ± 0.20^a	4.97 ± 0.84
Progesterone (ng/ml)	0.64 ± 0.04	0.47 ± 0.06^b	0.57 ± 0.14	0.44 ± 0.05^a
17-OH Progesterone (ng/ml)	1.35 ± 0.15	0.28 ± 0.08^a	0.61 ± 0.33	1.12 ± 0.30
Estradiol (pg/ml)	16.3 ± 0.7	10.0 ± 0^a	10.8 ± 0.08^a	19.2 ± 2.4
LH (mIU/ml)	12.7 ± 1.2	10.0 ± 1.0	8.0 ± 1.0	11.7 ± 1.8
FSH (mIU/ml)	7.6 ± 0.5	5.1 ± 0.7	6.4 ± 1.2	5.4 ± 0.9

Basal values are the means of six samples from each subject. All values are means ± SEM.
[a] $p < 0.005$ compared to basal mean result; [b] $p < 0.025$ compared to basal mean result

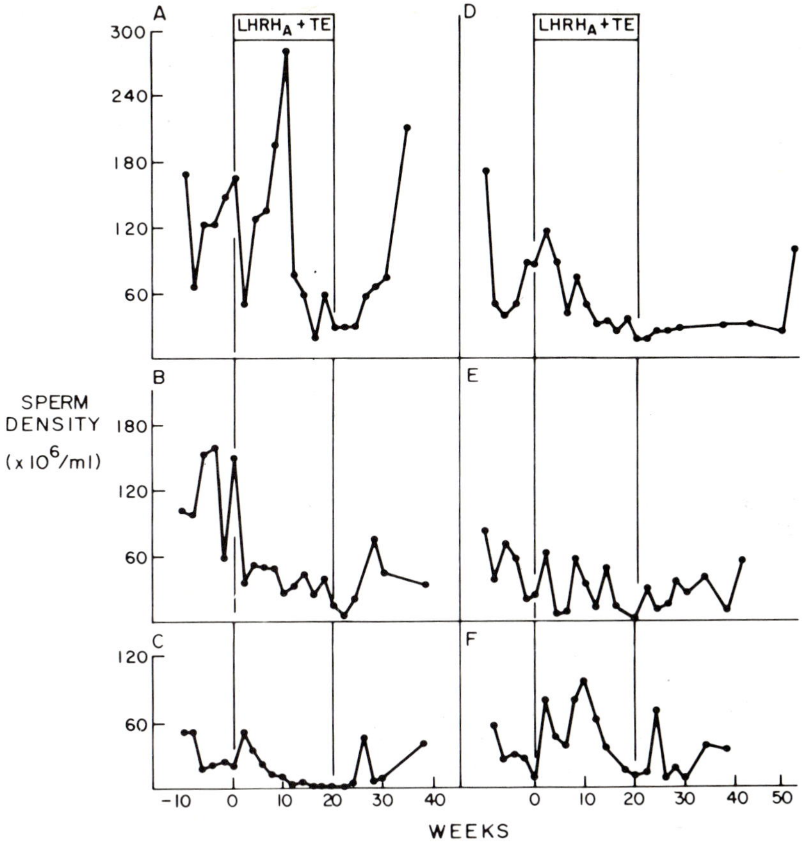

Figure 21.2 Individual sperm density results for subjects receiving LHRH-A and testosterone enanthate. Results shown are for basal, treatment and post-treatment periods.

group was 75 × 10^6/ml (range 26–106 × 10^6/ml), which was not significantly different from the mean sperm density of the 10-week interval comprising the latter 6 treatment weeks and first 4 recovery weeks (67 × 10^6/ml, range 24–128 × 10^6/ml). Thus, the addition of non-suppressive doses of testosterone enanthate to effective doses of LHRH-A is capable of eliminating diminished libido and potency, but does not modify LHRH-A's influence on sperm density.

PITUITARY AND GONADAL RESPONSES DURING ADMINISTRATION OF LHRH-A

The mechanism of action of LHRH-A remains uncertain. Preliminary studies performed in our laboratory, however, employing sampling of serum gonadotropins every 20 min and serum testosterone hourly, suggest a profound effect on the pituitary. In two subjects treated with 50 μg of LHRH-A daily, the normal pulsatile release of LH was abolished (Figures 21.3 and 21.4). Despite lowered testosterone concentration, mean gonadotropin levels were either unchanged or diminished (Table 21.3).

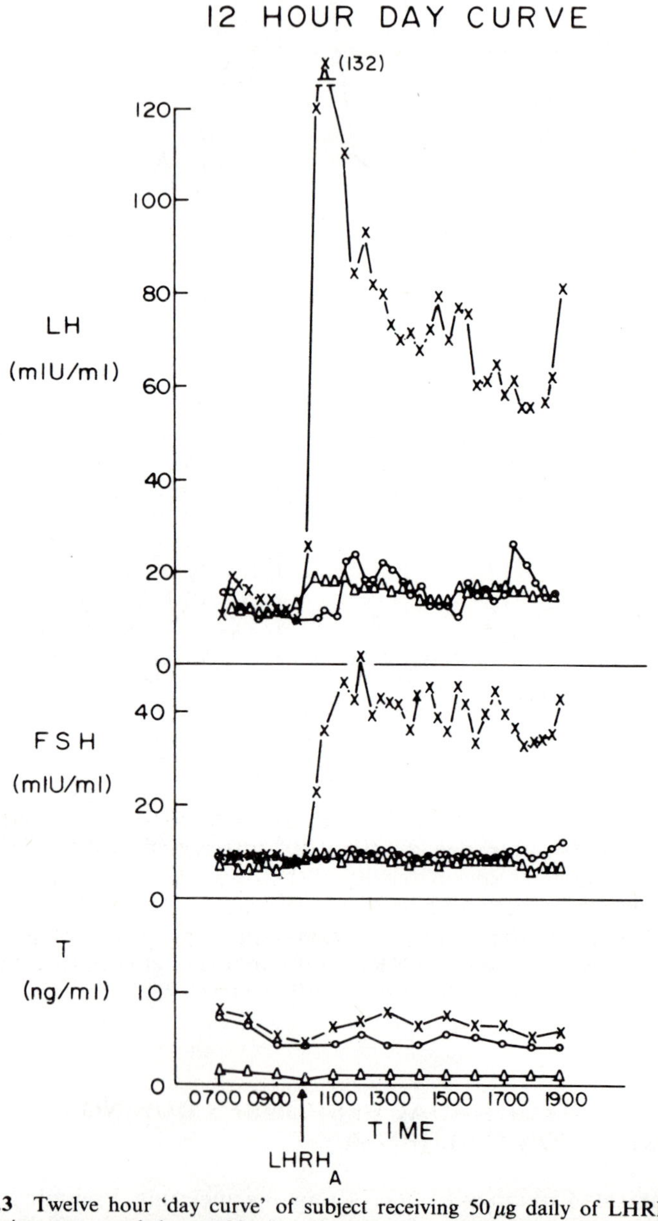

Figure 21.3 Twelve hour 'day curve' of subject receiving 50 μg daily of LHRH-A. Serum gonadotropins were sampled every 20 min and testosterone hourly. ○ = basal state, x = initial injection of LHRH-A, and Δ = 4 weeks of therapy. All injections were given at 09:30.

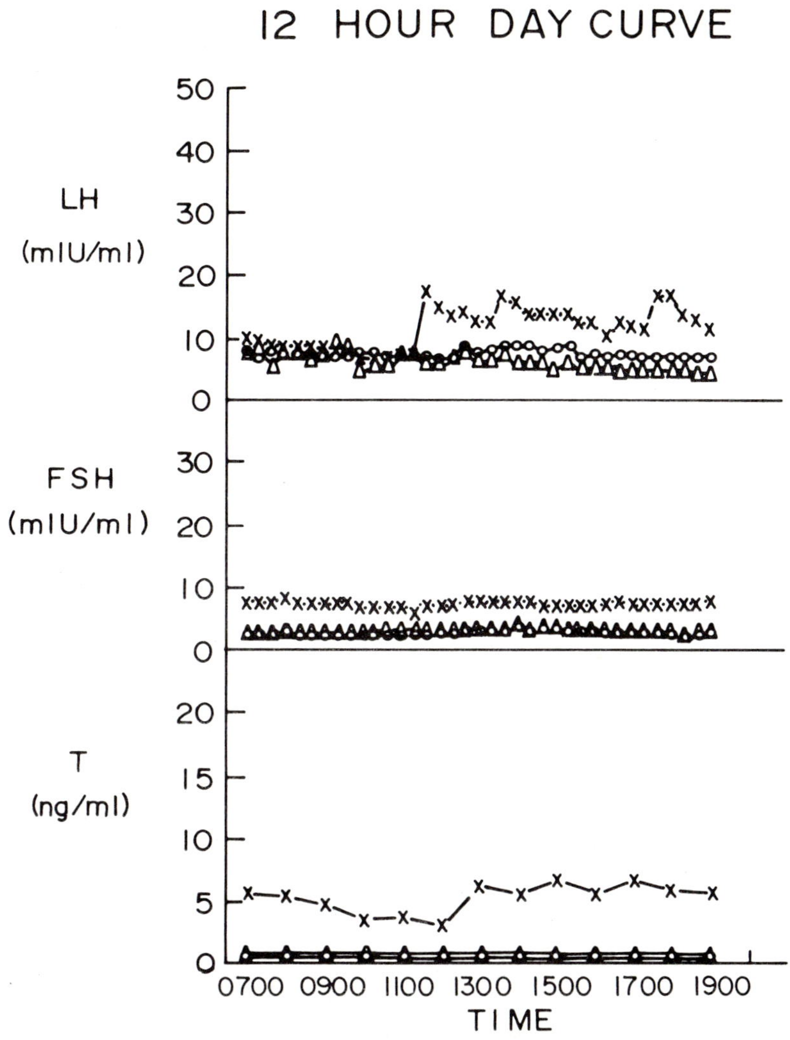

Figure 21.4 Twelve hour 'day curve' of subject receiving 50 μg daily of LHRH-A. Serum gonadotropins were sampled every 20 min and testosterone hourly. x = basal state, ○ = 4 weeks of therapy, and Δ = 8 weeks of therapy. All injections were given 20:00–22:00.

In order to assess the possible role of changes at the level of the Leydig cell, two other subjects treated with 50 μg daily of LHRH-A underwent 48 h constant infusion of human luteinizing hormone (obtained from the National Pituitary Agency) at 1.3 miu per minute for 48 h. Studies at 4 and 8 weeks (Table 21.4) indicate that the Leydig cell retains its responsiveness to exogenous gonadotropin in a manner similar to that observed in normal men.

Table 21.3 Mean hormonal concentrations during 12 h frequent sampling

Subject 1	*Pretreatment*	*Onset*	*4 Weeks*
LH (mIU/ml)	16 ±0.7	59 ±6	15 ±0.4
FSH (mIU/ml)	10 ±0.2	31 ±2.5	7.9 ±0.2
Testosterone (ng/ml)	4.9 ±0.2	6.5 ±0.3	1.0 ±0.05
Subject 2	*Pretreatment*	*4 Weeks*	*8 Weeks*
LH (mIU/ml)	11 ±0.5	7.3 ±0.1	5.9 ±0.7
FSH (mIU/ml)	7 ±0.1	2.6 ±0.1	3.1 ±0.1
Testosterone (ng/ml)	5.1 ±0.3	0.2 ±0.02	0.45 ±0.05

Table 21.4 Testosterone (T) concentrations during 48 h hLH infusion

		4 Weeks		*8 Weeks*	
Time (h)		*0*	*48*	*0*	*48*
Subject 1	T (ng/ml)	0.14	3.3	0.13	2.1
Subject 2	T (ng/ml)	0.08	2.7	0.08	2.0

These preliminary results indicate a marked alteration in the pituitary gonadotropin secretory pattern during chronic LHRH-A administration; acute injection of LHRH-A induces immediate and prolonged gonadotropin release, but this effect is attentuated with chronic administration. In addition to low ambient testosterone levels, there is a general flattening of the gonadotropin secretory curve and no evidence of spontaneous pulsations as seen in the basal state. The rise in plasma testosterone concentrations with infusion of exogenous human LH suggests that the Leydig cell maintains its responsiveness to the gonadotropin. If direct effects of LHRH-A at the Leydig cell occur, or if 'desensitization' of the Leydig cell to LHRH-A stimulated LH release is an important mechanism of action, one might expect blunted gonadal responsiveness to exogenous gonadotropin. However, this observation does not account for the failure of the Leydig cell to respond to the circulating LH present during LHRH-A administration. Alternative explanations include alterations in the bioactivity of the LH present, or attenuated gonadal response due to qualitative changes in the gonadotropin secretory pattern (i.e. loss of pulsations).

CONCLUDING REMARKS

LHRH agonist analogs, through complex, multiple, and only partially characterized mechanisms, produce reversible inhibition of spermatogenesis and testicular steroidogenesis in man. As single agents, LHRH agonists do not provide practical means of contraception because of associated loss of libido and potency; these latter effects are eliminated, however, by concomitant administration of low and non-suppressive doses of testosterone. Alterations in the dosage or schedule of administration of LHRH agonist, or the addition of testosterone in doses that independently suppress sperm count, might ultimately provide a practical means of reversible contraception in the human male.

References

Auclair, C., Kelly, P. A., Labrie, F., Coy, D. H. and Schally, A. V. (1977). Inhibition of testicular luteinizing hormone receptor level by treatment with a potent luteinizing hormone-releasing hormone agonist or human chorionic gonadotropin. *Biochem. Biophys. Res. Commun.*, **76,** 855

Bergquist, C., Nillius, S. J., Bergh, T., Skarin, G. and Wide, C. (1979). Inhibitory effects on gonadotropin secretion and gonadal function in men during chronic treatment with a potent stimulatory luteinizing hormone-releasing hormone analogue. *Acta Endocrinol.*, **91,** 601

Clayton, R. N., Katikineni, M., Chan, V., Dufau, M. L. and Catt, K. J. (1980). Direct inhibition of testicular function by gonadotropin-releasing hormone: Mediation by specific gonadotropin-releasing hormone receptors in interstitial cells. *Proc. Natl. Acad. Sci. USA*, **77,** 4459

Crowley, W. F., Vale, W., Beitins, I., Rivier, J., Rivier, C. and McArthur, J. W. (1979). Chronic administration of a long-acting agonist in hypogonadotropic hypogonadism: The critical nature of dosage, frequency, enhancement, extinction and restoration of gonadotropin responsiveness. *Endocrinology* (Suppl.), **103,** 76 (Abstract No. 16)

Crowley, W. F., Beitins, I. Z., Vale, W., Kliman, B., Rivier, J., Rivier, C. and McArthur, J. W. (1980). The biologic activity of a potent analogue of gonadotropin-releasing hormone in normal and hypogonadotropic men. *N. Engl. J. Med.*, **302,** 1052

Doelle, G., Linde, R., Alexander, N., Kirchner, F., Vale, W., Rivier, J. and Rabin, D. (1982). Intermittent long-term administration of a potent gonadotropin-releasing hormone agonist in normal men. *Int. J. Fertil.*, **27,** 234

Doelle, G. C., Alexander, A. N., Evans, R. M., Linde, R., Rivier, J., Vale, W., and Rabin, D. (1983). Combined treatment with an LHRH agonist and testosterone in man: reversible oligospermia without impotence. *J. Androl.*, **4,** 298

Heber, D. and Swerdloff, R. S. (1980). Male contraception: Synergism of gonadotropin-releasing hormone analog and testosterone in suppressing gonadotropin. *Science*, **209,** 936

Heber, D. and Swerdloff, R. S. (1981). Gonadotropin-releasing hormone analog and testosterone synergistically inhibit spermatogenesis. *Endocrinology*, **108,** 2019

Hsueh, A. J. W., Dufau, M. L. and Catt, K. J. (1976). Regulation of luteinizing hormone receptors in testicular interstitial cells by gonadotropin. *Biochem. Biophys. Res. Commun.*, **72,** 1145

Hsueh, A. J. W., Dufau, M. L. and Catt, K. J. (1977). Desensitization of testicular responses – negative control of LH/hCG receptors, cAMP production and steroidogenesis by exogenous hCG *in vivo*. *Proc. Natl. Acad. Sci. USA*, **74,** 592

Hsueh, A. J. W. and Erickson, G. F. (1979*a*). Extrapituitary action of gonadotropin-releasing hormone: Direct inhibition of ovarian steroidogenesis. *Science*, **204,** 854

Hsueh, A. J. W. and Erickson, G. F. (1979*b*). Extrapituitary inhibition of testicular function by luteinizing hormone releasing hormone. *Nature (Lond.)*, **281,** 66

Labrie, F., Bélanger, A., Cusan, L., Séguin, C., Pelletier, G., Kelly, P. A., Reeves, J. J., Lefebvre, F.-A., Lemay, A., Gourdeau, Y. and Raynaud, J.-P. (1980). Antifertility effects of LHRH agonists in the male. *J. Androl.*, **1,** 209

Lecomte, P., Wang, N.-G., Sundaram, K., Rivier, J., Vale, W. and Bardin, C. W. (1982). The antiandrogenic action of gonadotropin-releasing hormone and its agonists in the mouse kidney. *Endocrinology*, **110,** 1

Linde, R., Doelle, G. C., Alexander, N., Kirchner, F., Vale, W., Rivier, J. and Rabin, D. (1981). Reversible inhibition of testicular steroidogenesis and spermatogenesis by a potent gonadotropin-releasing hormone agonist in normal men. *N. Engl. J. Med.*, **305,** 663

National Coordinating Group on Male Antifertility Agents (1978). Gossypol – a new antifertility agent for males. *Chin. Med. J.*, **4,** 417

Paulsen, C. A., Leonard, J. M., Burgess, E. C. and Ospina, L. F. (1978). Male contraceptive development: Re-examination of testosterone enanthate as a single entity agent. In Patanelli,

D. J. (ed). *Hormonal Control of Male Fertility*, pp. 17–36. (DHEW Publication No. 78–1097) (NIH). (Bethesda, MD: US Department of Health, Education and Welfare)

Rippel, R. H. and Johnson, E. S. (1976). Inhibition of hCG induced ovarian and uterine weight augmentation of the immature rat by analogs of GnRH. *Proc. Soc. Exp. Biol. Med.*, **152,** 432

Rivier, C. and Vale, W. (1979). Hormonal secretion in male rats chronically treated with D-Trp^6,Pro^9-NEt-LRF. *Life Sci.*, **25,** 1065

Rivier, C., Rivier, J., Lasley, B. and Vale, W. (1980). Effects of D-Trp^6,Pro^9-NEt-LHRH on reproductive functions in the male rat. *Int. J. Fertil.*, **25,** 145

Sandow, J., von Rechenberg, W., Jerzabeck, G. and Stoll, W. (1978). Pituitary gonadotropin inhibition by a highly active analog of luteinizing hormone-releasing hormone. *Fertil. Steril.*, **30,** 205

Schearer, S. B. (1978). The use of progestins and androgens as a male contraceptive. In Patanelli, D. J. (ed.) *Hormonal Control of Male Fertility*, pp. 257–295. (DHEW Publication No. 78–1097) (NIH). (Bethesda, MD: US Department of Health, Education and Welfare)

Smith, R., Donald, R. A., Espiner, E. A., Stronach, S. G. and Edwards, I. A. (1979). Normal adults and subjects with hypogonadotropic hypogonadism respond differently to D-Ser(TBU)^6-LHRH-EA^{10}. *J. Clin. Endocrinol. Metab.*, **48,** 167

Steinberger, E. and Smith, R. D. (1977). Effect of chronic administration of testosterone enanthate on sperm production and plasma testosterone, follicle-stimulating hormone, and luteinizing hormone levels: A preliminary evaluation of a possible male contraceptive. *Fertil. Steril.*, **28,** 1320

Sundaram, K., Yung-Oing, C., Wang, N.-G., Bardin, C. W., Rivier, J. and Vale, W. (1981). Inhibition of the action of sex steroids by gonadotropin-releasing hormone (GnRH) agonists: A new biological effect. *Life Sci.*, **28,** 83

Tolis, G., Mehta, A., Comaru-Schally, A. M. and Schally, A. V. (1981). Suppression of androgen production by D-Tryptophan-6-Luteinizing Hormone-releasing hormone in man. *J. Clin. Invest.*, **68,** 819

Vale, W., Rivier, C., Brown, M. and Rivier, J. (1977). Pharmacology of thyrotropin releasing factor (TRF), luteinizing hormone releasing factor (LRF) and somatostatin. *Adv. Exp. Med. Biol.*, **87,** 123

Wiegelman, W., Solbach, H. G., Kley, H. K. and Kruskemper, H. L. (1977). LH- and FSH-response to long-term application of LHRH analogue in normal males. *Horm. Metab. Res.*, **9,** 521

SECTION VI

HUMAN THERAPEUTIC APPLICATIONS

22
LHRH therapy for hypogonadotropic hypogonadal men

A. HOFFMAN and W. F. CROWLEY Jr.

Idiopathic hypogonadotropic hypogonadism (IHH) is characterized by the failure or the arrest of the normal pubertal process in otherwise healthy adults. The disorder is congenital and deficiencies in olfactory function are frequently seen in the patients or their families (Kallmann *et al.*, 1944). In addition to anosmia, numerous other congenital abnormalities have been associated with IHH, including cleft lip and palate, and cryptorchidism (Santen and Paulsen, 1973*a*). Aside from the abnormalities in gonadotropin and testosterone secretion, hypothalamic and pituitary function are normal in these men (Winters *et al.*, 1978; Barden *et al.*, 1969). Recent studies indicate that this isolated gonadotropin deficiency in fact results from a lack of LHRH. Prolonged infusions of this peptide stimulate LH and FSH secretion in men with IHH (Yoshimoto *et al.*, 1975). Clomiphene citrate, an antiestrogen which normally causes the release of gonadotropins via the stimulation of hypothalamic LHRH, does not reliably elevate LH and FSH levels in these hypogonadal men (Hamilton *et al.*, 1973).

The goals of therapy in this group of patients are twofold: (1) the production of the physical changes seen in normal male puberty and (2) the induction of spermatogenesis. While virilization is easily achieved with the injection of long acting testosterone preparations, the initiation of spermatogenesis requires gonadotropin administration. With few exceptions, combination hCG and hMG therapy has allowed for both full virilization and the induction of fertility in men with gonadotropin deficiency (Bardin *et al.*, 1968; Mancini *et al.*, 1969; Santen and Paulsen, 1973*b*). Because of the expense of these drugs and the discomfort of the thrice weekly intramuscular injections used in this protocol, alternate forms of therapy are desirable. With the isolation and purification of LHRH, and the subsequent synthesis of long acting, superpotent LHRH analogs in the 1970s, it became possible to attack the problem of IHH at its source by providing patients having LHRH deficiency with hypothalamic hormone replacement therapy.

LHRH AND ANALOGS FOR THE INDUCTION OF PUBERTY: EARLY STUDIES

Native LHRH

Mortimer and his colleagues (1974) were the first to administer synthetic LHRH on a chronic basis to men with hypogonadotropic hypogonadism. They treated nine adult men who had a variety of hypothalamic–pituitary lesions (including four with IHH) with subcutaneous injections of LHRH, given as a bolus of 500 μg every 8 h for up to 26 weeks. On this regimen, serum gonadotropin and testosterone levels increased, but only two men exhibited serum testosterone concentrations that were within the normal adult range. None the less, all patients noted increased potency within 2 weeks of starting therapy, and testicular volume increased in all of the subjects. Spermatogenesis was achieved in two of the four patients with IHH.

Using a similar experimental design, two other groups were unable to induce pubertal changes or normal levels of serum testosterone in men with IHH (Happ *et al.*, 1975; Krabbe and Skakkeback, 1977) (Table 22.1). Infrequent subcutaneous injections of LHRH were unsuccessful in maintaining pubertal development (Van Loon and Brown, 1975; Brook and Dombey, 1979), and the administration of the drug by intranasal or intravenous routes also failed to induce puberty in men with IHH (Happ *et al.*, 1975; Hashimoto *et al.*, 1975).

Table 22.1 Chronic treatment of adult men with IHH using native LHRH

Study	*Dose/frequency of LHRH*	*Clinical changes*
Mortimer *et al.* (1974)	500 μg s.c. q 8 h	Increased potency within 7–14 days in all. Testis volume increased in all
Happ *et al.* (1975)	200 μg intranasal q 2 h × 8/d	No spermatogenesis
Van Loon and Brown (1975)	250–2000 μg s.c. q.d.	Increased libido. Developed antibody to LHRH, resulting in loss of response
Hashimoto *et al.* (1975) Hashimoto (1981)	200 μg i.v. q.d.	No clinical changes
Krabbe and Skakkebaek (1977)	200 μg s.c. q 8 h	No clinical changes
Brook and Dombey (1979)	500 μg s.c. b.i.d	Increased testicular volume. Good response initially
Skarin *et al.* (1982)	1–5 μg s.c. q 90 min	Normal testosterone Spermatogenesis, Fertility

LHRH analogs

Since native LHRH has a very short half-life, more potent analogs with a long duration of action were assessed for utility in treating IHH. The results of such

Table 22.2 The use of LHRH analogs to induce puberty in men

Study	*Analog*	*Dose/frequency*	*Duration*	*Clinical changes*
Tharandt *et al.*, 1977	[D-Leu^6,Pro^9-NHEt]LHRH	100 μg s.c. q.d.	2 months	No clinical changes
Smith *et al.*, 1979	[D-Ser(tBu)^6,Pro^9-NHEt]LHRH	1.25–5 μg s.c. q.d.	27–38 weeks	No change in testicular size. No pubertal changes
Guitelman *et al.*, 1979	[D-Leu^6,Pro^9-NHEt]LHRH	50 μg i.m. q.d.	60 d	All noted increased libido. Increased testicular size in two
Moore *et al.*, 1981	[D-Ser(tBu)^6,Pro^9-NHEt]LHRH	5 μg s.c. q 2 d	1–3 months	No clinical changes
Laron *et al.*, 1981	[D-Leu^6,Pro^9-NHEt]LHRH	10 μg i.m. q 2 d	6 months	Increased testicular size after 3 months, but no increase thereafter. Transient increases in LH and T
Crowley *et al.*, 1981	[D-Trp^6,Pro^9-NHEt]LHRH	10–50 μg s.c. q.d.	12–32 weeks	Transient increase in testicular size. No clinical changes
Morel *et al.*, 1982	[D-Ser(tBu)^6,Pro^9-NHEt]LHRH	348 μg q 2 d	3–6 months	Transient increase in testicular size. No clinical changes

studies are remarkably similar. Initially, serum LH levels may rise somewhat, but with continued treatment elevated gonadotropin levels cannot be sustained. Although transient increases in serum testosterone concentration were noted in several studies (Table 22.2), normal adult male levels were not reached.

In our experience also LHRH analog therapy was unsuccessful in inducing pubertal changes. Four adult men with IHH were treated with [D-Trp^6,Pro^9-NHEt]LHRH (LHRH-A) for as long as 16 weeks (Crowley *et al.*, 1980). Initially, they received 50 μg of LHRH-A subcutaneously every other day. Within 2 weeks, all four subjects complained of testicular discomfort, especially on those days when they received injections. Testicular size increased in three of the four subjects, reaching a plateau after 6–8 weeks of therapy (Figure 22.1). In one patient, an abdominal testis descended into the scrotum within 2 weeks of starting treatment. After 2 weeks of therapy, the LH but not the FSH response to LHRH-A was increased over the initial values, but serum testosterone levels did not rise.

Increasing the frequency of drug administration to daily injections of the same dose of LHRH-A resulted in decreased testicular volume and suppression of LH response to the analog. No change in serum testosterone was noted. In order to learn whether LHRH-A treatment had altered the ability of the testis to respond to gonadotropins, three subjects were treated with hCG

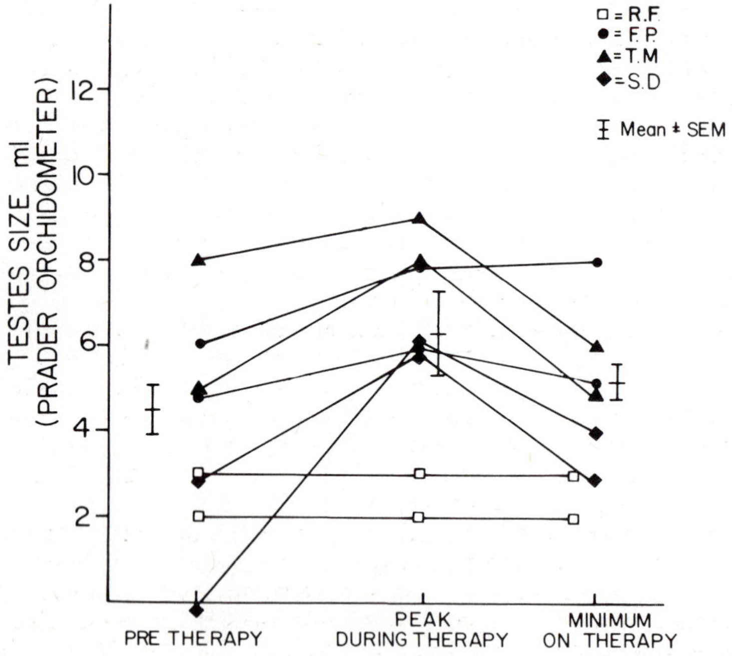

Figure 22.1 Testicular size in four hypogonadotropic males before treatment (pretherapy), with 50 μg LHRH-A on alternate days for 6–8 weeks (peak during therapy), and with 50 μg LHRH-A daily (minimum on therapy). All results are mean ± SEM (from Crowley *et al.*, 1981, by permission).

for 3 days while they were receiving daily LHRH-A therapy. Leydig cell responsiveness was assessed by measuring serum testosterone levels after the hCG injections. The peak post-hCG testosterone level during LHRH-A treatment was similar to that achieved prior to the initiation of LHRH-A therapy.

The daily dose of LHRH-A was subsequently lowered to 10 μg/day. No clinical changes could be discerned but LH responsiveness to LHRH-A was restored. Thus, while LHRH analog therapy may provide transient increases in serum LH and some testicular enlargement, prolonged treatment results in pituitary desensitization, and pubertal changes are not achieved.

NORMAL PHYSIOLOGY OF LHRH SECRETION

The failure of native LHRH and its analogs to induce puberty prompted a re-examination of the chronobiology of gonadotropin secretion. From early childhood onward, gonadotropins are released from the pituitary gland in episodic, pulsatile bursts (Jakacki *et al.*, 1982; Nankin and Troen, 1971; Naftolin *et al.*, 1972). LH release occurs every 90–120 min in adult men. Episodic LH discharge is also a feature of non-human primates (Wildt *et al.*, 1981).

The consequences of altering the pulsatile frequency of LHRH secretion were addressed in castrated rhesus monkeys (Belchetz *et al.*, 1978). Endogenous LHRH secretion was abolished by radio-frequency-induced lesions of the medial basal hypothalamus, and LHRH was administered via an intravenous catheter. Although continuous LHRH infusion did not produce a sustained increase in LH or FSH secretion, pulsatile administration of LHRH resulted in increased gonadotropin release. Reinstitution of continuous LHRH infusion led to suppression of LH and FSH levels. Moreover, when the frequency of LHRH pulses was altered in any way from the normal physiologic pattern of one pulse per hour in the rhesus, serum LH and FSH levels declined. Subsequently, puberty was induced in an infantile female rhesus using this protocol (Wildt *et al.*, 1980).

Protocols employing native LHRH in men called for infrequent administration of the hormone (usually 1–4 times each day). In the rhesus, such a regimen did not sustain normal gonadotropin secretion. Because the LHRH agonists have extended biological half-lives, their episodic use does not result in pulsatile LHRH activity. Instead, LHRH agonist administration can be likened to a continuous infusion of the native peptide, which depresses rather than stimulates gonadotropin release.

Recently, studies of pulsatile LHRH administration in men with IHH have shown that normal gonadotropin dynamics can be induced in humans. When 25 ng/kg doses of LHRH were infused intravenously every 2 hours for 5 days to four men with IHH, the pattern of gonadotropin secretion achieved was similar to that seen in normal puberty (Valk *et al.*, 1980). Despite the short duration of this study, small increases in plasma testosterone were achieved. In another study, two young boys with Kallmann's syndrome were given 40 μg of LHRH every 64 min for ten consecutive nights from a portable infusion pump (Jacobson *et al.*, 1979). Pulsatile LH secretion was achieved on this regimen, with one patient developing midpubertal levels of serum testosterone.

CHRONIC TREATMENT WITH PULSATILE LHRH

Induction of puberty

Six adult men with IHH (one with an acquired, adult-onset form of the syndrome) took part in our initial studies (Hoffman and Crowley, 1982). Testicular biopsies were obtained in most patients to eliminate the possibility of the Sertoli cell-only syndrome. Baseline gonadotropin status was evaluated by measuring serum LH and FSH every 20 min for 24 h. Following this initial monitoring period, the subjects were treated with 25 ng/kg of native LHRH, delivered subcutaneously every 2 h by the portable infusion pump. During each of the next 7 days, frequent gonadotropin measurements were obtained to monitor the effects of treatment. Although no response was noted after the first dose of LHRH, by day 7 serum LH concentration reached normal adult levels, and serum FSH was above the normal range (Figure 22.2). Normal adult testosterone levels were achieved in four patients by this time.

The subjects were then discharged from the hospital and instructed to wear

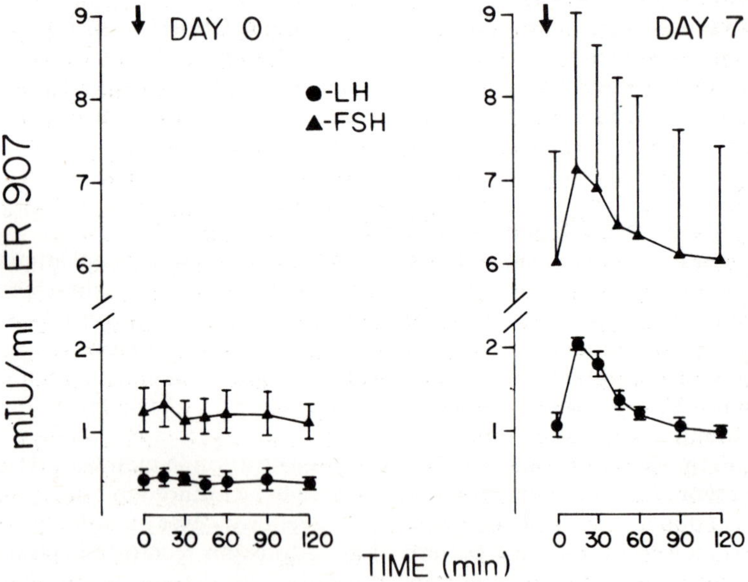

Figure 22.2 LH(●) and FSH (▲) responses to a bolus of 25 ng/kg LHRH at the beginning (day 0) and end (day 7) of 1 week of pulsatile LHRH therapy in six hypogonadotropic men. All results are expressed as mean ± SEM (from Crowley *et al.*, 1981, by permission).

the pump throughout the day and night. They returned to the hospital every 1–2 weeks thereafter for monitoring of gonadotropin levels. The serum LH concentration peaked by the fifth week of treatment and remained in the high to normal range thereafter; serum FSH concentration also remained above the normal adult male range throughout much of the treatment period. The four patients who attained normal serum testosterone levels within the first week of therapy maintained these levels for at least 3 months; midpubertal levels of testosterone were seen in the other two patients. In four subjects, the testes increased in size by an average of 100% during the first month of therapy. Maturation of spermatogenesis occurred in three patients after 4, 11 and 43 weeks of therapy, and one subject successfully impregnated his wife after 26 weeks of continuous LHRH therapy. Dramatic clinical changes were noted in all six subjects within the first 6–8 weeks of treatment, including the appearance of nocturnal emissions, spontaneous erections, transient tender gynecomastia and acne.

Effect of lowering the dose of LHRH

The very rapid pubertal maturation resulting from LHRH therapy is in marked contrast to the normal course of male puberty, which evolves over 2–4 years. To determine whether we could slow development by decreasing the LHRH dosage, six other men with IHH received 10 ng/kg of LHRH every 2 h for 12 weeks. In contrast to the findings with the higher dose, serum gonadotropins remained in the low normal range, with LH peaking at week 4, and FSH reaching its highest level after 2 weeks of treatment. The serum testosterone remained in the prepubertal range in all six men. Throughout the 12 weeks of therapy, LH and testosterone levels were significantly lower than in the men who received 25 ng/kg of LHRH. The FSH concentrations were also consistently lower in the subset of patients receiving 10 ng/kg of LHRH. None of these patients noted any emotional or psychologic changes associated with puberty, and none developed gynecomastia or dermatologic changes. All six men had an increase in testicular volume, with an average of 85% enlargement. Spermatogenesis was not achieved in any subject. These data suggest that in the initial stages of puberty, small amounts of LHRH are secreted by the hypothalamus, resulting in an increase in testicular size but no change in serum testosterone. Subsequently, more LHRH is released, resulting in midpubertal and adult levels of testosterone production.

Although large gonadotropin pulses appear necessary to stimulate the prepubertal testis, lesser amounts of LH and FSH may be required to maintain normal testicular activity in the mature, functioning gonad. In one patient from our initial study, normal serum testosterone levels were achieved within the first month of therapy with 25 ng/kg of LHRH, coincident with elevated levels of serum LH and FSH (Figure 23.3). After 9 months of treatment with 25 ng/kg of LHRH, the dose was reduced to 10 ng/kg, and then to 5 ng/kg, resulting in normalization of the gonadotropin levels. Serum testosterone concentration remained in the adult male range, and spermatogenesis ensued.

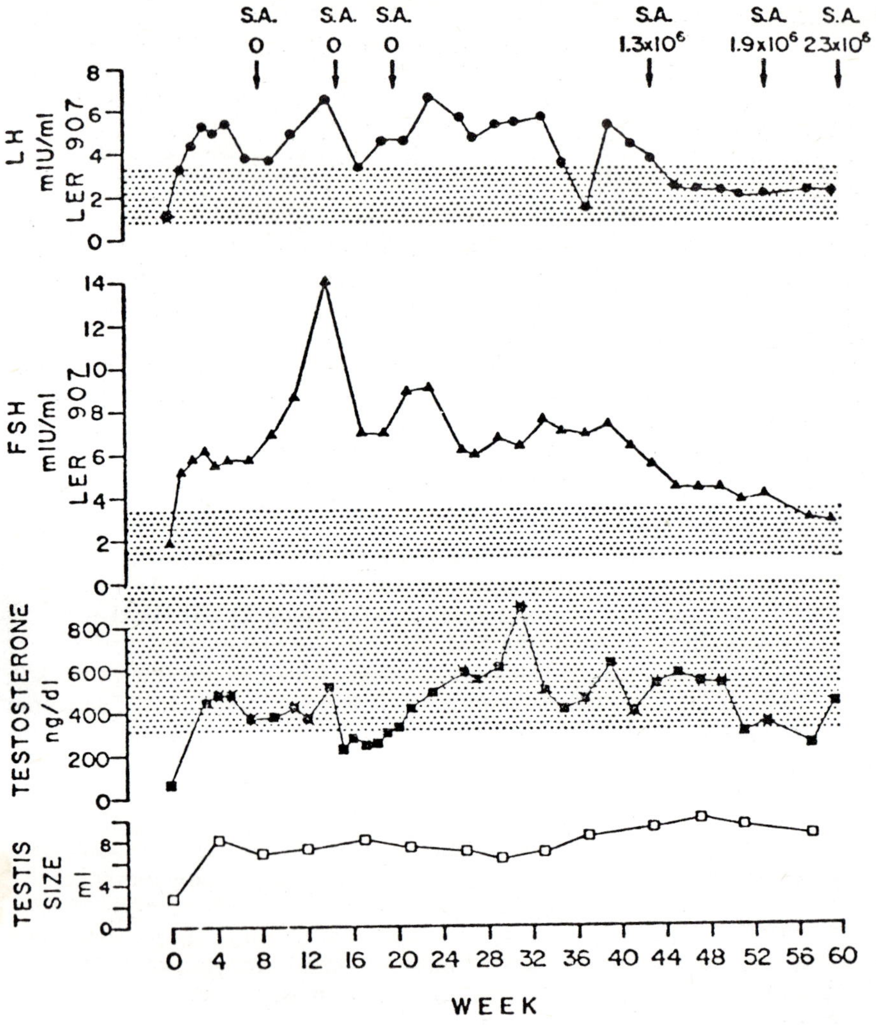

Figure 22.3 Course of long-term therapy in a single patient. LHRH was administered subcutaneously with Autosyringe (Flint). The doses (per kg body weight) were 25 ng (weeks 1–38), 10 ng (weeks 39–50), and 5 ng (weeks 51–59). The drug was delivered every 2 h, except during weeks 23–27, when it was administered every hour, and weeks 28–33, when it was administered every 90 min. The results of semen analysis (S.A.) are expressed as the number of sperm per milliliter of seminal fluid. The shaded area represents the range of normal values for adult men. Each measurement of luteinizing hormone (LH), follicle-stimulating hormone (FSH), and testosterone represents a value determined for a pool of 25 specimens obtained every 20 min over an 8 h period. Testis size is expressed as the average value for the patient's testes, as measured by a Prader orchidometer (from Hoffman and Crowley, 1982, with permission).

Alterations in pulse frequency

The effects of varying the frequency of LHRH administration were studied in four men with IHH who had been treated with 25 ng/kg of LHRH on a 2-hourly basis for 13–23 weeks. While the LHRH dosage was maintained at 25 ng/kg, the interdose interval was shortened from 120 to 60 min. When LHRH was given every hour, LH levels initially declined in two subjects, but were unchanged in the other two men; plasma FSH declined in all patients. No consistent changes in plasma testosterone concentrations were obtained. When LHRH is administered every 2 h, each injection is followed by the pulsatile release of LH. Increasing the administered pulse frequency to one per hour results in the failure of some LHRH pulses to elicit LH secretion (Figure 22.4). This breakdown in stimulus–response pattern was seen in all patients who received hourly boluses of LHRH.

Increasing the frequency of LHRH administration to every 30 min allowed mean LH levels to remain in the supraphysiologic range, but no regular pulsatile pattern is present, and many of the LHRH boluses are not followed by increases in serum LH (Figure 22.5). Plasma FSH declined below the detectability of the assay. The testosterone concentration continues to be

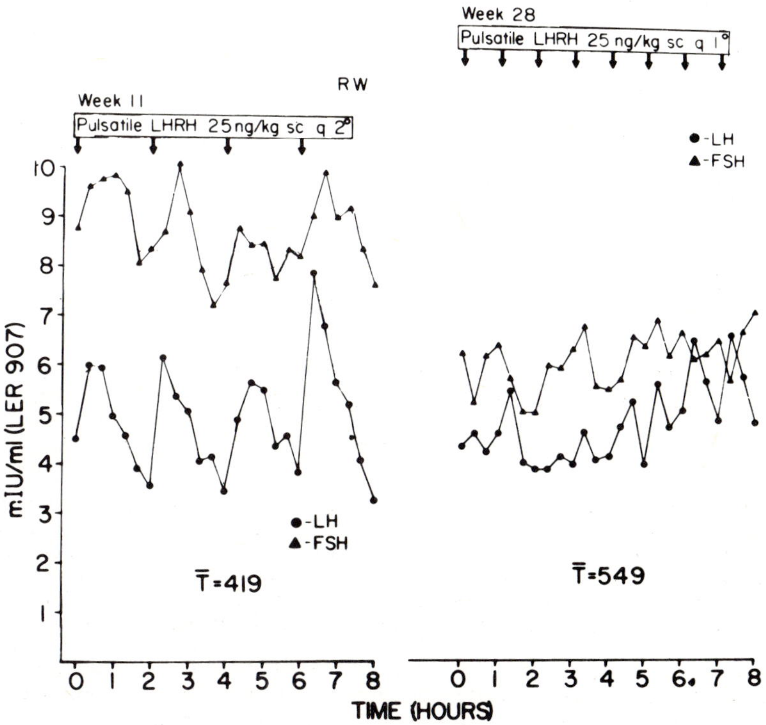

Figure 22.4 Gonadotropin pulsations in a man with IHH in response to LHRH 25 ng/kg (A) delivered every 2 h and (B) delivered every hour.

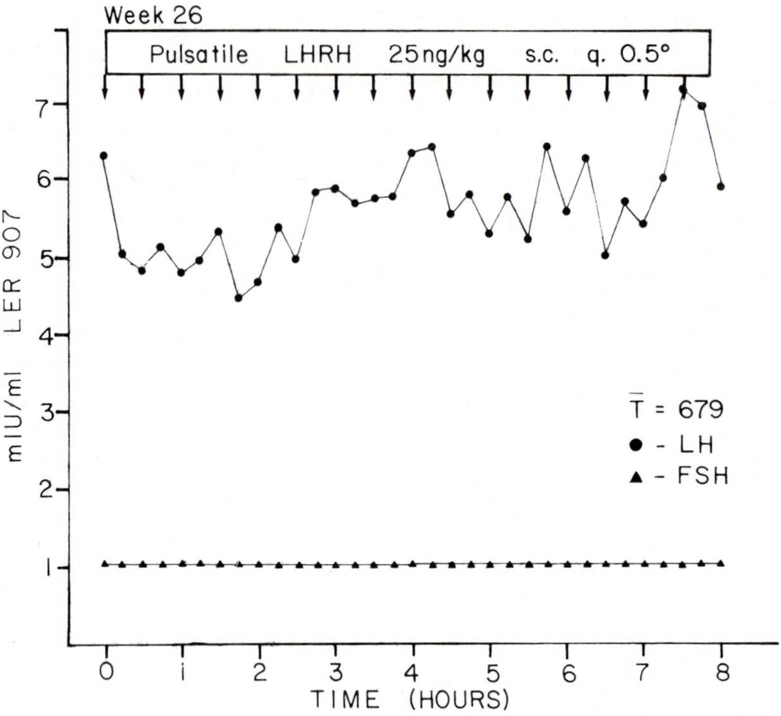

Figure 22.5 Gonadotropin levels in response to LHRH given every 30 min to a man with IHH.

within the normal range. This dissociated gonadotropin pattern, in which erratic, high amplitude LH pulses coexist with undetectable levels of FSH and normal levels of testosterone, persisted throughout the 7 weeks of treatment. This frequency of LHRH administration has thus resulted in isolated FSH deficiency.

When 25 ng/kg of LHRH was administered every 3 or 4 h, LH pulses of normal amplitude were noted following each LHRH injection. Plasma FSH levels, on the other hand, were often undetectable, and serum testosterone concentration fell to prepubertal levels. When the frequency of LHRH delivery is increased to every 2 h, normal testosterone levels and gonadotropin pulsations return.

Potential difficulties associated with LHRH treatment

Several patients failed to respond when treated on an every-2-hour basis with 25 ng/kg of LHRH. Increasing the dose to 100–200 ng/kg has induced pubertal changes in some of these men. Thus, there may be some men with IHH who are resistant to LHRH therapy. One subject initially responded well to LHRH, developing spermatogenesis and normal testosterone levels. His serum testosterone and gonadotropin levels slowly started to wane, however, and anti-LHRH antibodies were detected in his serum. Increasing the dose to 100 ng/kg had no beneficial effect. A similar observation has previously been reported (Van Loon and Brown, 1975).

When LHRH is given intravenously, a distinct high amplitude LHRH pulse is seen. Subcutaneous administration results in a more delayed hormone release, and peak serum LHRH levels are substantially lower than when the intravenous route is used. Intermittent subcutaneous injections may result in nearly constant LHRH blood levels and thereby cause pituitary desensitization. It is also possible that subcutaneous LHRH treatment may result in induction of local proteases as previously noted for insulin.

No extrapituitary effects of LHRH have been noted in men with IHH, and no significant side-effects have occurred. While LHRH can bind to specific hormone receptors in rodent gonads (Hsueh and Jones, 1981), receptors are not present on human testicular membranes. Leydig cell responsiveness to hCG is not altered by chronic LHRH analog treatment. Children who have been treated with large doses of LHRH analog for the treatment of precocious puberty revert to pretreatment gonadal function when the drug is discontinued (Comite *et al.*, 1981). Furthermore, LHRH-A is ineffective in suppressing testicular secretion in young boys with gonadotropin-independent precocious puberty.

CONCLUDING REMARKS

The ability of pulsatile LHRH therapy to induce all of the changes of normal puberty provides further evidence that IHH is a disorder of hypothalamic LHRH deficiency. The carefully timed treatment schedules required for successful LHRH replacement therapy have reinforced our concepts concerning the importance of pulsatility in the normal physiology of LHRH secretion. Only episodic LHRH secretion can elicit normal gonadotropin responses; frequent or continuous LHRH release causes rapid pituitary desensitization.

Hypothalamic hormone replacement therapy can now be given via externally-worn portable infusion pumps in order to stimulate virilization and spermatogenesis. In the near future, fully implantable computerized pumps will be able to provide lifelong LHRH therapy in men or women with IHH.

Acknowledgements

We are indebted to the staff of the General Clinical Research Center for their dedicated care of these patients; to Judith Donnelly and Steve Trigilio for outstanding technical assistance; to the National Pituitary Agency for the FSH antisera and standards; to Jean Rivier and Wylie Vale for their generous gift of the LHRH used in these studies and to Cheryl Sonnichsen for help in preparing this manuscript. This work is supported in part by NIH grants HD-15788 and RR 1066.

References

Bardin, C. W., Ross, G. T., Riskind, A. B., Cargille, C. M. and Lipsett, M. B. (1969). Studies of the pituitary–Leydig cell axis in young men with hypogonadotropic hypogonadism and hyposmia: Comparison with normal men, prepubertal boys and hypopituitary patients. *J. Clin. Invest.*, **48,** 2046

Belchetz, P. E., Plant, T. M., Nakai, Y., Keogh, E. J. and Knobil, E. (1978). Hypophyseal responses to continuous and intermittent delivery of hypothalamic gonadotropin-releasing hormone. *Science,* **202,** 631

Brook, C. G. D. and Dombey, S. (1979). Induction of puberty: long-term treatment with high-dose LHRH. *Clin. Endocrinol.,* **11,** 81

Comite, F., Cutler, G. B., Rivier, J., Vale, W. W., Loriaux, D. L. and Crowley, W. F. Jr. (1981). Short-term treatment of idiopathic precocious puberty with a long-acting analogue of luteinizing hormone-releasing hormone. *N. Engl. J. Med.,* **305,** 1546

Crowley, W. F. Jr., Beitins, I. Z., Vale, W., Kliman, B., Rivier, J., Rivier, C. and McArthur, J. W. (1980). The biologic activity of a potent analogue of a gonadotropin-releasing hormone in normal and hypogonadotropic men. *N. Engl. J. Med.,* **302,** 1052

Crowley, W. F. Jr., Vale, W., Rivier, J. and McArthur, J. W. (1981). LHRH in hypogonadotropic hypogonadism. In Zatuchni, G. I., Shelton, J. D., and Sciarra, J. J. (eds.) *LHRH Peptides as Female and Male Contraceptives,* pp. 321–333. (Philadelphia: Harper & Row)

Guitelman, A., Mancini, A. M., Aparicio, N. J., Tropea, L., Levalle, O. and Schally, A. V. (1979). Effect of D-leucine-6-luteinizing hormone-releasing hormone ethylamide in patients with hypogonadotropic hypogonadism with anosmia. *Fertil. Steril.,* **32,** 308

Hamilton, C. R., Henkin, R. I., Weir, G. and Kliman, B. (1973). Olfactory status and response to clomiphene in male gonadotrophin deficiency. *Ann. Intern. Med.,* **78,** 47

Happ, J., Neubauer, M., Egri, A., Demisch, K., Schoffling, K. and Beyer, J. (1975). GnRH therapy in males with hypogonadotrophic hypogonadism. *Horm. Metab.,* **7,** 526

Hashimoto, T. (1981). Failure of combined therapy with synthetic luteinizing hormone-releasing hormone and clomiphene citrate in patients with hypothalamic hypogonadism. *Fertil. Steril.,* **35,** 84

Hashimoto, T., Miyai, K., Onishi, T., Matsumoto, K. and Kumahara, Y. (1975). Comparison of short and long-term treatment with synthetic LH-releasing hormone and clomiphene citrate in male hypothalamic hypogonadism. *J. Clin. Endocrinol. Metab.,* **41,** 905

Hoffman, A. R. and Crowley, W. F. Jr. (1982). Induction of puberty in men by administration of low dose gonadotropin-releasing hormone. *N. Engl. J. Med.,* **307,** 1237

Hsueh, A. J. and Jones, P. B. (1981). Extrapituitary actions of gonadotropin-releasing hormone. *Endocr. Rev.,* **2,** 437

Jacobson, R. I., Seyler, L. E. Jr., Tamborlane, W. V. Jr., Gertner, J. M. and Genel, M. (1979). Pulsatile subcutaneous nocturnal administration of GnRH by portable infusion pump in hypogonadotropic hypogonadism: Initiation of gonadotropin responsiveness. *J. Clin. Endocrinol. Metab.,* **49,** 652

Jakacki, R. I., Kelch, R. P., Sauder, S. E., Lloyd, J. S., Hopwood, N. J. and Marshall, J. C. (1982). Pulsatile secretion of luteinizing hormone in children. *J. Clin. Endocrinol. Metab.,* **55,** 453

Kallmann, F. J., Schoenfeld, W. A. and Barrera, S. E. (1944). The genetic aspects of primary eunuchoidism. *Am. J. Ment. Def.,* **48,** 203

Krabbe, S. and Skakkebaek, N. E. (1977). Gonadotropin-releasing hormone (LH-RH) and human chorionic gonadotropin in the treatment of two boys with hypogonadotropin hypogonadism. *Acta Paediatr. Scand.,* **66,** 361

Laron, Z., Dickerman, Z., Ben Zeev, Z., Prager-Lewin, R., Comaru-Schally, A. M. and Schally, A. V. (1981). Long-term effect of D-Trp^6-luteinizing hormone-releasing hormone on testicular size and luteinizing hormone, follicle-stimulating hormone and testosterone levels in hypothalamic hypogonadotropic males. *Fertil. Steril.,* **35,** 328

Mancini, R. E., Seiguer, A. C. and Lloret, A. P. (1969). Effect of gonadotropins on the recovery of spermatogenesis in hypophysectomized patients. *J. Clin. Endocrinol.,* **29,** 467

Moore, M. P., Smith, R., Donald, R. A., Espiner, E. A. and Stronach, S. (1981). The effects of different dose regimes of D-$Ser(TBu)^6$-LHRH-EA^{10} (HOE 766) in subjects with hypogonadotrophic hypogonadism. *Clin. Endocrinol.,* **14,** 93

Morel, Y., Fournier, M., Mazenod, B., Tourniaire, J. and Mornex, R. (1982). Treatment of hypogonadotropic hypogonadal male patients with the luteinizing hormone-releasing hormone (LH-RH) analog D-Ser(TBu)^{6}EA^{10}LH-RH; transient disappearance of gonadotropin stimulation. *Fertil. Steril.*, **38,** 85

Mortimer, C. H., McNeilly, A. S., Fisher, R. A., Murray, M. A. F. and Besser, G. M. (1974). Gonadotrophin-releasing hormone therapy in hypogonadal males with hypothalamic or pituitary dysfunction. *Br. Med. J.*, **4,** 617

Naftolin, F., Yen, S. S. C. and Tsai, C. C. (1972). Rapid cycling of plasma gonadotrophins in normal men as demonstrated by frequent sampling. *Nature (New Biol.)*, **236,** 92

Nankin, H. R. and Troen, P. (1971). Repetitive luteinizing hormone elevations in serum of normal men. *J. Clin. Endocrinol.*, **33,** 558

Santen, R. J. and Paulsen, C. A. (1973*a*). Hypogonadotropic eunuchoidism. I. Clinical study of the mode of inheritance. *J. Clin. Endocrinol. Metab.*, **36,** 47

Santen, R. J. and Paulsen, C. A. (1973*b*). Hypogonadotropic eunuchoidism. II. Gonadal responsiveness to exogenous gonadotropins. *J. Clin. Endocrinol. Metab.*, **36,** 55

Skarin, G., Nillius, S. J., Wibell, L. and Wide, L. (1982). Chronic pulsatile low dose GnRH therapy for induction of testosterone production and spermatogenesis in a man with secondary hypogonadotropic hypogonadism. *J. Clin. Endocrinol. Metab.*, **55,** 723

Smith, R., Donald, R. A., Espiner, E. A. and Stronach, S. (1979). The effects of prolonged administration of D-Ser(TBu)^6-LH-RH-EA^{10} (HOE 766) in subjects with hypogonadotrophic hypogonadism. *Clin. Endocrinol.*, **11,** 553

Tharandt, L., Schulte, H., Benker, G., Hackenberg, K. and Reinwein, D. (1977). Treatment of isolated gonadotrophin deficiency in men with a more potent analogue of LH-RH. *Horm. Metab. Res.*, **9,** 342

Valk, T. W., Corley, K. P., Kelch, R. P. and Marshall, J. C. (1980). Hypogonadotropic hypogonadism: Hormonal responses to low dose pulsatile administration of gonadotropin-releasing hormone. *J. Clin. Endocrinol. Metab.*, **51,** 730

Van Loon, G. R. and Brown, G. M. (1975). Secondary drug failure occurring during chronic treatment with LHRH: Appearance of an antibody. *J. Clin. Endocrinol. Metab.*, **41,** 640

Wildt, L., Marshall, J. and Knobil, E. (1980). Experimental induction of puberty in the infantile female rhesus monkey. *Science*, **207,** 1373

Wildt, L., Hausler, A., Marshall, G., Hutchison, J. S., Plant, T. M., Belchetz, P. E. and Knobil, E. (1981). Frequency and amplitude of gonadotropin-hormone stimulation and gonadotropin secretion in the rhesus monkey. *Endocrinology*, **109,** 376

Winters, S. J., Mecklenburg, R. S. and Sherins, R. J. (1978). Hypothalamic function in men with hypogonadotrophic hypogonadism. *Clin. Endocrinol.*, **8,** 417

Yoshimoto, Y., Moridera, K. and Imura, H. (1975). Restoration of normal pituitary gonadotropin reserve by administration of luteinizing-hormone-releasing hormone in patients with hypogonadotropic hypogonadism. *N. Engl. J. Med.*, **292,** 242

23
Correction of infertility with LHRH agonists in the male

J. HAPP

The treatment of infertility due to hypogonadotropic hypogonadism, whether of hypophysial or hypothalamic origin, consisted hitherto of the application of gonadotropins. Gonadotropin therapy was also the initial treatment of cryptorchidism, unless mechanical causes made surgical treatment necessary. The achievement of complete testicular descent aims at preservation of testicular function and represents a prophylactic pro-fertility measure. Gonadotropins were also used in treatment of constitutional delay of puberty and in normogonadotropic oligoasthenoteratozoospermia (OAT syndrome). Cryptorchidism, delayed puberty and 'normogonadotropic' OAT syndrome are complex clinical pictures partly caused by mild testicular deficiency, secondary to disturbances at the pituitary or hypothalamic level. The success rate of an LHRH replacement therapy for these indications should represent the percentage of patients with gonadotropin deficiency of hypothalamic origin.

Positive therapeutic responses to LHRH were reported shortly after synthetic LHRH became available (Bergada *et al.*, 1973; Mortimer *et al.*, 1974). In hypogonadotropic eunuchoidism of different origins treated with LHRH, stimulation of endocrine testicular function and spermatogenesis were achieved. LHRH was also studied in treatment of idiopathic oligozoospermia or azoospermia. At first, therapeutic trials with LHRH in cryptorchidism were not successful (Bergada *et al.*, 1973). One year later, however, a very high success rate of LHRH therapy in cryptorchid boys was reported (Bartsch and Frick, 1974).

The duration of effect of a dose of LHRH is much shorter than that of human chorionic gonadotropin (hCG) and a higher frequency of administration of the former is necessary. Potent long acting analogs of LHRH were found, promising higher effectiveness and simplification of releasing hormone therapy (Happ *et al.*, 1977). For a short time, another course of simplifying treatment was followed by testing depot preparations (Happ *et al.*, 1980*c*).

The chronic application of high doses of LHRH leads to desensitization of the pituitary in rats and golden hamsters. These observations initiated systematic investigation of the inhibitory effects of high-dose LHRH therapy or of the application of potent LHRH analogs. This desensitization of the pituitary by overstimulation led to studies which showed the importance of pulsatility of stimulation of the pituitary (Belchetz *et al.*, 1978; Kelch *et al.*, 1980). Repetitive stimulation of gonadotropin secretion causes refractoriness of the pituitary when the intervals between doses are reduced below a critical value (Schneider and Dahlén, 1973). Pulsatile LHRH therapy was achieved by use of portable automatic infusion pumps with computerized timing (Jacobson *et al.*, 1979). Intranasal (i.n.) low-dose LHRH therapy applying multiple doses per day can also mimic the spontaneous episodic increases in the serum gonadotropins in normal subjects and can thus correct for a deficient LHRH secretion (Happ *et al.*, 1975).

CRYPTORCHIDISM

Clinical preconditions

Cryptorchidism may be caused by mechanical factors interfering with testicular descent or by primary or secondary testicular insufficiency. The heterogeneity of the syndrome of cryptorchidism causes considerable divergence in results of different clinical studies using hCG therapy, i.e. success rates between 20 and 90 % (Happ, 1984). The success rate of treatment with hCG should reflect the percentage of patients with cryptorchidism due to deficient gonadotropin secretion. The gonadotropin deficiency usually originates from hypothalamic disturbances because pituitary lesions are rare before puberty. LHRH replacement therapy therefore should show the same success rate as hCG treatment if optimal dosages are used.

Substances used, dosage and clinical effect

During the past 10 years, results have been published on a total of about 600 patients treated with LHRH or a potent analog of LHRH. Effectiveness of LHRH therapy was proved by double blind study (Illig *et al.*, 1977). The success rates are similar to those for hCG therapy and show the same variation (Happ, 1984). Relapses were rarely reported (Illig *et al.*, 1980). Intranasal (i.n.) application of 200 μg LHRH six times daily produces success rates between 22 and 64 % (Happ *et al.*, 1978*b*; Illig *et al.*, 1977, 1980; Hadziselimovic *et al.*, 1980; Cacciari *et al.*, 1982). Modifications of this dosage regimen as used by other authors did not significantly change the success rates (Happ, 1984). Treatment with parenteral high dosages of LHRH produced moderate or poor success rates, i.e. below 24 % (Bergada *et al.*, 1973; Bartolini *et al.*, 1980) whereas parenteral low-dose treatment resulted in success rates varying between 22 % and 78 % (Cacciari *et al.*, 1982; Bartsch and Frick, 1974). Results from urological or surgical departments did not markedly differ from those obtained by departments of endocrinology or pediatrics although urological and surgical departments usually have preselection of patients resulting in a high percentage of cases where mechanical factors are involved. Patients not responding to LHRH therapy generally reveal anatomical abnormalities at surgery (Bartolini *et al.*, 1980; Bartsch and Frick, 1974; Illig *et al.*, 1980). Thus, the success rate by medical treatment of cryptorchidism depends on the composition of the patient group.

Low-dose treatment with potent LHRH analogs also tended to produce higher success rates. For example, p.n. treatment with 25 μg of [D-Leu^6,Pro^9-NHEt]LHRH twice daily produced a success rate of 57 %, while 50 μg twice daily had only a 25 % success rate (Happ *et al.*, 1977, 1978*d*; Frick *et al.*, 1980) and no testicular descent was achieved with 100 μg [D-Ser(tBu)^6,Pro^9-NHEt]LHRH i.n. on alternate days, whereas with 25 μg on alternate days, the success rate was 40 % (Cacciari *et al.*, 1982).

Despite short treatment periods, some investigators reported good clinical results (Cacciari *et al.*, 1982; Bartolini *et al.*, 1980). In some of the studies (Happ *et al.*, 1978*b*,*d*), treatment was stopped as soon as complete testicular descent was diagnosed; the shortest successful treatment period was 7 days.

Hormonal effects

Whenever alterations of hormonal parameters were observed during treatment with LHRH or LHRH analog common trends to be recognized were stimulation of luteinizing hormone (LH) and testosterone (T) secretion as well as suppressive effects on follicle stimulating hormone (FSH) secretion. A decreased FSH response in stimulation tests (ΔFSH) was frequently seen by the end of the LHRH treatment (Bartolini *et al.*, 1980; Happ *et al.*, 1978*b*,*d*; Spona *et al.*, 1979; Illig *et al.*, 1980; Cacciari *et al.*, 1982). Basal serum concentration of FSH (FSH_b), however, was rarely found to be altered, possibly because of insufficient assay sensitivity. Similarly, changes in basal serum LH (LH_b), LH response (ΔLH) and basal serum T were infrequently seen. Some authors observed an increase in LH_b, ΔLH and/or T (Bergada *et al.*, 1973; Happ *et al.*, 1978*b*; Spona *et al.*, 1979; Illig *et al.*, 1980; Hadziselimovic *et al.*, 1980; Cacciari *et al.*, 1982).

If serum T did increase, then this increase was always small; therefore, androgenic effects and development of secondary sex characteristics with LHRH therapy or therapeutic use of LHRH agonists have not yet been observed. However, stimulated Leydig cell activity was demonstrated by testicular biopsies and therefore increased intratesticular T concentrations may be assumed (Bergada *et al.*, 1973; Hadziselimovic *et al.*, 1980).

The development of decreased FSH responsiveness, frequently observed in releasing hormone therapy in contrast to stimulatory effects on pituitary Leydig cell axis, indicates partial desensitization of the pituitary by the treatment. When 'low'-dose regimens were used (i.e. 200 μg LHRH i.n., six times daily) pituitary desensitization was restricted to FSH secretion. High doses caused desensitization affecting FSH as well as LH secretion (Bartolini *et al.*, 1980; Bergada *et al.*, 1973). A single daily dose of 50 μg i.n. of [D-Leu^6, Pro^9-NHEt]LHRH caused decreased basal secretion of LH and FSH in one study (Frick *et al.*, 1980) and the same total dose (25 μg twice daily) caused a decrease of FSH responsiveness only in another study (Happ *et al.*, 1978*d*). Although there is marked interindividual variation in development of pituitary desensitization phenomena, approximately 50 μg i.n. appears to be the critical dose of the analog for suppression of both gonadotropins.

Physiological dose levels

There is considerable interindividual variation of sensitivity to a given dose of LHRH and desensitization of the gonadotrophs develops gradually during treatment. This makes it difficult to predict behavior of the pituitary in an individual patient under treatment with a fixed 'physiological' dose derived from statistical evaluation of a clinical study (long term application). The physiological dose also may be found by testing the gonadotropin response to a single dose in the individual patient. The dose which does not exceed the normal range of the spontaneous fluctuations of serum gonadotropins can be considered physiological, provided that the frequency of application corresponds to the natural rhythm of hypothalamic activity. The difficulties in establishing a physiological dosage regimen by this method for a patient with decreased gonadotropin responsiveness to LHRH are evident. Establishment of a 'physiological' dosage regimen for long acting LHRH analogs also presents problems.

Doses ranging between 5 μg/m^2 and 100 μg of LHRH intravenously (i.v.) produced an increase of both gonadotropins significantly above basal serum concentrations (Roth *et al.*, 1972). Therefore, parenteral (i.m. or s.c.) single doses between 20 and 500 μg, used in four therapeutic studies (Happ, 1984), have to be regarded as supraphysiological. Single i.v. doses of LHRH exceeding 0.025 μg/kg body weight seem to represent supraphysiological stimuli (Kelch *et al.*, 1980).

Nasal absorption of LHRH in adults ranges between 1 and 4 % (Happ, 1984). Values as high as 10 % absorption have also been found (Happ *et al.*, 1981*c*). The absorption rate may depend on the galenic preparation. Thus, the i.n. doses of 200–500 μg of LHRH used for therapy of cryptorchidism also represent supraphysiological stimuli. Marked increases of serum LH and FSH were demonstrated (Hagberg and Westphal, 1982) after i.n. administration of 400 μg LHRH (Figure 23.1).

The stimulatory effect of a single 20 μg i.n. dose of [D-Leu^6,Pro^9-NHEt]LHRH in prepubertal boys was also tested (Happ *et al.*, 1978*a*). This dose may be regarded a supraphysiological dose, since serum LH and FSH levels were increased above the basal level for about 6 h. Higher doses effected marked increases in the serum gonadotropins (Figure 23.2) for up to 8 h (Frick *et al.*, 1980).

Dosage regimens which gave good clinical results (i.e. success rates higher than 30 %) did not lead to decreased basal serum LH or LH responsiveness. After 'high'-dose treatment, i.e. 200 or 500 μg LHRH i.m. daily (Bartolini *et al.*, 1980; Bergada *et al.*, 1973) or 50 μg [D-Leu^6,Pro^9-NHEt]LHRH i.n. once daily (Frick *et al.*, 1980), LH response tended to be decreased and success rates were below 30 %. However, no correlation was reported between a decreased LH response and treatment failures for individual patients. Therefore, despite

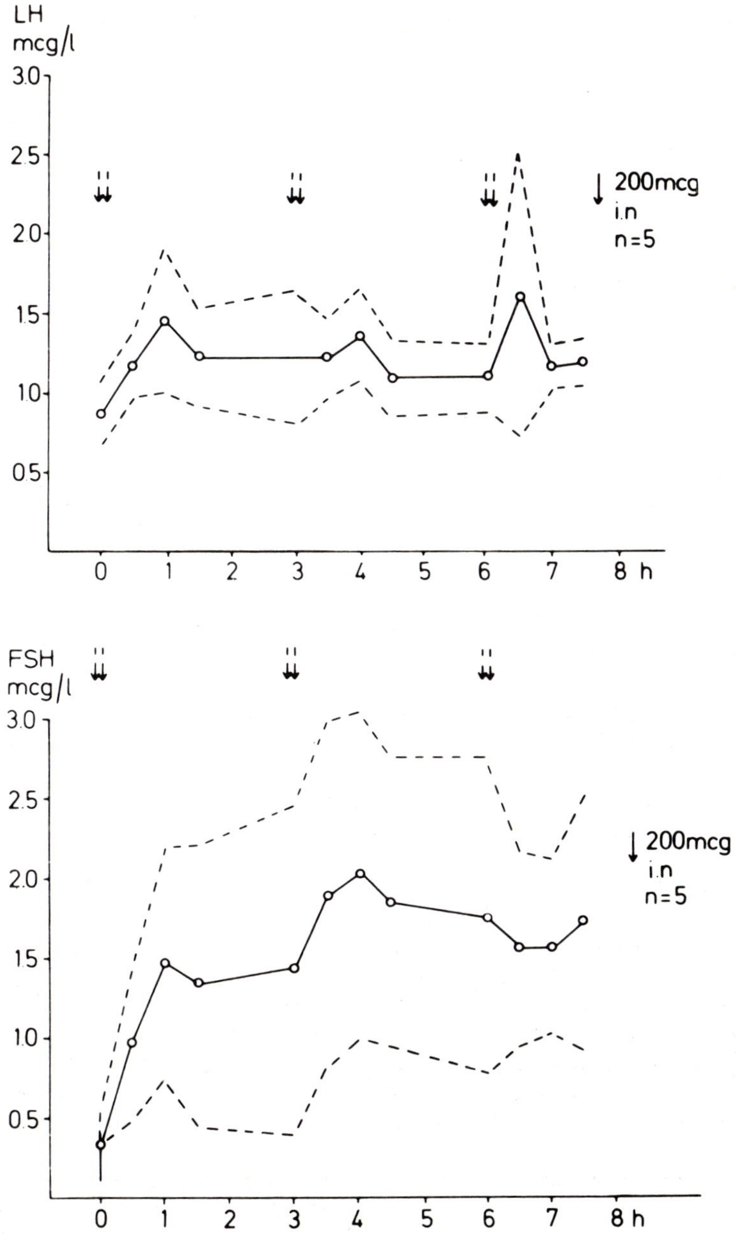

Figure 23.1 Serum LH and FSH after 400 μg LHRH administered (sprayed) intranasally (a single dose of 200 μg into each nostril) three times daily in five cryptorchid boys. Mean and SD are indicated (from Hagberg and Westphal, 1982, with permission).

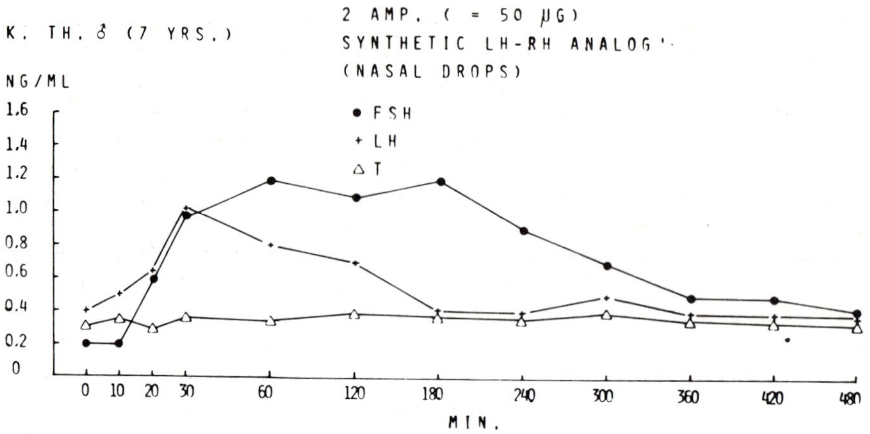

Figure 23.2 Serum FSH, LH and testosterone (T) after a single intranasal administration (drops) of [D-Leu^6,Pro^9-NHEt]LHRH in one of four cryptorchid boys tested (from Frick *et al.*, 1980, with permission).

decreased LH responsiveness to the treatment, LH secretion after each single dose must have been sufficient to maintain integrated serum LH within the effective range.

In adolescents or adults (Happ *et al.*, 1980*b*), serial LHRH tests during treatment with LHRH or analogs showed that pituitary desensitization begins about 4 weeks after the start of treatment. Desensitization of the gonadotropes is less of a problem in cryptorchidism treatment with LHRH since testicular descent is usually completed within 4 weeks of treatment. For cryptorchidism, high-dose treatment with LHRH analogs may not cause as many problems as in treatment of hypogonadism where much longer treatment periods are necessary.

Antibody formation

Formation of antibodies against LHRH or LHRH agonists, observed with LHRH therapy in an adult patient with idiopathic hypogonadotropic hypogonadism (Van Loon and Brown, 1975), was not reported to occur in treatment of cryptorchidism by releasing hormone therapy (Happ *et al.*, 1978*b*,*d*; Illig *et al.*, 1977).

IDIOPATHIC HYPOGONADOTROPIC HYPOGONADISM

Clinical preconditions

Idiopathic hypogonadotropic hypogonadism (IHH) may be attributed to deficient LHRH secretion if normal gonadotropin response to a test dose of LHRH proves normal functional capacity of the gonadotropes. Absent or diminished gonadotropin responsiveness may derive from disorders located at the pituitary level as well as in the hypothalamus. In some patients showing a decreased gonadotropin responsiveness, a normal result of the LHRH test is obtained after chronic stimulation with LHRH (Yoshimoto *et al.*, 1975). This demonstrates that unresponsiveness of the pituitary to LHRH was secondary to hypothalamic deficiency in those patients. A normal gonadotropin response, however, does not definitely exclude pituitary gonadotropic deficiency of minor degree since patients with pituitary tumors may present a normal LHRH test, especially when high test doses (above 50 μg) are used (Franchimont *et al.*, 1976). For diagnostic purposes we use 25 μg LHRH (i.v.) in adults. Combinations of LHRH deficiency and pituitary or primary testicular pathology were observed (Happ *et al.*, 1980*a*) which may present diagnostic problems or be responsible for ineffective releasing hormone therapy.

Substances used, dosage and clinical effects

Although stimulation of gonadotropin secretion during LHRH or LHRH analog treatment was generally observed in (approximately 120 published) patients with IHH or Kallmann's syndrome (KS), improvement of clinical findings was rarely reported. A change in androgen-dependent clinical parameters (libido, penile erections, ejaculations, pubic hair and penis growth) and stimulation of spermatogenesis were described (Bergada *et al.*, 1973; Mortimer *et al.*, 1974; Jaramillo *et al.*, 1978; Guitelman *et al.*, 1979).

A normal sperm count, however, occurred in only two IHH patients (Mortimer *et al.*, 1974; Happ *et al.*, 1980*b*,*c*). Many studies covered only 3 months and marked physical changes cannot be expected. Sperm count will not be normalized until 6 months of treatment since severe insufficiency of tubular function is usually present in patients with IHH. However, a number of patients treated up to 1 year showed no significant improvement of sperm count. The hormonal results of most studies suggest that failure of treatment is caused by insufficient hormonal response. The most promising clinical results were obtained with pulsatile LHRH therapy (Hoffman and Crowley, 1982).

Hormonal effects

Parallel changes in secretory behavior of LH and FSH usually occurred during releasing hormone therapy. In most cases, however, the initial increase in basal serum gonadotropins (LH_b, FSH_b) and/or gonadotropin responsiveness to a test dose of LHRH (ΔLH, ΔFSH) only lasted for several weeks and was not sustained under treatment (Rabin and McNeil, 1981; Happ *et al.*, 1978*c*, 1980*a*,*b*, 1981*a*,*b*,*c*; Krabbe and Skakkebaeck, 1977; Bergada *et al.*, 1973; Tharandt *et al.*, 1977; Hashimoto *et al.*, 1975; Laron *et al.*, 1981; Moore *et al.*, 1981). The most impressive changes were found in ΔLH of the patients. Transitory increase in gonadotropin responsiveness was generally obtained in patients showing a decreased ΔLH before treatment. In patients showing a normal ΔLH before treatment, a gradual decrease in gonadotropin responsiveness from approximately week 4 of treatment was observed.

A transitory decrease in gonadotropin responsiveness for the first few days of releasing hormone therapy (Happ *et al.*, 1975) may indicate exhaustion of the gonadotropin pool due to repeated stimulation before biosynthesis has normalized. Basal serum gonadotropins or gonadotropin responsiveness to LHRH frequently declined slowly during treatment. Secondary drug failure during treatment with LHRH or analogs generally cannot be ascribed to antibody formation since systematic testing usually led to negative results (Tharandt *et al.*, 1977; Happ *et al.*, 1978*b*,*d*). The phenomenon must result from desensitization of the pituitary especially when normal gonadotropin responsiveness before treatment disappears during therapy and serum testosterone (T) remains at subnormal levels.

Occurrence of decreasing gonadotropin responsiveness during treatment with LHRH seems to be mainly dependent on the dosage. Using i.n. LHRH therapy with daily doses between 1600 and 300 μg (Happ *et al.*, 1975, 1978*c*, 1980*a*,*c*, 1981*a*,*c*), the rate of occurrence of this phenomenon was lower than with parenteral therapy applying daily doses between 3000 and 200 μg (Rabin and McNeil, 1981; Mortimer *et al.*, 1974; Happ *et al.*, 1978*c*, 1980*c*; Krabbe and Skakkebaeck, 1977; Bergada *et al.*, 1973; Hashimoto *et al.*, 1975). However, the difference in the composition of the groups of patients must be taken into account. The groups of i.n. treated patients included a larger proportion of patients with delayed puberty (DP). Intermittent treatment with interposition of an interval of 2 weeks between treatment periods of 4 weeks could not prevent the occurrence of decreasing gonadotropin responsiveness (Happ *et al.*, 1980*b*, 1981*c*).

When utilizing the potent LHRH analog [D-Trp^6,Pro^9-NHEt]LHRH (10–50 μg i.n. or s.c. daily or on alternate days) decreased gonadotropin responsiveness was observed, especially with high dosages (Crowley *et al.*, 1983; Laron *et al.*, 1981). A similar study on [D-Ser(tBu)^6,Pro^9-NHEt]LHRH showed that parenteral dosages (1–5 μg s.c. daily) ten times smaller than the ones used with the other analog all led to decreased pituitary responsiveness (Moore *et al.*, 1981). Small i.n. doses of this analog (25–50 μg every other day), however, did not regularly lead to unresponsiveness of the pituitary (Happ *et al.*, 1981*b*; Mies *et al.*, 1982). The smallest risk of desensitization seems to be with [D-Leu^6,Pro^9-NHEt]LHRH (50–100 μg s.c. or i.m. daily, 100 μg i.n. daily), which is known as being the least potent of the three LHRH analogs used for treatment of IHH or DP (Tharandt *et al.*, 1977; Guitelman *et al.*, 1979; Happ *et al.*, 1977, 1980*c*).

Pulsatile LHRH therapy

Pulsatile LHRH therapy had a good stimulatory effect on gonadotropins (Jacobson *et al.*, 1979; Hetzel and Castillo, 1982; Vierhapper and Waldhäusl, 1983; Valk *et al.*, 1980; Crowley *et al.*, 1983; Happ *et al.*, 1983). The studies on supraphysiological dosages, however, were carried out over a short period (5–10 days) and did not exceed the critical duration when gonadotropin

Table 23.1 Pulsatile LHRH therapy in male patients with idiopathic hypogonadotropic hypogonadism or Kallmann's syndrome (IHH/KS) and delayed puberty (DP). Dosage regimens and hormonal changes under treatment

Daily dose, μg (applications × injected dose)	*Period* (days)	*Diagnosis and number of patients* (n)	*Patient age* (y)	LH_b	ΔLH	FSH_b	ΔFSH	T
440 s.c. (11 × 40)[a]	10	IHH/KS (2)	16–18	NC	+	+	+	(+)
320 i.v. (16 × 20)[b]	6	IHH/KS (7)	adult	NC	+	+	+	NC
180 s.c. (10 × 18)[c]	9	IHH/KS (1)	15	+	+	+	+	
50 s.c. (10 × 5)[c]	9	IHH/KS (1)	19	+	+	+	+	
20 i.v. (12 × 0.025/kg)[d]	5	IHH/KS (4)	20–34	+	(+)	+	+	NC
20 s.c. (12 × 0.025/kg)[e]	7	IHH/KS (6)	adult	(+)	+	+	+	+
20 s.c. (12 × 0.025/kg)[f]	up to 450	IHH/KS (6)	18–29	+		+		+
20 s.c. (10 × 2)[g]	90	IHH/KS (3), DP (1)	16–20	(+)	(+)	(+)	(+)	(+)

[a] Jacobson *et al.*, 1979 (inj. every 60 min within 10–12 h at night); [b] Hetzel and Castillo, 1982; [c] Vierhapper and Waldhäusl, 1983 (inj. every 90 min within 10 h at night); [d] Valk *et al.*, 1980; [e] Crowley *et al.*, 1983; [f] Hoffmann and Crowley, 1982; [g] Happ *et al.*, 1983

NC = no change

responsiveness begins to decrease (Happ *et al.*, 1980*b*). The longest follow-up of pulsatile low-dose LHRH therapy published (Hoffmann and Crowley 1982) covered a period of 15 months during which no signs of pituitary desensitization were observed (Table 23.1). In our own investigations (Happ *et al.*, 1983), the same observation was made in four patients treated for 3 months. However, normalization of serum T occurred only in two patients presenting normal ΔLH in LHRH tests from the beginning of the treatment. In Figure 23.3, development of Leydig cell function is shown for one of the two patients. Two other patients with decreased ΔLH before treatment showed slowly increasing gonadotropin responsiveness during treatment, whereas serum T was not changed during the 3 month period of treatment. Significant increase in testicular volumes and spermatogenesis under long term treatment was found in three of six IHH patients (Hoffmann *et al.*, 1982); although sperm counts remained low throughout the treatment, one patient fathered a child.

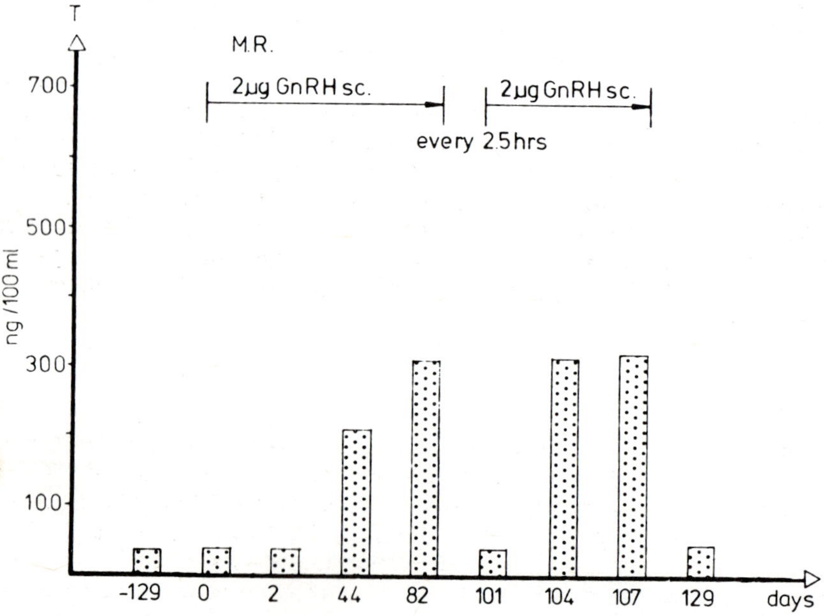

Figure 23.3 Serum testosterone (T) during pulsatile LHRH therapy in a male patient, 20 years of age, with Kallmann's syndrome: normalization of serum T during each treatment period, relapse to pretreatment stage after treatment.

OTHER INDICATIONS

Acquired hypogonadotropic hypogonadism

Releasing hormone therapy was also carried out in hypogonadotropic hypogonadism secondary to lesions of the hypothalamus and even of the pituitary gland. Patients with craniopharyngioma, with hypothalamic lesion due to tuberculous meningitis and with acromegaly were treated with LHRH (Mortimer *et al.*, 1974; Hashimoto *et al.*, 1975) or [D-Ser(tBu)^6,Pro^9-NHEt]LHRH (Moore *et al.*, 1981). For treatment of these patients, the investigators applied the same protocol as in treatment of patients with idiopathic hypogonadotropic hypogonadism (IHH) and qualitatively the same results were obtained. The groups of the patients with acquired hypothalamic hypogonadism, however, were too small to find statistical differences between the two forms of hypothalamic hypogonadism with regard to the efficiency of the treatment.

Delayed puberty

In treatment of delayed puberty (DP), there are two main problems to be considered: delimitation of constitutional DP from IHH before adult age if anosmia does not indicate Kallmann's syndrome and demarcation of therapeutic success from spontaneous pubertal development in patients with constitutional DP. A double-blind study on the efficiency of a LHRH analog in treatment of DP (50 μg [D-Ser(tBu)^6,Pro^9-NHEt]LHRH i.n. every other day) did not show a significant difference in hormonal and clinical response to the treatment compared with placebo (Mies *et al.*, 1982). However single cases could be demonstrated (Happ *et al.*, 1980*a*) showing normalization of serum T during low-dose p.n. LHRH therapy (200 μg six times daily) and a relapse to decreased serum T after termination of the treatment. This indicates effectiveness of the treatment in these patients. Desensitization of the pituitary also occurred in DP and was most frequently observed by us under high dosage LHRH agonist therapy.

Oligozoospermia

Patients with idiopathic normogonadotropic oligozoospermia (INO) were also treated with LHRH (parenteral daily doses between 100 and 1000 μg) or LHRH analogs (parenteral daily doses of 5–200 μg [D-Leu^6,Pro^9-NHEt]LHRH or 2 μg [D-Trp^6,Pro^9-NHEt]LHRH every other day). Some groups of investigators published disappointing results, others were rather optimistic about the efficiency of this kind of treatment. In azoospermic and oligozoospermic patients, improvement of sperm quality (sperm count, vitality and motility) was reported. High doses of [D-Leu^6,Pro^9-NHEt]LHRH did not influence the clinical parameters mentioned above (Schwarzstein *et al.*, 1978) whereas the results obtained by very low dosages of [D-Trp^6,Pro^9-NHEt]LHRH were promising (Levalle *et al.*, 1981).

Sexual impotence

During treatment of hypogonadal males with LHRH, some patients were noticed to have increased potency before their androgen secretion returned to normal (Bergada *et al.*, 1973; Mortimer *et al.*, 1974). This finding, together with the report that LHRH has a direct effect on central neurological mechanisms which resulted in stimulation of mating behavior in the rat, suggested that LHRH may stimulate libido in patients with sexual impotence (SI).

A double-blind cross-over trial of 500 μg LHRH or placebo subcutaneously every 8 h for 4 weeks in ten men, 25–75 years of age, with secondary SI resulted in some overall improvement in the libido score and a significant increase in spontaneous occurrence of erections during the treatment period (Davies *et al.*, 1976). Since sexual activity varies considerably from week to week and depends very much upon a number of external factors, convincing evidence for stimulation of libido and potency may not be obtained easily.

CONCLUDING REMARKS

There is good evidence of effectiveness of LHRH or potent LHRH analogs in treatment of different diseases originating from LHRH deficiency. The best results were obtained in treatment of cryptorchidism. For this indication, LHRH nasal spray was recently introduced into the German pharmaceutical market as a remedy.

Releasing-hormone therapy for cryptorchidism, especially by intranasal delivery, is highly effective, convenient and atraumatic. Treatment of maldescended testes with LHRH or potent analogs may be expected to be successful in patients in whom cryptorchidism is due to deficient gonadotropin secretion, generally resulting from hypothalamic disturbances. The clinical effect is mediated by stimulation of LH and possibly FSH. Stimulation of testicular tissues is more physiological than with hCG since androgenic side-effects were not seen. Potent long acting LHRH agonists, even by low-dose treatment, bring a higher risk of desensitization of the gonadotrophs. Larger clinical studies following the gonadotropin release of nasal dosage forms will soon be able to identify optimal dosage regimens. The antigenicity of analogs, however, must also be considered.

The reports on the efficiency of a releasing hormone therapy in hypothalamic eunuchoidism are crucial; only sporadic significant influence on spermatogenesis was observed, whereas stimulation of Leydig cell function was found more frequently. Occurrence of pituitary desensitization turned out to be the main problem in long term treatment of these patients and patients with idiopathic hypogonadotropic hypogonadism. Patients with Kallmann's syndrome were especially sensitive to this phenomenon. Since pituitary desensitization is known to be a typical reaction to supraphysiological dosage, particular interest has lately been focussed on the effectiveness of pulsatile low-dose LHRH therapy in treatment of patients with IHH and KS. This physiological form of replacement therapy reliably avoids desensitization and therefore appears to be the most promising approach to releasing hormone therapy in hypothalamic eunuchoidism but has the disadvantage of high technical costs compared to the convenient intranasal therapy with LHRH or its potent analogs.

Further studies are necessary to find out which role LHRH or its potent analogs may play in treatment of delayed puberty, idiopathic normogonadotropic oligozoospermia and sexual impotence.

Acknowledgements

Support was given by the Deutsche Forschungsgemeinschaft (DFG), grant no. BE 601/3. Nasal spray of LHRH (HOE 471) or buserelin (HOE 766) and Depot LHRH 20 were kindly supplied by Hoechst, Frankfurt. Leuprolide and [D-Trp^6,Pro^9-NHEt]LHRH were kindly supplied by Serono, Freiburg. Zyklomat^R pumps were kindly provided by Ferring, Kiel.

References

Bartolini, E., Barletta, D., Galli, P., Franchi, F., Gasperi, M., Luisi, M., Baldassari, S. and Fratta, M. (1980). Treatment of cryptorchidism with LHRH and orchidopexy: longitudinal study. In Cacciari, E. and Prader, A. (eds.) *Pathophysiology of Puberty*, pp. 257–263. (London: Academic Press)

Bartsch, G. and Frick, J. (1974). Therapeutic effects of luteinizing hormone releasing hormone (LH-RH) in cryptorchidism. *Andrologia*, **6**, 197

Belchetz, P. E., Plant, T. M., Nakai, Y., Koegh, E. J. and Knobil, E. (1978). Hypophyseal responses to continuous and intermittent delivery of hypothalamic gonadotropin-releasing hormone. *Science*, **202**, 631

Bergada, C., Mancini, R. E., Vilar, O., Rivarola, M. A., Calamera, J. C., Bianculli, C., Schally, A. V. and Kastin, A. J. (1973). Effect of chronic administration of synthetic LH-RH-FSH-RH on prepubertal boys and in hypogonadotropic hypogonadism. In Gual, C. and Rosemberg, E. (eds.) *Hypothalamic Hypophysiotropic Hormones, Physiological and Clinical Studies, Serono Health Foundation, Acapulco 1972*, pp. 299–301. (Amsterdam: Excerpta Medica)

Cacciari, E., Fréjàville, E. and Becca, A. (1982). Treatment of cryptorchidism by intranasal synthetic LHRH and its analogue D-Ser(TBU)^6-LHRH-EA^{10}. *Eur. J. Pediatr.*, **139**, 280

Crowley, W. F. Jr., Vale, W., Rivier, J. and McArthur, J. W. (1983). LHRH in hypogonadotropic hypogonadism. In Zatuchni, G. I., Shelton, J. D. and Sciarra, J. J. (eds.). *LHRH Peptides as Female and Male Contraceptives*, pp. 321–333. (Philadelphia: Harper & Row)

Davies, T. F., Mountjoy, C. Q., Gomes-Pan, A., Watson, M. J., Hanker, J. P., Besser, G. M. and Hall, R. (1976). A double blind cross over trial of gonadotropin releasing hormone (LHRH) in sexually impotent men. *Clin. Endocrinol.*, **5**, 601

Franchimont, P., Demoulin, A. and Bourguignon, J. P. (1976). The LH-RH test for clinical diagnosis. In Charro-Salgado, A. L., Fernández-Durango, R. and Lopez Del Campo, J. G. (eds.) *Basic Application and Clinical uses of Hypothalamic Hormones*, pp. 244–252. (New York: American Elsevier)

Frick, J., Daner, Ch., Kunit, G., Galva, G. and Bernroider, G. (1980). The effect of chronic administration of a synthetic LH-RH analogue intranasally in cryptorchid boys. *Int. J. Androl.*, **3**, 469

Guitelman, A., Mancini, A. M., Aparicio, N. J., Tropea, L., Levalle, O. and Schally, A. V. (1979). Effect of D-leucine-6-luteinizing hormone releasing hormone ethylamide in patients with hypogonadotropic hypogonadism with anosmia. *Fertil. Steril.*, **32**, 308

Hadziselimovic, F., Girard, J., Höcht, B., von der Ohe, M. and Stalder, G. (1980). Effect of LH-RH treatment on hypothalamic–pituitary–gonadal axis and Leydig cell ultrastructure in cryptorchid boys. *Horm. Res.*, **13**, 358

Hagberg, S. and Westphal, O. (1982). Treatment of undescended testes with intranasal application of synthetic LH-RH. *Eur. J. Pediatr.*, **139**, 285

Happ, J., Neubauer, M., Egri, A., Demisch, K., Schöffling, K. and Beyer, J. (1975). GnRH therapy in males with hypogonadotrophic hypogonadism. *Horm. Metab. Res.,* **7,** 526

Happ, J., Vogt, J., Weber, Th., Cordes, U., Krause, U., Callensee, W., Ermert, J. A., Kollmann, F. and Beyer, J. (1977). Therapeutic use of D-Leu[6]-des-Gly[10]-GnRH-ethylamide in normal human males and in prepubertal boys. *Acta Endocrinol.,* **84,** (Suppl. 208), 39

Happ, J., Depper, M., Weber, Th., Kollmann, F., Krause, U. and Beyer, J. (1978*a*). Gonadotropin secretion after D-leu[6]-des-Gly[10]-GnRH-ethylamide in normal human males and in prepubertal boys. In Voelter, W. and Gupta, D. (eds.) *Hypothalamic Hormones – Chemistry, Physiology and Clinical Applications, 2nd European Colloquium on Hypothalamic Hormones, Tübingen 1976,* pp. 589–598. (Weinheim, New York: Verlag Chemie)

Happ, J., Kollmann, F., Krawehl, C., Neubauer, M., Krause, U., Demisch, K., Sandow, J., von Rechenberg, W. and Beyer, J. (1978*b*). Treatment of cryptorchidism with pernasal gonadotropin releasing hormone therapy. *Fertil. Steril.,* **29,** 546

Happ, J., Neubauer, M., Egri, A., Demisch, K. and Beyer, J. (1978*c*). Gonadotropin releasing hormone (LHRH) therapy in human males with idiopathic hypogonadotropic hypogonadism. In Cortes-Prieto, J. and Semm, K. (eds.) *IV ESCO, Madrid, 1975,* pp. 516–520. (Madrid: Reproducción)

Happ, J., Weber, Th., Callensee, W., Ermert, J. A., Eshkol, A. and Beyer, J. (1978*d*). Treatment of cryptorchidism with a potent analog of the gonadotropin-releasing hormone. *Fertil. Steril.,* **29,** 552

Happ, J., Schmitz, V., Cordes, U., Krause, U., Atzpodien, W. and Beyer, J. (1980*a*). Treatment of delayed puberty by intranasal application of gonadotropin-releasing hormone (LHRH). *Int. J. Fertil.,* **25,** 247

Happ, J., Schmitz, V., Cordes, U., Krause, U. and Beyer, J. (1980*b*). Pernasal gonadotropin-releasing hormone therapy in male patients with hypogonadism of hypothalamic origin. Intra-individual comparison of continuous and intermittent treatment. In Cacciari, E. and Prader, A. (eds.) *Pathophysiology of Puberty,* pp. 373–384. (London: Academic Press)

Happ, J., Weber, Th., Cordes, U., Krause, U., Schramm, P. and Beyer, J. (1980*c*). Therapeutic use of gonadotropin-releasing hormone (LHRH) and a potent LHRH analog in male patients with idiopathic hypogonadotropic hypogonadism (IHH) or constitutional delay of puberty (DP). In Salvadori, B., Semm, K. and Vadorna, E. (eds) *Fertility and Sterility, V ESCO, Venice 1978,* pp. 187–191. (Rome: C.I.C., Edizioni Internationali Gruppo Editoriale Medico, Tipolitografia Aurelia 72)

Happ, J., Benner, A., Krause, U. and Beyer, J. (1981*a*). Treatment of delayed puberty by intranasal application of gonadotropin-releasing hormone (LHRH). Investigation of a new low-dose regimen. *Acta Endocrinol.,* **97** (Suppl. 243), abstr. 420

Happ, J., Benner, A., Krause, U. and Beyer, J. (1981*b*). Treatment of delayed puberty with a potent LHRH analog. Effectiveness of a low-dose regimen. *Acta Endocrinol.,* **96** (Suppl. 240), 112

Happ, J., Deigentasch, V., Schmitz, V., Krause, U., Beyer, J. and von der Ohe, M. (1981*c*). Intermittent pernasal gonadotropin-releasing hormone therapy in male patients with delayed puberty. In Voelter, W. and Weizel, G. (eds.) *Structure and Activity of Natural Peptides,* pp. 483–496. (Berlin: de Gruyter)

Happ, J., Ditscheid, W., Krause, U. and Beyer, J. (1983). Pulsatile gonadorelin (GnRH) therapy in male patients with Kallmann's syndrome or constitutional delay of puberty. In Leyendecker, G., Stock, H. and Wildt, L. (eds.) *Brain and Pituitary Peptides II – Pulsatile Administration of GnRH in Hypothalamic Failure – Basic and Chemical Aspects,* pp. 165–181. (Basel: Karger)

Happ, J. (1984). Gonadorelin (GnRH) therapy in cryptorchidism. In Kelâmi, A. and Pryor, J. P. (eds.) *Maldescensus Testis, Operative Andrology 2* (*Progress in Reproductive Biology and Medicine,* Vol. 10 and 11), pp. 88–96. (Basel: Karger)

Hashimoto, T., Miyai, K., Onishi, T., Matsumoto, K. and Kumanara, Y. (1975). Comparison of short and long-term treatment with synthetic LH-releasing hormone and clomiphene citrate in male hypothalamic hypogonadism. *J. Clin. Endocrinol. Metab.,* **41,** 905

Hetzel, W. D. and Castillo, O. (1982). Pulsatile LH-RH substitution in hypothalamo-hypogonadotropic men. *Acta Endocrinol.,* **99** (Suppl. 246), 86

Hoffmann, A. R. and Crowley, W. F. Jr. (1982). Induction of puberty in men by long-term pulsatile administration of low-dose gonadotropin-releasing hormone. *N. Engl. J. Med.*, **307,** 1237

Illig, R., Kollmann, F., Borkenstein, M., Kuber, W., Exner, G. U., Kellerer, K., Lunglmayr, L. and Prader, A. (1977). Treatment of cryptorchidism by intranasal synthetic luteinizing-hormone releasing hormone. Results of a collaborative double-blind study. *Lancet,* ii, 518

Illig, R., Bucher, H. and Prader, A. (1980). Success, relapse and failure after intranasal LHRH treatment of cryptorchidism in 55 prepubertal boys. *Eur. J. Pediatr.*, **133,** 147

Jacobson, R. I., Seyler, L. E. Jr., Tamborlane, W. V., Gertner, J. M. and Gemel, M. (1979). Pulsatile subcutaneous nocturnal administration of LHRH by portable infusion pump in hypogonadotropic hypogonadism: Initiation of gonadotropin responsiveness. *J. Clin. Endocrinol. Metab.*, **49,** 652

Jaramillo, C. J., Charro-Salgado, A. L., Fernandez-Cruz, A., Coy, D. H. and Schally, A. V. (1978). Clinical studies with D-Trp^6-luteinizing hormone-releasing hormone in men with hypogonadotropic hypogonadism. *Fertil. Steril.*, **30,** 430

Kelch, R. P., Corley, K. P., Valk, T. W. and Marshall, J. C. (1980). Quantitative estimation of gonadotropin-releasing hormone (GnRH) secretion during human puberty. In Cacciari, E. and Prader, A. (eds.) *Pathophysiology of Puberty*. Vol. 36, pp. 23–41. (London: Academic Press)

Krabbe, S. and Skakkebaeck, N. E. (1977). Gonadotropin-releasing hormone (LH-RH) and human chorionic gonadotropin in the treatment of two boys with hypogonadotropic hypogonadism. *Acta Paediatr. Scand.*, **66,** 361

Laron, Z., Dickerman, Z., Zeev, Z. B., Prager-Lewin, R., Comaru-Schally, A. M. and Schally, A. V. (1981). Long-term effect of D-Trp^6-luteinizing hormone-releasing hormone on testicular size and luteinizing hormone, follicle stimulating hormone, and testosterone levels in hypothalamic hypogonadotropic males. *Fertil. Steril.*, **35,** 328

Levalle, O., Tropea, L., Aparicio, N., Guitelman, A., Mancini, A., Comaru-Schally, A. M. and Schally, V. (1981). D-Tryptophan-6-LH-RH at low doses in the treatment of male subfertility. *Andrologia,* **13,** 207

Mies, R., Fischer, H. and von der Ohe, M. (1982). The efficiency of an LHRH analogue in the treatment of delayed puberty. *Acta Endocrinol.*, **99** (Suppl. 246), 90

Moore, M. P., Smith, R., Donald, R. A., Espiner, E. A. and Stronach, S. (1981). The effects of different dose regimens of D-Ser(TBU)^6-LHRH-EA^{10} (HOE 766) in subjects with hypogonadotropic hypogonadism. *Clin. Endocrinol.*, **14,** 93

Mortimer, C. H., McNeilly, A. S., Fisher, R. A., Murray, M. A. F. and Besser, G. M. (1974). Gonadotropin-releasing hormone therapy in hypogonadal males with hypothalamic or pituitary dysfunction. *Br. Med. J.*, **4,** 617

Rabin, D. and McNeil, L. W. (1981). Long-term therapy with luteinizing hormone-releasing hormone in isolated gonadotropin deficiency: failure of therapeutic response. *J. Clin. Endocrinol. Metab.*, **52,** 557

Roth, J. C., Kelch, R. P., Kaplan, S. K. and Grumbach, M. M. (1972). FSH and LH response to luteinizing hormone-releasing factor in prepubertal and pubertal children, adult males and patients with hypogonadotropic and hypergonadotropic hypogonadism. *J. Clin. Endocrinol. Metab.*, **35,** 926

Schneider, H. P. G. and Dahlén, H. G. (1973). Evidence for partial refractoriness of the human pituitary. *Acta Endocrinol.*, **72** (Suppl. 173), 86

Schwarzstein, L., Aparicio, N. H., Turner, D., de Turner, E. A., Premoli, F. and Schally, A. V. (1978): D-Leucine-6-luteinizing hormone-releasing hormone ethylamide in the treatment of normogonadotropic oligoasthenospermia. *Fertil. Steril.*, **29,** 332

Spona, J., Gleisbach, H., Happ, J., Kollmann, F., Torresani, T. and von der Ohe, M. (1979). Hormone serum levels during treatment of cryptorchidism by intranasal application of LH-RH. *Endocrinol Exp.*, **13,** 201

Tharandt, L., Schulte, H., Benker, G., Hackenberg, K. and Reinwein, D. (1977). Serum protein binding of 125-I-LH-RH and 125-I-6-D-leu-des-Gly-ethylamide-LH-RH (6-D-LH-RH) under treatment with the analogue in patients with isolated gonadotropin deficiency (IGD). *Acta Endocrinol.*, **84,** (Suppl. 208), 29

Valk, T. W., Corley, K. P., Kelch, R. P. and Marshall, I. C. (1980). Hypogonadotropic hypogonadism: hormonal responses to low-dose pulsatile administration of gonadotropin-releasing hormone. *J. Clin. Endocrinol. Metab.*, **51,** 730

Van Loon, G. R. and Brown, G. M. (1975). Secondary drug failure occurring during chronic treatment with LH-RH: appearance of an antibody. *J. Clin. Endocrinol. Metab.*, **41,** 610

Vierhapper, H. and Waldhäusl, W. (1983). Initiation of gonadotropin responsiveness in hypothalamic hypogonadism: comparison of pulsatile and continuous nocturnal subcutaneous administration of LH-RH. *Exp. Clin. Endocrinol.*, **81,** 249

Yoshimoto, Y., Moridera, K. and Imura, H. (1975). Restoration of normal pituitary gonadotropin reserve by administration of luteinizing hormone-releasing hormone in patients with hypogonadotropic hypogonadism. *N. Engl. J. Med.*, **292,** 242

24
LHRH analog therapy of precocious puberty

F. COMITE, G. B. CUTLER Jr and D. L. LORIAUX

INTRODUCTION

Puberty is initiated by the pulsatile secretion of gonadotropins, luteinizing hormone (LH) and follicle stimulating hormone (FSH). These gonadotropin pulsations, which result from the episodic release of LHRH from the hypothalamus, stimulate gonadal sex steroid secretion and the resulting secondary sexual changes of puberty (Boyar *et al.*, 1974). The normal pubertal age is 11 ± 2 years (mean ± 2SD) in females and 12 ± 2 years in males (Marshall and Tanner, 1969, 1970). Precocious puberty is the premature occurrence of sexual maturation. The presence in a girl of breasts or pubic hair before age 9, or menses before age 10, and the presence in a boy of testicular, pubic hair or penile development before age 10, suggests precocious puberty (Figure 24.1).

Precocious puberty adversely affects subsequent development in several ways. Adult stature may be compromised because of accelerated epiphyseal closure. Increased stature as a child may cause inappropriate expectations by the family and community concerning the child's psychological maturity. Adverse psychological effects of precocious puberty (including libido, the need for contraception and rejection by peers) may be profound for both the child and the family.

Precocious puberty may be classified as either true precocious puberty (TPP) or precocious pseudopuberty (PPP). True precocious puberty is mediated by hypothalamic–pituitary–gonadal activation. Precocious pseudopuberty is independent of hypothalamic–pituitary activation and generally arises from a gonadal or adrenal tumor or other rare disorders. Therapy of precocious pseudopuberty is directed at intercepting or removing the primary source of the abnormal sex steroid production (Comite *et al.*, 1983), which usually halts or reverses the pubertal process.

Although the underlying etiology of true precocious puberty is not always discernible, the differential diagnosis includes C.N.S. tumors (hypothalamic hamartomas, astrocytomas, gliomas, dermoid tumors, teratomas, subarachnoid cysts, pinealomas etc.), the McCune–Albright syndrome, von

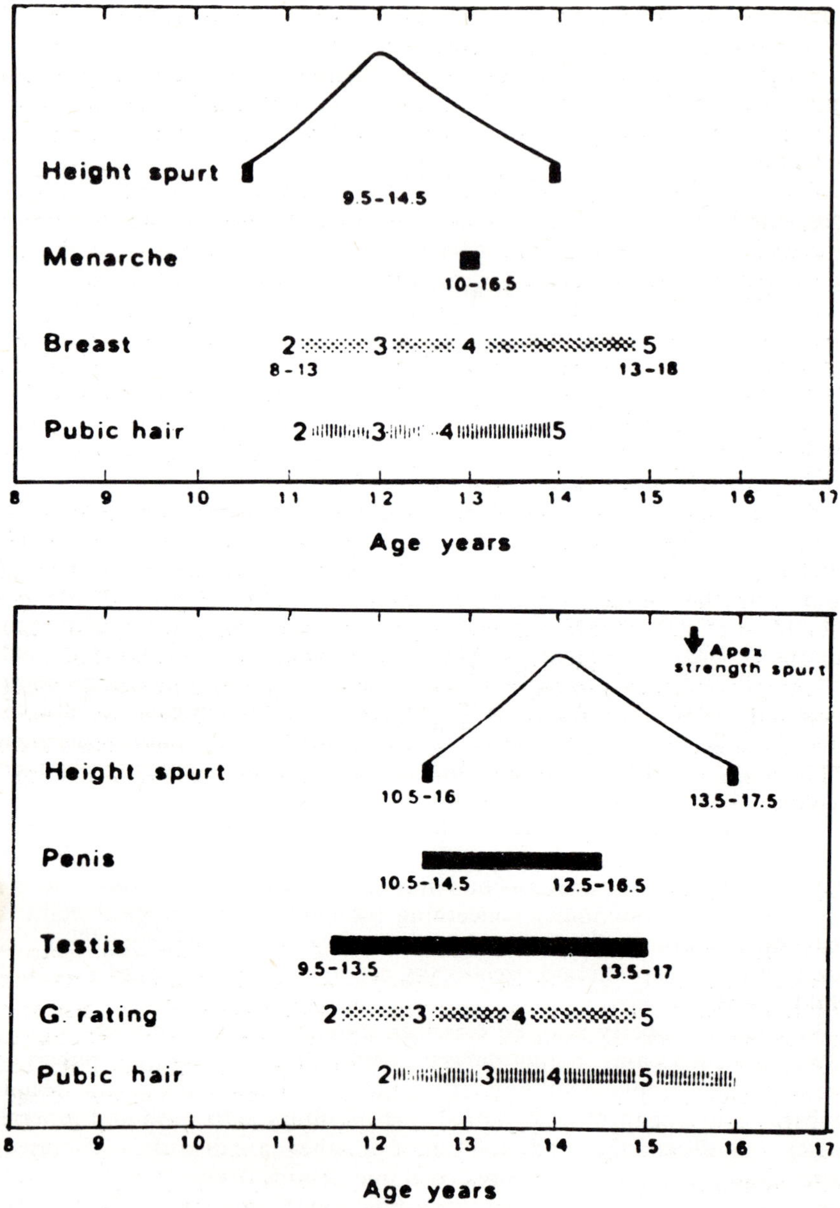

Figure 24.1 Diagrams of the sequence of the events at puberty. An average boy and girl represented in relation to the scale of ages: the range of ages within which some of the changes occur is indicated by the figures below them. (From Marshall and Tanner, 1970, by permission of *Archives of Diseases in Childhood.*)

Recklinghausen's disease, congenital adrenal hyperplasia (which can trigger early hypothalamic–pituitary–gonadal activation), familial and idiopathic precocious puberty (Styne and Grumbach, 1978).

Surgical treatment of hypothalamic hamartomas causing precocious puberty is usually not indicated and, even when undertaken, may not modify the ongoing pubertal process once the hypothalamic–pituitary axis has been activated.

Conventional therapy of true precocious puberty has been limited to the progestational agents, such as medroxyprogesterone acetate, to suppress gonadal secretion (Styne and Grumbach, 1978), or the use of the anti-androgen, cyproterone acetate, to antagonize the effects of sex steroids (Kauli *et al.*, 1976). These agents have not been uniformly successful in alleviating the progression of sexual maturation, and have had little effect on the rapid bone growth and early epiphyseal fusion that cause short stature as an adult (Lee, 1981). In addition, these drugs can have significant side-effects such as Cushingoid features, adrenal suppression and chromosomal breaks (Sadeghi-Nejad *et al.*, 1971; Mathews *et al.*, 1970; Kaplan *et al.*, 1968; Richman *et al.*, 1971; Camacho *et al.*, 1972; Rivarolo *et al.*, 1968).

An alternative approach to the therapy of true precocious puberty was suggested by the demonstration that the continuous administration of LHRH (Belchetz *et al.*, 1978; Brook and Dombey, 1979), or the intermittent administration of potent agonist analogs of LHRH (Happ *et al.*, 1978; Bergquist *et al.*, 1979*a,b*; Smith *et al.*, 1979; Linde *et al.*, 1981), will initially stimulate but subsequently inhibit the release of LH and FSH. This phenomenon appears to represent an uncoupling of LHRH receptor occupation and the pituitary response. This property of LHRH agonists suggested that these agents might be useful as a treatment for true precocious puberty. This chapter will describe the results of LHRH analog administration to children with true precocious puberty.

SHORT TERM THERAPY

The first group of children included five females with idiopathic true precocious puberty (Comite *et al.*, 1981*b*). The LHRH analog [D-Trp^6,Pro^9-NHEt]LHRH (LHRH-A) was given for 2 months. LHRH-A was dissolved in normal saline and 10% mannitol (Dermody and Reed, 1976). The parents were instructed to keep the preparation frozen until use. Subsequent studies have documented the short term stability of LHRH-A during repeated freezing and thawing, refrigeration, and mild heating (Winterer *et al.*, 1983). Each patient received LHRH-A at a dose of 4 μg/kg per day injected subcutaneously. During the 8th week of therapy, the patients were re-evaluated by the same protocol used before therapy. LHRH-A treatment was then discontinued in patients 1 to 3. These three patients returned during the 8th week after stopping therapy for a third inpatient evaluation identical to those performed before and during LHRH-A administration.

All the patients had measurable basal gonadotropin levels and a pubertal response to LHRH stimulation before therapy (Figure 24.2). After 8 weeks of treatment with LHRH-A, basal and peak gonadotropin levels fell signifi-

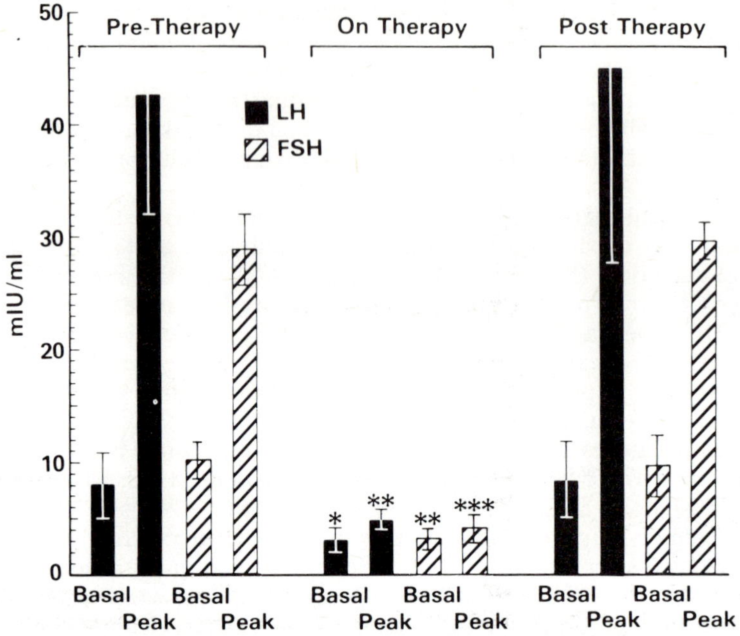

Figure 24.2 Effect of LHRH analog on basal and peak (LHRH-stimulated) gonadotropin levels in five girls with idiopathic precocious puberty (IPP). The basal LH and FSH values for each patient are means of 26 measurements performed at 20 min intervals from 10:00 a.m. to 2:00 p.m. and from 10:00 p.m. to 2:00 a.m. The peak values are the highest LH and FSH levels attained during the standard LHRH stimulation tests performed in each patient. The histograms represent the means + SEM of basal and peak values for each patient. The levels during therapy were measured during the 8th week of treatment. The post-therapy levels were measured in Patients 1–3, 8 weeks after discontinuation of LHRH-A treatment. Patients 4 and 5 continued to receive LHRH-A. (*) denotes $p < 0.025$, (**) $p < 0.01$, and (***) $p < 0.001$, as compared with pretreatment levels. (From Comite *et al.*, 1981*b*, by permission of *The New England Journal of Medicine.*)

cantly below pretreatment levels (Figure 24.2). Basal luteinizing hormone fell from 8 to 3 mIU/ml during treatment, and LHRH-stimulated peak luteinizing hormone fell from 43 to 5 mIU/ml. Basal follicle stimulating hormone declined from 10 to 3 and peak follicle stimulating hormone from 29 to 4 mIU/ml. Basal gonadotropins and the response to the LHRH stimulation test had returned to pretreatment levels 2 months after LHRH-A. Basal and peak luteinizing hormone were 8 and 45 mIU/ml. Basal follicle stimulating hormone was 10 and peak follicle stimulating hormone was 30 mIU/ml. Figure 24.3 shows the complete LHRH stimulation tests. LHRH-A completely suppressed the responses of luteinizing hormone and follicle stimulating hormone to exogenous LHRH. Two months after LHRH-A was discontinued, both the time course and the magnitude of the response to LHRH were nearly identical to the pubertal pattern observed before therapy.

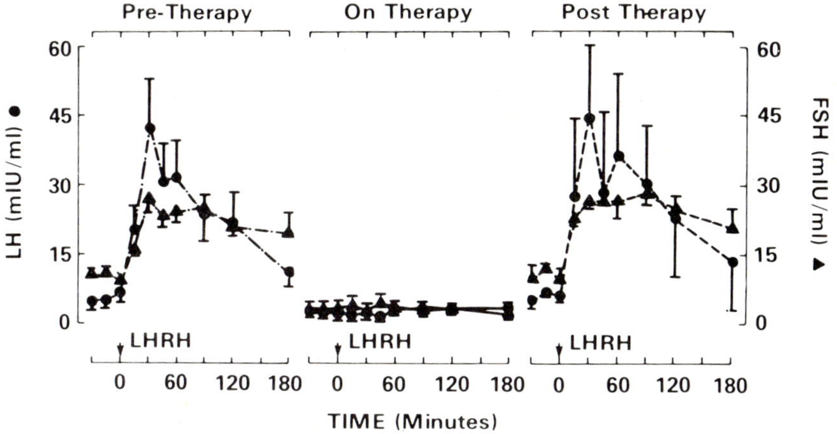

Figure 24.3 Effect of LHRH analog on gonadotropin response to exogenous LHRH in five girls with IPP. As in Figure 24.2, the post-therapy data are from Patients 1–3. (From Comite *et al.*, 1981*b*, by permission of *The New England Journal of Medicine*.)

Plasma estradiol concentrations also fell (from 28 to 16 pg/ml) by the 8th week of LHRH-A therapy. Two weeks after cessation of treatment, the level of plasma estradiol did not differ significantly from the pretreatment level. The maturation-index score decreased 25% after 8 weeks of treatment with LHRH-A – a change that did not reach statistical significance ($p = 0.09$). Two weeks after discontinuing LHRH-A, the maturation-index score had returned to the pretreatment value.

We measured adrenal androgen levels during treatment to determine whether LHRH-A influenced the adrenarchal component of puberty. The concentration of plasma dehydroepiandrosterone sulfate after 2 months of LHRH-A therapy was 19 μg/dl – not significantly different from the concentration before therapy (13 μg/dl).

INTERMEDIATE TERM THERAPY

The second study consisted of seven patients who were treated with LHRH-A continuously for 4 months (Comite *et al.*, 1981*a*) in order to assess clinical effects. Two children (one girl and one boy) had true precocious puberty secondary to a hypothalamic hamartoma while the remainder had idiopathic precocious puberty. Each patient was begun on LHRH-A at 4 μg/kg per day injected subcutaneously. All the patients returned to the NIH Clinical Center during the 4th month of treatment and were re-evaluated according to the same protocol as before therapy.

Following 4 months of LHRH-A, the levels of basal and stimulated gonadotropins were similar to those previously observed after 2 months of therapy (Figure 24.2). Plasma estradiol in the girls (Figure 24.4) fell from 37 to 13. The vaginal maturation-index score (MIS) (Figure 24.5) decreased

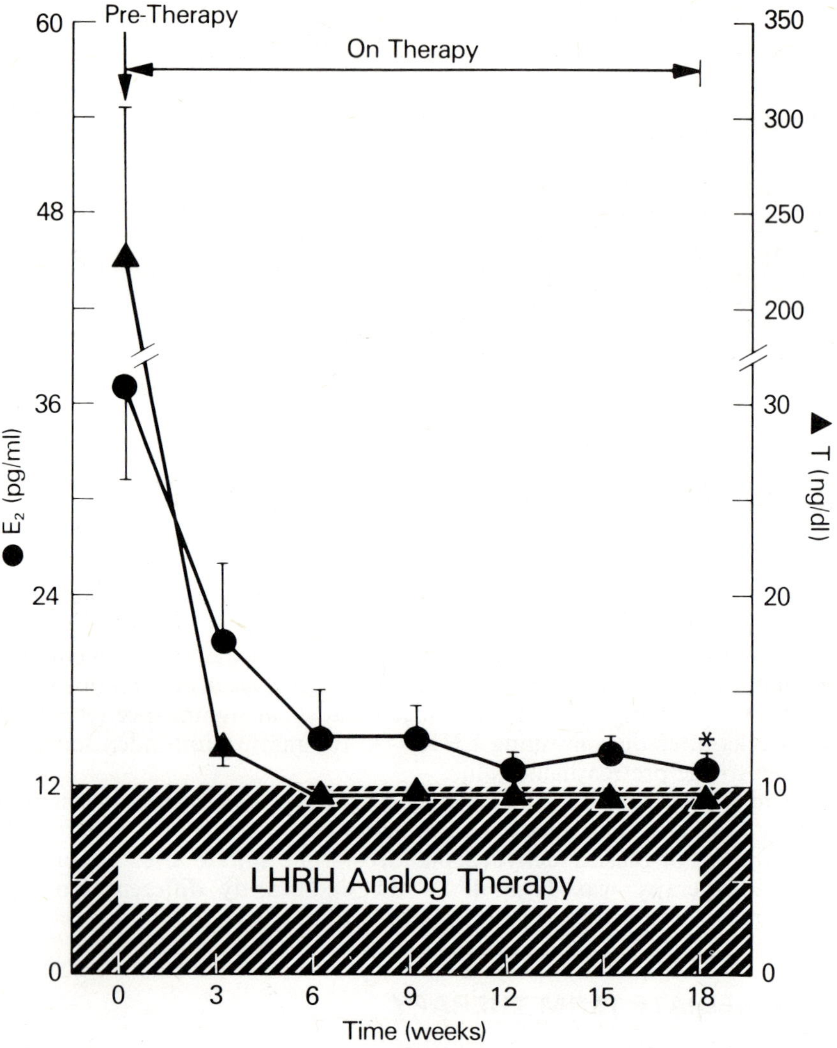

Figure 24.4 Effect of LHRH analog on plasma estradiol in six girls and plasma testosterone in one boy with true precocious puberty (TPP). Shaded area represents values below the detection limit of the assay. (*) denotes $p < 0.05$ as compared with pretreatment level.

significantly from 57 to 44, paralleling the fall in estradiol. Testosterone in the boy fell from 223 to < 10 by week 6 and remained < 10 throughout therapy (Figure 24.4).

Clinical changes (Table 24.1) included regression of breast size in four of the six girls, and loss of all pubic hair in two of the six girls. Testis size, measured by Prader orchidometer, regressed from 14 cc to 10 cc. No menses occurred during treatment.

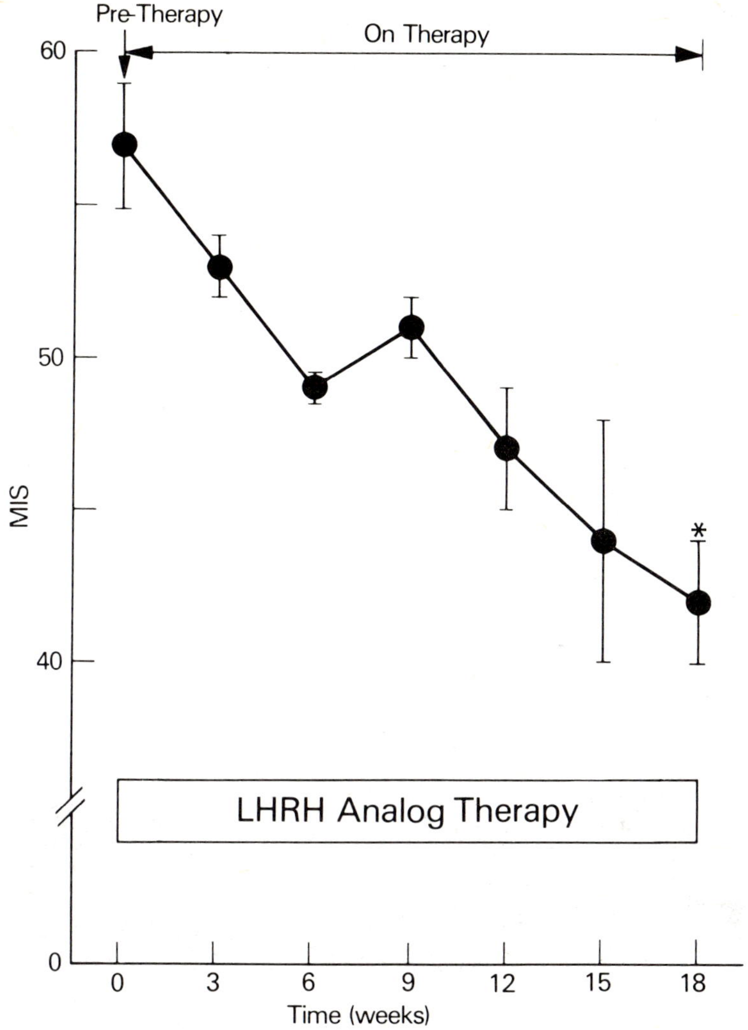

Figure 24.5 Effect of LHRH analog on vaginal maturation-index score in six girls with TPP. The vaginal maturation-index score, an index of estrogen effect on the vaginal mucosa, is calculated by adding the percentage superficial cells multiplied by 1.0 to the percentage of intermediate cells multiplied by 0.5 (Meisels, 1967). (*) denotes $p < 0.05$ as compared with pretreatment level.

LONG TERM THERAPY

Fifteen patients with true precocious puberty were treated for a period of 6–14 months with LHRH-A (Comite *et al.*, 1981*c*), a sufficient period for evaluation of changes in growth and bone age advancement. Growth parameters included linear growth velocity and bone age in all children, and ulnar growth

Table 24.1 Physical findings of seven patients with true precocious puberty before (pre) and after (on) 4 months of LHRH-A therapy

			Breast (Tanner Stage)		*Testes (cc)*		*Pubic hair (Tanner stage)*		*Menses*	
Patient	*Sex*	*Dx*	*Pre*	*On*	*Pre*	*On*	*Pre*	*On*	*Pre*	*On*
JN	F	HH	II	No change			II	No change	+	–
MH	F	IPP	III	↓[a]			III	No change	+	–
CJ	F	IPP	III	↓			II	I	–	–
TG	F	IPP	V	III			II	I	+	–
JS	F	IPP	III	↓			III	No change	–	–
KS	F	IPP	III	No change			III	No change	–	–
JE	M	HH			14	10	III	No change		

[a] = clinical decrease in breast size without change in Tanner Stage
HH = hypothalamic hamartoma; IPP = idiopathic precocious puberty

rate in seven of the 15 patients (Valk, 1971; Cassorla *et al*., 1981). The ulnar growth rate is determined by a measuring device which can detect changes in ulnar length over a 3-week period (Valk, 1971). It is an accurate and sensitive index of short term growth, and correlates well with long term linear growth.

Linear growth velocity (centimeters per year) prior to the onset of therapy in the 15 children was 13 cm/y and decreased significantly on treatment to 7 cm/y. The average growth rate on treatment did not differ significantly from the expected growth rate (7 cm/y) of normal children of the same age.

All patients had advanced bone age relative to their chronological age. Prior to therapy the rate of bone age advancement (years) per year of chronological age was 2.5. During therapy the bone age advanced 0.8 y per chronologic year.

Ulnar growth rate was determined in seven patients 2 months before and during LHRH-A administration (Figure 24.6). Ulnar growth rate (millimeters every 3 weeks) decreased from a pubertal rate of 1.00 to a prepubertal rate of 0.33 (Cassorla *et al*., 1981).

Secondary sexual characteristics showed continued improvement from the changes seen at 4 months. The females initially had Tanner II–V breasts and Tanner II–IV pubic hair (Tanner, 1978). Six of the girls had irregular vaginal bleeding. During LHRH-A therapy, breast size decreased in nine, and pubic hair in five of the 11 girls (Figure 24.7). No vaginal bleeding occurred during therapy. The males presented with Tanner II–IV pubic hair and testicular volumes of 10–25 ml. Facial hair was present in three of the boys. During LHRH-A therapy, facial and pubic hair decreased in three of the four boys (Figure 24.8). Testis size decreased from 15 to 10 ml.

Four children, who had been treated with LHRH-A continuously for 10 months, were taken off treatment at that time to assess the reversibility of treatment. Basal gonadotropins and the response to the LHRH stimulation test returned to pretreatment levels 2 months after discontinuing LHRH-A in the four patients.

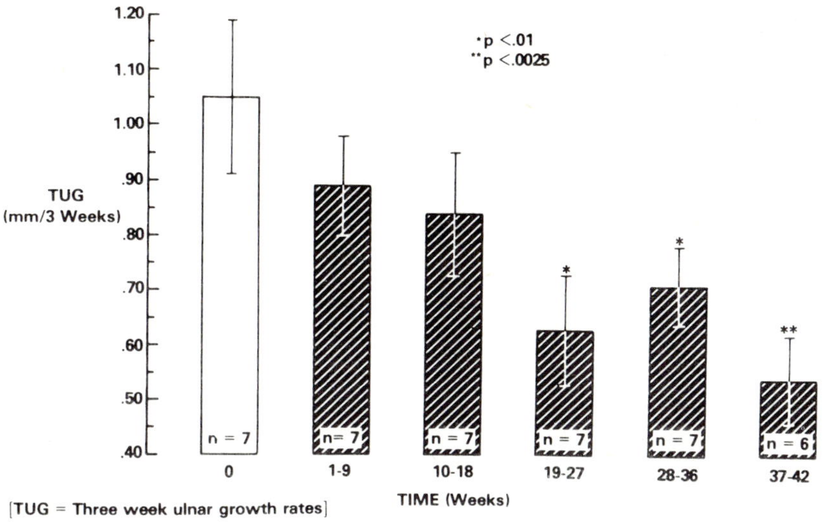

Figure 24.6 Effect of LHRH analog on ulnar growth rate in seven children with TPP. (*) denotes $p < 0.001$ as compared to pretreatment level. The histograms represent the means + SEM for each patient.

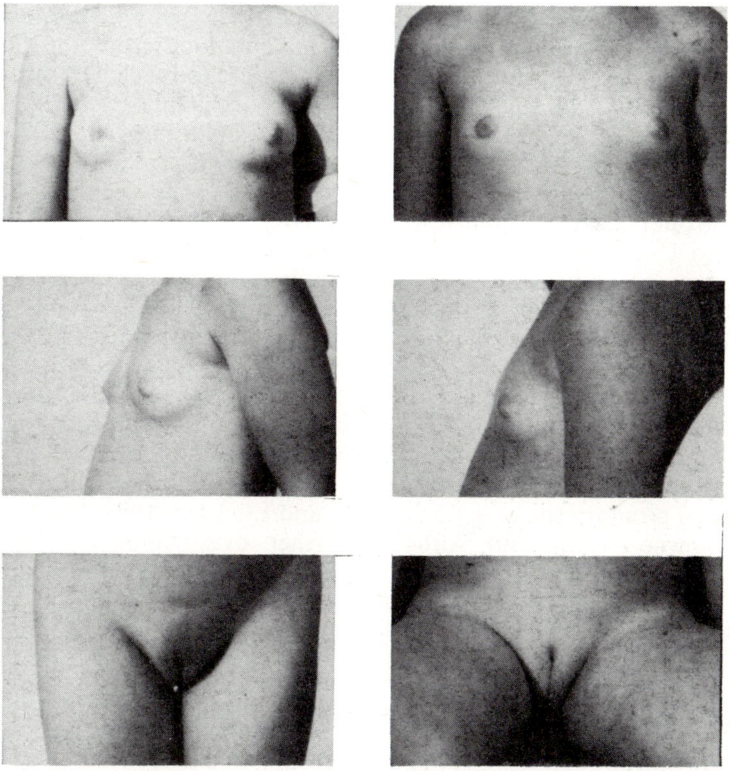

Figure 24.7 Effect of LHRH analog on breasts and pubic hair in a 5-year-old girl with IPP. In the left panel is pretreatment, and in the right panel is after 8 months of treatment.

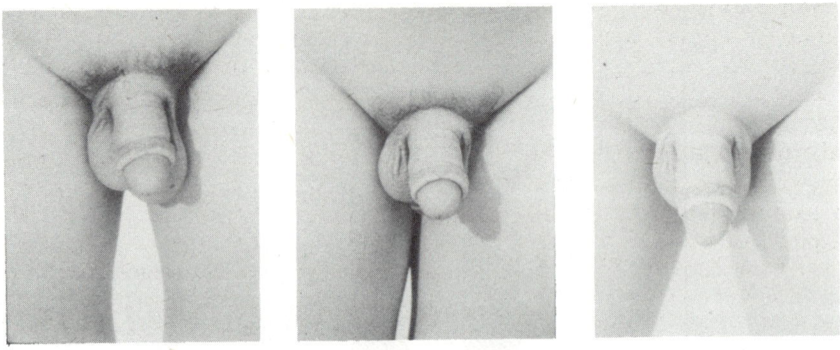

Figure 24.8 Effect of LHRH analog on testis and pubic hair in a 4-year-old boy with TPP secondary to a hypothalamic hamartoma. In the left panel is pretreatment, the center is after 6 months of treatment, and in the right panel is after 1 year of treatment.

DISCUSSION

General comments

Continuous administration of LHRH or intermittent administration of long acting LHRH analogs uncouples LHRH stimulation from the pituitary response and decreases pituitary gonadotropin secretion (Belchetz *et al.*, 1978; Comite *et al.*, 1981*b*; Rabin and McNeil, 1980; Wiegelmann *et al.*, 1979; Linde *et al.*, 1981; Davies *et al.*, 1977; Happ *et al.*, 1978; Bergquist *et al.*, 1979*b*; Vale *et al.*, 1977). The pituitary gonadotropins apparently require intermittent periods devoid of stimulation by LHRH or its analogs to maintain sustained gonadotropin release. Administration of LHRH-A daily over approximately 1 year to 15 patients produced continuous suppression of basal and peak gonadotropins and sex steroids to prepubertal levels. Secondary sexual characteristics regressed in all the children but to varying extents. Height velocity, bone age maturation and ulnar growth rate declined to the normal prepubertal rates.

Although these data provide convincing evidence that LHRH-A uncouples the pituitary response to LHRH, a direct effect on steroidogenesis at the gonadal level cannot be excluded. LHRH and its analogs can directly inhibit steroidogenesis by the ovary and testis in rats, in addition to exerting their effects at a pituitary site of action (Hsueh and Erickson, 1979; Clayton *et al.*, 1979; Bourne *et al.*, 1980). Although further investigation of this issue is needed, most investigators have concluded that the principal mechanism by which LHRH-A lowers sex steroid secretion is inhibition of pituitary gonadotropin release.

Use of LHRH-A as a diagnostic test

The uniformity of the response of gonadotropins and sex steroids to LHRH-A in true precocious puberty suggests that LHRH-A administration may provide a useful diagnostic test in the diagnosis of true precocious puberty. Failure of suppression during an adequate trial (4–6 weeks) of LHRH-A suggests that the diagnosis is unlikely to be true precocious puberty. We encountered one 5-year-old girl with precocious puberty and the McCune–Albright syndrome (*café-au-lait* pigmentation, polyostotic fibrous dysplasia and precocious puberty) in whom LHRH-A administration for 10 months did not significantly alter serum gonadotropins. Basal gonadotropins ranged from < 1 to 3 mIU/ml and LHRH-stimulated gonadotropins remained < 3 mIU/ml. Despite low gonadotropins, estradiol levels (in pg/ml) were 64 pretherapy, 893 at 3 weeks, 31 at 10 weeks, 220 at 13 weeks, 28 at 18 weeks, 814 at 25 weeks and 55 at 38 weeks. Estradiol levels appeared to correlate with an ovarian cyst (pelvic ultrasound). The left ovarian cyst was 2.0 cm at 0 weeks, 0.3 cm at 10 weeks, 0.4 cm at 18 weeks, 3.4 cm at 25 weeks, and 1.8 cm at 38 weeks (Comite *et al.*, 1981*d*). The failure of LHRH-A to alter cyclical ovarian cyst enlargement and estradiol secretion, despite suppressed gonadotropin levels, suggests a pseudopuberty mechanism for the precocious puberty in this patient. LHRH-A did not appear to inhibit steroidogenesis at the ovarian level in this patient.

LHRH antagonist analogs

We have used an LHRH agonist rather than an antagonist in our studies. Although both agonist and antagonist analogs of LHRH can inhibit gonadotropin secretion, only the agonist analogs have been shown to produce profound gonadotropin suppression with a single daily injection. However, the development of increasingly potent antagonist analogs of LHRH suggests that in the future it may be possible to compare LHRH agonists and antagonists in the therapy of precocious puberty (Rivier *et al.*, 1980).

Routes of administration

Currently, LHRH-A is administered via a subcutaneous route in children with precocious puberty. An alternate route would be via an intranasal spray. This would require an analog to be sufficiently soluble to dissolve 10–20 fold larger doses (since absorption across the nasal mucosa is generally about 5 %) in volumes suitable for a nasal spray (0.5 ml or less).

Intranasal LHRH analog administration suppresses ovulation in women (Bergquist *et al.*, 1979*b*) and lowers gonadotropins and testosterone in men with cancer of the prostate. Application of intranasal LHRH-A delivery to children with precocious puberty might be similarly effective.

CONCLUDING REMARKS

LHRH analog treatment of true precocious puberty appears very promising. No serious adverse effects have been seen in any children. Full recovery of gonadotropins and sex steroids was observed in all subjects in whom

LHRH- A administration has been discontinued. Regression of secondary sexual characteristics was noted in the majority of patients within several months of treatment. Preliminary results suggests that LHRH-A has been effective in decreasing linear and ulnar growth to normal prepubertal rates and in slowing the rapid bone maturation. Full assessment of the merits of this new therapy must await investigation of long term LHRH analog treatment on pubertal progression and ultimate adult stature.

Acknowledgements

We are indebted to Karen Hench, R. N., Ann McNemar, R. N., M. N. and the Clinical Center at the National Institutes of Health for their invaluable assistance in these studies. We gratefully acknowledge Barbara Filmore, Jeannie Combs, Mary Hall, Judy Aabel and Elizabeth Salvati for their technical assistance, and the referring physicians, associates, and fellows involved in this study for their support.

References

Belchetz, P. E., Plant, T. M., Nakai, U., Keogh, E. J. and Knobil, E. (1978). Hypophysial responses to continuous and intermittent delivery of hypothalamic gonadotropin-releasing hormone. *Science,* **202,** 631

Bergquist, C., Nillius, S. J. and Wide, L. (1979*a*). Reduced gonadotropin secretions in postmenopausal women during treatment with a stimulatory LRH analogue. *J. Clin. Endocrinol. Metab.,* **49,** 472

Bergquist, C., Nillius, S. J. and Wide, L. (1979*b*). Intranasal gonadotropin-releasing hormone agonist as a contraceptive. *Lancet,* **2,** 215

Bourne, G. A., Regiani, S., Payne, A. H. and Marshall, J. C. (1980). Testicular GnRH receptors – characterization and localization on interstitial tissue. *J. Clin. Endocrinol. Metab.,* **51,** 407

Boyar, R. M., Rosenfield, R. S., Kapan, S., Finkelstein, J. W., Roffwarg, H. P., Weitzman, E. D. and Hellman, L. (1974). Human puberty: Simultaneous augmented secretion of luteinizing hormone and testosterone during sleep. *J. Clin. Invest.,* **54,** 609

Brook, C. G. D. and Dombey, S. (1979). Induction of puberty: long-term treatment with high dose LHRH. *Clin. Endocrinol.,* **11,** 81

Camacho, A. M., Williams, D. L. and Montalvo, J. M. (1972). Alterations of testicular histology and chromosomes in patients with constitutional sexual precocity treated with medroxyprogesterone acetate. *J. Clin. Endocrinol.,* **34,** 279

Cassorla, F., Comite, F., Skerda, M., Valk, I. M., Cutler, G. B. Jr. and Loriaux, D. L. (1982). Ulnar growth deceleration in children with idiopathic precocious puberty (IPP) treated with an LHRH analog. *Society for Pediatric Research,* Washington D.C., April

Clayton, R. N., Harwood, J. P. and Catt, K. J. (1979). Gonadotropin-releasing hormone analogue binds to luteal cells and inhibits progesterone production. *Nature (Lond.),* **282,** 90

Comite, F., Crowley, W. F., Jr., Rivier, J., Vale, W. W., Loriaux, D. L. and Cutler, G. B. Jr. (1981*a*). Luteinizing-hormone releasing hormone analog therapy of true precocious puberty. In Grumbach, M. M. (ed.) *Second International Conference on the Control of the Onset of Puberty.* Serono Symposia, Stresia, Italy. (In press)

Comite, F., Cutler, G. B. Jr., Rivier, J., Vale, W. W., Loriaux, D. L. and Crowley, W. F. Jr. (1981*b*). Short-term treatment of idiopathic precocious puberty with a long-acting analogue of luteinizing hormone-releasing hormone. *N. Engl. J. Med.,* **305,** 1546

Comite, F., Hench, K., McNemar, A. and Dwyer, A. (1982). LHRH analog therapy in 15 children with true precocious puberty: effect on somatic growth and bone maturation. *Endocrine Society,* San Francisco, June

Comite, F., Shawker, T. H., Crowley, W. F. Jr., Loriaux, D. L. and Cutler, G. B., Jr. (1981*d*). Mechanism of precocious puberty in McCune–Albright Syndrome (MAS). Presented at *First Joint Meeting of the Lawson Wilkins Pediatric Endocrine Society and the European Society for Pediatric Endocrinology,* Geneva, Switzerland, No. 59

Comite, F., Schiebinger, R. J., Albertson, B. D., Cassorla, F. G., Vander Ven, K., Cullen, T. F., Loriaux, D. L. and Cutler, G. B. Jr. (1984). Isosexual precocious pseudopuberty secondary to a feminizing adrenal tumor. *J. Clin. Endocrinol. Metab.,* (In press)

Davies, T. F., Gomez-Pan, A., Watson, M. J., Mountjoy, C. Q., Hanker, J. P., Besser, G. and Hally, R. (1977). Reduced 'gonadotropin response to releasing hormone' after chronic administration to impotent men. *Clin. Endocrinol.,* **6,** 213

Dermody, W. C. and Reed, I. R. (1976). Effect of storage on LHRH. *N. Engl. J. Med.,* **295,** 173

Happ, J., Scholz, P., Weber, T., Corles, U., Schramm, P., Neubauer, M. and Beyer, J. (1978). Gonadotropin secretion in eugonadotropic human males and postmenopausal females under long-term application of a potent analog of gonadotropin-releasing hormone. *Fertil. Steril.,* **30,** 674

Hsueh, A. T. W. and Erickson, G. F. (1979). Extrapituitary action of gonadotropin-releasing hormone: direct inhibition of ovarian steroidogenesis. *Science,* **204,** 854

Kaplan, S. A., Ling, S. M. and Irani, N. G. (1968). Idiopathic isosexual precocity: Therapy with medroxyprogesterone acetate. *Am. J. Dis. Child.,* **116,** 591

Kauli, R., Pertzelan, A., Prager-Lewin, R., Günebaum, M. and Laron, Z. (1976). Cyproterone acetate in treatment of precocious puberty. *Arch. Dis. Child.,* **51,** 202

Lee, P. A. (1981). Medroxyprogesterone therapy for sexual precocity in girls. *Am. J. Dis. Child.,* **135,** 443

Linde, R., Dochle, G. C., Alexander, N., Kirchner, F., Vale, W., Rivier, J. and Rabin, D. (1981). Reversible inhibition of testicular steroidogenesis and spermatogenesis by a potent gonadotropin-releasing hormone agonist in normal men: an approach toward the development of a male contraceptive. *N. Engl. J. Med.,* **305,** 663

Marshall, W. A. and Tanner, J. M. (1970). Variations in the pattern of pubertal changes in boys. *Arch. Dis. Child.,* **45,** 13

Marshall, W. A. and Tanner, J. M. (1969). Variations in the pattern of pubertal changes in girls. *Arch. Dis. Child.,* **42,** 291

Mathews, J. H., Abrams, C. A. L. and Morishima, A. (1970). Pituitary–adrenal function in ten patients receiving medroxyprogesterone acetate for true precocious puberty. *J. Clin. Endocrinol.,* **30,** 653

Meisels, A. (1967). That maturation value. *Acta Cytol.,* **11,** 249

Rabin, D. and McNeil, L. W. (1980). Pituitary and gonadal desensitization after continuous luteinizing hormone-releasing hormone infusion in normal females. *J. Clin. Endocrinol. Metab.,* **51,** 873

Richman, R. A., Underwood, L. E., French, F. S. and Van Wyk, J. J. (1971). Adverse effects of large doses of medroxyprogesterone (MPA) in idiopathic isosexual precocity. *J. Pediatr.,* **79,** 963

Rivier, C., Rivier, J. and Vale, W. (1980). Antireproductive effects of a potent gonadotropin-releasing hormone in the male rat. *Science,* **210,** 93

Rivarolo, M. A., Camacho, A. M. and Migeon, C. J. (1968). Effect of treatment with medroxyprogesterone acetate (Provera) on testicular function. *J. Clin. Endocrinol.,* **28,** 679

Sadeghi-Nejad, A., Kaplan, S. L. and Grumbach, M. M. (1971). The effect of medroxyprogesterone acetate on adrenocortical function in children with precocious puberty. *J. Pediatr.,* **78,** 616

Smith, R., Donald, R. A., Espiner, E. A. and Stronach, S. (1979). The effects of prolonged administration of D-Ser(TBU)6-LH-RH-EA[10] (HOE 766) in subjects with hypogonadotropic hypogonadism. *Clin. Endocrinol.,* **11,** 553

Styne, D. M. and Grumbach, M. M. (1978). Puberty in the male and female; its physiology and disorders. In Yen, S. S. C. and Jaffe, R. B. (eds) *Reproductive Endocrinology: Physiology, Pathophysiology and Clinical Management,* pp. 234–35. (Philadelphia: Saunders)

Tanner, J. M. (1978). *Growth at Adolescence,* pp. 28–39. (Oxford: Blackwell)

Valk, I. M. (1971). Accurate measurement of the length of the ulna and its application in growth hormone. *Growth,* **36,** 297

Vale, W., Rivier, C., Brown, M. and Rivier, J. (1977). Pharmacology of thyrotropin releasing factor (TRF), luteinizing hormone releasing hormone (LRH), and somatostatin. *Adv. Exp. Med. Biol.*, **87,** 123

Wiegelmann, W., Solbach, H. G., Kley, H. K. and Kruskemper, H. L. (1977). LH and FSH response to long-term application of LH-RH analogue in normal males. *Horm. Metab. Res.*, **9,** 521

Winterer, J., Chatterji, D., Comite, F., Decker, M. H., Loriaux, D. L., Gallelli, J. F. and Cutler, G. B. Jr. (1983). Thermal stability of a long-acting analogue of luteinizing hormone releasing hormone (D-Trp^6-Pro^9-NEt-LHRH). *Contraception,* **27,** 195

25
LHRH analogs for human mammary carcinoma

H. A. HARVEY, A. LIPTON and D. T. MAX

The pioneering demonstration in 1890 by Sir George Beatson (Beatson, 1896) that metastatic breast cancer in women could be successfully palliated by surgical castration led to the use of endocrine therapy for this disease. Today, hormonal therapy is a safe, simple and highly effective means of controlling advanced breast cancer in patients whose tumors are estrogen receptor rich (McGuire *et al.*, 1977). The endocrine ablative techniques of hypophysectomy and adrenalectomy are giving way to the use of antiestrogens and other non-surgical estrogen-suppressive techniques (Kiang *et al.*, 1980; Harvey *et al.*, 1979; Santen *et al.*, 1981). The use of steroid hormones continues to be an effective therapy (Kennedy, 1974). Approximately 100 000 women undergo mastectomy for breast cancer each year in the United States. One third of these patients will have hormone-dependent tumors as defined by the presence of estrogen receptors. Sixty per cent of these women will ultimately develop metastatic disease. Thus, a large number of women become candidates for palliative endocrine therapy. An even larger number of patients would require this type of treatment if the use of hormones as an adjunct to surgery becomes accepted (Meakin, 1980; Fisher *et al.*, 1981). It is a common clinical observation that two or more forms of endocrine therapy may be used sequentially to the benefit of the patient with advanced disease. Thus, the addition of new forms of endocrine treatment with unique mechanisms of therapeutic action might potentially add to the clinician's armamentarium and have a wide application. The LHRH analogs, a new class of compounds, provide such an intriguing possibility.

ANIMAL STUDIES AND RATIONALE

The chronic administration of LHRH analogs produces a paradoxical inhibition of pulsatile LH and FSH secretion by the pituitary leading to suppression of gonadal steroidogenesis. The DMBA (7,12-dimethylbenzanthracene) induced rat mammary carcinoma is a hormonally sensitive tumor and was used in the first studies of a therapeutic effect of chronically administered LHRH analogs.

A 50% response rate was reported in Sprague–Dawley rats bearing DMBA induced tumors following the chronic daily subcutaneous injection of the LHRH agonist [D-Leu^{6},Pro^{9}-NHEt]LHRH (Johnson *et al.*, 1976; DeSombre *et al.*, 1976). The effects of the potent agonist [D-Ser (tBu)^{6},AzaGly^{10}]LHRH on DMBA induced rat mammary tumors were also studied (Nicholson *et al.*, 1978). This agent was administered twice daily by intramuscular injection over 3 weeks. Animals with strongly estrogen receptor (ER) positive tumors exhibited a high rate of regression similar to that seen following either oophorectomy or treatment with tamoxifen. The elevation of plasma LH and FSH levels was followed by decreased circulating estradiol concentrations and thus the inhibition of tumor growth resulted from estrogen withdrawal. The administration of [D-Leu^{6},Pro^{9}-NHEt]LHRH in both the DMBA and *N*-Nitrosomethylurea induced rat mammary carcinoma models led to similar conclusions (Rose and Pruitt, 1979, Pruitt, *et al.*, 1979). Treatment with [D-Ala^{6},Pro^{9}-NHEt]LHRH inhibited the growth of mouse mammary carcinoma inoculated into immunosuppressed weanling hamsters (Corbin *et al.*, 1980). This analog also inhibited tumor growth in the DMBA rat model (Turcot-Lemay *et al.*, 1981). It was therefore proposed that superagonists of LHRH could be used to induce a functional castration in women with metastatic breast cancer (Nicholson *et al.*, 1978; Corbin, 1982).

The primary mechanism by which LHRH analogs lead to regression of estrogen dependent mammary tumors in animals is by the inhibition of ovarian production of estrogens. The superagonists of LHRH also may have direct gonadal or end-organ effects (Sundaram *et al.*, 1981). There is evidence that the growth of mammary carcinoma in these rodent tumor systems may depend on other hormones such as prolactin or growth hormone (Sterental *et al.*, 1963; Arafah *et al.*, 1980). The importance of these hormones in controlling the growth of human breast carcinoma has not been clearly established. (Manni *et al.*, 1979).

CLINICAL EXPERIENCE

One multicenter trial has evaluated the safety and endocrine effects of [D-Leu^{6},Pro^{9}-NHEt]LHRH (leuprolide) in a group of postmenopausal patients with advanced breast cancer (Harvey *et al.*, 1981). Patients received the analog in a dose of 1–10 mg by daily s.c. injection. A total of 72 patients was studied. The first 31 patients had undergone extensive prior treatment with chemotherapy, multiple forms of endocrine therapy and all had far-advanced disease. Subsequent patients were chosen to be of better performance status and had not received more than two previous endocrine manipulations. There was no clinical or laboratory evidence of side-effects. There was an initial rise followed by a persistent decline of both plasma FSH and LH (Figure 25.1). Ten per cent of the patients had an objective partial response of soft tissue metastases (defined as > 50% decrease in measurable disease) for a median duration of 20 weeks. Twenty-two per cent of all women experienced stabilization of their disease. This low level of objective tumor response is not surprising, as any biologic activity of the analog in this group of patients defies

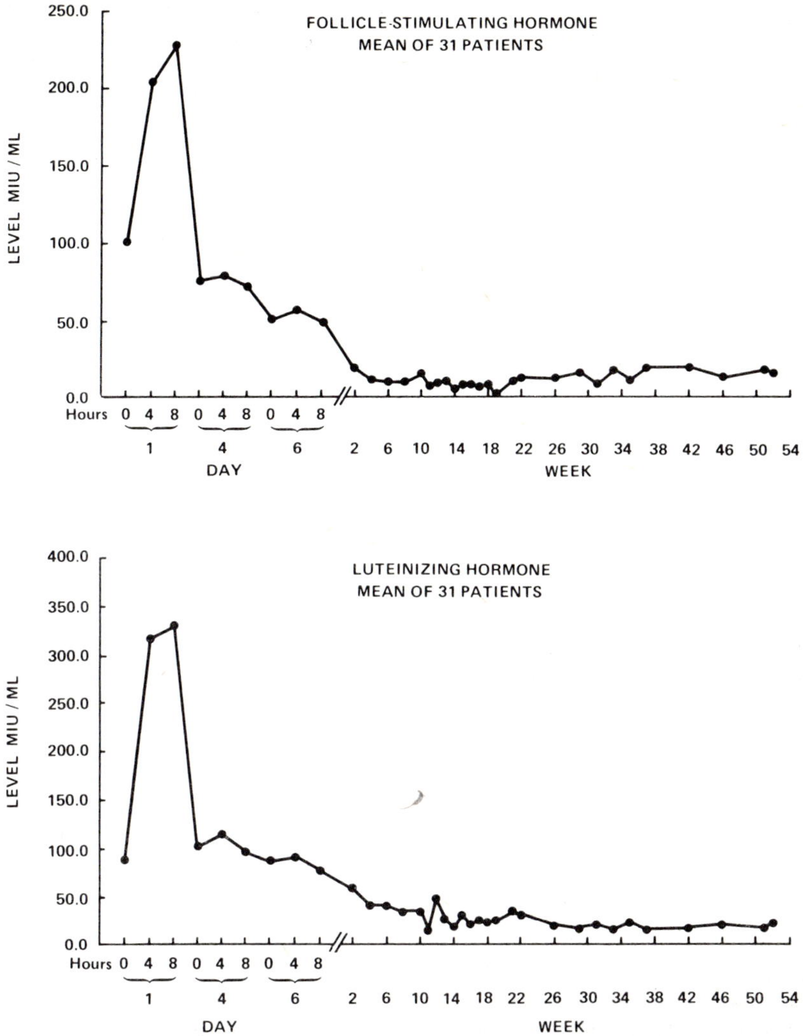

Figure 25.1 Serum FSH and LH levels in 31 breast cancer patients treated with [D-Leu^6,Pro^9-NHEt]LHRH (1 mg s.c. daily).

a facile explanation, since responders could not be distinguished from non-responders on the basis of plasma estrone, estradiol, cortisol or other hormone levels (Schneir *et al.*, 1981).

In another study, four premenopausal patients were treated with [D-Ser (tBu)^6,Pro^9-NHEt]LHRH (buserelin). The analog was administered by intravenous infusion over 8 h on 7 successive days in three patients and as a constant i.v. infusion for 3 days in the fourth patient (Klijn & De Jong, 1982). The intravenous dose of the analog was 3 mg/day. Following the infusion period medication was continued intranasally by 200–400 μg administered three times daily. No side-effects were noted from these doses of the analog. Plasma LH and FSH levels were markedly suppressed after about 2 weeks of treatment. Plasma estradiol fell to castrate levels in all patients, although two of them showed transient elevations periodically. Two patients experienced clinically useful objective tumor regression and a third had stabilization of her disease through the follow-up period of 20 weeks.

Observations in three premenopausal patients treated by the present authors also illustrate the potential therapeutic role for the LHRH analogs in advanced breast cancer. The first patient had several lytic bone metastases. Treatment with leuprolide in a dose of 5 mg s.c. daily led to partial healing of some of these lesions, as demonstrated by the skull radiographs (Figure 25.2). This response lasted for 34 weeks. On progression, the patient was treated with tamoxifen with a further satisfactory clinical response. A second patient with a malignant pleural effusion and progressive vertebral metastases was considered not to be a good surgical risk to undergo oophorectomy because of severe heart disease. She received leuprolide 1 mg s.c. daily and achieved excellent stabilization and increasing sclerosis of bone disease for a period of 88 weeks. The final patient had rapid progression of both soft tissue and visceral metastases. All three patients developed amenorrhea shortly after the start of therapy with this LHRH analog. In the two responding patients plasma estrone and estradiol levels were reduced to castrate levels. The third patient showed no significant change of these hormones from pretreatment values. Table 25.1 summarizes the clinical data on these three premenopausal patients. Preliminary analysis of a further study in 30 patients suggests a frequency of positive response with this analog comparable to that expected for oophorectomy or antiestrogen therapy (Harvey and Max, unpublished observations).

FUTURE DIRECTIONS

Large scale clinical trials are needed to confirm a therapeutic role for the LHRH analogs in the overall management of human breast cancer and other hormonally dependent tumors. These trials must establish optimal dosage and schedules. Complete suppression of plasma estrogens may not be achievable in some patients and may not always be a prerequisite for optimal tumor response. The reversibility of the estrogen suppression following long term therapy with the agonist in cancer patients has not yet been addressed. The cessation of therapy following a response to chronic analog administration may be associated with a tumor flare, as has been noted in some animal studies. It remains to be established whether successful medical castration will predict for or preclude success of subsequent hormonal manipulations. Future studies should involve randomized comparisons of LHRH analogs against oophorectomy and tamoxifen in premenopausal women with ER positive metastatic breast cancer. Subsequent studies should then examine an optimal sequence of therapy and also the benefit of LHRH analogs in combination with other forms of hormonal therapy (e.g. antiestrogens or

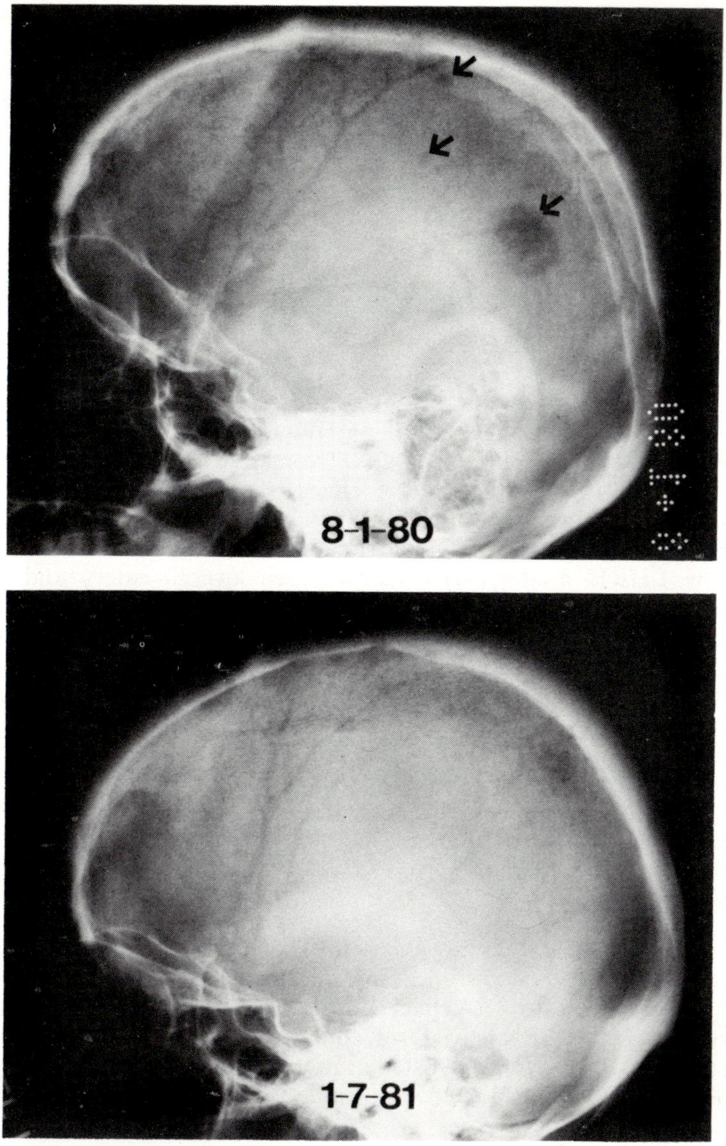

Figure 25.2 Skull radiographs of Patient 1 (see text).

progestins) or chemotherapy. Finally, the LHRH analogs could have a potential role as adjuvant therapy following mastectomy in young women with ER positive primary tumors and a high risk of developing recurrent disease.

Table 25.1 Hormonal and clinical features in premenopausal patients with advanced breast cancer treated with [D-Leu[6],Pro[9]-NHEt]LHRH

Patient	*Age* (y)	*Hormonal values decrease from pretreatment levels (day 56)*				*Metastasis site*	*Response (duration)*
		LH	*FSH*	E_1	E_2		
1	52	86%	83%	28%	38%	Bone	Partial (34 weeks)
2	43	53%	23%	57%	68%	Bone; pleura	Stable (88 weeks)
3	50	0	0	18%	0	Bone; skin	Progression

CONCLUDING REMARKS

Evidence from the study of hormone-dependent mammary carcinomas in animal model systems suggests a therapeutic role for the LHRH analogs in treating breast cancer in premenopausal women. These studies indicate that the mechanism of this therapeutic effect is the suppression of ovarian production of estrogen resulting from the inhibition of pituitary gonadotropins. Early clinical trials of 'medical castration' in breast cancer patients using the LHRH analogs demonstrate their overall safety and hint at therapeutic efficacy but are too preliminary to be conclusive. Yet this class of peptide compounds offers great promise as a new and useful therapeutic tool in the management of estrogen-dependent human tumors. Further clinical trials must establish an effectiveness of the LHRH analogs comparable to available antiestrogens or the simple endocrine ablative procedures currently used in managing breast cancer. The widespread acceptance of analogs of LHRH in this new therapeutic role will also critically depend on the development of convenient dose schedules and drug formulations at acceptable cost.

Acknowledgements

The authors wish to acknowledge the collaboration of the following investigators who provided clinical information on their patients: George C. Escher, Mark A. Hardy, Michael L. Glode, Albert Segaloff, Richard L. Landau and Harvey Schneir. Dr Kenneth Roberts performed hormonal assays and Mrs Judy Weigel assisted in preparation of the manuscript. Drug for studies with leuprolide was kindly supplied by TAP Pharmaceuticals/Abbott Laboratories.

References

Arafah, B. M., Manni, A. and Pearson, O. H. (1980). Effect of hypophysectomy and hormone replacement on hormone receptor levels and the growth of 7,12-dimethylbenz (a) anthracene-induced mammary tumors in the rat. *Endocrinology*, **107**, 1364

Beatson, G. W. (1896). On the treatment of inoperable cases of carcinoma of the mamma: suggestions for a new method of treatment with illustrative cases. *Lancet*, **2**, 104, 162

Corbin, A. (1982). From contraception to cancer: A review of the therapeutic applications of LHRH analogues as antitumor agents. *Yale J. Biol. Med.*, **55**, 27

Corbin, A., Rosanoff, E. and Bex, F. J. (1980). LHRH and LHRH-like synthetic agonists: paradoxical antifertility effects and their therapeutic relevance to steroid dependent tumors. In Iacobelli, S., Lindner, H. R., King, R. J. B. and Lippman, M. E. (eds.) *Progress in Cancer Research and Therapy,* Vol. 14: *Hormones and Cancer,* pp. 533–540. (New York: Raven Press)

DeSombre, E. R., Johnson, E. S. and White, W. F. (1976). Regression of rat mammary tumors effected by a gonadoliberin analog. *Cancer Res.,* **36,** 3830

Fisher, B., Redmond, C., NSAB investigators (1981). Treatment of primary breast cancer with chemotherapy and tamoxifen. *N. Engl. J. Med.,* **305,** 1

Harvey, H. A., Santen , R. J., Osterman, J., Samojlik, E., White, D. S. and Lipton, A. (1979). A comparative trial of transsphenoidal hypophysectomy and estrogen suppression with aminoglutethimide in advanced breast cancer. *Cancer,* **43,** 2207

Harvey, H. A., Lipton, A., Santen, R. J., Escher, G. C., Hardy, M. N., Glode, L. M., Segaloff, A., Landau, R. Z., Schneir, H. and Max, D. T. (1981). Phase II study of a gonadotropin-releasing hormone analogue (Leuprolide) in postmenopausal advanced breast cancer patients. *Proc. Am. Assoc. Cancer Res./Am. Soc. Clin. Oncol.,* **22,** 444 (abstract).

Johnson, E. S., Seely, J. H., White, W. F. and DeSombre, E. R. (1976). Endocrine-dependent rat mammary tumor regression: use of a gonadotropin releasing hormone analog. *Science,* **194,** 329

Kennedy, B. J. (1974). Hormonal therapies in breast cancer. In Yarbro, J. W., Bornstein, R. S. and Mastrangelo, M. J. (eds.) *Seminars in Oncology.* Vol. 1:2, pp. 119–130. (New York: Grune & Stratton)

Kiang, D. T., Frenning, D. H., Vosika, G. J. nd Kennedy, B. J. (1980). Comparison of tamoxifen and hypophysectomy in breast cancer treatment. *Cancer,* **45,** 1322

Klijn, J. G. and De Jong, F. H. (1982). Treatment with a luteinizing-hormone-releasing-hormone analogue (buserelin) in premenopausal patients with metastatic breast cancer. *Lancet,* **1,** 1213

McGuire, W. L., Horwitz, K. B., Pearson, O. H. and Segaloff., A. (1977). Current status of estrogen and progesterone receptors in breast cancer. *Cancer,* **39,** 2934

Manni, A., Pearson, O. H., Brodkey, J. and Marshall, J. S. (1979). Transphenoidal hypophysectomy in breast cancer. Evidence for an individual role of pituitary and gonadal hormones in supporting tumor growth. *Cancer,* **44,** 2330

Meakin, J. W. (1980). Is there a place for adjuvant endocrine therapy of breast cancer? *Rec. Results Cancer Res.,* **71,** 178

Nicholson, R. I., Finney, E. J. and Maynard, P. V. (1978). Activity of a new analogue of luteinizing hormone releasing hormone, ICI118630, on the growth of rat mammary tumours. *J. Endocrinol.,* **79,** 51P–52P

Nicholson, R. I. and Maynard, P. V. (1979). Antitumor activity of ICI118630, a new potent luteinizing hormone-releasing hormone agonist. *Br. J. Cancer,* **39,** 268

Pruitt, B., Rose, D. P. and Bryan, G. T. (1979). Hormone dependence of N-nitrosomethyl-urea (NMU)-induced rat mammary tumors: response to two modes of antiestrogen therapy. *Proc. Am. Assoc.Cancer Res.,* **20,** 87 (abstract)

Rose, D. P. and Pruitt, B., (1979). Modification of the effect of a gonadoliberin analog on 7,12-dimethy-benz(a)-anthracene-induced rat mammary tumors by hormone replacement. *Cancer Res.,* **39,** 3968

Santen, R. J., Worgul, T. J., Samojlik, E., Interrante, A., Boucher, A. E., Lipton, A., Harvey, H. A., White, D. S., Smart, E., Cox, C. and Wells, S. A. (1981). Randomized trial comparing surgical adrenalectomy with aminogluthimide plus hydrocortisone in women with advanced breast carcinoma. *N. Engl. J. Med.,* **305,** 545

Schneir, H. E., Landau, R. L., Max, D., Harvey, H. A., Lipton, A., Escher, C., Hardy, M.A., Glode, M. L. and Segaloff, A. (1981). The endocrine effect of chronic treatment with a gonadotropin releasing hormone analogue. The Endocrine Society 63rd annual meeting. *Endocrinology,* **108,** Suppl. 369 (abstract)

Sterental, A., Dominguez, J. M., Weissman, C. and Pearson, O. H. (1963). Pituitary role in the estrogen dependency of experimental mammary cancer. *Cancer Res.,* **23,** 481

Sundaram, K., Cao, Y. O. and Wang, N. G. (1981). Inhibition of the action of steroids by gonadotropin-releasing hormone (GnRH) agonists: a new biological effect. *Life Sci.,* **28,** 83

Turcot-Lemay, L., Cusan, L., Séguin, C., Kelly, P. and Labrie, F. (1981). Effect of an LHRH analog on growth and hormone receptor levels in DMBA-induced mammary tumors in the rat. *J. Receptor Res.,* **2,** 135

26
Buserelin therapy for prostatic carcinoma

N. FAURE, A. LEMAY, G. TOLIS, F. LABRIE, A. BÉLANGER and A. T. A. FAZEKAS

The synthesis of potent LHRH analogs was achieved with the aim of developing compounds of longer duration of action and greater potency than the native decapeptide for use in the treatment of infertility or hypothalamic hypogonadal states. However, these new molecules have potent antireproductive effects first noticed during toxicity trials in animals: disruption of estrous cycles, interference with implantation, interruption of pregnancy and, in the male, involution of the prostate and seminal vesicles and impaired spermatogenesis.

The disrupted secretion of pituitary LH (inappropriately high levels with loss of the pulsatile pattern) induced by the potent agonists was followed by inhibitory effects on gonadal LH receptor number and activity. The loss of gonadotropin receptors along with a probable direct action of the LHRH agonist at the gonadal level led to a marked decrease in testicular steroidogenesis in the rat (Arimura *et al.*, 1979; Auclair *et al.*, 1977; Bélanger *et al.*, 1980*a*). The inhibition of gonadal function led to a number of potential applications of LHRH agonists. A clinical application under intensive study is cancer of the prostate.

HORMONAL DEPENDENCE OF PROSTATIC CANCER

Prostatic carcinoma is the third cause of death by cancer in men. Growth and maintenance of the prostate is dependent on the presence of circulating androgens. It is generally accepted that the majority of carcinomas of the prostate are androgen dependent at least in part. The introduction of hormonal manipulation (Huggins *et al.*, 1941) revolutionized the treatment of the disease with a 70% positive, if temporary, response. However, conventional therapies have major drawbacks: castration has an adverse psychological impact; the use of high doses of estrogens is often associated with cardiovascular effects, limiting hormonal therapy to the late stages of the disease (Bailar *et al.*, 1970; Hedlund *et al.*, 1980).

The majority of patients have advanced disease when the diagnosis of prostatic carcinoma is first made. Palliative therapy is thus of major importance since the majority of patients cannot be treated by radical surgery. Significant improvements in survival in this disease would require the development of new approaches for early detection of the disease, new prophylactic measures or the development of new forms of therapy. Suppression of testicular androgens secondary to the paradoxical inhibition by chronic LHRH agonist treatment could be a valuable approach.

SENSITIVITY TO LHRH AGONIST IN MEN

Dose–response studies

Prolonged treatment with repetitive administration of LHRH agonists in men is associated with a loss of responsiveness of the gonadotropes to the neurohormone (Hashimoto *et al.*, 1975; Davies *et al.*, 1977). The administration of a potent LHRH agonist, [D-Ser(tBu)^6,Pro^9-NHEt]LHRH (buserelin) subcutaneously (s.c.) at the daily dose of 5 μg for 1 week led to decreased serum testosterone levels (Smith *et al.*, 1979). When the same LHRH analog was administered once intranasally, a transient rise of steroid levels on the day of its administration was followed by a loss of diurnal variation and a decrease of serum testosterone and dihydrotestosterone levels on days 2 and 3. This was followed by a return to normal cyclicity and levels at later time intervals (Bélanger *et al.*, 1980*b*). The importance of using a maximal dose of LHRH analogs for efficient inhibitory effects at the testicular level has been demonstrated in male rats (Labrie *et al.*, 1978).

Thirty-six volunteers (six per group) received, after informed consent, a single dose of 50, 100, 200, 500 , 1250 or 2500 μg of buserelin by nasal spray. The intranasal (i.n.) route of administration of the potent LHRH agonist buserelin was chosen because of its ease of application and potential widespread use in clinical investigations. Blood samples were collected at various time intervals to measure the extent and duration of the LH response. The serum LH response is minimal and of a very short duration at the two lowest doses used, while a near-maximal effect is obtained at the 200 μg dose, usually 2 h after its administration (Figure 26.1). A longer duration of action of the peptide is seen with increasing doses, the elevation from baseline levels being still significant after 8 and 14 h for the 1250 and 2500 μg doses, respectively.

Site of action of testicular suppression

Figure 26.2 shows the effect of increasing doses of intranasal buserelin on serum levels of testosterone. The administration of buserelin is followed by a loss of the diurnal cyclicity of circulating androgens at all doses studied. After 200 μg or more of buserelin i.n., an initial rise in testosterone levels is followed by a decrease of the level of the steroid during post-treatment days 1–3. Thereafter, there is a return to normal circadian cyclicity. A similar pattern has

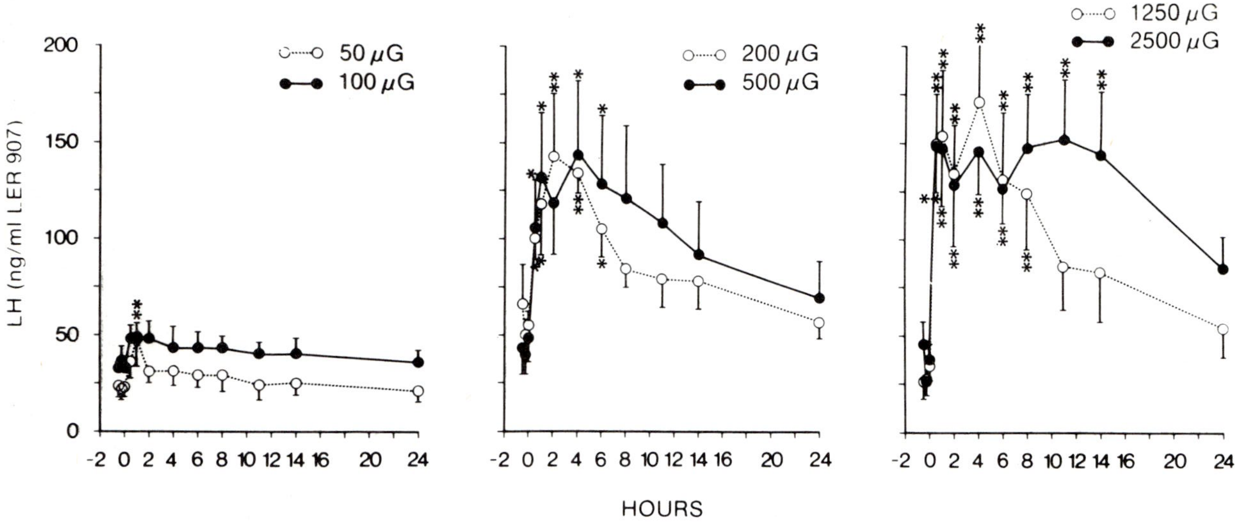

Figure 26.1 Effect of single intranasal administration of increasing doses of buserelin in young adult men on serum LH levels. Data are expressed as means ±SEM of values obtained from six subjects per group.*, $p<0.05$;**, $p<0.01$.

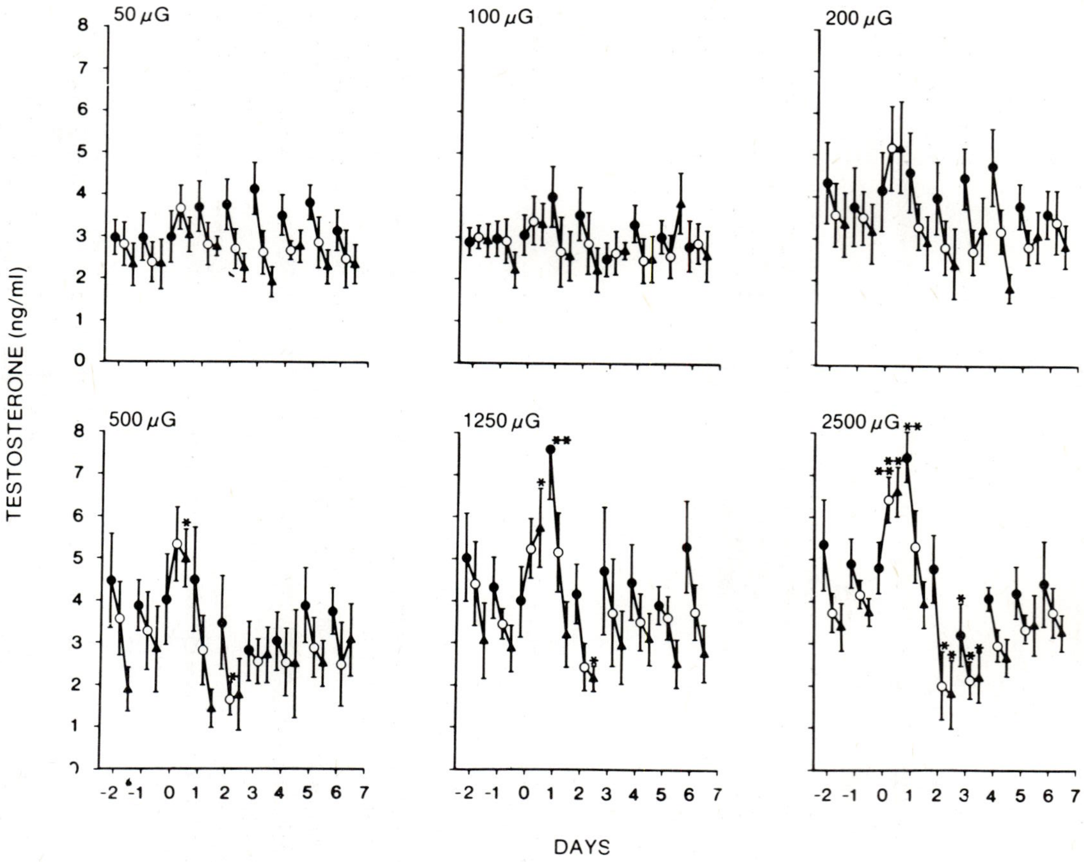

Figure 26.2 Effect of single intranasal administration of increasing doses of buserelin in young adult men on serum testosterone levels measured at 08:00 (●——●), 15:00 (○——○) and 22:00 (▲——▲)h. Serum testosterone levels were measured on 2 pretreatment, 1 treatment and 6 post-treatment days.

been obtained on serum 17 OH-progesterone levels. On the other hand there were no significant changes in serum levels of the steroid precursors pregnenolone and progesterone.

Unchanged levels of pregnenolone, in the presence of decreased 17α OH-progesterone and testosterone concentrations, suggest that a block of 17-hydroxylase and 17, 20 desmolase activity takes place in the human testis. The time-course of action on serum 17 OH-progesterone and testosterone levels in men resembles that found in the rat. A blockade of testicular 17α-hydroxylase and 17,20-desmolase activities has been demonstrated in this species following an acute dose of LHRH agonist (Bélanger *et al.*, 1979, 1980*a*).

Thus the acute inhibitory effects in the human might also be due to the blockade of steroid biosynthesis. No data are available on possible down regulation of testicular gonadotropin receptors under similar conditions. A possible direct action of LHRH on testis appears unlikely since no LHRH receptors could be identified in the human testis (Clayton and Huhtaniemi, 1982).

TESTICULAR ANDROGEN INHIBITION WITH LHRH AGONISTS IN MEN

Chronic administration to normal men

Daily treatment of normal adult men with 5 μg of buserelin s.c. for 1–17 weeks resulted in decreased serum testosterone levels (Happ *et al.*, 1978; Bergquist *et al.*, 1979; Smith *et al.*, 1979). Daily s.c. injections of [D-Trp^6,Pro^9-NHEt]LHRH were administered to men for 6–10 weeks to evaluate its antispermatogenic potential. A consistent and reversible inhibition of testosterone levels was obtained (Linde *et al.*, 1981). The induction of functional castration in male transsexuals (Tolis *et al.*, 1981) by administration of [D-Trp^6]LHRH for periods of 2–6 months supports the use of LHRH agonists for therapy of prostatic carcinoma.

Chronic administration to men with cancer of the prostate

Buserelin was administered at the dose of 200 and 500 μg twice daily i.n. for 9–34 weeks to patients with a histologic diagnosis of cancer of the prostate. At the end of the various treatment periods, serum testosterone was unchanged by the 200 μg dose but was inhibited by 71% at the 500 μg dose level. The decreases began after a delay of 2–5 weeks. The time-course and the maximal degree of inhibition was variable between different subjects and ranged from no change or a slight stimulation in a few cases to a 92% inhibition (Faure *et al.*, 1982).

Because of the high interindividual variation of the steroidogenic blockade after i.n. administration of the peptide, a daily subcutaneous dose of 50 μg was evaluated. Testosterone levels were 60–75% inhibited after only 1 week of treatment (Figure 26.3). The plasma LH levels were elevated for 1 month, then

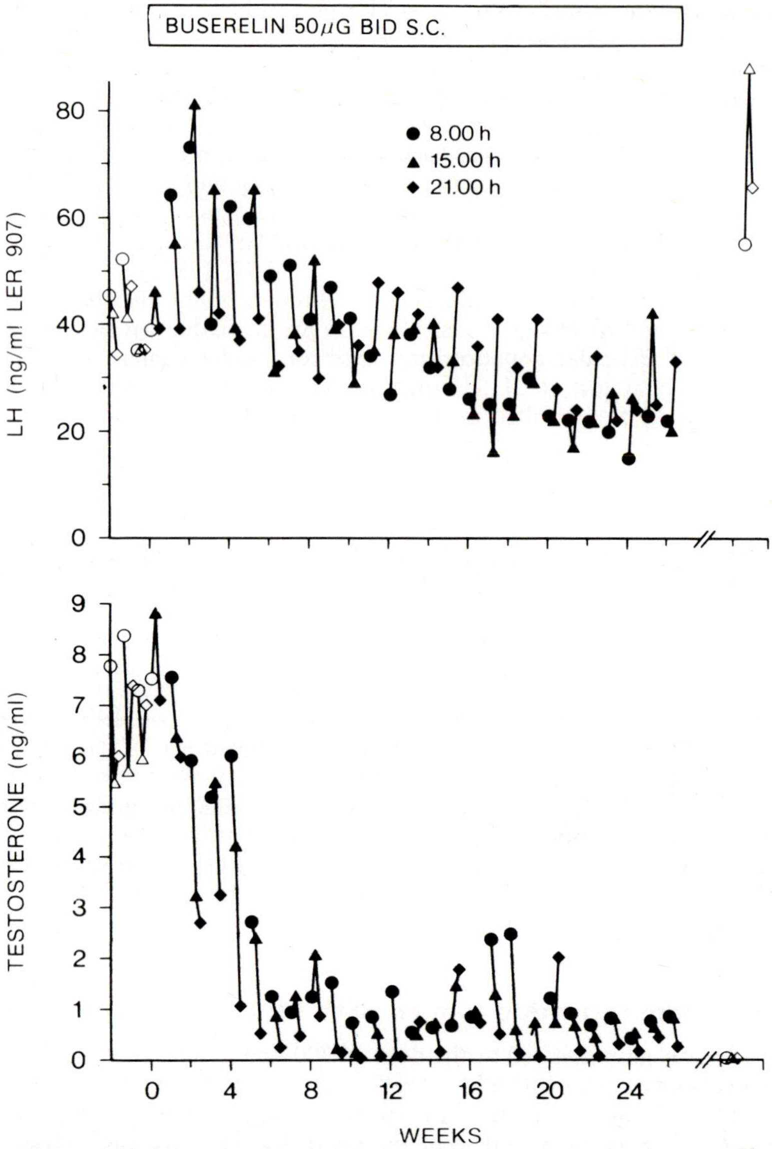

Figure 26.3 Effect of daily subcutaneous administration of 50 μg buserelin on serum testosterone and LH levels in a patient with cancer of the prostate. Open symbols represent values obtained before buserelin treatment and closed symbols values obtained during the 15-week treatment period.

decreased to normal. There was no effect on serum LH and testosterone levels measured 7 h after administration of buserelin.

A group of eight patients was treated for periods varying between 4 and 32 weeks. At this dose, the treatment leads to an approximately 75% inhibition of serum testosterone levels as early as 2 weeks after beginning of the treatment and maximal inhibition to 10–15% of control is achieved at 3–4 weeks up to the last time interval studied (32 weeks). Figure 26.4 shows serum basal LH (A) and testosterone (B) levels measured in this group of patients. Testosterone is

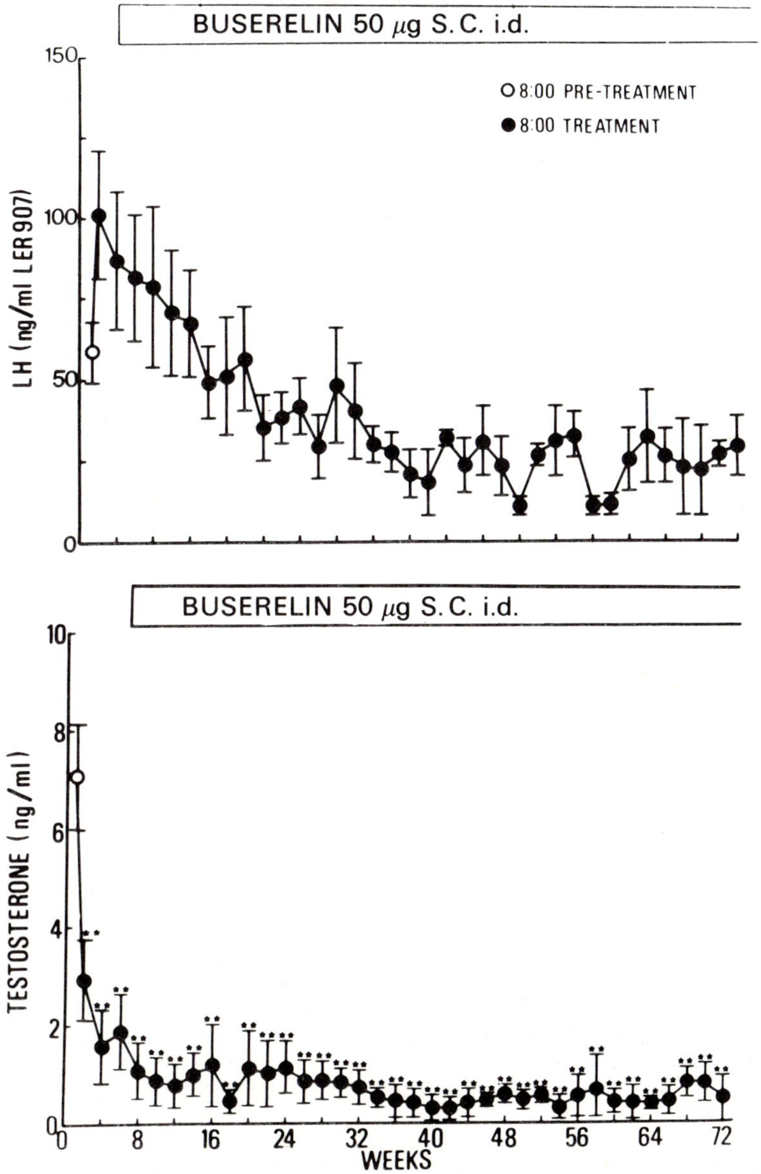

Figure 26.4 Mean ± SEM basal serum LH(A) and testosterone (B) before (—O—) and during (—●—) treatment with 50 μg daily, subcutaneous buserelin in 10 patients with prostatic carcinoma. **, $p < 0.01$.

decreased to 1.09 ± 0.45 ng/ml after 8 weeks and remains around 1 ng/ml during the whole treatment period.

After a transient rise on the first days of treatment, serum 17β-estradiol levels decreased in most subjects. Serum pregnenolone levels fluctuated during treatment without the establishment of a definite pattern. Plasma levels of 17 OH-progesterone and 5α-dihydrotestosterone were decreased to 41% and 30% of control values, respectively (Faure *et al.*, 1982).

Despite a decrease of preinjection plasma androgen levels, most of the injections of the agonist elicit a small response 8–12 h after administration. Similar acute responses are seen for LH levels even after a few months of daily administration of buserelin. The daily small response in testosterone levels probably results from these LH elevations.

Chronic i.n. administration of buserelin almost completely abolishes the acute LH response to the peptide. The reversibility of the pituitary desensitization is shown by the return of the LH responsivity 1 month after cessation of treatment (Figure 26.5).

Similar results are being reported for other analogs. Chronic daily subcutaneous injections of [D-Leu^6,Pro^9-NHEt]LHRH (leuprolide) induced a 98% reduction of testosterone levels in 50 prostate cancer patients treated over an 11 week period (Warner *et al.*, 1982). In another group of patients treated subcutaneously or intranasally with [D-Trp^6]LHRH or buserelin, a

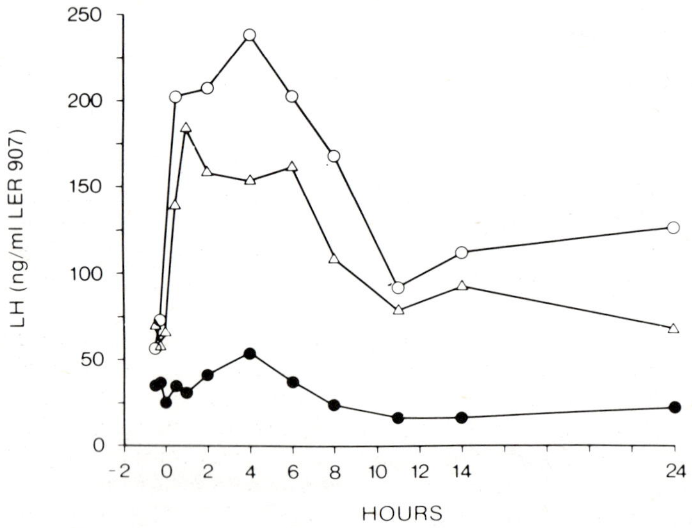

Figure 26.5 Effect of chronic (3 months) twice daily intranasal administration of 200 μg buserelin on the plasma LH response to buserelin in a patient with cancer of the prostate. LH levels following the first administration (○——○), after 3 months of treatment (●——●), and 1 month post-treatment (△——△) are shown.

75 % suppression of plasma testosterone levels was noted from the 3rd week of treatment which was maintained until the end of treatment (Tolis *et al.*, 1982).

Combinations of subcutaneous and intranasal administration

Subcutaneous injections for the first few days of therapy may be used to obtain a rapid inhibition of testicular steroidogenesis followed by the use of the more convenient i.n. insufflation to keep the circulating androgens low. The efficacy of such a combined regimen was recently demonstrated (Borgmann *et al.*, 1982): patients were treated with 1 mg twice daily of buserelin s.c. for 3 days, followed by 0.6 to 1.2 mg of buserelin i.n. in three daily doses. Serum testosterone fell below 1 ng/ml within 3 weeks and remained in the castrated range for the 6 months of the study. A 0.4 mg dose i.n. once daily was not sufficient to sustain testosterone suppression.

This combination of s.c. and i.n. administration of buserelin was used in our more recent study of prostatic carcinoma therapy. Eighteen patients have been treated for periods of 1–5 months with 500 μg s.c. every 8 h followed by 400 μg i.n. every 8 h. The inhibition of testosterone levels is more rapid and more profound with the combined treatment. The basal testosterone levels are below 1 ng/ml after only 4 months of treatment, in 13 out of 18 patients (Figure 26.6).

REGRESSION OF CLINICAL SYMPTOMS OF PROSTATE CANCER

LHRH agonist alone

A rapid decrease in symptomatology related to prostate cancer as well as an improvement of the objective signs was reported after treatment of patients having either stage C or D prostatic cancer (Tolis *et al.*, 1982). The treatment period varied between 6 weeks and 12 months. In all patients with stage C, there was a decrease in signs of prostatism, along with a decrease in the size of the primary tumor in half of the patients. Three of four stage D patients experienced a decrease in bone pain and use of analgesics. After 10 months of treatment of one patient, the bone scan that had previously shown diffuse osteoblastic lesions became practically normal.

Buserelin treatment by the combination s.c. and i.n. regimen described above has now been extended to a larger group of patients, all of whom had stage C and D prostatic cancer. The follow up period has ranged from 2 to 28 months, 38 % of patients having been treated for more than 12 months. Preliminary subjective evaluation indicates that symptoms of prostatism were decreased in 73 % of cases and that bone pain was decreased in intensity in 56 % of patients. Prostate volume, measured by ultrasonography, was decreased in nine of 13 patients. Bone scans were positive in 20 patients before buserelin treatment: stabilization of the metastatic process was found in 47 % of the cases and an improvement in another 25 %, followed for periods of 4–24

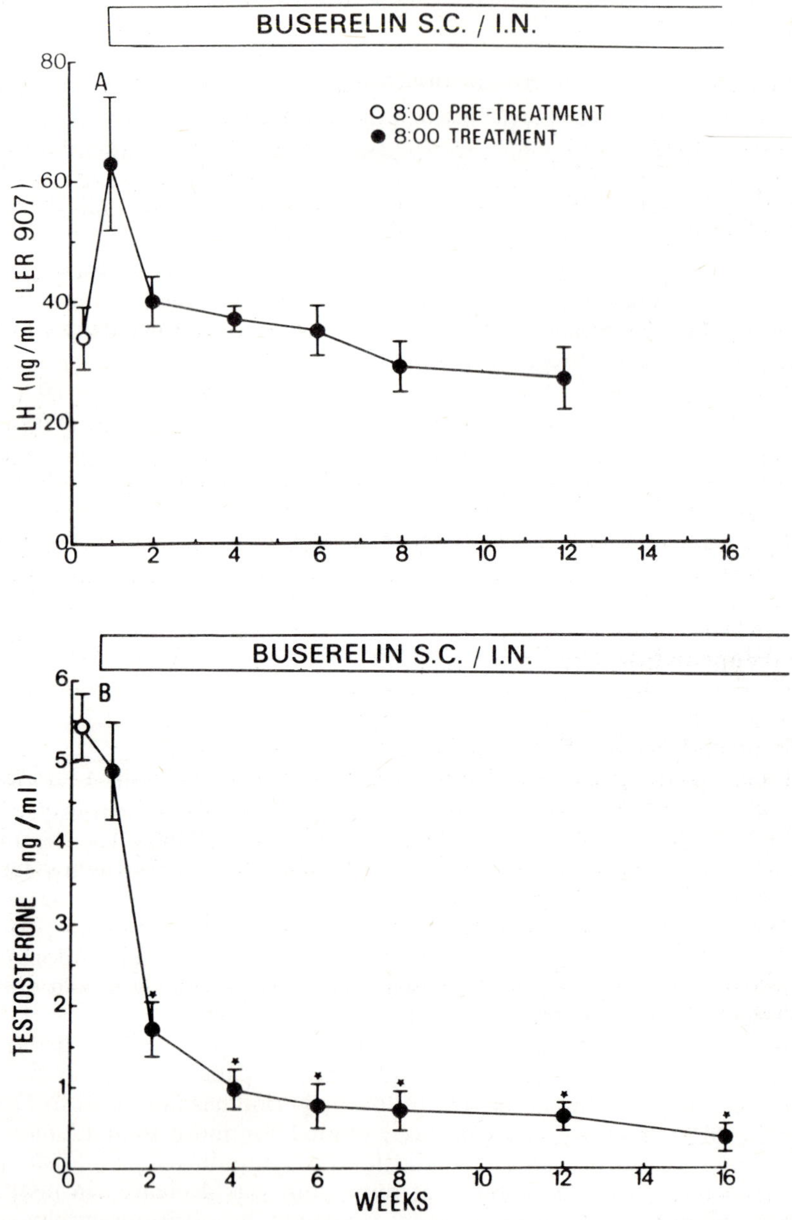

Figure 26.6 Mean ± SEM basal LH (A) and testosterone (B) in 12 patients with stage D prostatic carcinoma who were treated daily with buserelin (500 μg subcutaneously every 8 h for 7 days followed by 400 μg intranasally every 8 h). *, $p < 0.01$.

months. Three of the four patients with pathological lymph nodes showed a decrease of the node after 4–20 weeks of treatment. The prostatic acid phosphatase was found to be elevated in 19 patients: it decreased to normal or by more than half in 42 %.

No side-effect which could be attributed to treatment with buserelin was noticed except those related to decreased androgen secretion, such as gradual decrease in potency in 87 % of those patients who were sexually active at the beginning of treatment. Hot flashes were noticed more frequently in patients treated subcutaneously than in patients treated intranasally, reflecting the more efficient androgen inhibition with the former route of administration.

Combination treatment with buserelin and an antiandrogen

Pure antiandrogens can neutralize the action of androgens from all sources and thus theoretically represent the ideal form of therapy. However, a secondary increase of gonadotropin and androgen secretion results from such treatment and the need arises for progressively higher doses of the drug in order to neutralize the rising androgen levels efficiently (Neumann *et al.*, 1977; Geller *et al.*, 1981).

The combination of an LHRH analog and an antiandrogen has been shown in the rat to be more effective in diminishing prostate or seminal vesicle weight than either treatment alone (Séguin *et al.*, 1981). Furthermore, combination of an LHRH agonist and a pure antiandrogen avoids the limitations of treatment with the antiandrogen alone (Neumann *et al.*, 1977; Raynaud *et al.*, 1977). High doses of available antiandrogens are hepatotoxic. Lower doses of the antiandrogens may be required for combination treatment because of the low levels of androgens which remain to be neutralized after LHRH agonist treatment. The long term use of antiandrogens alone is known to be associated with an escape phenomenon because of the absence of androgen negative feedback at the pituitary level (Neumann *et al.*, 1977; Raynaud *et al.*, 1977). The pituitary being already desensitized by the LHRH agonist, the antiandrogens should then keep their optimal effectiveness.

Owing to its ease of application and lack of secondary effects as well as complete neutralization of androgenic influence, this combined treatment with an LHRH agonist and an antiandrogen is promising as judged from preliminary studies in men.

CONCLUDING REMARKS

Our studies were aimed at evaluating the effect of chronic treatment with the LHRH agonist buserelin in patients with cancer of the prostate. Following our dose-range finding study, a practical regimen was applied and we could obtain an inhibition of testicular androgens biosynthesis sufficiently complete to act as a medical castration. Clinical results are still preliminary but indicate a potential beneficial effect at an advanced stage of the disease.

Such a therapeutic regimen could also be used to identify the hormone-resistant tumors during the first 3–6 months of therapy before eventually proceeding to a more definitive procedure. The efficacy of LHRH agonist treatment as a palliative endocrine therapy remains to be established by long term studies on a large series of patients comparing conventional treatment with buserelin alone or combined with an antiandrogen. The possibility of a beneficial effect on long term survival by starting the hormonal treatment at an early stage of the disease, before metastatic dissemination, is an open question that will be very difficult to resolve.

Acknowledgement

This work has been supported by a grant from the National Cancer Institute of Canada.

References

Arimura, A., Serafini, P., Talbot, S. and Schally, A. V. (1979). Reduction of testicular luteinizing hormone/human chorionic gonadotropin receptors by D-Trp^6-luteinizing hormone-releasing hormone in hypophysectomized rats. *Biochem. Biophys. Res. Commun.*, **90,** 687

Auclair, C., Kelly, P. A., Labrie, F., Coy, D. H. and Schally, A. V. (1977). Inhibition of testicular LH/hCG receptor level by treatment with a potent LHRH agonist or hCG. *Biochem. Biophys. Res. Commun.*, **76,** 855

Bailar, J. C., Byar, D. P. and Veterans Administration Cooperative Urological Research Group (1970). Estrogen treatment for cancer of the prostate. *Cancer,* **26,** 257

Bélanger, A., Auclair, C., Séguin, C., Kelly, P. A. and Labrie, F. (1979). Down-regulation of testicular androgen biosynthesis and LH receptor levels by an LHRH agonist: role of prolactin. *Mol. Cell. Endocrinol.*, **13,** 47

Bélanger, A., Auclair, C., Ferland, L. and Labrie, F. (1980*a*). Time-course of the effects of treatment with a potent LHRH agonist on testicular steroidogenesis and gonadotropin receptor levels in the adult rat. *J. Steroid. Biochem.*, **13,** 191

Bélanger, A., Labrie, F., Lemay, A., Caron, S. and Raynaud, J. P. (1980*b*). Inhibitory effects of a single intranasal administration of [D-Ser-(TBU)^6,des-Gly-NH_2^{10}]LHRH agonist, on serum steroid levels in normal adult men. *J. Steroid. Biochem.*, **13,** 123

Bergquist, C., Nillius, S. J., Bergh, T., Skarin, G. and Wide, L. (1979). Inhibitory effects on gonadotropin secretion and gonadal function in men during chronic treatment with a potent stimulatory luteinizing hormone-releasing hormone analogue. *Acta Endocrinol.*, **91,** 601

Borgmann, V., Hardt, W., Schmidt-Gollwitzer, M., Adenauer, H. and Nagel, R. (1982). Sustained suppression of testosterone production by the LHRH agonist buserelin in patients with advanced prostate carcinoma. *Lancet,* **1,** 1097

Clayton, R. N. and Huhtaniemi, I. T. (1982). Absence of gonadotropin-releasing hormone receptors in human gonadal tissue. *Nature* (*Lond.*), **299,** 56

Davies, T. F., Gomez-Pan, A., Watson, M. J., Mountjoy, C. Q., Hanker, J. P., Besser, G. M. and Hall, R. (1977). Reduced gonadotropin response to releasing hormone after chronic administration to impotent men. *Clin. Endocrinol.*, **6,** 213

Faure, N., Labrie, F., Lemay, A., Bélanger, A., Gourdeau, Y., Laroche, B. and Robert, G. (1982). Inhibition of serum androgen levels by chronic intranasal and subcutaneous administration of a potent luteinizing hormone-releasing hormone (LH-RH) agonist in adult men. *Fertil. Steril.*, **37,** 416

Geller, J., Albert, J., Yen, S. S. C., Geller, S. and Loza, D. (1981). Medical castration with megestrol acetate and minidose of diethylstilbestrol. *Urology Suppl.*, **17,** 27

Happ, J., Scholz, P., Weber, T., Cordes, U., Schramm, P., Neubauer M. and Beyer, J. (1978). Gonadotropin secretion in eugonadotropic human males and post-menopausal females under long-term application of a potent analogue of gonadotropin-releasing hormone. *Fertil. Steril.*, **30,** 674

Hashimoto, T., Miyar, K., Vozumi, T., Mori, S., Watanabe, M. and Kumahara, Y. (1975). Effect of prolonged LH-releasing hormone administration on gonadotropin response in patients with hypothalamic and pituitary tumors. *J. Clin. Endocrinol. Metab.,* **41,** 712

Hedlund, P. O., Gustafson, H. and Sjogren, S. (1980). Cardiovascular complications to treatment of prostate cancer with estramustine phosphate (estracyt) or conventional estrogen. A follow-up of 212 randomized patients. *Scand. J. Urol. Nephrol. Suppl.,* **55,** 103

Huggins, C., Steven, R. E. and Hodges, C. V. (1941). Studies on prostatic cancer, II; The effects of castration on advanced carcinoma of the prostate gland. *Arch. Surg.,* **43,** 209

Labrie, F., Auclair, C., Cusan, L., Kelly, P. A., Pelletier, G. and Ferland, L. (1978). Inhibitory effects of LHRH and its agonists on testicular gonadotropin receptors and spermatogenesis in the rat. In Hansson, V., (ed.) Endocrine Approach to Male Contraception, *Int. J. Androl.* (Suppl. 2), pp. 303–318

Linde, R., Doelle, G. C., Alexander, N., Kirchner, F., Vale, W., Rivier, J. and Rabin, D. (1981). Reversible inhibition of testicular steroidogenesis and spermatogenesis by a potent GNRH agonist in normal men. *N. Engl. J. Med.,* **305,** 663

Neumann, F., Graf, K. J., Hasans, H., Schenck, B. and Steinbeck, H. (1977). Central actions of antiandrogens. In Martini, L. and Motta, M. (eds.) *Androgens and Antiandrogens,* pp. 163–177. (New York: Raven Press)

Raynaud, J. P., Azadian-Boulanger, G., Bonne, C., Perronet, J. and Sakiz, E. (1977). Present trends in antiandrogen research. In Martini, L. and Motta, M. (eds.) *Androgens and Antiandrogens,* pp. 281–293. (New York: Raven Press)

Séguin, C., Cusan, L., Bélanger, A., Kelly, P. A., Labrie, F. and Raynaud, J. P. (1981). Additive inhibitory effects of treatment with an LHRH agonist and an antiandrogen on androgen-dependent tissues in the rat. *Mol. Cell. Endocrinol.,* **21,** 37

Smith, R., Donald, R. A., Espiner, E. A., Stronach, S. G. and Edwards, I. A. (1979). Normal adults and subjects with hypogonadotropic hypogonadism respond differently to [D-Ser(TBU)^6,des-Gly-NH_2^{10}]LHRH-EA. *J. Clin. Endocrinol. Metab.,* **48,** 167

Tolis, G., Mehta, A., Comaru-Schally, A. M. and Schally, A. V. (1981). Suppression of androgen production by D-Tryptophan-6-luteinizing hormone-releasing hormone in man. *J. Clin. Invest.,* **68,** 819

Tolis, G., Ackman, D., Stellos, A., Mehta, A., Labrie, F., Fazekas, A. T. A., Comaru-Schally, A. M. and Schally, A. V. (1982). Tumor growth inhibition in patients with prostatic carcinoma treated with luteinizing hormone-releasing hormone agonists. *Proc. Natl. Acad. Sci. USA,* **79,** 1658

Warner, B., Santen, R. and Demers, L. (1982). Effects of [D-Leu^6,Des-Gly NH_2^{10}, Pro-ethylamide^9]-GnRH (Leuprolide) on steroidogenesis when used to treat prostatic carcinoma. *J. Androl.,* **3,** 14

27
Leuprolide therapy for prostatic carcinoma

R. J. SANTEN, B. WARNER, L. M. DEMERS, M. DUFAU and J. A. SMITH Jr.

Seventy thousand new cases of prostate carcinoma are diagnosed in the United States yearly (Silverberg and Holleb, 1982). At presentation approximately three quarters of these tumors are androgen-dependent. This estimate is based upon the observation that lowering of androgen levels by surgical or pharmacologic means produces objective tumor regression in approximately 75% of patients (Schirmer *et al.*, 1965). Nuclear androgen receptors are usually demonstrable in the tumors of men responding to hormonal manipulation (Ekman *et al.*, 1979; Ghanadian *et al.*, 1981). Several non-surgical methods of inhibiting the synthesis of androgens or their cellular action have been utilized in the treatment of prostatic carcinoma. Pharmacologic amounts of estrogen are frequently administered to suppress the release of LH by the pituitary and thereby inhibit androgen production (Johnson *et al.*, 1975). Induction of accelerated cardiovascular disease or of thrombophlebitis, particularly with higher estrogen doses, complicates this mode of treatment. Antiandrogens such as cyproterone acetate (Rost *et al.*, 1981) and flutamide (Stoliar and Albert, 1974) show promise as means of antagonizing androgen action at a cellular level and thus producing tumor regression. These antihormonal agents require further evalution before wide clinical application is appropriate. Orchiectomy is also used to lower androgen levels acutely. This treatment effects regression in men with androgen-dependent tumors but is not acceptable to many patients.

The above considerations highlight the need for development of a non-toxic, specific inhibitor of androgen biosynthesis for use in men with prostatic carcinoma. The ability of the LHRH agonist analogs to reduce testosterone production in animals and in normal men suggested that these compounds would be logical candidates for treating prostatic cancer.

INHIBITION OF ANDROGEN BIOSYNTHESIS

Standard LHRH agonist doses

LHRH agonists produce reproductive atrophy in the male rodent by suppressing testosterone production. These effects occur with doses ranging from 0.001 to 1 μg/300 g rat (Rivier *et al.*, 1979) and with injection schedules varying from twice daily to three times weekly. Investigators initially emphasized the fact that relatively small doses of LHRH agonists inhibited testosterone and produced virtually no systemic toxicity (Rivier *et al.*, 1979; Labrie *et al.*, 1980*a*). Based upon these observations, doses of LHRH agonists were chosen for clinical trials which approximated those used in the rodent if calculated on a per meter squared basis (Freireich *et al.*, 1966). The mode of administration included daily subcutaneous injections or insufflation by nasal spray. With the latter method, approximately 1–5% of the compound is absorbed (London *et al.*, 1972; Dahlen *et al.*, 1974).

Doses of either 100 μg/day of [D-Trp^6]LHRH subcutaneously, 50 μg/day of [D-Ser(tBu)^6,Pro^9-NHEt]LHRH (buserelin) subcutaneously or 500 μg/day of buserelin by nasal spray twice daily were administered to ten men with prostatic carcinoma (Tolis *et al.*, 1982). The investigators observed a fall in testosterone to 65 ng/dl during treatment for up to 16 weeks. When 50 μg/day of buserelin was administered subcutaneously, testosterone declined to 128 ng/dl in eight normal men (Faure *et al.*, 1982). The degree of testosterone suppression achieved in these patients with prostatic carcinoma was less than that observed in normal men given 50 μg/day (Linde *et al.*, 1981). Testosterone levels as low as 24 ng/dl were observed in eight men receiving [D-Trp^6,Pro^9-NHEt]LHRH for 10 weeks. Suppression of testosterone to similar levels occurred in four transsexuals given [D-Trp^6,Pro^9-NHEt]LHRH for up to 8 weeks (Tolis *et al.*, 1981).

Mega-dose LHRH-A therapy

From rodent studies (Warner *et al.*, 1983), we and others (personal communication, records of the Abbott Corporation) observed that the dose-response curve for [D-Leu^6,Pro^9-NHEt]LHRH (leuprolide) extends well beyond the 0.001–1 μg range of LHRH agonists used in the majority of prior studies. For example, 200 μg of [D-Leu^6,Pro^9-NHEt]LHRH produced significantly greater suppression of seminal vesicle and prostatic weight and of testosterone levels than 40 μg administered subcutaneously daily. Neither dose inhibited prostatic or seminal vesicle weight to the same extent as induced by surgical castration. These considerations led the Abbott Study Group (see Appendix) to choose very high ('mega') doses of [D-Leu^6,Pro^9-NHEt]LHRH for treatment of men with prostatic carcinoma. Extrapolations from the rodent data on a mg/m^2 basis indicated that administration of 1000 and 10 000 μg subcutaneously daily (Freireich *et al.*, 1966) in men would approximate the 40 and 200 μg daily dose in rodents.

In contrast to data obtained in the rodent, no difference in effect was noted between the 1000 and 10 000 μg doses in men. Testosterone increased initially

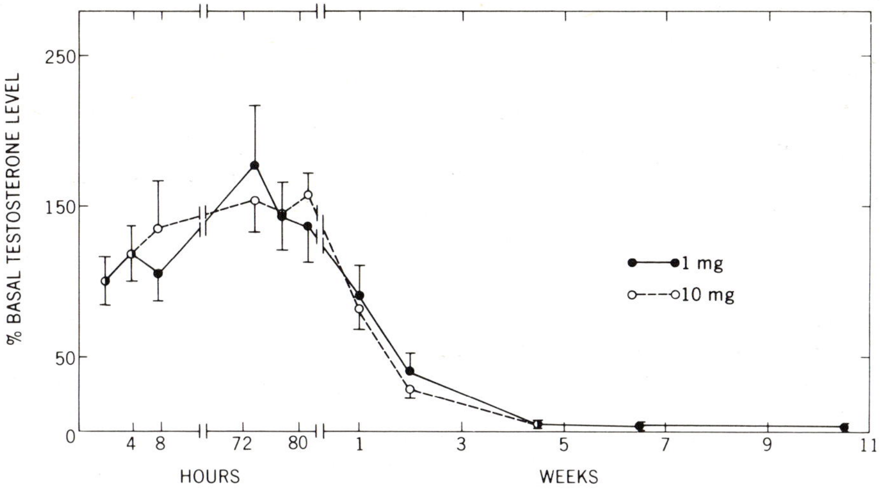

Figure 27.1 Dose-response effects of 1 mg and 10 mg of [D-Leu^6,Pro^9-NHEt]LHRH on serum testosterone expressed as percent of basal mean values. Data points represent the mean ±SEM.

to 150–170% of basal on the third day of drug administration with both doses (Figure 27.1) and then reached maximally suppressed levels by the fourth week to 5% of basal. Since neither testosterone (nor any other hormonal parameter measured) differed between the 1000 and 10 000 μg groups, all subsequent data were pooled to facilitate presentation.

Men were divided into two categories: those with no prior treatment (non-castrate) and those given DES (non-castrate DES) up to 2 weeks before receiving LHRH agonist. In response to injections of [D-Leu^6,Pro^9-NHEt]LHRH, testosterone initially increased over 3 days to peak at 656 ng/dl on day 3 in the non-castrate group and 464 ng/dl in the non-castrate DES patients (Figure 27.2). During chronic treatment (i.e. week 11), the concentrations of this androgen were profoundly suppressed to castrate levels (Figure 27.3). The concentrations of dihydrotestosterone paralleled those of testosterone with an acute rise from basal levels in both the previously untreated group and those receiving DES previously (Figure 27.2). This steroid then fell to levels similar to those observed in castrate men (Figure 27.3). Mega-dose LHRH agonist therapy thus produces the hormonal equivalent of castration. The use of standard doses produced a similar suppression of testosterone in some studies (Linde *et al.*, 1981) but not in others (Tolis *et al.*, 1982; Faure *et al.*, 1982). Direct comparison of groups of patients treated with both mega and standard doses of the same analog is indicated.

An alternative, recently reported approach utilized initial mega-dose LHRH agonist treatment followed by maintenance with standard amounts (Borgmann *et al.*, 1982). Patients were treated with 1000 μg of buserelin twice daily subcutaneously for 1 week and then with 400 μg, three times daily intranasally (estimated absorption is 1–5% of dose). This regimen suppressed testosterone to castrate levels in three patients observed for 24 weeks. Thus,

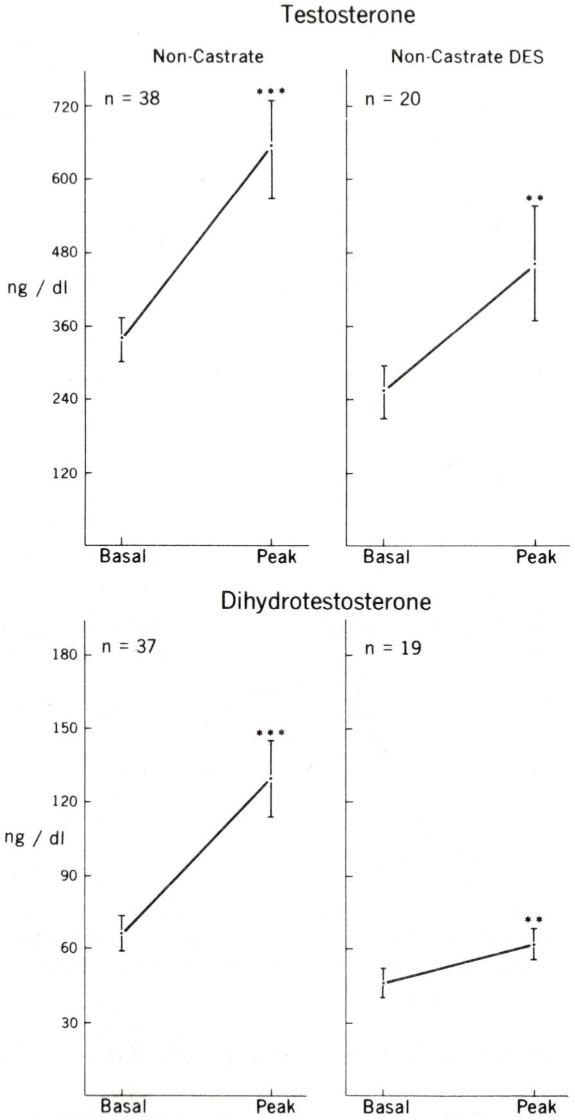

Figure 27.2 Testosterone and dihydrotestosterone levels following acute administration of [D-Leu[6],Pro[9]-NHEt]LHRH subcutaneously daily. The basal levels and the peak level following injection (i.e. 8–80 h, see Figure 27.1) are shown. Two groups of patients, those previously untreated (non-castrate) and those given DES (diethylstilbestrol) until 2 weeks prior to study are included (non-castrate DES). Data points indicate the mean ± SEM. *, $p < 0.05$, **, $p < 0.01$, ***, $p < 0.001$, n = number of subjects.

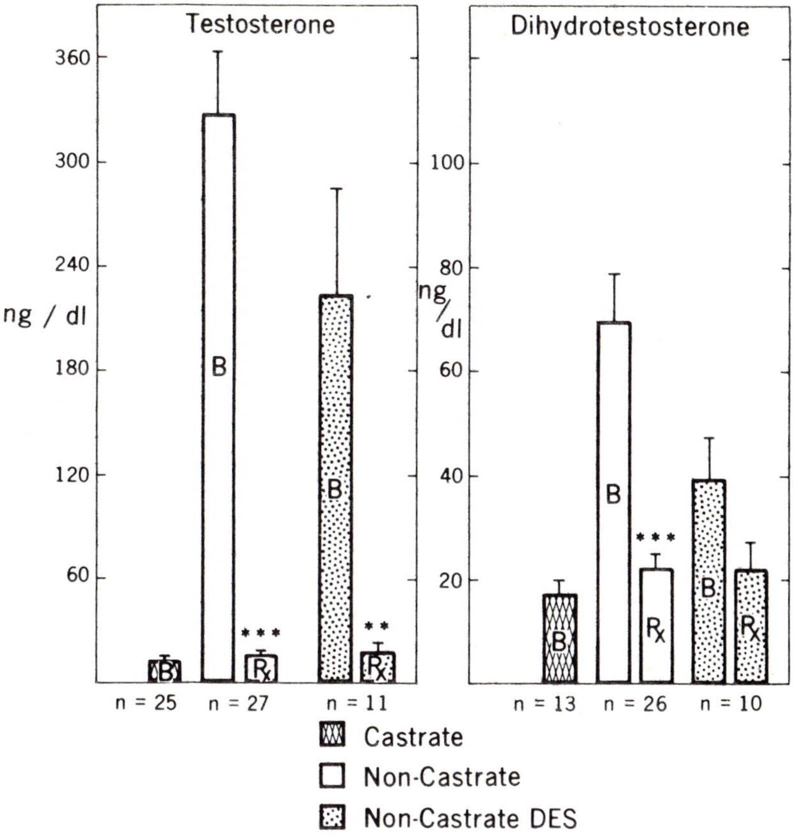

Figure 27.3 Testosterone and dihydrotestosterone levels measured basally (B) in the castrate men and on the eleventh week of treatment (Rx) in the non-castrate and non-castrate-DES group.

profound testosterone suppression may be achieved rapidly with mega-dose treatment and maintained by lower doses given chronically.

INHIBITION OF GONADOTROPIN SECRETION

Standard dose therapy

In intact male rodents, LH levels remain constant or even rise during chronic administration of LHRH agonists even though testosterone concentrations are suppressed. Only in castrate rats do LH levels uniformly decline during administration of standard doses of LHRH agonists (Tcholakian *et al.*, 1978; Labrie *et al.*, 1978, 1980*a,b*; Rivier *et al.*, 1979; Clayton *et al.*, 1980). In intact men with prostatic carcinoma, no consistent decline in LH was observed during daily administration of 50 μg of buserelin subcutaneously (Faure *et al.*,

1982). A 50% decrease in LH was observed in eight normal men given [D-Trp[6],Pro[9]-NHEt]LHRH (Linde *et al.*, 1981). A 20–39% decrease in LH was found in four transsexuals given [D-Trp[6]]LHRH (Tolis *et al.*, 1981). These studies indicate that LH is not completely suppressed with standard doses of LHRH agonist.

Mega-dose LHRH agonist treatment

Men given 1000 or 10 000 μg of [D-Leu[6],Pro[9]-NHEt]LHRH by injections experienced an initial increase in LH which peaked during the first day of treatment (Figure 27.4). This acute stimulation occurred in castrate as well as intact untreated and intact, DES pretreated, men. At 11 weeks, plasma LH levels were at the limit of assay sensitivity (8 miu/ml) in all three groups (Figure 27.5). In order to quantitate the exact level of LH suppression, two additional methods of quantitating LH were utilized as means of markedly enhancing assay sensitivity: (1) the LH *in vitro* bioassay and (2) radioimmunoassay of 40-fold urinary concentrates. The LH bioassay (rat interstitial cell testosterone assay) can detect LH levels equivalent to 0.4 miu/ml in the corresponding radioimmunoassay, an 80-fold enhancement of assay sensitivity (Dufau *et al.*, 1976; Solano *et al.*, 1979). When assayed by this method, LH levels fell to < 0.4 miu/ml in 7 out of 9 intact men with prostatic carcinoma treated with mega-dose [D-Leu[6],Pro[9]-NHEt]LHRH (leuprolide) (Figure 27.6) and by 10- and 30-fold in the other two.

Such profound decrements in LH were also detected by the radioimmunoassay of 40-fold urinary concentrates for LH (Kulin *et al.*, 1975). During chronic administration of mega-dose leuprolide in six men with prostatic cancer, urinary LH excretion averaged 64 miu/h in previously untreated, non-castrate men. This represents levels 20-fold lower than the mean in normal men and is similar to that observed in prepubertal boys.

Radioimmunoassay of plasma FSH levels in treated men indicated patterns very similar to those for LH (Figures 27.4 and 27.5), although a sensitive urinary method revealed a lesser degree of suppression of FSH than of LH. During chronic treatment in previously untreated non-castrate men, FSH excretion was at the lower limit of the normal adult male range.

DIRECT GONADAL EFFECTS

Studies in male rats identified GnRH receptors in the testis (Bourne *et al.*, 1980; Clayton *et al.*, 1980) and a direct inhibitory action of LHRH or its analogs on Leydig cell function (Hsueh and Jones, 1981). With standard amounts of LHRH agonist in men, the degree of decline in testosterone appears greater than that of LH in some studies (Faure *et al.*, 1982). With mega-dose LHRH agonist administration, however, the degree of suppression of LH is sufficient to fully explain the fall in testosterone levels observed.

LHRH agonists can alter intratesticular steroidogenic enzymes in rats. These effects may result from a direct action of these compounds or indirectly

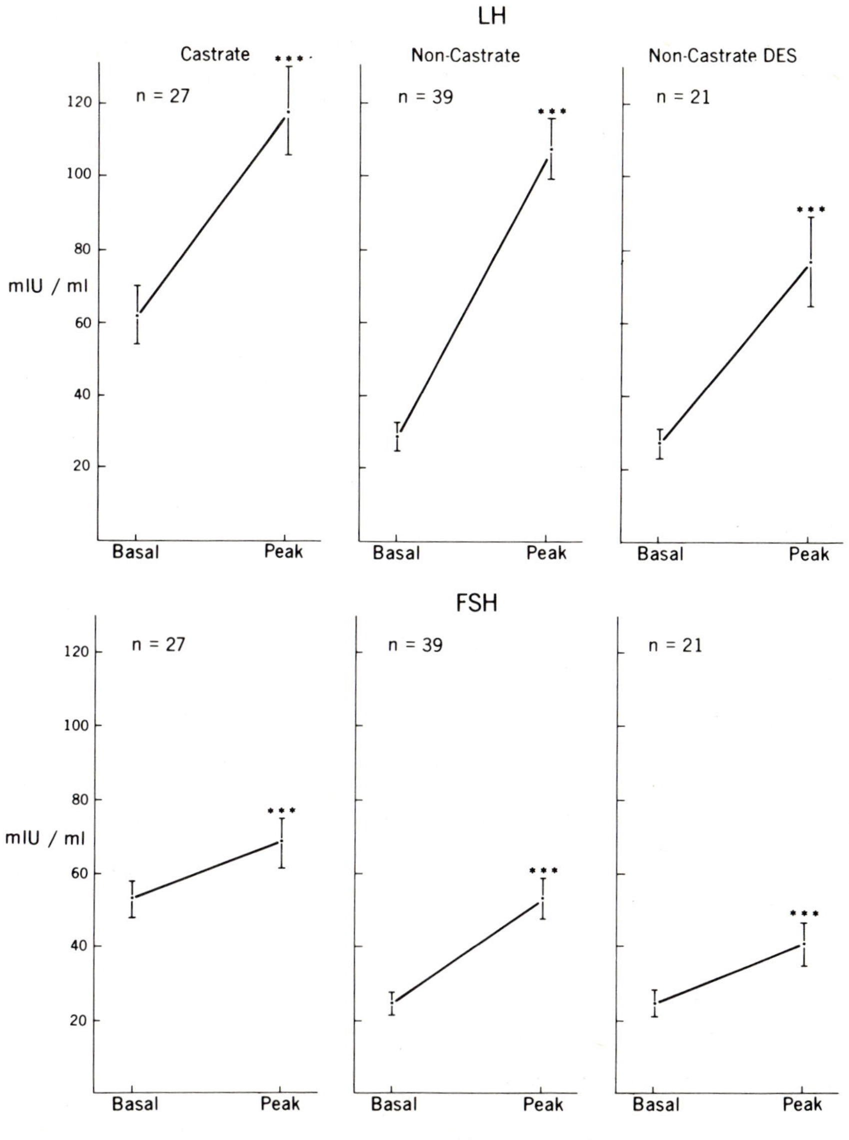

Figure 27.4 LH and FSH levels following acute administration of [D-Leu[6],Pro[9]-NHEt]LHRH subcutaneously daily. The basal levels and peak following the injections (i.e. 8 h after initial injection) are shown. Three groups of patients, those previously untreated (non-castrate), those given DES until 2 weeks prior to study (non-castrate DES), and castrate men are included.

through alterations of LH secretion. Inhibition of 17,20-lyase and of 17α-hydroxylase and stimulation of 5α-reductase and 3-ketoreductase are observed (Labrie *et al.*, 1980). In male rats, this produces an increase in plasma progesterone with concomitant reduction in 17α-hydroxyprogesterone and

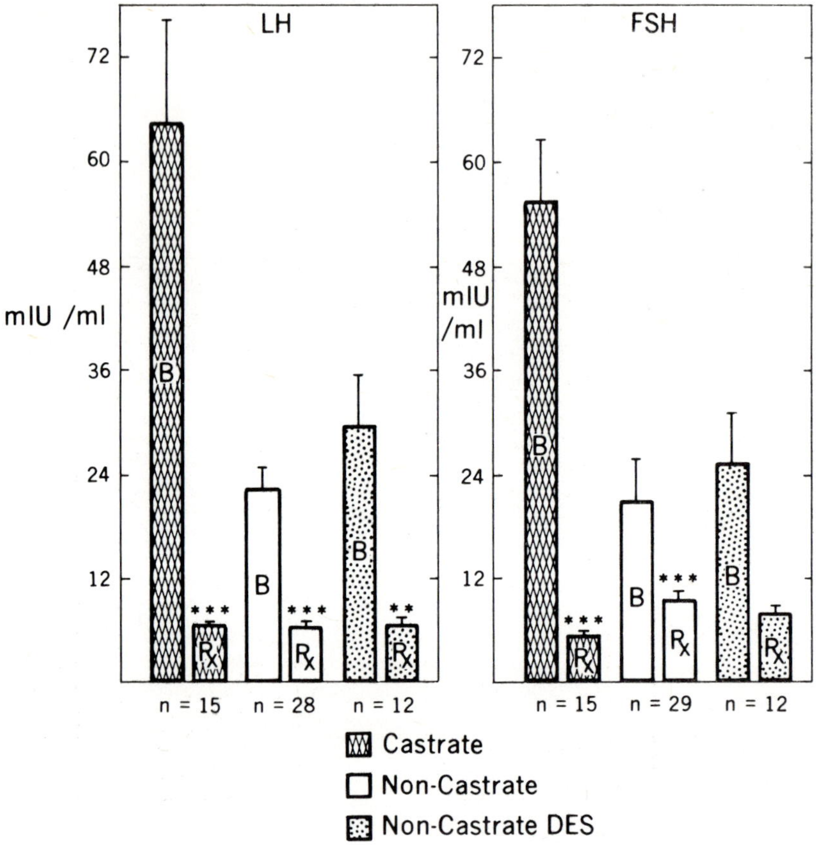

Figure 27.5 LH and FSH levels basally and on week 11 of treatment. Castrate, non-castrate and non-castrate-DES groups are shown.

testosterone. The stimulation of the distal metabolic enzymes (5α-reductase and 3-ketoreductase) causes a lesser reduction of dihydrotestosterone than of testosterone and an increase in 3α-androstanediol.

Levels of 17α-hydroxyprogesterone, predominantly a testicular steroid in men (de la Torre *et al.*, 1981), fell in patients treated with mega-dose LHRH agonist therapy whereas progesterone remained unchanged. Dihydrotestosterone concentrations declined to a lesser extent than did those of testosterone (Figure 27.3). Considered together, these data suggest at best only a minor direct effect of the LHRH agonists on testicular enzymes.

SPECIFICITY OF PITUITARY SUPPRESSION

Under a variety of circumstances, hypothalamic releasing factors can non-specifically stimulate the secretion of pituitary hormones other than those

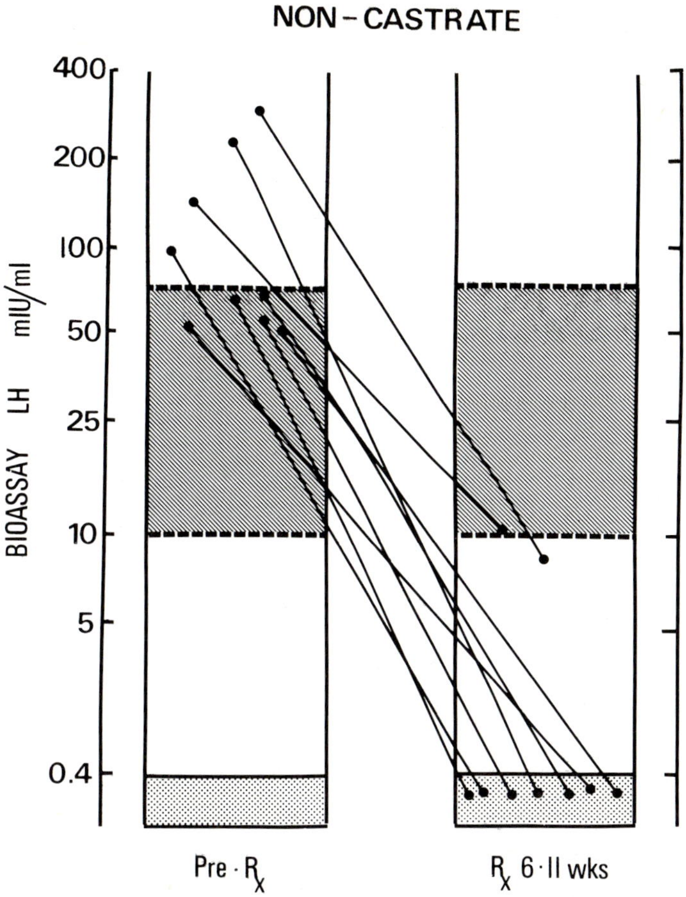

Figure 27.6 Bioassay (RICT) of LH in 9 men measured prior to treatment and in a single sample obtained during the 6th–11th weeks of treatment. The lines connect the basal and treatment values. In two patients LH levels were still measurable during therapy. In the remaining 7 men (closed circles), LH fell to undetectable titers during treatment.

released by their specific target cells (Warner and Santen, 1981). This raises the possibility that the LHRH agonists may affect the level of pituitary hormones other than LH and FSH. Thus, it was pertinent to examine the plasma levels of pituitary hormones other than LH or FSH in patients with prostatic carcinoma receiving [D-Leu^6,Pro^9-NHEt]LHRH. With mega-dose therapy, no significant alteration of plasma prolactin or cortisol (as a reflection of ACTH) occurred during chronic drug administration. Taken together, these data emphasize the specifiity of the LHRH agonists to inhibit gonadotropin secretion and to produce a selective 'medical hypophysectomy'.

REGRESSION OF PROSTATIC CANCER TISSUE

Standard-dose GnRH-A therapy

A pilot trial, including ten patients treated with either 100 μg of [D-Trp^6] LHRH or 50 μg of buserelin subcutaneously daily or 500 μg of buserelin twice daily by nasal spray demonstrated the antitumor efficacy of standard doses of LHRH agonist (Tolis *et al.*, 1982). Antitumor activity was observed in two of four patients with metastatic disease. In addition, patients with stage C disease associated with elevated acid phosphatase levels experienced a normalization of acid phosphatase during treatment (Tolis *et al.*, 1982).

Mega-dose GnRH-A therapy

A multicenter Phase II clinical trial using 1000–10 000 μg/day of [D-Leu^6, Pro^9-NHEt]LHRH in men with metastatic or locally invasive, inoperable prostatic carcinoma has been conducted (Smith and the Abbott Leuprolide Prostatic Cancer Study Group, 1982; Glode, 1982). To allow comparison with other forms of treatment, standard criteria developed by the National Prostatic Cancer Project for scoring responses objectively were utilized (Schmidt *et al.*, 1980). Table 27.1 details the criteria required for patient entry and follow-up. The patient population consisted of 59 previously untreated patients with prostatic carcinoma; 27 men who had received diethylstilbestrol (or Tace in two patients) and later experienced progressive disease; and 31 subjects who underwent surgical castration as initial treatment and whose tumors were progressing at entry into study. Responses were scored after 4 months of therapy.

The greatest frequency of responses occurred in the men with no prior treatment. Fifty-three per cent of these experienced a measurable objective regression of tumor after 4 months of therapy. An additional 34% of these patients had objectively stable disease whereas 13% progressed. Subjective relief of pain or improvement of performance score lasting at least 10 weeks also occurred in 91% of these previously untreated men. Improvement in bone scan or healing of blastic metastases on X-ray were observed and provided the most convincing evidence of drug efficacy. The frequency of responses observed in these previously untreated men is comparable to those reported in similar groups of men treated with surgical orchiectomy or high-dose diethylstilbestrol.

The second group of men receiving mega-dose LHRH agonist therapy had previously been treated with diethylstilbestrol (or Tace in two patients) before entering study. In these men, 19% experienced objective tumor regression, 33% objectively stable disease and 48% progression of cancer at the end of 10 weeks. It should be noted that four of the five men with objective responses had not shown disease progression while on estrogens and some received suboptimal estrogen treatment. Fifty-six per cent of men noted a subjective relief of symptoms. However, by the end of 4 months, 64% of patients had experienced objective tumor progression. Prior studies have also indicated an

Table 27.1 Clinical criteria for study entry and scoring of responses

Entry into study
Required:
Measurable or evaluable disease including at least two of the following:
peri-prostatic disease
osteoblastic or osteolytic metastases
elevated acid phosphatase
objective evidence of ureteral obstruction
measurable soft tissue metastases
Exclusions:
history of adrenalectomy or hypophysectomy
previous or concurrent malignancy other than prostate cancer
life-threatening medical disease

Response criteria
Objective regression:
(1) At least one tumor mass, if present, is reduced by >50% in cross-sectional area
(2) Elevated acid phosphatase, if present, returned to normal
(3) Osteolytic lesions, if present, underwent recalcification in one or more, but not necessarily in all
(4) Osteoblastic lesions, if present, did not progress
(5) If hepatomegaly is a significant indicator, there must be at least a 30% reduction in liver size indicated by a change in the measurements, and at least a 30% improvement of all pretreatment abnormalities of liver function, including bilirubin (mg %) and SGOT
(6) There may be no increase in any other lesion and no new areas of malignant disease may appear
(7) No significant cancer-related deterioration in weight (>10%), symptoms, or performance status
Objectively stable:
All of the following criteria:
(1) No new lesions occurred and no measurable lesions increased more than 25% in cross-sectional area
(2) Elevated acid phosphatase, if present, decreased, though need not have returned to normal
(3) Osteolytic lesions, if present, did not appear to worsen
(4) Osteoblastic lesions, if present, remained stable
(5) Hepatomegaly, if present, did not appear to worsen by more than a 30% increase in the measurements, and hepatic abnormalities did not worsen including bilirubin mg % and SGOT
(6) No significant cancer-related deterioration in weight (>10%), symptoms, or performance status
Objective Progression (or also Relapse after Adequate Therapy):
Any of the following criteria:
(1) Significant cancer-related deterioration in weight (>10%), symptoms, or performance status
(2) Appearance of new areas of malignant disease
(3) Increase in any previously measurable lesion by >25% in cross-sectional area

approximately 20% response rate to surgical orchiectomy in men previously treated with other hormonal methods (Schirmer *et al.*, 1965).

The known physiology of the LHRH agonists would suggest that previously orchiectomized men would not respond to administration of this compound. Data analysis indicated that this was the case since no patient in this category had objective disease regression, 6% experienced objectively stable disease and 94% had disease progression at the end of 4 months. Only 23% in this group experienced subjective relief of symptoms. It can be considered that these 31 previously orchiectomized men provided a basis for comparison with the patients who had no prior therapy. The lack of objective changes and relative infrequency of subjective improvement in the castrated group serves to strengthen the validity of the favorable responses observed in the previously untreated men.

The possibility of dose-response differences in clinical parameters was next addressed. Evaluation of tumor responses to the 1000 (64 patients) and 10 000 μg (58 patients) LHRH agonist doses revealed no dose-related differences among the various groups studied. This would be expected because no greater suppression of the androgens in men receiving 10 000 μg/day was observed than in men receiving 1000 μg/day of LHRH agonist.

Testosterone levels transiently increase upon initiation of LHRH agonist therapy. Administration of exogenous androgens to men with prostatic carcinoma frequently causes an acute worsening or 'flare' of tumor progression. For these reasons, each investigator was alerted to look for tumor flare upon initiation of leuprolide therapy. Objective signs suggesting this phenomenon occurred in three of 87 non-castrate men. Ten per cent of subjects in the previously untreated group initially experienced an increase in bone pain which subsided by the second week of treatment. As expected, the decrease in bone pain paralleled the reduction in serum testosterone levels.

CONCLUDING REMARKS

Administration of LHRH agonists in men with prostatic cancer produces definite antitumor effects. Controlled, randomized trials of LHRH agonist versus surgical orchiectomy and versus diethylstilbestrol are now required to establish relative frequency and duration of responses, frequency of side-effects and relative toxicities. Studies of standard versus mega-dose LHRH agonist administration will be necessary.

Acknowledgements

The authors wish to acknowledge the excellent secretarial assistance of Mrs Marlene Thompson in preparing this manuscript. Dr Michael Glode provided the urines for the radioimmunoassay of urinary LH and FSH. The study reported in this review was conducted as a collaborative trial under the direction of TAP Pharmaceuticals, Abbott Laboratories. The investigators participating in this study are listed in the Appendix.

References

Borgmann, V. Hardt, W., Schmidt-Gollwitzer, M., Adenauer, H. and Nagel, R. (1982). Sustained suppression of testosterone production by the luteinizing-hormone releasing-hormone agonist buserelin in patients with advanced prostate carcinoma. *Lancet*, **1**, 1097

Bourne, G. A., Regiani, S., Payne, A. H. and Marshall, J. C. (1980). Testicular GnRH receptors – Characterization and localization on interstitial tissue. *J. Clin. Endocrinol. Metab.*, **51**, 407

Clayton, R. N., Katikineni, M., Chan, V., Dufau, M. L. and Catt, K. J. (1980). Direct inhibition of testicular function by gonadotropin-releasing hormone: Mediation by specific gonadotropin-releasing hormone receptors in interstitial cells. *Proc. Natl. Acad. Sci. USA*, **77**, 4459

Clayton, R. N. (1982). Gonadotropin-releasing hormone modulation of its own pituitary receptors: Evidence for biphasic regulation. *Endocrinology*, **111**, 152

Dahlen, H. G., Keller, E. and Schneider, H. P. G. (1974). Linear dose dependent LH release following intranasally sprayed LRH. *Horm. Metab. Res.*, **6**, 510

de la Torre, B., Sjoberg, B., Hedman, M., Bartfai, G. and Diczfalusy, E. (1981). A study of the short-term variation and interrelationship of plasma hormone levels reflecting pituitary adrenocortical and testicular function in fertile men. *Int. J. Androl.*, **4**, 532

Dufau, M. L., Pock, R., Neubauer, A. and Catt, R. J. (1976). In vitro bioassay of LH in human serum: The rat interstitial cell testosterone (RICT) assay. *J. Clin. Endocrinol. Metab.*, **42**, 958

Ekman, P., Snochowski, M., Zetterberg, A., Hogberg, B. and Gustafsson, J.-A. (1979). Steroid receptor content in human prostatic carcinoma and response to endocrine therapy. *Cancer*, **44**, 1173

Faure, N., Labrie, F., Lemay, A., Bélanger, A., Gourdeau, Y., Laroche, B. and Robert, G. (1982) Inhibition of serum androgen levels by chronic intranasal and subcutaneous administration of a potent luteinizing hormone-releasing hormone (LH-RH) agonist in adult men. *Fertil. Steril.*, **37**, 416

Freireich, E. J., Gehan, E. A., Rall, D. P., Schmidt, L. H. and Skipper, H. E. (1966). Quantitative comparison of toxicity of anticancer agents in mouse, rat, hamster, dog, monkey, and man. *Cancer Chemother. Rep.*, **50**, 219

Ghanadian, R., Auf, G., Williams, G., Davis, A. and Richards, B. (1981). Predicting the response of prostatic carcinoma to endocrine therapy. *Lancet*, **2**, 1418

Glode, L. M. (1982). Leuprolide therapy of advanced prostatic cancer. *Proceedings of the ASCO Annual Meeting*, April 25–27, St. Louis, MO

Hsueh, A. J. W. and Jones, P. B. C. (1981). Extrapituitary actions of gonadotropin-releasing hormone. *Endocr. Rev.*, **2**, 437

Johnson, D. E., Kaesler, K. E. and Ayala, A. G. (1975). Megestrol acetate for treatment of advanced carcinoma of the prostate. *J. Surg. Oncol.*, **7**, 9

Kulin, H. E., Bell, P. M., Santen, R. J. and Ferber, A. J. (1975). Integration of pulsatile gonadotropin secretion by timed urinary measurements: An accurate and sensitive 3-hour test. *J. Clin. Endocrinol. Metab.*, **40**, 783

Labrie, F., Auclair, C., Cusan, L., Kelly, P., Pelletier, G. and Ferland, L. (1978). Inhibitory effect of LHRH and its agonists on testicular gonadotrophin receptors and spermatogenesis in the rat. *Int. J. Androl.* (Suppl. 2), 303

Labrie, F., Cusan, L., Séguin, C., Bélanger, A., Pelletier, G., Reeves, J., Kelly, P. A., Lemay, A. and Raynaud, J. P. (1980*a*). Antifertility effects of LHRH agonists in the male rat and inhibition of testicular steroidogenesis in man. *Int. J. Fertil.*, **25**, 157

Labrie, F., Bélanger, A. Cusan, L., Séguin, C., Pelletier, G., Kelly, P. A., Reeves, J. J., Lefebvre, F.-A., Lemay, A., Gourdeau, Y. and Raynaud, J.-P. (1980*b*). Antifertility effects of LHRH agonists in the male. *J. Androl.*, **1**, 209

Linde, R., Doelle, G. C., Alexander, N., Kirchner, F., Vale, W., Rivier, J. and Rabin, D. (1981). Reversible inhibition of testicular steroidogenesis and spermatogenesis by a potent gonadotropin-releasing hormone agonist in normal men. *N. Engl. J. Med.*, **305**, 663

London, D. R., Butt, W. R., Lynch, S. S., Marshall, J. C., Owusu, S., Robinson, W. R. and Stephenson, J. M. (1972). Hormonal responses to intranasal luteinizing hormone-releasing hormone. *J. Clin. Endocrinol. Metab.*, **37**, 829

Rivier, C., Rivier, J. and Vale, W. (1979). Chronic effects of [D-Trp^6,Pro^9-NEt] luteinizing hormone-releasing factor on reproductive processes in the male rat. *Endocrinology*, **105**, 1191

Rost, A., Schmidt-Gollwitzer, M., Hantelmann, W. and Brosig, W. (1981). Cyproterone acetate, testosterone, LH, FSH, and prolactin levels in plasma after intramuscular application of cyproterone acetate in patients with prostatic cancer. *Prostate*, **2**, 315

Schirmer, H. K. A., Murphy, G. P. and Scott, W. W. (1965). Hormone therapy of prostatic cancer and the clinical course of the disease. *Urol. Digest*, **4**, 15

Schmidt, J. D., Scott, W. W., Gibbons, R., Johnson, D. E., Prout, G. R. Jr., Loening, S., Soloway, M., deKernion, J., Pontes, J. E., Slack, N. H. and Murphy, G. P. (1980). Chemotherapy programs of the National Prostatic Cancer Project (NPCP). *Cancer*, **45**, 1937

Silverberg, E. and Holleb, A. I. (1982). Cancer Statistics. *CA-A Cancer J. Clinicians,* **32,** 15

Smith, J. A. and the Abbott Leuprolide Prostatic Cancer Study Group (1982). Leuprolide in metastatic cancer. *Proceeding of the American Urological Association Annual Meeting,* Kansas City

Solano, A. R., Dufau, M. L. and Catt, K. J. (1979). Bioassay and radioimmunoassay of serum luteinizing hormone in the male rat. *Endocrinology,* **105,** 372

Stoliar, B. and Albert, D. J. (1974). SCH 13521 in the treatment of advanced carcinoma of the prostate. *J. Urol.,* **111,** 803

Tcholakian, R., de la Cruz, A., Chowdhury, M., Steinberger, A., Coy, D. and Schally, A. (1978). Unusual antireproductive properties of the analog [D-Leu^{6},des-gly-NH_2^{10}]-luteinizing hormone-releasing hormone ethylamide in male rats. *Fertil Steril.,* **30,** 600

Tolis, G., Mehta, A., Comaru-Schally, A. M. and Schally, A. V. (1981). Suppression of androgen production by D-tryptophan-6-luteinizing hormone-releasing hormone in man. *J. Clin. Invest.,* **68,** 819

Tolis, G., Ackman, D., Stellos, A., Mehta, A., Labrie, F., Fazekas, A. T. A., Comaru-Schally, A. M. and Schally, A. V. (1982) Tumor growth inhibition in patients with prostatic carcinoma treated with luteinizing hormone-releasing hormone agonists. *Proc. Natl. Acad. Sci. USA,* **79,** 1658

Warner, B. A. W. and Santen, R. J. (1981). Response to TRH in FSH secreting adenomas, an example of hormone cross-talk. *Lancet,* **2,** 42

Warner, W., Worgul, T. J., Drago, J., Demers, L., Dufau, M., Max, D., Santen, R. J. and members of the Abbott Study Group (1983). Effect of very high-dose D-Leu^{6}-GnRH proethylamide on the hypothalamic-pituitary testicular axis in patients with prostatic cancer. *J. Clin. Invest.,* **71,** 184

Appendix

N. L. Block and M. A. Eisenberger, University of Miami Hospitals and Clinical Center, Miami, FL 33136; R. J. Correa and R. S. Gibbons, Department of Urology, The Mason Clinic, Seattle, WA 98111; A. G. Glass, Department of Oncology, Permanente Clinic, Portland, OR 97232; H. A. Harvey and A. Lipton, Department of Medicine, Division of Oncology, The Milton S. Hershey Medical Center of The Pennsylvania State University, Hershey, PA 17033; L. M. Glode and J. N. Wettlaufer, University of Colorado, Denver, CO 80262; J. A. Smith, Division of Urology, University of Utah Medical Center, Salt Lake City, UT 88413; G. H. Sokol, Department of Radiation Oncology, Tampa General Hospital, Tampa, FL 33606; M. T. Resnick and H. B. Muss, Section of Hematology/Oncology, Bowman Gray School of Medicine, Winston-Salem, NC 27103; P. R. Band, Institut du Cancer de Montréal, Center Hospitalier Nôtre-Dame, Montréal, Québec, Canada H21 4MI; H. Schneir, VA Hospital, Sepulveda, CA 91343; D. Heber and J. Rajfer, Clinical Research Center, Harbor General Hospital, UCLA, Torrance, CA 90509; B. S. Stein, Temple University Hospital, Philadelphia, PA 19140; A. F. Greco, Oncology Division, Vanderbilt University School, Nashville, TN 37232; and J. N. Hueser, Boone Clinic, Columbia, MO 65201.

SECTION VII

DIAGNOSTIC APPLICATIONS OF LHRH

28
Diagnostic uses of LHRH

Z. LARON, R. PRAGER-LEWIN and Z. DICKERMAN

LH and FSH, known to be secreted already in utero and in early infancy (Faiman and Winter, 1971), activate the production of both male and female gonadal hormones (Forest *et al.*, 1973; Bidlingmaier and Knorr, 1978). In the clinic LHRH is most frequently used for diagnostic purposes, to test the integrity of the hypothalamic–pituitary–gonadal axis. Experience in many clinics has led to a number of test procedures which are based on common principles but differ in the dosage employed and the mode of administration. The physiological basis for the LHRH test is the ability of LHRH, whether administered intravenously or intramuscularly, to induce secretion of the pool of pituitary LH and FSH which in normal circumstances is readily releasable. This review of diagnostic procedures emphasizes the experience gained in our clinic during the past 10 years in performing several thousand LHRH tests, mainly in children.

ASSESSMENT OF MATURATION STAGE IN CHILDHOOD

Several methods have been used to measure the gonadotropins released in response to an LHRH challenge. Although a few clinics use the urinary gonadotropin determination (Reiter *et al.*, 1977), the more accurate and less cumbersome plasma radioimmunoassay (RIA) determination of LH and FSH is the assay method used in most clinics. Performance of i.v. LHRH tests in large numbers of prepubertal and pubertal children of both sexes by several investigators (Garnier *et al.*, 1974; Kelch *et al.*, 1976; Dickerman *et al.*, 1976*a*) has revealed that, despite a wide distribution of individual plasma LH and FSH values, mean values of basal and peak levels show a definite pattern for each sex in the different pubertal stages (Table 28.1). Of particular interest is the sharp rise in plasma FSH in prepubertal girls (Dickerman *et al.*, 1979). We found the dose of 50 $\mu g/m^2$ given in one i.v. bolus adequate for the discrimination between various degrees of responsiveness, but other groups have used doses from 25 to 1000 μg, often without adjustment according to body surface or weight. In girls after menarche and in mature females it is advised that the test be done in the follicular phase (Lemarchand-Beraud *et al.*, 1975) unless there are specific indications otherwise.

Table 28.1 Plasma LH and FSH levels in boys and girls at different pubertal stages during LHRH test

Pubertal stage	Boys[a]				Girls[a]			
	LH (mIU/ml)		*FSH* (mIU/ml)		*LH* (mIU/ml)		*FSH* (mIU/ml)	
	Basal	*Peak*	*Basal*	*Peak*	*Basal*	*Peak*	*Basal*	*Peak*
1A[b]	0.54 ±0.1	1.3±0.17	0.6 ±0.2	1.5 ±0.5	0.5 ±0.1	1.6 ±0.2	0.9 ±0.1	8.0 ±1.0
1B[b]					0.9 ±0.2	1.8 ±0.3	0.7 ±0.1	6.5 ±0.9
2	0.83 ±0.06	5.9 ±0.4	1.0 ±0.4	2.4 ±0.9	0.6 ±0.3	3.6 ±2.3	1.9 ±0.9	8.7 ±3.7
3	0.8 ±0.17	6.4 ±0.3	1.9 ±0.6	3.0 ±1.0	0.9 ±0.1	9.7 ±0.9	1.4 ±0.5	3.4 ±1.2
4	1.34 ±0.2	14.9 ±2.2	2.1 ±0.8	3.0 ±1.0	1.6 ±0.2	13.5 ±2.0	2.0 ±0.7	4.5 ±1.6
5	1.9 ±0.4	14.2 ±2.2	2.6 ±1.0	4.5 ±1.6	2.3 ±0.3	13.8 ±2.1	2.5 ±0.9	4.8 ±1.8

[a] Values given are mean ±SD. The dose of LHRH was 50 $\mu g/m^2$ i.v.
[b] According to the FSH response to LHRH two subgroups were distinguished

Due to the short duration of the i.v. LHRH test (90–120 min) only minor changes in sexual hormones are registered and these are of a degree which is insufficient to be of any more value than the basal levels in reaching a diagnosis.

Although the mechanism of the maturation of the gonadal axis has not yet been clarified (Grumbach *et al.*, 1974) recent evidence indicates that in both sexes an important role is played by changes in endogenous estradiol secretion (Dickerman *et al.*, 1982; Gurewitz *et al.*, 1982).

DELAYED PUBERTY

Delayed puberty, i.e. the lack of appearance of secondary sexual signs at the expected age, is more frequent in boys. It often occurs as a hereditary trait and can be considered a physiological aberration. There is also a phenomenon of 'slow puberty', i.e. the appearance of secondary sexual characteristics at the expected age but with a slower progression than in most children. Both forms are accompanied by a delay in, or slowing of, the pubertal growth spurt which can cause psychological tension and concern in both the youngsters and their parents. The performance of an LHRH test and proof of a positive response (Laron and Dickerman, 1977; Dickerman *et al.*, 1977; Savage *et al.*, 1981; Bourguignon *et al.*, 1982) provides reassurance that normal puberty can be achieved, with or without pharmacological acceleration (Galatzer *et al.*, 1977).

HYPOGONADOTROPIC HYPOGONADISM

Hypogonadotropic hypogonadism can be caused either by a derangement in LHRH secretion or a defect in the gonadotropin-secreting pituitary cells. Making the differential diagnosis is often difficult, particularly if the LHRH deficiency is suspected to be total rather than partial. A response of LH and FSH which is inadequate for age can be considered evidence for a deficit in the hypothalamic or pituitary axis. By analogy with other hormonal axes, it may be assumed that if the deficiency is partial or of relatively short duration there will be at least a slight rise in LH and/or FSH in response to LHRH. A single rapid intravenous bolus is unlikely to be adequate to stimulate a normal pituitary when the deficiency is hereditary or longstanding. Therefore, various changes in the standard i.v. LHRH test have been proposed, including i.v. infusion of LHRH (Reiter *et al.*, 1977; Dickerman *et al.*, 1977), priming by repeated intramuscular injections of LHRH (Dickerman *et al.*, 1976*b*; Fernandez-Castaner *et al.*, 1982) and the use of a superactive LHRH analog (Laron *et al.*, 1981*a*; Vaughan Williams *et al.*, 1982). The response of LH and/or FSH to any of these stimuli suggests that the deficiency is at the hypothalamic and not the pituitary level whereas a lack of response in repeated tests indicated pituitary failure.

Although experience with the new superactive LHRH analogs as diagnostic aids is still limited, we found that the administration of five daily i.m. injections

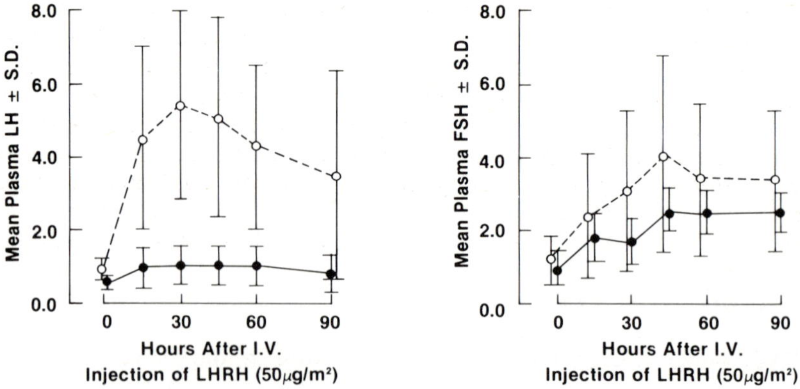

Figure 28.1 Plasma LH and plasma FSH in five patients before (●——●) and after (○--○) five daily i.m. injections of 100 μg LHRH.

of synthetic LHRH consecutively at a dose of 100 μg/day was superior to two consecutive daily i.m. injections of [D-Trp^6]LHRH at a dose of 50–100 μg/day in promoting the gonadotropin response during the standard i.v. LHRH test (50 μg/m^2). Whereas all ten patients responded by an LH rise to the repeated i.m. priming with natural LHRH (5 × 100 μg), only four of ten responded to the priming with the LHRH analog [D-Trp^6]LHRH, (2 × 50–100 μg).

The LHRH test is also helpful in diagnosing a gonadotropin deficiency when it is suspected to be one of multiple pituitary hormone deficiencies (MPHD) (Laron, 1981). We prefer to perform a combined test, e.g. (insulin tolerance test) ITT plus LHRH, with the insulin (0.05–0.1 u/kg) and LHRH injected together i.v. in a single bolus. In accordance with the indications it is also possible to combine the LHRH with an oral glucose tolerance test, e.g. in cases of acromegaly, or with clonidine (Laron *et al.*, 1983), e.g. in cases with growth retardation.

In normal children there is some response of LH and FSH to LHRH even in the prepubertal period and a failure of plasma LH and FSH to rise in response to repeated LHRH tests after priming is very suggestive of gonadotropin deficiency, even at an early age. An intrauterine deficiency of gonadotropins may result in undescended testes and micropenis as signs of hypogonadism which may be apparent in early childhood. At birth basal gonadotropins are usually elevated, and the determination of basal LH and FSH at this time may avert the performance of subsequent LHRH tests.

PRIMARY GONADAL DYSFUNCTION

In partial primary testicular failure of various etiologies, including unilateral cryptorchidism, the basal level of LH may be within normal limits but the response to the LHRH test is exaggerated (Laron *et al.*, 1975, 1980). This over-responsiveness may be detected even prepubertally (Dickerman *et al.*,

1978). In various syndromes associated with progressive gonadal failure, such as Bloom syndrome (Kauli *et al.*, 1977*a*), Reifenstein syndrome (Flatau *et al.*, 1975), Klinefelter's syndrome (Topper *et al.*, 1982), gonadal dysgenesis in females (Laron, 1975) and ataxia telangiectasia (Zadik *et al.*, 1978), repeated LHRH tests are helpful in assessing the progression of the gonadal dysfunction and aid in defining the stage at which sex hormone replacement therapy should be initiated. Among patients with these syndromes the LHRH test will also help in uncovering the exceptional cases who do not undergo gonadal degeneration (Laron *et al.*, 1982) and those very rare cases who develop precocious puberty.

IRREGULAR AND PRECOCIOUS PUBERTY

The LHRH test performed consecutively at different ages is helpful in the differential diagnosis and grading of central precocious puberty (Kauli *et al.*, 1975, 1977*b*, 1978; Marilus *et al.*, 1981). In this disorder the basal and peak LH and FSH levels correspond to the pubertal stage and not to the chronological age. In precocious thelarche, and even more so in precocious adrenarche, the gonadotropin response corresponds to the chronological and not to the skeletal age. It is noteworthy that in cases of untreated congenital virilizing adrenal hyperplasia the pattern of the LH and FSH response to LHRH may correspond to the stage of precocious sexual development and advanced bone age and not to the chronological age (Pertzelan *et al.*, 1978).

The LHRH test is of particular clinical importance in monitoring the treatment of precocious puberty with the superactive LHRH analog [D-Trp^6]LHRH (Laron *et al.*, 1981*b*; Crowley *et al.*, 1981; Kauli *et al.*, 1984), the purpose of which is to suppress the secretion of gonadotropins. The aim is to find the minimal daily dose of [D-Trp^6]LHRH which will suppress the response of LH and FSH to i.v. LHRH and this is achieved by the periodic performance of the test.

OTHER INDICATIONS

It has been reported that an unspecific response to LHRH, such as that of growth hormone, may be indicative of a disturbance at the neurotransmitter–hypothalamus level. This has been found in untreated adolescent schizophrenia (Gil-Ad *et al.*, 1981), with a normalization of the response (i.e. no rise in hGH) after therapy, and also in some patients with Klinefelter's syndrome (Dickerman *et al.*, 1981).

CONCLUDING REMARKS

As a diagnostic and therapeutic aid the i.v. LHRH test is an indispensable tool in the evaluation of normal and abnormal developmental stages and pathological conditions of the hypothalamo–pituitary–gonadal axis.

Acknowledgements

The authors are indebted to Ayerst International, Canada; Ferring AG, Malmo; and Serono, Roma, for their generous supply of LHRH for investigational purposes. Professor A. V. Schally and Dr A. M. Comaru-Schally, New Orleans, kindly supplied the [D-Trp[6]]LHRH.

References

Bidlingmaier, F. and Knorr, D. (1978). *Oestrogens.* In Laron, Z. (ed.) *Pediatric and Adolescent Endocrinology.* Vol. 4, pp. 48–58. (Basel: Karger)

Bourguignon, J. P., Vanderschueren-Lodeweyckx, M., Wolter, R., Malvaux, P., Craen, M., Du Caju, M. V. L., Ernould, C. and Franchimont, P. (1982). Hypopituitarism and idiopathic delayed puberty: A longitudinal study in an attempt to diagnose gonadotropin deficiency before puberty. *J. Clin. Endocrinol. Metab.,* **54,** 733

Crowley, W. Jr., Comite, F., Vale, W., Rivier, J., Loriaux, D. L. and Cutler, G. B. (1981). Therapeutic use of pituitary desensitization with a long-acting LHRH agonist: a potential new treatment for idiopathic precocious puberty. *J. Clin. Endocrinol. Metab.,* **52,** 370

Dickerman, Z., Prager-Lewin, R. and Laron, Z. (1976*a*). Response of plasma LH and FSH to synthetic LHRH in children at various pubertal stages. *Am. J. Dis. Child.,* **130,** 634

Dickerman, Z., Prager-Lewin, R. and Laron, Z. (1976*b*). The effect of repeated injections of synthetic luteinizing hormone releasing hormone on the response of plasma luteinizing hormone and follicle stimulating hormone in young hypogonadotrophic hypogonadal patients. *Fertil. Steril.,* **7,** 162

Dickerman, Z., Laron, Z., Prager-Lewin, R. and Mulder, J. (1977). Influence of the mode of administration of LHRH on the response of plasma LH and FSH in various disorders of puberty. *Israel J. Med. Sci.,* **13,** 313

Dickerman, Z., Landman, J., Prager-Lewin, R. and Laron, Z. (1978). Evaluation of testicular function in prepubertal boys by means of the LHRH test. *Fertil. Steril.,* **29,** 655

Dickerman, Z., Prager-Lewin, R. and Laron, Z. (1979). The plasma FSH and LH response to synthetic LHRH in normal prepubertal girls – a re-evaluation. *Acta Endocrinol.,* **91,** 14

Dickerman, Z., Rachmel, A., Gil-Ad, I., Prager-Lewin, R., Galatzer, A. and Laron, Z. (1981). Rise in plasma growth hormone in response to exogenous LRH in Klinefelter's syndrome. *Clin. Endocrinol.,* **15,** 403

Dickerman, Z., Gurewitz, R., Peleg, S., Keret, R., Gidali, A. and Laron, Z. (1982). Dynamics of basal pituitary gonadotropin secretion and responsiveness to LRH following estradiol benzoate in normal boys. *Hormone Res.,* **16,** 115

Faiman, C. and Winter, J. S. D. (1971). Sex differences in gonadotropin concentrations in infancy. *Nature (Lond.),* **232,** 130

Fernandez-Castaner, M., Martinez de Osaba, M. J. and Vilardell, E. (1982). Insuffisance hypophysaire post-traumatique. *Ann. Endocrinol. (Paris)* **43,** 213

Flatau, E., Josefsberg, Z., Prager-Lewin, R., Markman Halabe, E., Kaufman, H. and Laron, Z. (1975). Response to LHRH and HCG in two brothers with the Reifenstein syndrome. *Helv. Paediatr. Acta,* **30,** 377

Forest, M. G., Cathiard, A. M. and Bertrand, J. A. (1973). Evidence of testicular activity in early infancy. *J. Clin. Endocrinol. Metab.,* **37,** 148

Galatzer, A., Kaufman, V. and Laron, Z. (1977). Psychological aspects of delayed puberty in boys. In Chiumello, G. and Laron, Z. (eds.) *Recent Progress in Pediatric Endocrinology, Proceedings of the Serono Foundation Symposia No. 12,* pp. 153–155. (London: Academic Press)

Garnier, P. E., Chaussain, J. L., Binet, E., Schlumberger, A. and Job, J. C. (1974). Effect of synthetic luteinizing hormone (LHRH) on the release of gonadotropins in children and adolescents. VI. Relations to age, sex and puberty. *Acta Endocrinol.,* **77,** 422

Gil-Ad, I., Dickerman, Z., Weitzman, R., Weitzman, A., Tyano, S. and Laron, Z. (1981). Abnormal growth hormone response to LRH and TRH in male adolescent schizophrenics. *Am. J. Psychiatry,* **138,** 357

Grumbach, M. M., Roth, J. C., Kaplan, S. L. and Kelch, R. P. (1974). Hypothalamic pituitary regulation of puberty: Evidence and concepts derived from clinical research. In Grumbach, M. M., Grave, G. D. and Mayer, F. E. (eds.) *The Control of Onset of Puberty*, p. 115. (New York: Wiley)

Gurewitz, R., Dickerman, Z., Peleg, S., Keret, R., Gidali, A. and Laron, Z. (1982). Dynamics of basal pituitary gonadotropin secretion and responsiveness to LRH following estradiol benzoate in normal girls. *Hormone Res.*, **16**, 174

Kauli, R., Prager-Lewin, R., Keret, R. and Laron, Z. (1975). The LH response to LHRH in children with true isosexual precocious puberty treated with cyproterone acetate. *Clin. Endocrinol.*, **4**, 305

Kauli, R., Prager-Lewin, R., Kaufman, H. and Laron, Z. (1977*a*). Gonadal function in Bloom's syndrome. *Clin. Endocrinol.*, **6**, 285

Kauli, R., Prager-Lewin, R., Keret, R. and Laron, Z. (1977*b*). The LH and FSH response to LHRH in girls with true precocious puberty treated with cyproterone acetate. *Eur. J. Pediatr.*, **125**, 205

Kauli, R., Prager-Lewin, R. and Laron, Z. (1978). Pubertal development in the Prader–Labhert–Willi syndrome. *Acta Paediatr. Scand.*, **67**, 763

Kauli, R., Pertzelan, A., Ben Zeev, Z., Kaufman, H., Prager-Lewin, R., Comaru-Schally, A. M., Schally, A. V. and Laron, Z. (1984). Treatment of precocious puberty with a superactive LHRH analog (D-TRP^6-LHRH) in combination with cyproterone acetate. *Clin. Endocrinol.*, (In press)

Kelch, R. P., Markovs, M. and Huss, J. (1976). LH and FSH responsiveness to intravenous gonadotropin-releasing hormone (Gn-RH) in children with hypothalamic or pituitary disorders. *J. Clin Endocrinol. Metab.*, **42**, 1104

Laron, Z. (1975). Influence of endocrine equilibrium on the response to LHRH in children. In Franchimont, P. (ed.) *Some Aspects of Hypothalamic Regulation of Endocrine Function (Symposia Medica Hoechst 7)*, pp. 125–127. (Stuttgart, New York: Schattauer)

Laron, Z. (1981). Clinical aspects of pituitary dwarfism and related conditions. In Daughaday, W. H. (ed.) *Endocrine Control of Growth*, pp. 175–205. (New York: Elsevier-North Holland)

Laron, Z., Dickerman, Z., Prager-Lewin, R., Keret, R. and Halabe, E. (1975). Plasma LH and FSH response to LRH in boys with compensatory testicular hypertrophy. *J. Clin. Endocrinol. Metab.*, **40**, 977

Laron, Z. and Dickerman, Z. (1977). Usefulness of the LHRH test in the choice of therapy in delayed puberty in boys. In Chiumello, G. and Laron, Z. (eds.) *Recent Progress in Pediatric Endocrinology, Proceedings of the Serono Foundation Symposia No. 12*, pp. 139–151. (London: Academic Press)

Laron, Z., Dickerman, Z., Ritterman, I. and Kaufman, H. (1980). Follow-up of boys with unilateral compensatory testicular hypertrophy. *Fertil. Steril.*, **33**, 297

Laron, Z., Dickerman, Z., Ben Zeev, Z., Prager-Lewin, R., Comaru-Schally, A. M. and Schally, A. V. (1981*a*). Long term effect of D-TRP^6-LHRH in testicular size and LH, FSH and testosterone levels in hypothalamic hypogonadotrophic males. *Fertil. Steril.*, **35**, 328

Laron, Z., Kauli, R., Ben Zeev, Z., Comaru-Schally, A. M. and Schally, A. V. (1981*b*). D-TRP^6 analogue of LHRH in combination with cyproterone acetate to treat precocious puberty. *Lancet*, **2**, 955

Laron, Z., Dickerman, Z., Zamir, R. and Galatzer, A. (1982). Paternity in Klinefelter's syndrome – a case report. *Arch. Androl.*, **8**, 149

Laron, Z., Topper, E. and Gil-Ad, I. (1983). Oral clonidine – a simple, safe and effective test for growth hormone secretion. In Laron, Z. and Butenandt, O. (eds.) *Evaluation of Growth Hormone Secretion, Pediatric and Adolescent Endocrinology*, Vol. 12. pp. 103–121, (Basel: Karger) (In press)

Lemarchand-Beraud, T., Reymond, M., Rappaport, G., Magrini, G. and Gomez, J. (1975). Action des stéroïdes sexuels sur les réponses LH et FSH au LH RH chez le sujet normal. *Pathol. Biol.*, **23**, 917

Marilus, R., Dickerman, Z., Kaufman, H., Varsano, I. and Laron, Z. (1981). Addison's disease associated with precocious sexual development in a boy. *Acta Paediatr. Scand.*, **70**, 587

Pertzelan, A., Laron, Z., Adler Bier, M., Prager-Lewin, R. and Kaufman, H. (1978). Gonadotrophin release in untreated congenital virilizing adrenal hyperplasia. *Arch. Dis. Child.*, **53**, 305

Reiter, E. O., Root, A. W. and Duckett, G. E. (1977). LH and FSH levels in urine and serum of prepubertal and pubertal children receiving a 3 hour infusion of LHRH. *J. Clin. Endocrinol. Metab.*, **44**, 56

Savage, M. O., Preece, M. A., Cameron, N., Jones, J., Theintz, G., Penfold, J. L. and Tanner, J. M. (1981). Gonadotrophin response to LHRH in boys with delayed growth and adolescence. *Arch. Dis. Child.*, **56**, 552

Topper, E., Dickerman, Z., Prager-Lewin, R., Kaufman, H., Maimon, Z. and Laron, Z. (1982). Puberty in 24 patients with Klinefelter's syndrome. *Eur. J. Pediatr.*, **139**, 8

Vaughan Williams, C. A., McNeilly, A. S. and Baird, D. T. (1982). Assessment of pituitary secretory capacity in women with hypogonadotrophic hypogonadism by using a long acting synthetic analogue of luteinizing hormone releasing factor. *Br. J. Obstet. Gynaecol.*, **89**, 738

Zadik, Z., Lewin, S., Prager-Lewin, R. and Laron, Z. (1978). Gonadal dysfunction in patients with ataxia telangiectasia. *Acta Paediatr. Scand.*, **67**, 477

SECTION VIII

APPLICATIONS IN ANIMALS

29
Actions of LHRH and its analogs in lower vertebrates

L. W. CRIM

Pituitary gonadotropic hormone function in lower vertebrates is under stimulatory control by the brain (Ball, 1981). Gonadal regression results from the isolation or the removal of specific neurosecretory brain centres in reptiles, amphibians and fish. Extracts of both fish and sheep hypothalamus increase gonadotropin release from mature carp pituitaries incubated *in vitro* (Breton *et al.*, 1972). Injections of synthetic LHRH into carp and trout increase circulating gonadotropin levels (Breton and Weil, 1973; Crim and Cluett, 1974). The high doses of LHRH required to elicit gonadotropin release from the fish pituitary lead to speculation that the structures of mammalian and fish LHRH are different.

LHRH-LIKE ACTIVITY IN BRAIN OF LOWER VERTEBRATES

Early work on the structure of LHRH in lower vertebrates suffered from lack of good assay methods for the detection and quantification of the hormone. Frog pituitaries release gonadotropin *in vitro* in response to hypothalamic extracts and LHRH treatment (Thornton and Geschwind, 1974). *In vitro* bioassays for fish LHRH have now been developed (Breton *et al.*, 1975; *De* Vlaming and Vodicnik, 1975; Crim and Evans, 1980). The stimulation of adenyl cyclase activity in the ventral lobe of the dogfish pituitary has been used to evaluate LHRH activity in extracts of the dogfish brain (Deery and Jones, 1975). LH release from rat pituitaries *in vitro* was used to determine the LHRH activity in cod hypothalami (Barnett *et al.*, 1979); similarly, LH release from cultured ovine anterior pituitary cells was used to estimate the activity of extracts of the teleost hypothalami (King and Millar, 1980).

Antibodies to LHRH have been used for the immunohistochemical localization of LHRH in the brains of reptiles, amphibia and fishes (Nozaki and Kobayashi, 1979; Peter, 1982). Recently, radioimmunoassays for LHRH have been developed and have aided the purification and characterization of LHRH from lower vertebrates.

Frog sympathetic ganglia contain a substance structurally related to but chemically separable from synthetic mammalian LHRH (Eiden and Eskay, 1980). However, frog brain contains LHRH-like material which shares chemical and immunological similarities with mammalian LHRH (King and Millar, 1979). There is immunological and chromatographic evidence of heterogeneity between mammalian LHRH and a group of LHRHs similar to one another which are obtained from the hypothalami of birds, reptiles and the fishes (King and Millar, 1980). LHRHs have been partially characterized and are shown to be chromatographically distinguishable from synthetic mammalian LHRH in four different species of fish including tilapia (King and Millar, 1980), the goldfish and cod (Barnett *et al.*, 1982) and the winter flounder (Idler and Crim, 1984). The immunological behavior of fish LHRHs with region-specific LHRH antisera suggested that fish LHRHs differ from mammalian LHRH by at least one amino acid substitution near the peptide C-terminus (King and Millar, 1980; Barnett *et al.*, 1982). Possibly, fish LHRHs may also differ structurally from each other since immunoreactive LHRH obtained from tilapia and winter flounder hypothalami elute more quickly than mammalian LHRH on reverse phase high performance liquid chromatography. In contrast, codfish and goldfish LHRHs are retained more strongly, suggesting that the latter peptides are relatively more hydrophobic. Recently, the decapeptide amino acid sequence of chicken LHRH was found to differ from mammalian LHRH at position 8, replacing arginine with a glutamine residue (King and Millar, 1982). During preparation of this chapter the structure of salmon LHRH was reported as [Trp^7,Leu^8]LHRH (Sherwood *et al.*, 1983).

GONADOTROPIN-RELEASE INHIBITING HORMONE

In addition to LHRH activity, the goldfish brain appears to contain a factor which inhibits gonadotropin release (Peter and Paulencu, 1980). Although the chemical nature of this inhibitory substance is unknown, dopamine inhibits the release of gonadotropic hormone in the goldfish (Chang and Peter, 1983).

ACTIONS OF LHRH AND ITS ANALOGS

In the green turtle LHRH administration stimulates modest increases in both plasma gonadotropins and progesterone (Licht, 1980). However, treatment of the olive ridley sea turtle with either synthetic LHRH or the agonistic LHRH analog, [D-His(Bzl)^6,Pro^9-NHEt]LHRH, does not increase plasma gonadotropin or the steroid levels in either sex (Licht *et al.*, 1982).

LHRH induces spermiation in the frog, *Hyla regella* (Licht, 1974). Since LHRH fails to induce spermiation in hypophysectomized frogs, the hormone appears to act at the pituitary level to release gonadotropin. LHRH restores spermatogenesis in hypophysectomized-pituitary grafted newts (Mazzi *et al.*, 1974) and induces ovulation in female crested newts (Vellano *et al.*, 1974). Repetitive LHRH injections induce ovulation in the toad, *Xenopus laevis* (Thornton and Geschwind, 1974). Recent studies have explored the actions of

LHRH and also agonist and antagonist analogs of LHRH in the bullfrog, *Rana catesbeiana* (Daniels and Licht, 1980; McCreery *et al.*, 1982). Compared with the release profile of LH and FSH using synthetic LHRH, the agonist analog, [D-His(Bzl)^6,Pro^9-NHEt]LHRH has approximately a 45-fold greater potency and the duration of action is prolonged. Repeated daily injections of the analog induce ovulation but at relatively high doses of the LHRH agonist, plasma gonadotropin levels are reduced, suggesting that the frog pituitary becomes desensitized under certain conditions. In male frogs the stimulation of gonadotropin release by LHRH can be suppressed by pretreatment with an LHRH antagonist, [N-Ac-Δ^3-Pro^1,D-pCl-Phe^2,D-Trp^{3,6},N-MeLeu^7]LHRH.

There have been attempts to induce captive fish to spawn by administering either mammalian or fish pituitary hormone preparations (Harvey and Hoar, 1979). Such procedures have been successful in some cases; however, pituitary hormones are expensive to prepare and difficult to store properly with maintenance of biological activity, and may cause harmful side-effects in brood stock fishes (antibody formation, excess water absorption). As an alternative, LHRH was shown to be an effective spawning agent in female fish, inducing ovulation in the ayu, *Plecoglossus altivelis* (Hirose and Ishida, 1974). Large doses of LHRH also have been used to induce ovulation in a variety of other teleost fishes including goldfish, plaice and goby, the Japanese medaka, and various carp species (Lam, 1982). LHRH and also the LHRH analogs, [D-Ala^6,Pro^9-NHEt]LHRH or [D-Ser(tBu)^6,Pro^9-NHEt]LHRH, evoke oocyte maturation but not ovulation in the European carp (Sokolowska *et al.*, 1978; Weil *et al.*, 1980; Breton *et al.*, 1984). LHRH stimulates release of gonadotropin in coho salmon but smaller doses of [D-Ala^6,Pro^9-NHEt] LHRH trigger increased gonadotropin secretion and stimulate oocyte maturation as well (Van Der Kraak *et al.*, 1983).

Induction of spawning in male and female Chinese carp has been accomplished with [D-Ala^6,Pro^9-NHEt]LHRH which is reported to be 100-fold more potent than LHRH administration in these fish (Anon, 1977*b*). This LHRH analog also induces ovulation in *Hypophthalmichthys molitrix* (Billard *et al.*, 1984) and it has been used to advance ovulation in coho salmon following primary injections of gonadotropic hormone (Donaldson *et al.*, 1981; Sower *et al.*, 1982). [D-Trp^6,Pro^9-NHEt]LHRH accelerates ovulation and synchronizes spawning in groups of landlocked Atlantic salmon (Crim *et al.*, 1983*a*). This LHRH analog was implanted intraperitoneally in pelleted form, which is designed for prolonged release of small amounts of the peptide hormone (Kent *et al.*, 1980). The same pelleted LHRH analog was also used recently to advance ovulation in rainbow trout which were held in cold water ($< 2°C$) prior to spawning normally in the spring (Crim *et al.*, 1983*b*). At low environmental temperatures ($0°C$) pelleted LHRH analog can be used to advance spawning in the winter flounder, a marine species (Figure 29.1). In the goldfish, LHRH and [D-Ala^6,Pro^9-NHEt]LHRH analog induce only a low percentage ($< 50\%$) of mature fish to ovulate (Lin *et al.*, 1984). Pelleted [D-Trp^6,Pro^9-NHEt]LHRH administration does not improve the rate of ovulation in goldfish despite significantly elevated plasma gonadotropin levels over several days (Sokolowska *et al.*, 1984). Gonadotropin release inhibiting

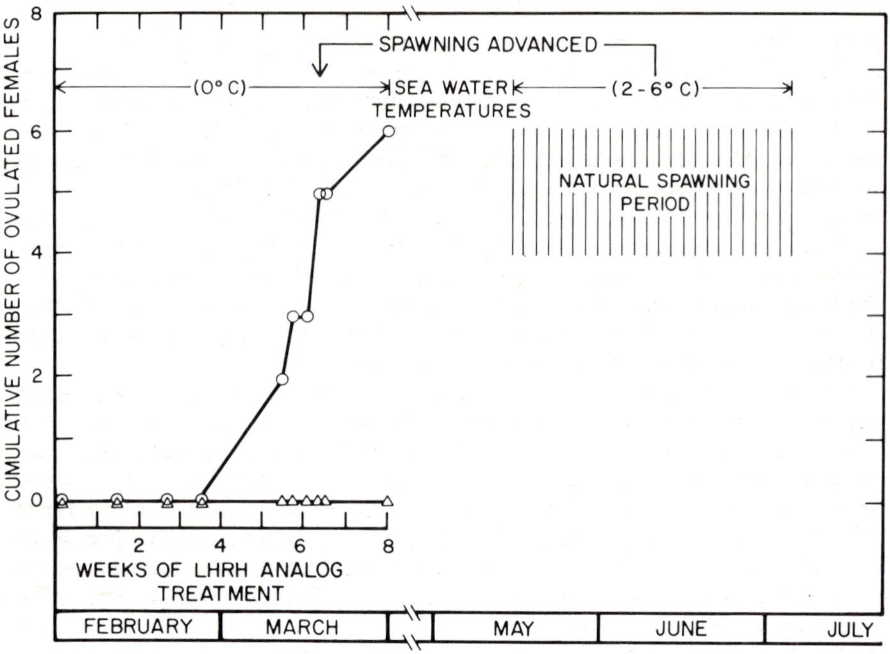

Figure 29.1 The influence of pelleted [D-Trp^6,Pro^9-NHEt]LHRH on acceleration of ovulation in female winter flounder held in the laboratory at ambient temperatures. Treated females (○———○) were implanted with a single cholesterol pellet containing 125 μg LHRH analog. Sham control females (△———△) received surgical procedures only.

factor in goldfish is thought to play a role in timing the ovulatory surge of gonadotropin. A recent paper suggests that gonadotropin release inhibitory factor may reduce the effectiveness of LHRH treatment and that a significant improvement in ovulatory performance to LHRH can be achieved by pretreating mature goldfish with a dopamine antagonist, pimozide (Chang and Peter, 1983).

In males, [D-Ala^6,Pro^9-NHEt]LHRH stimulates spermiation in carp (Anon, 1977*a*) and pelleted [D-Nal(2)^6,Pro^9-NHEt]LHRH treatment increases milt collection in landlocked salmon (Crim *et al.*, 1983*a*). Both of the above LHRH analogs advance the onset of spermiation and also increase the quantity of collectable milt in the male landlocked salmon (Weil and Crim, 1983). Milt collection can be difficult in the European carp and [D-Ala^6,Pro^9-NHEt]LHRH has been successfully used to stimulate the spermiation response of this fish (F. Takashima, C. Weil and R. Billard, personal communication).

In relation to seasonal reproductive development the fish pituitary may undergo fluctuations in LHRH responsitivity. In the adult fish pituitary cyclic seasonal changes in LHRH sensitivity occur in trout (Crim and Cluett, 1974; Weil *et al.*, 1978), carp (Weil *et al.*, 1975) and in the goldfish (Lin *et al.*, 1984). A renewal of ovarian growth and development is stimulated in the sexually regressed Japanese medaka by frequent injections of LHRH over a six week period (Chan, 1977). Ovarian growth is stimulated by pelleted [D-Trp^6,Pro^9-NHEt]LHRH administration in the landlocked salmon but in male salmon this hormone treatment during the time of rapid reproductive development inhibits the expected increases in testes weight (Crim *et al.*, 1983*a*). These data suggest that the paradoxical effects of LHRH noted for mammals can be expected in fish but that in the latter the results of LHRH treatment may depend upon the time of year. [D-Ala^6,Pro^9-NHEt]LHRH treatment suppresses the reproductive system of goldfish undergoing seasonal gonadal recrudescence (Lin *et al.*, 1984). An LHRH antagonist, [D-Phe^{2,6}, Phe^3]LHRH inhibits LHRH-stimulated gonadotropin release in trout (Crim *et al.*, 1981) but the ability of LHRH antagonist to interfere with reproductive events in fish has not been demonstrated.

LHRH sensitivity of the fish pituitary gland may also change in accordance with different stages of the life cycle. Although repeated LHRH injections accelerate sexual development of neonatal platyfish (Bao and Kallman, 1982), juvenile rainbow trout do not show signs of premature reproductive development or pituitary stimulation following prolonged administration of pelleted [D-Trp^6,Pro^9-NHEt]LHRH (Crim and Evans, 1983). The same pelleted LHRH agonist fails to initiate reproductive development in the juvenile milkfish (C. Marte and L. W. Crim, unpublished results). Since some juvenile fish appear to be unresponsive to LHRH, these data suggest that the pituitary LHRH responsitivity in sexually regressed adults and that of juvenile fishes may be dissimilar.

OPTIMIZATION OF LHRH THERAPY

LHRH has usually been dissolved in saline and injected into the dorsal lymph sac of frogs or directly into the perivisceral cavity of fish. Lower doses of LHRH are required if injected into the intracranial cavity of fish (Anon, 1975; Lam *et al.*, 1975; Sokolowska *et al.*, 1978) but this is of questionable practicality. In goldfish [D-Ala^6,Pro^9-NHEt]LHRH stimulates prolonged release of gonadotropin; furthermore, double injections spaced by 3 h potentiate the LHRH stimulatory effect (Lin *et al.*, 1984). Pelleted preparations of LHRH analogs have induced chronic gonadotropin increases for at least 30 days in the plasma of salmon (Crim *et al.*, 1983*a*). The stimulation of spermiation in male landlocked salmon was equivalent when LHRH agonist was administered via solid pelleted implants or by frequent injections of solutions in saline. Injections of LHRH agonist in 40 % propylene/glycol were less effective (Weil and Crim, 1983).

CONCLUDING REMARKS

LHRH and its analogs clearly possess biological activity in many lower vertebrates. To achieve biological responses in these animals relatively large doses of LHRH seem to be required. LHRHs are detectable in lower vertebrate brain and evidence of their heterogeneity compared with mammalian LHRH is accumulating. Availability of LHRH analogs improves the ability to manipulate the reproductive cycle of lower vertebrates. A knowledge of the structure(s) of LHRH in lower vertebrates may lead to development of analogs specifically for use in these animals. Delivery systems for LHRH administration are needed for long term, continuous hormone treatment or for pulsatile delivery. Finally, more trials with inhibitory analogs of LHRH are required to evaluate the capacity of these substances to regulate reproductive events.

Acknowledgement

This research was supported by Natural Sciences and Engineering Research Council of Canada grants A9729 and A7277. Marine Sciences Research Laboratory Contribution Number 497.

References

Anon (Conference on Application of Hormones to Economic Fish) (1975). *Kexue Tonghoe,* **20,** 43 (Fishery Marine Service Translation Series No. 4186)

Anon (The Fukien–Kiangsu–Chekiang–Shanghai Cooperative Group for Artificial Reproduction of Freshwater Economic Fishes) (1977*a*). A further investigation on the stimulatory effect of a synthetic analogue of hypothalamic luteinizing hormone releasing hormone (LRH-A) on spawning in 'Domestic Fishes'. *Acta Biochem. Biophys. Sinica,* **9,** 12

Anon (Cooperative Team for Hormonal Application in Pisciculture) (1977*b*). A new highly effective ovulating agent for fish reproduction. Practical application of LH-RH analogue for the induction of spawning of farm fishes. *Sci. Sinica.,* **20,** 469

Ball, J. N. (1981). Hypothalamic control of the pars distalis in fishes, amphibians and reptiles. *Gen. Comp. Endocrinol.,* **44,** 135

Bao, I. Y. and Kallman, K. D. (1982). Genetic control of the hypothalamo-pituitary axis and the effect of hybridization on sexual maturation (Xiphophorus, Pisces, Poeciliidae). *J. Exp. Zool.,* **220,** 297

Barnett, F. H., Jackson, I. M. D., Sohn, J. and Reichlin, S. (1979). Novel large molecular weight luteinizing hormone releasing hormone in teleost fish brain. *Endocrinology,* **104,** 148A

Barnett, F. H., Sohn, J., Reichlin, S. and Jackson, I. M. D. (1982). Three luteinizing hormone-releasing hormone like substances in a teleost fish brain: none identical with the mammalian LH-RH decapeptide. *Biochem. Biophys. Res. Commun..* **105,** 209

Billard, R., Marcel, J., Matéi, D. and Rusu, C. (1984). Induction de l'ovulation par un analogue du LH-RH chez *Hypophthalmichthys molitrix* (Poisson Téléostéen) placé dans diverses conditions d'environnement. *Bull. Cere. Pisc. (Romania),* (In press)

Breton, B., Weil, C., Jalabert, B. and Billard, R. (1972). Activité réciproque des facteurs hypothalamiques de bélier (*Ovis aries*) et de poissons téléostéen sur la sécrétion *in vitro* des hormones gonadotropes G-HG et LH respectivement par les hypophyses de carpe et de bélier. *C.R. Acad. Sci. Ser. D.,* **274,** 2530

Breton, B. and Weil, C. (1973). Effets du LH/FSH-RH synthétique et d'extraits hypothalamiques de carpe sur la sécrétion d'hormone gonadotrope *in vivo* chez la carpe (*Cyprinus carpio* L.). *C.R. Acad. Sci. Ser. D.,* **277,** 2061

Breton, B., Jalabert, B. and Weil, C. (1975). Characterisation partielle d'un facteur hypothalamique de libération des hormones gonadotropes chez la carpe (*Cyprinus carpio* L.). Etude *in vitro. Gen. Comp. Endocrinol.,* **25,** 405

Breton, B., Jalabert, B., Bieniarz, I., Sokolowska, M. and Epler, P. (1984). The effects of synthetic LH-RH and analog (D6 Serine Ethylamide 10 Gn-RH) on gonadotropin plasma levels, and oocyte sensitization to 17α-Hydroxy-20β-Dihydroprogesterone induced vesicle germinal breakdown. *Aquaculture* (In press)

Chan, K. S. K. (1977). Effect of synthetic luteinizing hormone-releasing hormone (LH-RH) on ovarian development in Japanese medaka, *Oryzias latipes*. *Can. J. Zool.*, **55,** 155

Chang, J. P. and Peter, R. E. (1983*a*). Effects of dopamine on gonadotropin release in female goldfish, *Carassius auratus*. *Neuroendocrinology*, **36,** 351

Chang, J. P. and Peter, R. E. (1983*b*). Effects of pimozide and des-Gly^{10},[D-ala^{6}] luteinizing hormone-releasing hormone ethylamide on serum gonadotropin concentrations, germinal vesicle migration and ovulation in female goldfish, *Carassius auratus*. *Gen. Comp. Endocrinol.* **52,** 30

Crim, L. W. and Cluett, D. M. (1974). Elevation of plasma gonadotropin concentration in response to mammalian gonadotropin releasing hormone (GRH) treatment of the male brown trout as determined by radioimmunoassay. *Endocr. Res. Commun.*, **1,** 101

Crim, L. W. and Evans, D. M. (1980). LH-RH stimulated gonadotropin release from the rainbow trout pituitary gland: An *in vitro* assay for detection of teleostean gonadotropin releasing factor(s). *Gen. Comp. Endocrinol.*, **40,** 283

Crim, L. W. and Evans, D. M. (1983). Influence of testosterone and/or luteinizing hormone releasing hormone analogue on precocious sexual development in the juvenile rainbow trout. *Biol. Reprod.*, **29,** 137

Crim, L. W., Evans, D. M., Coy, D. H. and Schally, A. V. (1981). Control of gonadotropic hormone release in trout: influence of synthetic LH-RH and LH-RH analogues *in vivo* and *in vitro*. *Life Sci.*, **28,** 129

Crim, L. W., Evans, D. M. and Vickery, B. H. (1983*a*). Manipulation of the seasonal reproductive cycle of the landlocked salmon (*Salmo salar*) by LHRH analogues administered at various stages of gonadal development. *Can. J. Fish. Aquat. Sci.*, **40,** 61

Crim, L. W., Sutterlin, A. M., Evans, D. M. and Weil, C. (1983*b*). Accelerated ovulation by pelleted LHRH analogue treatment of spring-spawning rainbow trout (*Salmo gairdneri*) held at low temperature. *Aquaculture*, **35,** 299

Daniels, E. and Licht, P. (1980). Effects of gonadotropin-releasing hormone on the levels of plasma gonadotropins (FSH and LH) in the bullfrog, *Rana catesbeiana*. *Gen. Comp. Endocrinol.*, **42,** 455

Deery, D. J. and Jones, A. C. (1975). Effects of hypothalamic extracts, neurotransmitters and synthetic hypothalamic releasing hormones on the adenyl cyclase activity of the pituitary of the dogfish (*Scyliorhinus canicula* L.). *J. Endocrinol.*, **64,** 49

De Vlaming, V. L. and Vodicnik, M. J. (1975). Effects of photoperiod-temperature regimes on pituitary gonadotrophs, pituitary gonadotropin potency and hypothalamic gonadotropin releasing activity in the teleost *Notemigonus crysoleucas*. *J. Thermal Biol.*, **1,** 119

Donaldson, E. M., Hunter, G. A. and Dye, H. M. (1981). Induced ovulation in coho salmon (*Oncorhynchus kisutch*). II. Preliminary study of the use of LH-RH and two high potency LH-RH analogues. *Aquaculture*, **26,** 129

Eiden, L. E. and Eskay, R. L. (1980). Characterization of LRF-like immunoreactivity in the frog sympathetic ganglia: non-identity with LRH decapeptide. *Neuropeptides*, **1,** 29

Harvey, B. J. and Hoar, W. S. (1979). *The Theory and Practice of Induced Breeding in Fish*. (Ottawa: The International Development Research Centre)

Hirose, K. and Ishida, R. (1974). Induction of ovulation in the ayu, *Plecoglossus altivelis* and LH-releasing hormone (LH-RH). *Bull. Jpn. Soc. Sci. Fish.*, **40,** 1235

Idler, D. R. and Crim, L. W. (1984). Gonadotropin releasing factor(s) (GtH-RF) from hypothalamus of winter flounder. In Lofts, B. (ed.) *Proceedings of the Ninth International Symposium on Comparative Endocrinology*. (Hong Kong: University of Hong Kong Press) (In press)

Kent, J. S., Vickery, B. H. and McRae, G. I. (1980). The use of a cholesterol matrix pellet implant for early studies on the prolonged release in animals of agonist analogues of luteinizing hormone releasing hormone. Presented at *7th International Symposium* (*Controlled Release of Bioactive Materials*), Fort Lauderdale, Florida

King, J. A. and Millar, R. P. (1979). Heterogeneity of vertebrate luteinizing releasing hormone. *Science*, **206,** 67

King, J. A. and Millar, R. P. (1980). Comparative aspects of luteinizing hormone-releasing hormone structure and function. *Endocrinology*, **106,** 707

King, J. A. and Millar, R. P. (1982). Structure of chicken hypothalamic luteinizing hormone-releasing hormone. II. Isolation and characterization. *J. Biol. Chem.*, **257,** 10729

Lam, T. J. (1982). Application of endocrinology to fish culture. *Can. J. Fish. Aquat. Sci.*, **39,** 111

Lam, T. J., Pandey, S. and Hoar, W. S. (1975). Induction of ovulation in goldfish by synthetic luteinizing hormone-releasing hormone (LH-RH). *Can. J. Zool.*, **53,** 1189

Licht, P. (1974). Induction of sperm release in frogs by mammalian gonadotropin-releasing hormone. *Gen. Comp. Endocrinol.*, **23,** 352

Licht, P. (1980). Evolutionary and functional aspects of pituitary gonadotropins in the green turtle, *Chelonia mydas. Am. Zool.*, **20,** 565

Licht, P., Owens, D. W., Cliffton, K. and Penaflores, C. (1982). Changes in LH and progesterone associated with the nesting cycle and ovulation in the olive ridley sea turtle, *Lepidochelys olivacea. Gen. Comp. Endocrinol.*, **48,** 247

Lin, H.-R., Peter, R. E., Nahorniak, C. S. and Bres, O. (1984). Actions of the superactive analogue Des-Gly[10][D-Ala[6]]LRH ethylamide (LRH-A) on gonadotropin secretion in goldfish. In Lofts, B. (ed.) *Proceedings of the Ninth International Symposium on Comparative Endocrinology*. (Hong Kong: University of Hong Kong Press) (In press).

McCreery, B. R., Licht, P., Barnes, R., Rivier, J. E. and Vale, W. W. (1982). Actions of agonistic and antagonistic analogs of gonadotropin releasing hormone (Gn-RH) in the bullfrog *Rana catesbeiana. Gen. Comp. Endocrinol.*, **46,** 511

Mazzi, V., Vellano, C., Colucci, D. and Merlo, A. (1974). Gonadotropin stimulation by chronic administration of synthetic luteinizing hormone-releasing hormone in hypophysectomized pituitary grafted male newts. *Gen. Comp. Endocrinol.*, **24,** 1

Nozaki, M. and Kobayashi, H. (1979). Distribution of LHRH-like substance in the vertebrate brain as revealed by immunohistochemistry. *Arch. Histol. Jpn.*, **42,** 201

Peter, R. E. (1982). Nature, localization and actions of neurohormones regulating gonadotropin secretion in teleosts. In Richter, C. J. J. and Goos, H. J. Th. (eds.) *Proceedings of the International Symposium on Reproductive Physiology of Fish*, pp. 30–40. *Pudoc: Wageningen*

Peter, R. E. and Paulencu, C. R. (1980). Involvement of the preoptic region in gonadotropin release-inhibition in goldfish, *Carassius auratus. Neuroendocrinology*, **31,** 133

Sherwood, N., Eiden, L., Brownstein, M., Spiess, J., Rivier, J. and Vale, W. (1983). Characterization of a teleost gonadotropin-releasing hormone. *Proc. Natl. Acad. Sci. U.S.A.*, **80,** 2794

Sokolowska, M., Popek, W. and Bieniarz, K. (1978). Synthetic releasing hormones LH/FSH-RH and LH-RH: effect of intracerebral and intramuscular injections on female carp (*Cyprinus carpio* L.) maturation. *Ann. Biol. Anim. Biochim. Biophys.*, **18,** 963

Sokolowska, M., Peter, R. E., Nahorniak, C. S., Pan, C. H., Chang, J. P., Crim, L. W. and Weil, C. (1983). Induction of ovulation in goldfish, *Carassius auratus*, by pimozide and analogues of LH-RH. *Aquaculture*, **36,** 71

Sower, S. A., Schreck, C. B. and Donaldson, E. M. (1982). Hormone-induced ovulation of coho salmon (*Oncorhynchus kisutch*) held in seawater and fresh water. *Can. J. Fish. Aquat. Sci.*, **39,** 627

Thornton, V. F. and Geschwind, I. I. (1974). Hypothalamic control of gonadotropin release in amphibia: evidence from studies of gonadotropin release *in vitro* and *in vivo*. *Gen. Comp. Endocrinol.*, **23,** 294

Van Der Kraak, G., Lin, H.-R., Donaldson, E. M., Dye, H. M. and Hunter, G. A. (1982). Effects of LH-RH and des-Gly[10][D-Ala[6]]LH-RH-ethylamide on plasma gonadotropin levels and oocyte maturation in adult female coho salmon (*Oncorhynchus kisutch*). *Gen. Comp. Endocrinol.*, **49,** 470

Vellano, C., Bona, A., Mazzi, V. and Colucci, D. (1974). The effect of synthetic luteinizing hormone releasing hormone on ovulation in the crested newt. *Gen. Comp. Endocrinol.*, **24,** 338

Weil, C., Breton, B. and Reinaud, P. (1975). Etude de la réponse hypophysaire à l'administration de Gn-RH exogène au cours du cycle reproducteur annuel chez la carpe *Cyprinus carpio* L. *C. R. Acad. Sci. 280D*, 2469

Weil, C., Billard, R., Breton, B. and Jalabert, B. (1978). Pituitary response to LH-RH at different stages of gametogenesis in the rainbow trout (*Salmo gairdneri*). *Ann. Biol. Anim. Biochim., Biophys.*, **18,** 863

Weil, C., Fostier, A., Horvath, L., Marlot, S. and Berscenyl, M. (1980). Profiles of plasma gonadotropin and 17β-estradiol in the common carp, *Cyprinus carpio* L., as related to spawning induced by hypophysation or LH-RH treatment. *Reprod. Nutr. Devel.*, **20,** 1041

Weil, C. and Crim, L. W. (1983). Administration of LHRH analogues in various ways: effect on the advancement of spermiation in prespawning landlocked salmon, *Salmo salar. Aquaculture* **35,** 103

30
LHRH and analogs in relation to livestock

B. D. SCHANBACHER

Since its structural elucidation and synthesis, luteinizing hormone releasing hormone (LHRH) has been utilized extensively in most domestic species of livestock. On the other hand, evaluation of the *in vivo* effects of the LHRH analogs in these same species has been limited to only a few studies. The commercial availability of LHRH and its analogs and an increased awareness of how these peptide hormones can affect mammalian reproduction has prompted investigations into the utility of these preparations for large animal medicine. Application of these peptide hormones to the livestock industry involves both their profertility and antifertility properties.

PROFERTILITY EFFECTS

Seasonal anestrum

Seasonal breeding prevails in many wild and domestic species, including sheep. Seasonality of reproduction is insured in sheep by neuroendocrine and endocrine changes within the hypothalamo–pituitary–gonadal axis in response to changing photoperiod (Karsch *et al*, 1980; Lincoln and Short, 1980; Haynes and Schanbacher, 1983). Although exposure of ewes (Hackett and Wolynetz, 1982) and rams (Schanbacher, 1979) to artificially shortened photoperiods has proven successful in systems aimed at producing lambs out-of-season, the hormonal approach is preferred (Gordon, 1963).

Induction of ovulation in anestrous sheep with crude hypothalamic extracts provided initial evidence that a neural factor was required for follicular development and ovulation (Domanski and Kochman, 1968). Since then, LHRH has been used to regulate tonic LH secretion in seasonally anestrous ewes (McNatty *et al.*, 1981; Wheaton and Mullett, 1982). High frequency, low dose LHRH treatment regimens (Figure 30.1) have proven most effective for ovulation induction in anestrous ewes (McLeod, 1982; McNatty *et al.*, 1982). Normal ovarian cyclicity and successful reproduction are critically dependent on the frequency and amplitude of hypothalamic LHRH release and provide

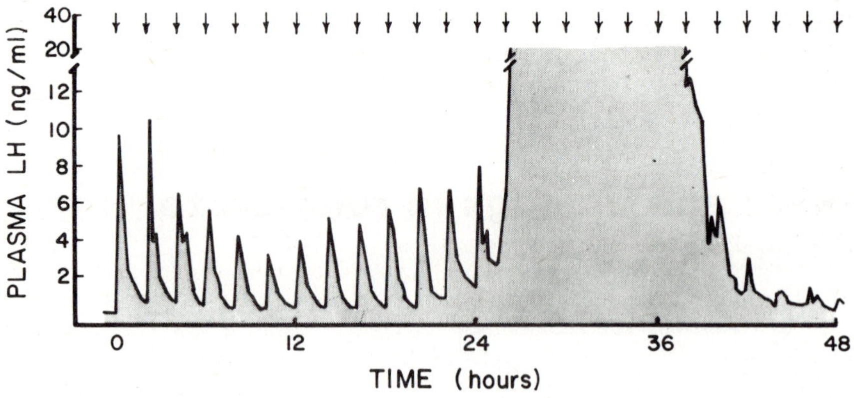

Figure 30.1 Plasma LH concentrations in a seasonally anestrous ewe in response to intravenous injections of 75 ng LHRH at 2 h intervals for 48 h. The arrows denote the times of LHRH injection. Note the ovulatory LH surge between 26 and 40 h. Redrawn from McLeod, 1982.

incentive for the development of a simple LHRH delivery system for use in anestrous sheep.

Postpartum anestrum

Early re-establishment of reproductive activity after parturition in beef and dairy cattle is necessary to minimize the costs of brood-cow maintenance. While several environmental and physiological factors can disrupt regular once-a-year calving intervals, suckling and lactation themselves are thought to contribute most to the duration and variability in intervals from calving to estrus and ovulation (Wetteman *et al.*, 1978). Exogenous LHRH has been used to enhance gonadotropin secretion and return postpartum anestrous cows to active reproduction cows (Riley *et al.*, 1981; Walters *et al.*, 1982).

LHRH administration to postpartum dairy cows with large follicles results in the development of corpora lutea with prominent ovulation papilla within 3 days of treatment (Garverick *et al.*, 1980). Several studies have shown that the postpartum anestrous beef and/or dairy cow responds to LHRH administration (Britt *et al.*, 1974; Garverick *et al.*, 1980; Lofstedt *et al.*, 1981; Walters *et al.*, 1982). Ovulation, however, is not always accompanied by behavioral estrus.

Ovarian cysts

Persistent ovarian follicular cysts are a common reproductive problem in dairy cattle (Short, 1962; Al-Dahashn and David, 1977). Repeated doses of LHRH (100 μg) to cystic cows produces an LH response similar to the preovulatory surge and initiates normal cycles (Kittok *et al.*, 1973; Bierschwal *et al.*, 1975; Cantley *et al.*, 1975). LHRH is effective therapeutically in cows with ovarian cysts because of its ability to luteinize the outermost portion of the theca interna and thereby enhance testosterone and progesterone secretion at the expense of estradiol-17β (Kesler *et al.*, 1981; Brown *et al.*, 1982; Hernandez-Ledezma *et al.*, 1982).

Delayed puberty

Pubertal development is associated with decreased sensitivity of the hypothalamus and pituitary to gonadal steroid feedback and increased gonadotropin secretion (Foster *et al.*, 1978). Increased frequency and/or amplitude of LH secretory pulses in response to an increased output of LHRH is responsible for the increased circulating gonadotropin levels observed in pubertal age bulls (Lacroix and Pelletier, 1979; Schanbacher, 1982*a*). Prepubertal gonadal activation can be achieved in rats (Moger, 1982), rhesus monkeys (Wildt *et al.*, 1980) and estradiol-implanted pubertal-age bull calves (Schanbacher *et al.*, 1982) by treatment with repeated small-dose injections of LHRH.

Testicular growth, spermatogenesis and testosterone secretion in young bulls are inhibited by low levels of exogenous estradiol (Schanbacher, 1981). Initiation of pulsatile LH release by hourly LHRH pulse infusion not only overcomes the estrogen-induced inhibition of LH and testosterone secretion in these animals (Schanbacher *et al.*, 1982), but stimulates spermatogenesis and increases testes size (Table 30.1). Attempts to initiate pubertal development in young bulls with continuous or low frequency LHRH treatment, (Haynes *et al.*, 1977; Schanbacher, unpublished data) however, have not met with success. In view of the pituitary refractoriness which develops following continuous exposure to LHRH (Bremner *et al.*, 1980), initiation of pubertal development in estrogen-treated bull calves (Schanbacher *et al.*, 1982) must be attributed to the ability of exogenously administered LHRH to mimic the pulsatile pattern of LH release required of young pubertal-age bulls.

Table 30.1 Testes weight and total daily sperm production (mean ±SEM) in three sham-treated control bulls, three bulls implanted with an estradiol-17β (E_2) capsule and three E_2 implanted bulls receiving LHRH by hourly pulse infusion

Treatment	*Body weight* (kg)	*Testes weight* (g)	*Total daily sperm production* ($\times 10^9$)
Control	328 ± 12	352 ± 26^a	3.3 ± 0.9^a
E_2-implanted	306 ± 8	105 ± 14^b	0.0
E_2-implanted, LHRH infused	313 ± 7	254 ± 12^c	1.2 ± 0.3^b

[a,b,c] Means without a common superscript differ significantly ($p<0.01$). From Schanbacher *et al*, 1982

ANTIFERTILITY EFFECTS

Paradoxical effects

Administration of amounts of LHRH and its agonists which are substantially higher than are needed to stimulate gonadotropin release interfere with normal reproductive function. Such interference includes suppression of gonadotropin and gonadal steroid secretion, inhibition of ovulation, luteal function and pregnancy in the female, inhibition of libido and spermatogenesis in the male and delayed onset of puberty in both males and females (Vickery, 1982). These seemingly paradoxical effects may be mediated at pituitary and/or gonadal sites (Reeves *et al.*, 1980; Séguin *et al.*, 1981), and suggest the utility of LHRH analogs for non-surgical castration, contraception and treatment of steroid-dependent neoplasms.

LHRH analogs in females

The LHRH analogs, [D-Ala^6,Pro^9-NHEt]LHRH and [D-Leu^6,Pro^9-NHEt]LHRH are 50 times more potent than synthetic LHRH in stimulating LH release in anestrous ewes (Rippel *et al.*, 1975; Kinder *et al.*, 1976). Both analogs increased the total LH released, mean peak LH and duration of the LH release compared to that obtained with LHRH. Although the results of this early work suggested that the LHRH analogs might prove useful in increasing ovulation in farm animals, subsequent reports have failed to demonstrate a beneficial effect of [D-Leu^6,Pro^9-NHEt]LHRH in anestrous ewes (Frandle *et al.*, 1977) or [D-Ala^6,Pro^9-NHEt]LHRH in synchronized breeding cows (Chipepa *et al.*, 1977). Infusion or repeated injections of [D-Leu^6,Pro^9-NHEt]LHRH to the prepubertal lamb caused decreased pituitary LH content and release with an associated decrease in pituitary LHRH receptors (Mayar *et al.*, 1978).

Inhibition of estrus and ovulation in the rat (Johnson *et al.*, 1976; Vickery and McRae, 1980) by agonistic analogs of LHRH suggested that similar treatment of feedlot heifers may induce functional castration. Suppression of estrus was achieved in young, mature cycling heifers weighing 250–300 kg by subcutaneous implantation of compacted cholesterol pellets containing [D-Trp^6,Pro^9-NHEt]LHRH (Herschler and Vickery, 1981). The estrus- and ovulation-suppressive effects of this treatment were not associated with a change in live weight gain or food intake compared to controls. The antireproductive effect of [D-Trp^6,Pro^9-NHEt]LHRH was reversible since estrus was re-established 16–19 days after pellet removal. Thus, the agonistic analogs of LHRH may have potential for (1) inducing reversible non-surgical castration in feedlot heifers and (2) synchronizing estrus in breeding females.

LHRH analogs in males

In male rats, chronic treatment with long acting analogs of LHRH decreases testicular weights, inhibits spermatogenesis, causes a decline in testicular receptors for LH and reduces serum testosterone levels (Sandow *et al.*, 1978). The temporary nature of this inhibition suggests that functional castration might be reversibly imposed in the male of domestic species.

Chronic treatment of boars with [D-Ala^6,Pro^9-NHEt]LHRH indeed produced inhibition of testicular function (Greger *et al.*, 1984). Decreased serum concentrations of testosterone and the boar taint steroid, 5α-

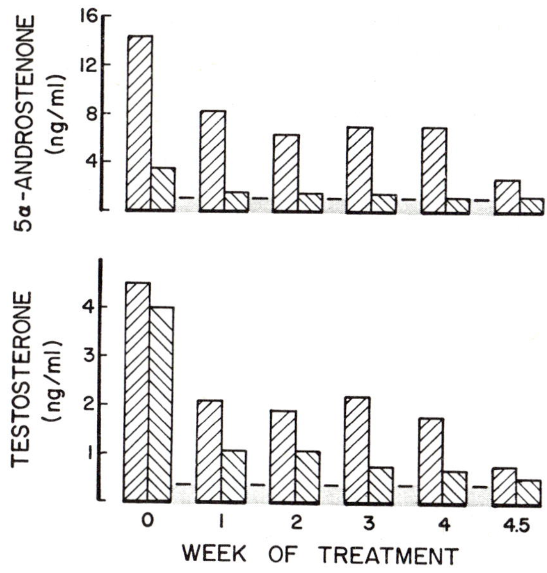

Figure 30.2 Serum concentrations of testosterone and 5α-androsten-3-one in two sexually mature boars (boar 1, ▨; boar 2, ▧) treated daily (s.c. injection) with 100 μg [D-Ala[6],Pro[9]-NHEt]LHRH for 31 days. The broken line depicts hormone levels observed in castrates. Redrawn from Greger *et al*, 1984.

androstenone (Figure 30.2), were associated with a reduction in testicular size after 30 days of treatment. These data suggest that the LHRH agonists could be used to reduce the objectionable taint associated with intact boars and that surgical castration may be unnecessary. Similar studies aimed at suppressing gonadal steroid secretion in males of other domestic species, as well as evaluating the antifertility effects of such treatment, are yet to be reported.

LHRH immunoneutralization

The effects of immunoneutralization of endogenous LHRH in rodents have demonstrated the importance of this decapeptide in normal reproductive function (Fraser, 1975). Mature male and female rats and rabbits, immunized against LHRH, produced antibodies specific to LHRH. The response to LHRH immunoneutralization included low to non-detectable gonadotropin levels, testicular involution, aspermatogenesis, low serum testosterone levels and atrophy of the seminal vesicles and prostate in males and disruption of estrous cyclicity and reduction in the weights of the ovaries and uteri of females.

LHRH immunoneutralization provides a useful investigative tool for the study of neuroendocrine factors which control reproduction and has been shown to induce functional gonadectomy in the monkey (Hodges and Hearn, 1977), dog (English *et al.*, 1983; Schanbacher *et al.*, 1983), ewe (Clarke *et al.*,

Table 30.2 Testes weight, antibody titers and concentrations of LH, FSH and testosterone in serum of ram lambs actively immunized against LHRH

Treatment[a]	*Testes weight* (g)	*Antibody titers* (%)[b]	*Serum LH* (ng/ml)	*Serum FSH* (ng/ml)	*Serum testosterone* (ng/ml)
Intact	342 ±21	N.D.	2.0 ±0.2	101 ±9	2.4 ±0.5
Intact-BSA	318 ±21	N.D.	2.1 ±0.2	81 ±10	2.3 ±0.3
Intact-LHRH	68 ±26	40 ±5	0.6 ±0.04	56 ± 3	0.35 ±0.04
Castrate	–	N.D.	12.8 ±2.7	376 ±28	0.3 ±0.1

[a] Intact-BSA: ram lambs immunized against BSA. Intact-LHRH: ram lambs immunized against an LHRH-albumin conjugate
[b] Percentage of ^{125}I-LHRH specifically bound in serum diluted 1:10^4. From Schanbacher, 1982*b*

1978; Jeffcoate *et al.*, 1978), ram (Jeffcoate *et al.*, 1982; Schanbacher, 1982*b*) and bull (Robertson *et al.*, 1979; Jeffcoate *et al.*, 1982). Immunized ram lambs, for example, produced sufficient LHRH antibody titer to suppress serum LH, FSH, and testosterone and prevent testicular development (Table 30.2). The consistent response observed in lambs shows the utility of this approach to non-surgical castration and provides the incentive which industry needs to make LHRH 'immunocastration' a reality for both livestock producer and veterinarian.

Evidence exists for natural reversal of the gonadectomy effect imposed by LHRH immunoneutralization (Jeffcoate *et al.*, 1982). Alternatively, treatment with immunologically distinct analogs of LHRH may effectively reverse the inhibitory effects imposed by LHRH immunization (Fraser and Sandow, 1977). These authors reported that the potent LHRH analog, [D-Ser(tBu)^6,Pro^9-NHEt]LHRH, was able to induce LH and FSH release in LHRH immunized adult male rats. A large dose of LHRH, however, was ineffective in this regard. The most useful information derived from LHRH immunization studies may be (1) the non-invasive elucidation of the biochemical and neuroendocrine mechanisms governing reproduction and (2) identification of important uses of LHRH agonists and antagonists for the clinician and researcher.

CONCLUDING REMARKS

Although the basic chemistry and physiology of LHRH and its analogs have been thoroughly investigated in the research laboratory (Sandow *et al.*, 1978), their therapeutic value as profertility and antifertility agents in man and animals with normal and abnormal gynecological and andrological conditions is only now being scrutinized and evaluated. For the livestock producer and veterinarian, synthetic LHRH can be used as a profertility drug to stimulate gonadotropin secretion and improve the chances for reproductive success or it can be administered in a way to take advantage of its antifertility properties. Utilization of the potent agonistic and antagonistic analogs of LHRH to selectively inhibit gonadal steroid secretion and gamete production should prove effective as a reliable and reversible method for controlling reproduction in animals destined for slaughter and for those temporarily removed from the breeding stock.

References

Al-Dahashn, S. Y. A. and David, J. S. E. (1977). Histological examination of ovaries and uteri from cows with cystic ovaries. *Vet. Rec.*, **101,** 342

Bierschwal, C. J., Garverick, H. A., Martin, C. E., Youngquist, R. S., Cantley, T. C. and Brown, M. D. (1975). Clinical response of dairy cows with ovarian cysts to GnRH. *J. Anim. Sci.*, **41,** 1660

Bremner, W. J., Findlay, J. K., Lee, V. W. K., deKretser, D. M. and Cumming, I. A. (1980). Feedback effects of the testis on pituitary responsiveness to luteinizing hormone-releasing hormone infusions in the ram. *Endocrinology*, **106,** 329

Britt, J. H., Kittok, R. J. and Harrison, D. S. (1974). Ovulation, estrus and endocrine response after GnRH in early postpartum cows. *J. Anim. Sci.*, **39,** 915

Brown, E. M., Elmore, R. G., Garverick, H. A. and Kesler, D. J. (1982). Gonadotropin releasing hormone treatment of dairy cows with ovarian cysts. II. Histology of ovarian cyst walls. *Theriogenology*, **17,** 689

Cantley, T. C., Garverick, H. A., Bierschwal, C. J., Martin, C. E. and Youngquist, R. S. (1975). Hormonal response of dairy cows with ovarian cysts to GnRH. *J. Anim. Sci.*, **41,** 1666

Chipepa, J. A. S., Kinder, J. E. and Reeves, J. J. (1977). Synchronized breeding in cattle using $PGF_{2\alpha}$ and LHRH/FSHRH stimulatory analogs. *Theriogenology*, **8,** 25

Clarke, I. J., Fraser, H. M. and McNeilly, A. S. (1978). Active immunization of ewes against luteinizing hormone releasing hormone and its effects on ovulation and gonadotrophin, prolactin and ovarian steroid secretion. *J. Endocrinol.*, **78,** 39

Domanski, E. and Kochman, K. (1968). Induction of ovulation in sheep by intraadenohypophysial infusion of hypothalamic extracts. *J. Endocrinol.*, **42,** 383

English, H. F., Schanbacher, B. D., Gross, D., Walker, M. F., Falvo, R. E. and Santen, R. J. (1983). Animal model of isolated gonadotropin deficiency: II. Morphological responses to LHRH immunoneutralization. *J. Androl.*, **4,** 240

Foster, D. L., Mickelson, I. H., Ryan, K. D., Coon, G. A., Drongowski, R. A. and Holt, J. A. (1978). Ontogeny of pulsatile luteinizing hormone and testosterone secretion in male lambs. *Endocrinology*, **102,** 1137

Frandle, K. A., Kinder, J. E., Coy, D. H., Schally, A. V., Reeves, J. J. and Estergreen, V. L. (1977). Plasma progestins in anestrous ewes treated with D-Leu^{6} desGlyNH_2^{1} ^{10}-LHRH ethylamide. *J. Anim. Sci.*, **45,** 486

Fraser, H. M. (1975). Effects of antibodies to luteinizing hormone releasing hormone on reproductive functions in rodents. In Nieschlag, E. (ed.) *Immunization with Hormones in Reproduction Research*, pp. 107–116. (Amsterdam: North Holland)

Fraser, H. M. and Sandow, J. (1977). Gonadotrophin release by a highly active analogue of luteinizing hormone releasing hormone in rats immunized against luteinizing hormone releasing hormone. *J. Endocrinol.*, **74,** 291

Garverick, H. A., Elmore, R. G., Vaillancourt, D. H. and Sharp, A. J. (1980). Ovarian response to gonadotropin-releasing hormone in postpartum dairy cows. *Am. J. Vet. Res.*, **41,** 1582

Gordon, I. (1963). The induction of pregnancy in the anoestrous ewe, by hormonal therapy. *J. Agric. Sci. Camb.*, **60,** 77

Greger, D. L., Stricklin, W. R., Haaland, M. A., Vickery, B. H. and Kushinsky, S. (1984). Reduction of boar taint steroid (5α-androst-16-en-3-one) and testosterone in serum of boars treated with an LHRH agonist. Submitted for publication

Hackett, A. J. and Wolynetz, M. S. (1982). Reproductive performance of confined sheep in an accelerated controlled program under two lighting regimes. *Theriogenology*, **18,** 621

Haynes, N. B., Hafs, H. D. and Manns, J. G. (1977). Effect of chronic administration of gonadotrophin releasing hormone and thyrotrophin releasing hormone to pubertal bulls on plasma luteinizing hormone, prolactin and testosterone concentration, the number of epididymal sperm and body weight. *J. Endocrinol.*, **73,** 227

Haynes, N. B. and Schanbacher, B. D. (1983). The control of reproductive activity in the ram. In Haresign, W. (ed.) *Sheep Production*, pp. 441–465. (London: Butterworth)

Hernandez-Ledezma, J. J., Garverick, H. A., Elmore, R. G., Brown, E. M. and Kesler, D. J. (1982). Gonadotropin releasing hormone treatment of dairy cows with ovarian cysts. III. Steroids in ovarian follicular fluid and ovarian cyst fluid. *Theriogenology*, **17**, 697

Herschler, R. C. and Vickery, B. H. (1981). Effects of (D-Trp^6-Des Gly^{10}-Pro $NH_2{}^9$)-Luteinizing hormone-releasing hormone ethylamide on the estrous cycle, weight gain, and feed efficiency in feedlot heifers. *Am. J. Vet. Res.*, **42**, 1405

Hodges, J. K. and Hearn, J. P. (1977). Effects of immunization against luteinizing hormone releasing hormone on reproduction of the marmoset monkey (*Callithrix jacchus*). *Nature (Lond.)*, **265**, 747

Jeffcoate, I. A., Foster, J. P. and Crighton, D. B. (1978). Effect of active immunization of ewes against synthetic luteinizing hormone releasing hormone. *Theriogenology*, **10**, 323

Jeffcoate, I. A., Lucas, J. M. S. and Crighton, D. B. (1982). Effects of active immunization of ram lambs and bull calves against synthetic luteinizing hormone releasing hormone. *Theoriogenology*, **18**, 65

Johnson, E. S., Gendrich, R. L. and White, W. F. (1976). Delay of puberty and inhibition of reproductive processes in the rat by a gonadotrophin releasing hormone agonist analog. *Fertil. Steril.*, **27**, 853

Karsch, F. J., Goodman, R. L. and Legan, S. J. (1980). Feedback basis of seasonal breeding: test of an hypothesis. *J. Reprod. Fertil.*, **58**, 521

Kesler, D. J., Elmore, R. G., Brown, E. M. and Garverick, H. A. (1981). Gonadotropin releasing hormone treatment of dairy cows with ovarian cysts. I. Gross ovarian morphology and endocrinology. *Theriogenology*, **16**, 207

Kinder, J. E., Adams, T. E., Nett, T. M., Coy, D. H., Schally, A. V. and Reeves, J. J. (1976). Serum gonadotropin concentrations and ovarian response in ewes treated with analogs to LH-RH/FSH-RH. *J. Anim. Sci.*, **42**, 1220

Kittok, R. J., Britt, J. H. and Convey, E. M. (1973). Endocrine response after GnRH in luteal phase cows and cows with ovarian follicular cysts. *J. Anim. Sci.*, **37**, 985

Lacroix, A. and Pelletier, J. (1979). LH and testosterone release in developing bulls following LH-RH treatment. Effect of gonadectomy and chronic testosterone propionate pre-treatment. *Acta Endocrinol.*, **91**, 719

Lincoln, G. A. and Short, R. V. (1980). Seasonal breeding: Nature's contraceptive. *Recent Prog. Horm. Res.*, **36**, 1

Lofstedt, R. M., Manns, J. G., Murphy, B. D., Humphrey, W. D. and Mapletoft, R. J. (1981). Influence of GnRH infusion on endocrine parameters and duration of postpartum anestrus in beef cows. *Theriogenology*, **15**, 359

McLeod, B. J. (1982). Plasma luteinizing hormone and ovarian follicle development in the ewe. *Ph D Thesis*, University of Nottingham

McNatty, K. P., Gibb, M., Dobson, C. and Thurley, D. C. (1981). Evidence that changes in tonic luteinizing hormone secretion regulate the growth of the preovulatory follicle in the ewe. *J. Endocrinol.*, **90**, 375

McNatty, K. P., Ball, K., Gibb, M., Hudson, N. and Thurley, D. C. (1982). Induction of cyclic ovarian activity in seasonally anoestrous ewes with exogenous GnRH. *J. Reprod. Fertil.*, **64**, 93

Mayar, M. Q., Tarnavsky, G. K. and Reeves, J. J. (1978). Pituitary responsiveness following infusion or repeated injections of [D-Leu^6,des Gly -$NH_2{}^{10}$]-LHRH-ethylamide in prepubertal ewes. *J. Anim. Sci.*, **47**, 235

Moger, W. H. (1982). Impact of pulsatile administration of gonadotropin-releasing hormone on the pituitary-testicular axis of the immature rat. *J. Androl.*, **3**, 256

Reeves, J. J., Séguin, C., Lefebvre, F. A., Kelly, P. A. and Labrie, F. (1980). Similar LHRH binding sites in the rat anterior pituitary and ovary. *Proc. Natl. Acad. Sci. USA*, **77**, 5567

Riley, G. M., Peters, A. R. and Lamming, G. E. (1981). Induction of pulsatile LH release, FSH release and ovulation in postpartum acyclic beef cows by repeated small doses of Gn-RH. *J. Reprod. Fertil.*, **63**, 559

Rippel, R. H., Johnson, E. S., White, W. F., Fujino, M., Fukuda, T. and Kobayashi, S. (1975). Ovulation and gonadotropin-releasing activity of [D-Leu^6,Des Gly$NH_2{}^{10}$, Pro-Ethylamide^9]-GnRH. *Proc. Soc. Exp. Biol. Med.*, **148**, 1193

Robertson, I. S., Wilson, J. C. and Fraser, H. M. (1979). Immunological castration in male cattle. *Vet. Rec.*, **105**, 556

Sandow, J., von Rechenberg, W. V., Konig, W., Hahn, M., Jerzabek, G. and Fraser, H. (1978). Physiological studies with highly active analogues of LHRH. In Gupta, D. and Voelter, W. (eds.) *Hypothalamic Hormones – Chemistry, Physiology and Clinical Applications*, pp. 307–326. (Weinheim: Verlag Chimie)

Schanbacher, B. D. (1979). Increased lamb production with rams exposed to short daylengths during the nonbreeding season. *J. Anim. Sci.*, **49,** 927

Schanbacher, B. D. (1981). Importance of the episodic nature of luteinizing hormone secretion for normal development of the bovine testis during puberty: Interference with oestradiol-17β. *J. Endocr.*, **88,** 393

Schanbacher, B. D. (1982*a*). Hormonal interrelationships between hypothalamus, pituitary and testis of rams and bulls. *J. Anim. Sci.* (Suppl. II) **55,** 56

Schanbacher, B. D. (1982*b*). Response of ram lambs to active immunization against testosterone and luteinizing hormone-releasing hormone. *Am. J. Physiol.*, **242,** E201

Schanbacher, B. D., D'Occhio, M. J. and Kinder, J. E. (1982). Initiation of spermatogenesis and testicular growth in oestradiol-17β-implanted bull calves with pulsatile infusion of luteinizing hormone releasing hormone. *J. Endocrinol.*, **93,** 183

Schanbacher, B. D., English, H. F., Gross, D., Santen, R. J., Walker, M. F. and Falvo, R. E. (1983). Animal model of isolated gonadotropin deficiency: I. Hormonal responses to LHRH immunoneutralization. *J. Androl.*, **4,** 233

Séguin, C., Bélanger, A., Cusan, L., Pelletier, G., Reeves, J.J., Lefebvre, F.-A., Kelly, P. A. and Labrie, F. (1981). Relative importance of the adenohypophyseal and gonadal sites of inhibitory action of LHRH agonists. *Biol. Reprod.*, **24,** 889

Short, R. V. (1962). Steroid concentrations in normal follicular fluid and ovarian cyst fluid from cows. *J. Reprod. Fertil.*, **4,** 27

Vickery, B. H. (1982). Antigonadotropic, antisteroidogenic and antisteroidal activities of agonist analogs of luteinizing hormone-releasing hormone as revealed by their antireproductive activities. In Agarwal, M. K.(ed.) *Hormone Antagonists*, pp. 623–657. (Berlin: de Gruyter)

Vickery, B. H. and McRae, G. I. (1980). Synchronization of oestrus in adult female rats by utilizing the paradoxical effects of an LH-RH agonist. *J. Reprod. Fertil.*, **60,** 399

Walters, D. L., Short, R. E., Convey, E. M., Staigmiller, R. B., Dunn, T. G. and Kaltenback, C. C. (1982). Pituitary and ovarian function in postpartum beef cows. III. Induction of estrus, ovulation and luteal function with intermittent small-dose injections of GnRH. *Biol. Reprod.*, **26,** 655

Wetteman, R. P., Turman, E. J., Wyatt, R. D. and Totusek, R. (1978). Influence of suckling intensity on reproductive performance of range cows. *J. Anim. Sci.*, **47,** 342

Wheaton, J. E. and Mullett, M. A. (1982). Effects of progesterone treatment on basal and LH-RH-induced plasma LH concentrations in anoestrous and ovariectomized sheep. *J. Reprod. Fertil.*, **64,** 325

Wildt, L., Marshall, G. and Knobil, E. (1980). Experimental induction of puberty in the infantile rhesus monkey. *Science*, **207,** 1373

SECTION IX

METABOLIC PARAMETERS

31
Enzymatic degradation of LHRH and analogs

G. FLOURET, M. A. STETLER-STEVENSON, F. A. CARONE and D. R. PETERSON

The plasma level of LHRH is determined by the amount of released hypothalamic hormone entering the general circulation and by clearance from plasma by distribution to the extracellular fluid, accumulation in tissues, degradation or excretion. The plasma level of exogenous LHRH, or an LHRH analog, is determined by its rate of entry into the general circulation from the site of administration and by its plasma clearance.

When injected intravenously, tritiated LHRH (^{3}H-LHRH) underwent plasma clearance with a half-life of about 7 min in female rats although only 15 % of the radioactivity was recovered in the urine after 60 min (Redding and Schally, 1973). ^{3}H-LHRH is distributed in the extracellular fluid and then is concentrated in various organs. A tissue to plasma ratio (T/P) greater than 1 has been found in kidney, liver, pineal, and posterior and anterior pituitary, indicating accumulation of LHRH in these organs. A T/P lower than 1 has been found in hypothalamus, cerebral cortex or muscle, indicating no hormone accumulation by these organs. As shown by autoradiography, the skin, intestinal wall and bladder also accumulate ^{3}H-LHRH (Dupont *et al.*, 1974). The large tissue mass and high vascularity of the liver or kidney coupled with their capacity to accumulate ^{3}H-LHRH suggest that they might be the major sites for the inactivation and/or excretion of the hormone. The hypothalamus may contain degrading enzymes involved in the regulation of hormone release (Schally *et al.*, 1969), and the anterior pituitary may control the duration of hormone action through enzymatic inactivation at the receptor (Clayton and Shakespear, 1978).

Studies on the enzymatic inactivation of LHRH have been done either *in vivo*, or *in vitro* with organ homogenates, subcellular particles or isolated peptidases, employing labeled or unlabeled hormone and/or selected analogs.

IN VITRO STUDIES

Brain and pituitary homogenates

Rat hypothalamic extracts contain a peptidase which inactivates LHRH. The activity of this peptidase is decreased by gonadectomy and is returned to normal levels by treatment with estradiol or androgen (Griffiths *et al.*, 1975). Such treatment also causes changes in gonadotropin secretion, exerted partly through action on the hypothalamus, and may be mediated by changes in hypothalamic peptidase activity. However, in studies with extracts of homogenized mediobasal hypothalamus or frontal cortex, there was no change in apparent K_m values or in specific activity of the soluble enzymes either in intact or in castrated male rats (Loudes *et al.*, 1978).

Rat hypothalamic extracts were incubated with LHRH containing [pGlu-3-^{3}H]LHRH as a marker and the breakdown products were analyzed by electrophoresis and amino acid analysis (Koch *et al.*, 1974). The major breakdown product was pGlu-His-Trp-Ser-Tyr-Gly (metabolite 6, Figure 31.1), and a minor product was Glu-His-Trp-Ser-Tyr-Gly. Since Leu-Arg-Pro-Gly-NH_2 was also isolated and characterized by comparison to a standard, it was concluded that the initial site of cleavage of LHRH was at the Gly^6–Leu^7 bond. Anterior pituitary homogenates also cleave the hormone to metabolite 6 and to Glu-His-Trp-Ser-Tyr-Gly (Fridkin *et al.*, 1977).

Rat brain homogenates were incubated with LHRH or one of several LHRH analogs and the rate of release of amino acids was determined by amino acid analysis (Marks and Stern, 1974). The results suggested an initial

AMINO ACID SEQUENCE	CODE
pGlu	1
pGlu-His	2
pGlu-His-Trp	3
pGlu-His-Trp-Ser	4
pGlu-His-Trp-Ser-Tyr	5
pGlu-His-Trp-Ser-Tyr-Gly	6
pGlu-His-Trp-Ser-Tyr-Gly-Leu	7
pGlu-His-Trp-Ser-Tyr-Gly-Leu-Arg	8
pGlu-His-Trp-Ser-Tyr-Gly-Leu-Arg-Pro	9
pGlu-His-Trp-Ser-Tyr-Gly-Leu-Arg-Pro-Gly	10
pGlu-His-Trp-Ser-Tyr-Gly-Leu-Arg-Pro-Gly-NH_2	LHRH, H

Figure 31.1 Peptide sequences for LHRH and its pyroglutamyl metabolites.

breakdown of LHRH at Tyr^5–Gly^6 and Gly^6–Leu^7 bonds by a neutral brain peptidase, followed by sequential action of amino- and carboxypeptidases. A slower acting enzyme removed glycineamide from the C-terminus. Incubation of [Pro^9-NHEt]LHRH did not release Pro, incubation of [D-Ala^6,Pro^9-NHEt]LHRH gave no cleavage products, and incubation of [D-Ala^6]LHRH released C-terminal amino acids, suggesting that analogs with a blocked C-terminus had greater potency because of resistance to enzymatic degradation.

Pituitary homogenates also degrade LHRH (Koch *et al.*, 1974; Kochman *et al.*, 1975), and this enzymatic action may play a physiological role in the fine control of the amount of hormone binding to specific receptors (Koch *et al.*, 1977). The increased resistance of [D-Ala^6]LHRH and [D-Trp^6]LHRH to LHRH-degrading peptidases from rat hypothalamus or anterior pituitary correlates with their increased biological potency (Koch *et al.*, 1977).

Incubation of a rat hypothalamic homogenate with LHRH produced on thin layer chromatography (TLC) a spot which co-migrated with metabolite 6, and the biological activity of [D-Ser(tBu)^6,Pro^9-NHEt]LHRH and [D-Leu^6,Pro^9-NHEt]LHRH decreased more slowly than that of LHRH during incubation, suggesting that the primary site of LHRH cleavage was Gly^6–Leu^7 (Kelly *et al.*, 1979).

Contrary to the above findings, incubation of [pGlu-^{3}H]LHRH with bovine brain and pituitary homogenates, and analysis of radiolabeled fragments by co-chromatography with peptide standards produced metabolites 1, 5 and 9, but not 6 (Bauer *et al.*, 1979). In addition, when [pGlu-3,4-^{3}H]LHRH was incubated with homogenates of rat brain and of anterior pituitary, and the incubates were analyzed at various times by HPLC, metabolites 1, 5 and 9 were the initial breakdown products and metabolites 2, 3 and 4 were secondary breakdown products (Flouret, G., Carone, F. A., Stetler-Stevenson, M. A., Gulczynski, B., Nakamura, S. and Peterson, D., unpublished).

Pituitary membranes

^{125}I-LHRH, incubated with plasma membranes prepared from rat anterior pituitary, lost immunoreactivity in proportion to membrane concentration. To avoid ligand breakdown, the highly potent [D-Ser(tBu)^6,Pro^9-NHEt] LHRH (buserelin) was employed in other binding studies (Clayton and Shakespear, 1978). The enzymatic content of plasma membranes and homogenate differ, as ^{125}I-labeled buserelin is degraded by pituitary plasma membranes at one twenty-seventh the rate of ^{125}I-labeled LHRH and by a pituitary homogenate at one third the rate of LHRH. The physiological action of sex steroids at the pituitary level may alter the concentration of surface peptidases on pituitary gonadotropes, and the enzymatic action may be an important factor in determining the potency and duration of action of LHRH and its analogs (Clayton *et al.*, 1977). However, as the enzyme could be embedded on the outer or inner side of the cell membrane, it is not conclusive that it plays a role in hormone binding. Binding studies with rat anterior pituitary membranes have demonstrated that ^{125}I-labeled buserelin has 60 times greater binding affinity than LHRH, and 50 times greater biological effect than the hormone in the release of LH from anterior pituitary cells in culture (Reeves *et al.*, 1980). Therefore, the increased potency of this and similar analogs featuring D-amino acids at position 6 may relate to higher binding potency, and analog resistance to enzymatic degradation may be of lesser importance than was previously suggested (Reeves *et al.*, 1977). In other binding studies the receptor affinity of buserelin was between seven and eight times that of LHRH whereas the biological activity in an *in vivo* assay was 130 times higher (Clayton and Catt, 1980). The enhanced potency of the analog *in vivo* may thus be the result of both high affinity for receptors and decreased peptide degradation either in the peripheral circulation or at the level of the pituitary gland. The low affinity binding of LHRH to pituitary membranes may represent binding to a membrane associated peptidase (Heber *et al.*, 1978; Clayton *et al.*, 1979).

Pituitary and brain enzymes

A postproline-cleaving-enzyme has been isolated and purified from rabbit brain (Orlowski *et al.*, 1979), bovine brain (Hersh and McKelvy, 1979) and bovine anterior pituitary (Knisatschek and Bauer, 1979). Incubation of LHRH with postproline-cleaving-enzyme resulted in metabolite 9 and Gly-NH_2. A general role was suggested for postproline-cleaving-enzyme in the inactivation of brain neuropeptides containing proline (Wilk *et al.*, 1979). Because LHRH appears to be inactivated by more than one mechanism, the physiological significance of the prolyl endopeptidase is not clear, and it would be helpful to determine the cellular site of the enzyme and its substrates.

Three enzymes have been isolated from bovine brain and pituitary homogenates: pyroglutamate aminopeptidase, which cleaves LHRH to pGlu (Bauer *et al.*, 1979); postproline-cleaving-enzyme, which cleaves LHRH to metabolite 9 (Knisatschek and Bauer, 1979); a non-chymotrypsin-like endopeptidase which hydrolyses LHRH preferentially at Tyr^5–Gly^6 and the resulting N-terminal pentapeptide at the His^2–Trp^3 bond (Horsthemke and Bauer, 1980). The endopeptidase was the most active of the three enzymes isolated. Evidence was obtained that substituents at positions 'remote' to the site of enzymatic attack alter the rate of cleavage (Horsthemke and Bauer, 1981). Thus, incubations with pyroglutamate amino peptidase showed that [Pro^9-NHEt]LHRH and [D-Ser(tBu)^6,Pro^9-NHEt]LHRH were degraded more slowly than LHRH and [D-Ser(tBu)^6]LHRH respectively. This is probably due to steric interactions between the C- and N-termini. Incubations with LHRH degrading endopeptidase showed that analogs containing D-amino acids at position 6 are not cleaved at Tyr^5–Gly^6 or His^2–Trp^3. Even modifications at positions remote from Tyr^5–Gly^6, e.g. [D-Phe^2]LHRH, decrease degradation by endopeptidase. [Pro^9-NHEt]LHRH and other ethylamide analogs are degraded very slowly by postproline-cleaving-enzyme. H⌣wever, modifications in positions remote from the scissile peptide bond also influence the degradation by this enzyme, either decreasing (e.g. [D-Ala^6]LHRH) or increasing (e.g. [D-Phe^2,D-$Trp^{3,6}$]LHRH) the rate of hydrolysis. [D-Ser^4]LHRH is recovered intact after incubation with rat brain homogenates (Flouret, G., Carone, F. A., Stetler-Stevenson, M. A., Gulczynski, B., Nakamura, S. and Peterson, D., unpublished). There is no strict colinearity between biological activity of LHRH analogs and resistance to degradation by endopeptidase and postproline-cleaving-enzyme; hence other factors, such as increased receptor binding or stimulation, must be considered (Horsthemke *et al.*, 1981).

Liver, gonad and lung homogenates and blood

As shown by radioimmunoassay and/or bioassay, LHRH is slowly degraded by rat, guinea pig, chicken, dog, sheep and human plasma, (Bennett and Martin, 1979), rat serum being 2–5-fold more active than human serum (Benuck and Marks, 1976). Blood probably plays a negligible role in the degradation of this hormone, since after injection LHRH has a half-life of 2–12 min depending on the species (Bennett and McMartin, 1979).

Incubation of [(^{3}H)Trp^3,(^{14}C)Pro^9]LHRH with rat liver homogenates gave products consistent with cleavage at Tyr^5–Gly^6 (Hudson *et al.*, 1976). We have corroborated the latter preliminary findings by studying the cleavage of LHRH by rat liver homogenates as a function of time, which showed metabolites 5 and 9 to be the initial products and metabolites 2, 3 and 4 to increase in concentration with time (Flouret, G., Carone, F. A., Stetler-Stevenson, M. A., Gulczynski, B., Nakamura, S. and Peterson, D., unpublished).

[pGlu-3,4-^{3}H]LHRH incubated with a rat testis homogenate showed with time the initial appearance of metabolites 3 and 5, and subsequently metabolites 2 and 4. With a rat ovary homogenate, metabolites 3, 5 and 9 formed initially and metabolites 2, 4 and 7 formed subsequently. With a rat lung homogenate, metabolites 3, 5 and 7 formed initially and metabolites 2, 4 and 9 formed subsequently (Flouret, G., Carone, F. A., Stetler-Stevenson, M. A., Gulczynski, B., Nakamura, S. and Peterson, D., unpublished).

Kidney homogenates and isolated renal tubules

The kidney is a regulator of plasma levels of peptide hormones. The half-life and metabolic clearance rate for LHRH are prolonged in individuals with chronic renal failure (Pimstone *et al.*, 1977). Small linear peptides undergo glomerular filtration and are hydrolyzed in the proximal tubule by brush border enzymes; other segments of the nephron are not important (Carone *et al.*, 1982). The metabolites produced may be reabsorbed or excreted in the urine.

Assuming conventional proteolytic patterns, ten pyroglutamic acid-containing (and hence labeled) metabolites can be produced in the kidney from [pGlu-3,4-^{3}H]LHRH (Figure 31.1). We were unable adequately to separate LHRH and metabolites 1–10 on either thin layer electrophoresis (TLE) at various time periods and several pH conditions or on TLC with 20 different solvent systems, using either silica gel or microcellulose as the chromatographic medium (Stetler-Stevenson *et al.*, 1980). Usually, peptides

3–7 moved as one group, and peptides 8–10 and LHRH (arginyl peptides) moved as another group. These experiments underscore the usefulness of having standards of all predicted metabolites and a chromatographic method which resolves all of them, in order to be able to identify the enzymatic breakdown products.

The mixture of metabolites 1–10 and LHRH was separated by HPLC (Figure 31.2). Glu-His, Glu-His-Trp and Glu-His-Trp-Ser separate from their pyroglutamyl counterparts on our HPLC system. We analyzed the chymotryptic products of cleavage of [pGlu-3,4-^{3}H]LHRH by co-injecting an aliquot of the incubate plus 'cold' standards 1–10 and LHRH, in order to test the viability of our method. We detected only radioactivity which co-

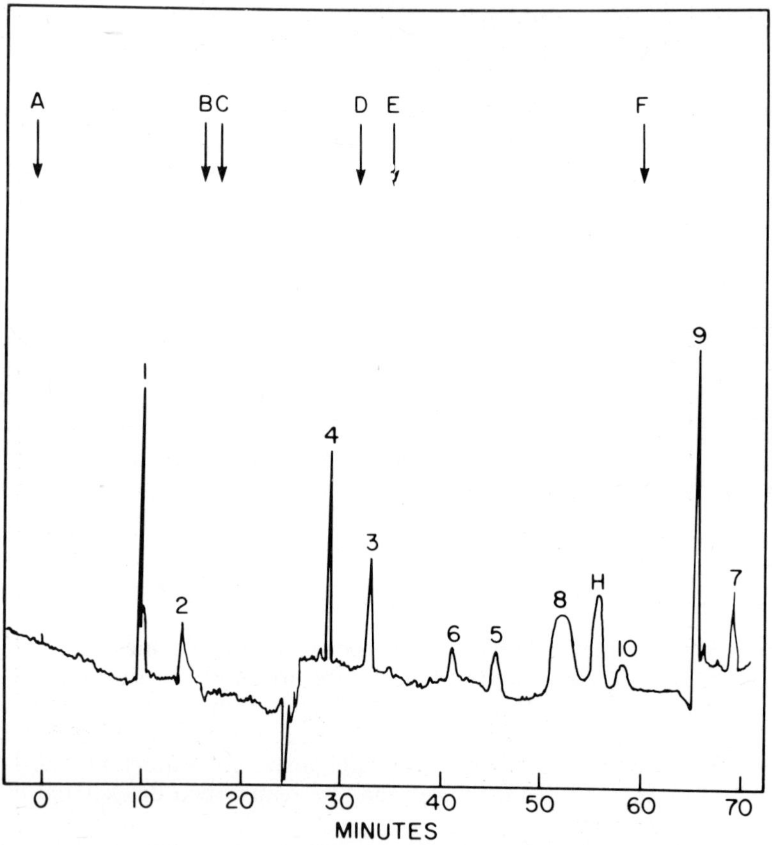

Figure 31.2 Typical elution pattern of LHRH (LHRH = H) and N-terminal peptide fragments 1–10 from a micro-Bondapak-C_{18} column, employing combinations of water (solvent A) and 60% of CH_3CN-40% of 0.5% H_3PO_4 (solvent B). Initial conditions: 100% solvent A at a flow rate of 0.3 ml/min; A = point of injection; B = rate increased from 0.3 ml/min to 1.5 ml/min; C = initiation of 3 min linear gradient from 0 to 20% solvent B; D = initiation of 5 min linear gradient from 20 to 25% solvent B; E = rate increased from 1.5 ml/min to 1.9 ml/min; F = initiation of 2 min linear gradient from 25 to 35% solvent B.

eluted with standards of fragments 3 and 5 (Stetler-Stevenson *et al.*, 1981*c*); we had previously isolated 3 and 5 after chymotryptic cleavage of LHRH followed by gel filtration, and had verified their structure by amino acid analysis (White *et al.*, 1973). The advantages of this method are: (1) rapid analysis, (2) detection of all predicted pGlu products, (3) sensitivity of the analysis in the pmole range using tritiated LHRH with specific activity of about 30 Ci/mmol, (4) feasibility of rate studies, useful to determine initial site(s) of cleavage and (5) ability to analyze tritiated LHRH metabolites in urine and in serum, in the presence of degradation products of endogenous LHRH, or other amino acids, or peptides normally found in these fluids.

A study of the cleavage of [pGlu-3,4-^{3}H]LHRH by rat kidney homogenates as a function of time (Figure 31.3) showed that metabolites 4, 5 and 6 were the major initial products and that metabolites 1, 2 and 3 were subsequent products (Flouret, G., Carone, F. A., Stetler-Stevenson, M. A., Gulczynski, B., Nakamura, S. and Peterson, D., unpublished).

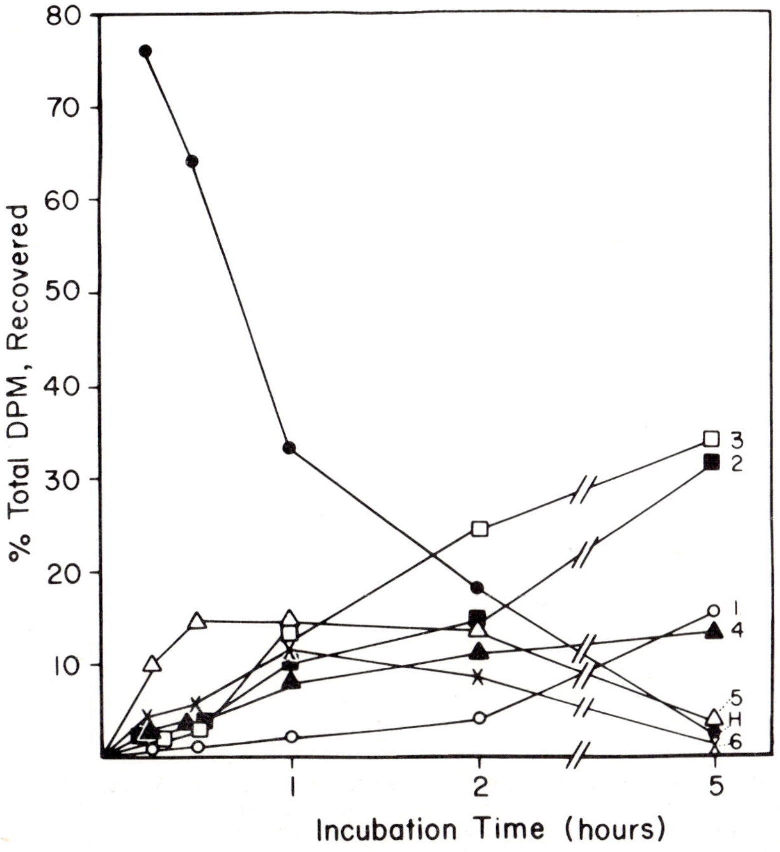

Figure 31.3 Percentage of total radioactivity corresponding to LHRH and N-terminal peptides measured in the incubation mixture of [pGlu-3,4-^{3}H]LHRH and rat renal homogenates as a function of time.

[pGlu-3,4-^{3}H]LHRH was microperfused *in vitro* (Stetler-Stevenson *et al.*, 1981*b*) by standard techniques (Burg *et al.*, 1966) into proximal straight tubule segments isolated from rabbit kidney (Figure 31.4). Reabsorption of radiolabel was measured, and labeled products were identified by HPLC. The results showed that: (1) the luminal collection fluid had 94% of the radioactivity perfused, with two thirds of the label corresponding to metabolites 2, 3 and 4, and one third to intact hormone, (2) the bathing medium had 5% of the radioactivity perfused, with the label consisting of metabolites 1, 2, 3 and 4, and (3) there was only trace label in the tubular cells.

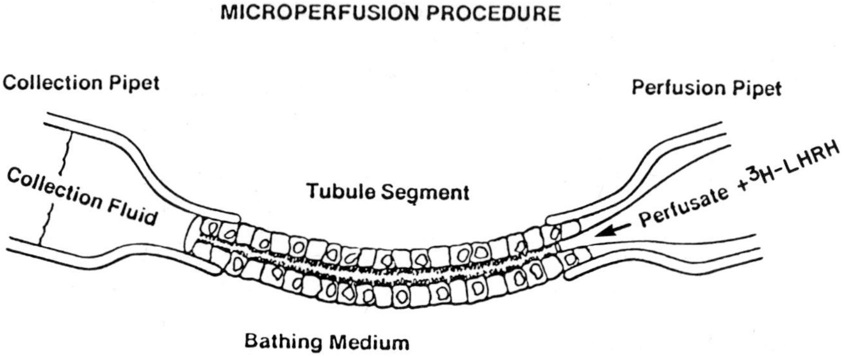

Figure 31.4 Scheme of the procedure for microperfusion of an isolated rabbit renal tubular segment *in vitro*.

LHRH may be initially hydrolyzed at the luminal brush border of the proximal tubule. Incubation of tritiated hormone with isolated brush border membranes from rabbit cortical portions of the kidney yielded only metabolites 2, 3 and 4, the same metabolites which appeared in luminal fluid. A partial reabsorption of metabolites 2–4 followed by further intracellular hydrolysis could follow, as indicated by the appearance of metabolite 1 in bathing medium (Figure 31.5). Metabolites 2–4, found in collection fluid, could be liberated directly from LHRH by separate brush border endopeptidases, or alternatively metabolite 4 might form first and serve as a precursor for metabolites 3 and then 2 via carboxypeptidase removal of C-terminal amino acids.

The absence of LHRH in bathing medium indicates that once LHRH undergoes glomerular filtration it is not reabsorbed intact and is irreversibly lost from the circulation. Peptide fragments were reabsorbed into the bathing medium, which is the equivalent of the extracellular fluid. Previously, microperfusion of proximal renal tubules with small linear peptides had resulted in the recovery of labeled amino acids and not peptides in the bathing medium (Carone and Peterson, 1980). Pyroglutamyl peptide metabolites are probably immune to attack by some peptidases and may be reabsorbed intact.

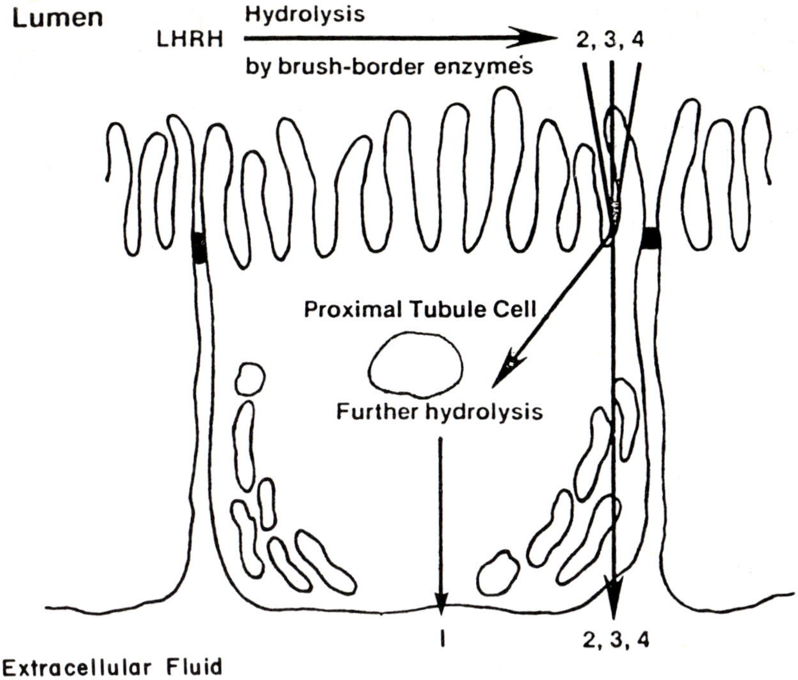

Figure 31.5 Proposed scheme of LHRH degradation and handling by epithelial cells lining the renal tubule. (From Stetler-Stevenson *et al.*, 1981*a*, reproduced by permission of Pierce Chemical Company.)

IN VIVO STUDIES

A circulating peptide may be processed in an organ by various mechanisms: (1) it may be degraded by cell surface enzymes, (2) it may be internalized by the tissue and hydrolyzed, and either the intact peptide and/or the metabolites may eventually be released back into the circulation, and (3) it may be filtered in the kidney glomerulus and then be hydrolyzed by brush border enzymes in the proximal tubule, and the intact peptide and/or its metabolites may be excreted in the urine or some of the metabolites may be absorbed and re-enter the circulation.

In connection with the latter mechanism, when [pGlu-3,4-^{3}H]LHRH (Stetler-Stevenson *et al.*, 1981*a*) was microinfused *in vivo* into proximal tubules of the rat kidney (Gottschalk *et al.*, 1965), metabolites 2, 3 and 4 and intact LHRH were recovered in urine. On the other hand, microinfusion into distal tubules resulted in the recovery of intact hormone alone. After intravenous injection of tritiated LHRH in man, pyroglutamic acid and pGlu-His were found in the urine (Redding *et al.*, 1973).

In another experimental design, the tritiated hormone was presented to the renal artery of rats *in vivo*, and the labeled products were characterized in the renal venous blood and in the urine of filtering kidneys, and in the renal venous blood of non-filtering kidneys. Non-filtering kidneys had the left ureter ligated 3 days prior to the experiment (Figure 31.6). At the time of the experiment, the right renal artery and vein were ligated and tritiated hormone was injected into the aorta above the renal artery while the aorta was occluded distally by applying brief external pressure. Renal venous blood and urine were collected during single vascular and tubular transit times. In filtering kidneys, metabolites 2, 3 and 4 appeared in the urine; however, metabolites 2, 3 and 4 and, in addition, pyroglutamic acid, appeared in renal venous blood. In non-filtering kidneys only intact LHRH was detected in the renal venous blood. Since LHRH would have come in contact with peritubular membranes and interstitial and endothelial cells in the non-filtering kidney, it follows that these structures did not degrade detectable amounts of LHRH during a single renal vascular transit. These *in vivo* findings support the mechanism for handling of LHRH by the proximal tubule suggested by *in vitro* studies (Stetler-Stevenson *et al.*, 1983). The formation of metabolites 5 and 6 in rat kidney homogenates but not in the intact renal tissue indicates that some intracellular peptidases are present in compartments inaccessible to circulating LHRH.

When tritiated hormone was injected into the carotid artery and blood was

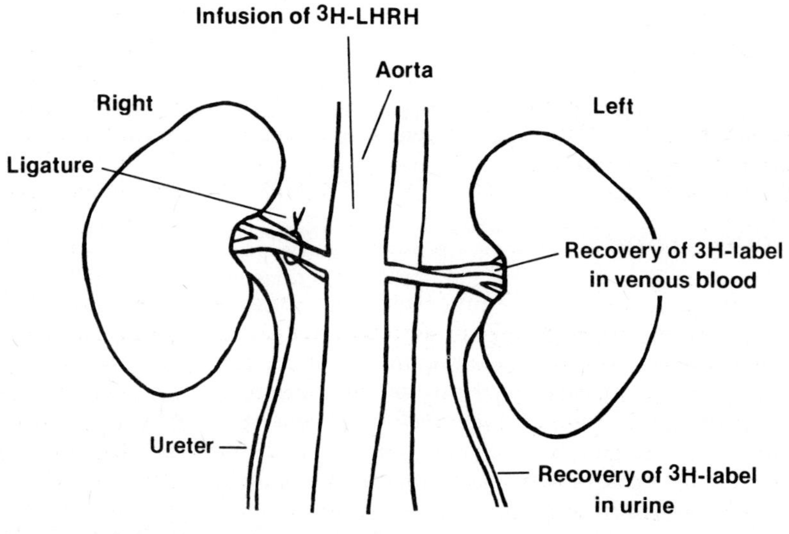

KIDNEY	URINE	VENOUS BLOOD
Filtering	2,3,4, LHRH	1,2,3,4, LHRH
Non-Filtering	0	LHRH

Figure 31.6 Recovery of LHRH and pyroglutamyl metabolites in urine and venous blood of filtering and non-filtering kidneys during a single tubular or vascular transit following infusion of [pGlu-3,4-^{3}H]LHRH into the aorta. (From Carone *et al.*, 1982, reproduced by permission of the *Journal of Laboratory and Clinical Medicine*.)

recovered from the contralateral jugular vein after one transit through the brain, 87% of the label recovered corresponded to LHRH and 13% to metabolites 2, 3 and 4. Metabolites 5 and 9 (found after incubation of LHRH with brain homogenates) may therefore form initially, and metabolite 9 may then be cleaved to metabolite 5 which in turn is converted by other enzymes and/or carboxypeptidase to metabolites 2, 3 and 4. Alternatively, LHRH may be exposed only to endopeptidase(s) cleaving at positions 2, 3 and/or 4, and to a carboxypeptidase, but not to enzymes cleaving at position 5 and 9 (Flouret, G., Carone, F. A., Stetler-Stevenson, M. A., Gulczynski, B., Nakamura, S. and Peterson, D., unpublished). Tritiated LHRH does not accumulate in hypothalamic or cerebral cortical tissue (Redding and Schally, 1973) but is nevertheless degraded by the brain.

LHRH does not accumulate in skeletal muscle and abdominal muscle homogenates do not inactivate LHRH (Redding and Schally, 1973). When [pGlu-3,4-^{3}H]LHRH was injected into the rat femoral artery, only intact hormone was recovered in femoral venous blood. Therefore, during one transit of LHRH through the leg, neither the vascular endothelium nor the muscle cells metabolized the hormone (Stetler-Stevenson *et al.*, 1983).

Injection of tritiated LHRH into the jugular vein, and sampling of blood in the aorta after one transit through the lungs, showed no breakdown of the hormone. There was no breakdown of the LHRH during one vascular transit through the liver and there was only a trace of radioactivity in bile following injection of tritiated LHRH (Flouret, G., Carone, F. A., Stetler-Stevenson, M. A., Gulczynski, B., Nakamura, S. and Peterson, D., unpublished). Only brain and kidney degrade substantial amounts of LHRH during a single vascular transit, which suggests that these organs are major sites for the breakdown of circulating LHRH. However, LHRH may accumulate in tissues and undergo slow degradation which would not be detected by these studies.

LHRH had a half-life ($T_{\frac{1}{2}}$) of 2–12 min depending on the species (Bennett and McMartin, 1979). After single bolus injection in human volunteers, the $T_{\frac{1}{2}}$ for disappearance of LHRH using radioimmunoassay was 4.8 min (Arimura *et al.*, 1974) and 5.3 min (Jeffcoate *et al.*, 1974). Using the technique of continuous intravenous infusion of LHRH with cessation of infusion when a constant plasma level is attained, the $T_{\frac{1}{2}}$ for LHRH in man was found to be 5.5–8 min (Pimstone *et al.*, 1977) and 7.8 min (Barron *et al.*, 1982). By similar methodology, the superactive analog [D-Trp^{6}]LHRH had a $T_{\frac{1}{2}}$ of 18.8 $\pm$ 1.8 (SEM) and a metabolic clearance rate of 503.4 $\pm$ 196.4 min versus 1766.6 $\pm$ 404.3 ml/min for LHRH (Barron *et al.*, 1982). The decreased metabolic clearance and longer half-life of the analog may be due in part to a decreased rate of degradation. There was no difference in $T_{\frac{1}{2}}$ for LHRH and some superactive LHRH analogs after i.v. administration of a single bolus to sheep (Swift and Crighton, 1979).

CONCLUDING REMARKS

The design of active LHRH analogs has not been guided by metabolic studies, but rather metabolic studies have been used to rationalize the high biological activity of some analogs. Attempts to correlate analog potency with resistance to degradation by tissue homogenates or by purified tissue peptidases must be cautiously evaluated, as these enzymes probably are compartmentalized and might not come in contact with LHRH or its analogs under physiological conditions. The resistance of some LHRH analogs having D-amino acids at position 6 to degradation by rat brain or pituitary homogenates as proof of the existence of a peptidase cleaving LHRH at Gly^6–Leu^7 is of questionable validity. Indeed, the postulated enzyme has not been isolated to date. Additionally, several LHRH analogs substituted with D-amino acids have inhibitory effects on three different bovine brain peptidases cleaving peptide bonds 'remote' to the site of substitution (Horsthemke *et al.*, 1981) and [D-Ser^4]LHRH is not cleaved by rat brain homogenates (Flouret, G., Carone, F. A., Stetler-Stevenson, M. A., Gulczynski, B., Nakamura, S. and Peterson, D., unpublished). Incubations of LHRH with several organ homogenates suggest that metabolite 5, rather than metabolite 6, is one of the earliest metabolites detected as a function of time. Studies with the kidney tubule *in vitro* and *in vivo* demonstrate that, after glomerular filtration, LHRH is cleaved to metabolite 4 as the longest pyroglutamyl peptide and that LHRH is not reabsorbed intact. Additionally, injection of LHRH into the arterial circulation of various organs showed that brain and kidney are major sites in the degradation of LHRH during a singular transit time, yielding metabolite 4 as the longest pyroglutamyl peptide rather than metabolites 5 or 6. Thus, in the design of metabolically resistant, long acting analogs of LHRH, the substitution of unnatural amino acids at position 4 may prove effective.

Acknowledgements

We gratefully acknowledge support in part by Grant HD-08669 from the National Institute of Child Health and Human Development, and by Grants AM-27646 and AM-14610 from the National Institute of Arthritis, Metabolism and Digestive Diseases.

References

Arimura, A., Kastin, A. J., Gonzalez-Barcena, D., Siller, J., Weaver, R. E. and Schally, A. V. (1974). Disappearance of LH-releasing hormone in man as determined by radioimmunoassay. *Clin. Endocrinol.*, **3,** 421

Barron, J. L., Millar, R. and Searle, D. (1982). Metabolic clearance and plasma half-disappearance time of D-Trp^6 and exogenous luteinizing hormone-releasing hormone. *J. Clin. Endocrinol. Metab.*, **54,** 1169

Bauer, K., Horsthemke, B., Knisatschek, H., Norvak, P. and Kleinhauf, H. (1979). Degradation of luliberin (LH-RF) by brain and pituitary tissue enzymes. *Z. Physiol. Chem.*, **360,** 229

Bennett, H. P. J. and McMartin, C. (1979). Peptide hormones and their analogues: distribution, clearance from the circulation and inactivation in vivo. *Pharmacol. Rev.*, **30,** 247

Benuck, M. and Marks, N. (1976). Differences in the degradation of hypothalamic releasing factors by rat and human serum. *Life Sci.*, **19,** 1271

Burg, J. J., Grantham, M., Abramow, M. and Orloff, J. (1966). Preparation and study of fragments of single nephrons. *Am. J. Physiol.*, **210,** 1293

Carone, F. A. and Peterson, D. R. (1980). Hydrolysis and transport of small peptides by the proximal tubule. *Am. J. Physiol.*, **238,** F151

Carone, F. A., Peterson, D. R. and Flouret, G. (1982). Renal tubular processing of small peptide hormones. *J. Lab. Clin. Med.*, **100,** 1

Clayton, R. N., Shakespear, R. A. and Marshall, J. C. (1977). Luteinizing hormone releasing hormone degrading activity associated with a purified pituitary plasma membrane fraction. *J. Endocrinol.*, **73,** 34P

Clayton, R. N. and Shakespear, R. A. (1978). [D-Serine $(Bu^t)^6$] luteinizing hormone releasing $hormone_{1-9}$ ethylamide: enhanced biological activity because of resistance to degradation. *J. Endocrinol.*, **77,** 34P

Clayton, R. N., Shakespear, R. A., Duncan, J. A. and Marshall, J. C. (1979). Luteinizing hormone-releasing hormone inactivation by purified pituitary plasma membranes: effects on receptor-binding studies. *Endocrinology*, **104,** 1484

Clayton, R. N. and Catt, K. J. (1980). Receptor-binding affinity of gonadotropin-releasing hormone analogs: analysis by radioligand-receptor assay. *Endocrinology*, **106,** 1154

Dupont, A., Labrie, F., Pelletier, G., Puviani, R., Coy, D. H., Coy, E. J. and Schally, A. V. (1974). Organ distribution of radioactivity and disappearance of radioactivity from plasma after administration of (^{3}H)luteinizing hormone-releasing hormone to mice and rats. *Neuro-endocrinology*, **16,** 65

Fridkin, M., Hazum, E. Baram, T., Lindner, H. R. and Koch, Y. (1977). Hypothalamic and pituitary LRF-degrading enzymes: characterization, purification and physiological role. In Goodman, M. and Meienhofer, J. (eds.) *Peptides*, pp. 193–196. (New York: Halsted Press)

Gottschalk, C. W., Morel, F. and Myelle, M. (1965). Tracer microinjection studies of renal tubular permeability. *Am. J. Physiol.*, **209,** 173

Griffiths, E. C., Hooper, K. C., Jeffcoate, S. L. and Holland, D. T. (1975). The effects of gonadectomy and gonadal steroids on the activity of hypothalamic peptidases inactivating luteinizing hormone-releasing hormone (LH-RH). *Brain Res.*, **88,** 384

Heber, D., Marshall, J. C. and Odell, W. D. (1978). GnRH membrane binding: identification, specificity and quantification in nonpituitary tissues. *Am. J. Physiol.*, **235,** E227

Hersh, L. B. and McKelvey, J. F. (1979). Enzymes involved in the degradation of thyrotropin releasing hormone (TRH) and luteinizing hormone releasing hormone (LHRH) in bovine brain. *Brain Res.*, **168,** 553

Horsthemke, B. and Bauer, K. (1980). Characterization of a nonchymotrypsin-like endopeptidase from anterior pituitary that hydrolyzes luteinizing hormone-releasing hormone at the tyrosyl-glycine and histidyl-tryptophan bonds. *Biochemistry*, **19,** 2867

Horsthemke, B., Knisatschek, H., Rivier, J., Sandow, J. and Bauer, K. (1981). Degradation of luteinizing hormone-releasing hormone and analogs by adenohypophyseal peptidases. *Biochem. Biophys. Res. Commun.*, **100,** 753

Hudson, D., Pickering, A., McLoughlin, J. L., Matthews, E., Sharpe, R., Fink, G., MacIntyre, I. and Szelke, M. (1976). The synthesis and metabolic fate of 3-(^{3}H)Trp, 9-(^{14}C)Pro-LHRH. *V International Congress of Endocrinology, Hamburg, July 18–24.* Abstract 43, p. 18

Jeffcoate, S. L., Greenwood, R. H. and Holland, D. T. (1974). Blood and urine clearance of luteinizing hormone releasing hormone in man measured by radioimmunoassay. *J. Endocrinol.*, **60,** 305

Kelly, J. A., Griffiths, E. C., Jeffcoate, S. L. and Hopkinson, C. R. N. (1979). Hypothalamic inactivation of luliberin (luteinizing-hormone-releasing hormone). *Biochem. Soc. Trans.*, **7,** 76

Knisatschek, H. and Bauer, K. (1979). Characterization of 'thyroliberin-deamidating enzyme' as a post-proline-cleaving enzyme. *J. Biol. Chem.*, **254,** 10936

Koch, Y., Baram, T., Chobsieng, P. and Fridkin, M. (1974). Enzymic degradation of luteinizing hormone-releasing hormone (LHRH) by hypothalamic tissue. *Biochem. Biophys. Res. Commun.*, **61,** 95

Koch, Y., Baram, T., Hazum, E. and Fridkin, M. (1977). Resistance to enzymic degradation of LHRH analogues possessing increased biological activity. *Biochem. Biophys. Res. Commun.*, **74,** 488

Kochman, K., Kerdelhue, B., Zor, U. and Jutisz, M. (1975). Studies of enzymatic degradation of luteinizing hormone-releasing hormone by different tissues. *FEBS Lett.*, **50,** 190

Loudes, C., Joseph-Bravo, P., Leblanc, P. and Kordon, C. (1978). Specific activity of LHRH and TRH degrading enzymes in various tissues of normal and castrated male rats. *Biochem. Biophys. Res. Commun.*, **83,** 921

Marks, N. and Stern, F. (1974). Enzymatic mechanisms for the inactivation of luteinizing hormone-releasing hormone (LHRH). *Biochem. Biophys. Res. Commun.*, **61,** 1458

Orlowski, M., Wilk, E., Pearce, S. and Wilk, S. (1979). Purification and properties of a prolyl endopeptidase from rabbit brain. *J. Neurochem.*, **33,** 461

Pimstone, B., Epstein, S., Hamilton, S. M., LeRoith, D. and Hendricks, S. (1977). Metabolic clearance and plasma half disappearance time of exogenous gonadotropin releasing hormone in normal subjects and in patients with liver disease and chronic renal failure. *J. Clin. Endocrinol. Metab.*, **44,** 356

Redding, T. W. and Schally, A. V. (1973). The distribution, half-life and excretion of tritiated luteinizing hormone-releasing hormone (LHRH) in rats. *Life Sci.*, **12,** 23

Redding, T. W., Kastin, A. J., Gonzalez-Barcena, D., Coy, D. H., Coy, E. J., Schalch, D. S. and Schally, A. V. (1973). The half-life, metabolism and excretion of tritiated luteinizing hormone-releasing hormone (LHRH) in man. *J. Clin. Endocrinol. Metab.*, **37,** 626

Reeves, J. J., Tarnavsky, G. K., Becker, S. R., Coy, D. and Schally, A. V. (1977). Uptake of iodinated luteinizing hormone releasing hormone analogs in the pituitary. *Endocrinology*, **101,** 540

Reeves, J. J., Seguin, C., Lefebvre, F. A., Kelly, P. A. and Labrie, F. (1980). Similar luteinizing hormone-releasing hormone binding sites in rat anterior pituitary and ovary. *Proc. Natl. Acad. Sci. USA*, **77,** 5567

Schally, A. V., Bowers, C. Y., Carter, W. H., Arimura, A., Redding, T. W. and Saito, M. (1969). Effect of actinomycin D on the inhibitory response of estrogen on LH release. *Endocrinology*, **85,** 290

Stetler-Stevenson, M. A., Yang, D. C., McCartney, L., Peterson, D., Lipkowski, A. and Flouret, G. (1980). On the metabolic breakdown products of LHRH by renal tissue. In Brunfeldt, K. (ed.) *Peptides*, pp. 725–730. (Copenhagen: Scriptor)

Stetler-Stevenson, M. A., Carone, F., Flouret, G. and Peterson, D. (1981*a*). On the metabolic breakdown of LHRH by renal tissue. In Rich, D. H. and Gross, E. (eds.) *Peptides*, pp. 821–824. (Rockford, IL: Pierce Chemical Co.)

Stetler-Stevenson, M. A., Flouret, G. and Peterson, D. R. (1981*b*). Handling of luteinizing hormone-releasing hormone by renal proximal tubular segments in vitro. *Am. J. Physiol.*, **241,** F117

Stetler-Stevenson, M. A., Yang, D. C., Lipkowski, A., McCartney, L., Peterson, D. and Flouret, G. (1981*c*). An approach to the elucidation of metabolic breakdown products of the luteinizing hormone-releasing hormone. *J. Med. Chem.*, **24,** 688

Stetler-Stevenson, M. A., Flouret, G., Nakamura, S., Gulczynski, B. and Carone, F. A. (1983). In vivo metabolism of tritiated LHRH by the whole kidney and individual tubules of rats. *Am. J. Physiol.*, **244,** F628

Swift, A. D. and Crighton, D. B. (1979). Relative activity, plasma elimination and tissue degradation of synthetic luteinizing hormone releasing hormone and certain of its analogues. *J. Endocrinol.*, **80,** 141

White, W. T., Hedlund, M. T., Rippel, R. H., Arnold, W. and Flouret, G. R. (1973). Chemical and biological properties of gonadotropin releasing hormone synthesized by the solid-phase method. *Endocrinology*, **93,** 96

Wilk, S., Benuck, M., Orlowski, M. and Marks, N. (1979). Degradation of luteinizing hormone-releasing hormone (LHRH) by brain prolyl endopeptidase with release of des-glycinamide LHRH and glycinamide. *Neurosci. Lett.*, **14,** 275

32
Metabolism of [D-Trp^6]LHRH

J. BARRON, E. GRIFFITHS, G. TSALACOPOULOS and R. P. MILLAR

Superactive analogs of LHRH have enhanced LH releasing activity relative to the natural peptide both *in vivo* and *in vitro* (Vale *et al.*, 1977; Sandow and Konig, 1978). The enhanced biological activity is apparently due to a greater resistance to degradation (Sandow *et al.*, 1978) and to a higher binding affinity for LHRH receptors (Clayton and Catt, 1980). However, the relative contribution of these two factors in increasing biological activity is not clear.

LHRH is degraded by enzymes present in many tissues (Vale *et al.*, 1977; Sandow and Konig, 1978; Bennett and McMartin, 1978), including pituitary membranes (Clayton *et al.*, 1979; Elkabes *et al.*, 1981). It is uncertain whether the enzymes studied play an important part in physiological regulation. Hypothalamic peptidase inactivation of LHRH is altered by the steroid milieu (Griffiths *et al.*, 1975) and LHRH degrading enzymes may regulate the amount of hormone released or the amount reaching the target site. However, a number of hypothalamic enzymes not associated with LHRH metabolism are also altered by physiological manipulation (Bauer *et al.*, 1980).

A pituitary endopeptidase that cleaves the Tyr–Gly bond of LHRH has been characterized (Horsthemke and Bauer, 1980, 1981). Substitution of Gly by D-amino acids results in protection of the 5–6 bond from enzymatic degradation *in vitro* (Vale *et al.*, 1977; Sandow and Konig, 1978; Bennett and McMartin, 1978) and a reduced clearance rate in humans *in vivo* when compared with LHRH (Barron *et al.*, 1982). This promotes enhanced gonadotropic hormone releasing activity which is possibly further increased by the replacement of the C-terminal glycinamide by an ethylamide (Vale *et al.*, 1977).

The stability of LHRH and analogs in the circulation may be important in determining the biological response. *In vitro* studies have shown that human plasma has very low LHRH degrading activity (Swift and Crighton, 1979; Koch *et al.*, 1974) while homogenates of brain, pituitary, gonad, liver, kidney and lung from rats and sheep rapidly inactivate LHRH (Swift and Crighton, 1979; Vale, *et al.*, 1977; Sandow and Konig, 1978). The plasma clearance of LHRH in dogs was slightly impaired by occlusion of the renal blood supply, but grossly impaired following occlusion of the hepatic blood supply (Sandow and Konig, 1978). The clearance of exogenous LHRH is impaired in persons with renal disease but is not significantly affected in patients with hepatic disease (Pimstone *et al.*, 1977). Renal clearance of LHRH is due to metabolism by the proximal tubules following glomerular filtration (Carone *et al.*, 1982). Thus the liver and the kidney may be sites of LHRH removal.

DEGRADATION OF LHRH AND [D-TRP^{6}]LHRH *IN VITRO*

LHRH degrading activity by two subcellular fractions prepared from brain tissue was investigated. Tissues obtained from adult male rats, killed by decapitation, were homogenized. Two subcellular fractions, consisting of a postmitochondrial supernatant and a particulate fraction containing microsomes, lysosomes and mitochondria were prepared (Griffiths *et al.*, 1979). Aliquots of the subcellular fractions containing 150 μg protein were incubated with LHRH or [D-Trp^{6}]LHRH. Enzymatic activity was terminated by boiling for 10 min. The residual [D-Trp^{6}]LHRH was measured using antiserum 69, which is directed towards the middle of the molecule and requires the D-Trp residue for binding. Antiserum 1076, which requires residues Ser^{4}–Leu^{7} of LHRH for effective binding, was used to assay LHRH in the presence of [D-Trp^{6}]LHRH (Barron *et al.*, 1982).

LHRH was degraded more rapidly than [D-Trp^{6}]LHRH by the brain tissues examined (Table 32.1). Using hypothalamic supernatant and particulate fractions, the degradation of LHRH was more rapid than of [D-Trp^{6}]LHRH and was biphasic for both peptides (Figure 32.1). When LHRH and [D-Trp^{6}]LHRH were incubated together, the degradation of LHRH was slower, a finding in agreement with that of previous workers (Millar *et al.*, 1978; Sandow *et al.*, 1979).

The extent to which tissues catabolize LHRH or its analogs *in vivo* is difficult to assess. In the majority of the studies to date, the degradation of LHRH and analogs has been compared using tissue homogenates (Vale *et al.*, 1977; Swift and Crighton, 1979). Although LHRH may come in contact with degrading enzymes from these tissues *in vivo*, studies on the degradation of LHRH and analogs during perfusion of intact tissues such as the kidney (Carone *et al.*, 1982) must be performed before conclusions are drawn on a catabolic role for different tissues.

Table 32.1 Comparison of the degradation of LHRH and [D-Trp^{6}] LHRH by supernatant and particulate fractions (Mean ± SD, n = 4)

	Degradation (ng/min)			
	Supernatant		*Particulate*	
	LHRH	[D-Trp^{6}]LHRH	LHRH	[D-Trp^{6}]LHRH
Hypothalamus	6.61 ± 0.03	0.31 ± 0.01	2.55 ± 0.15	0.10 ± 0.05
Pituitary	4.82 ± 0.05	0.74 ± 0.02	0.67 ± 0.26	0.11 ± 0.03
Thalamus	4.84 ± 0.39	1.02 ± 0.05	0.60 ± 0.05	0.09 ± 0.01
Cortex	5.63 ± 0.05	0.81 ± 0.02	2.07 ± 0.19	0.09 ± 0.02
Cerebellum	4.61 ± 0.33	0.40 ± 0.03	3.88 ± 0.04	0.27 ± 0.02

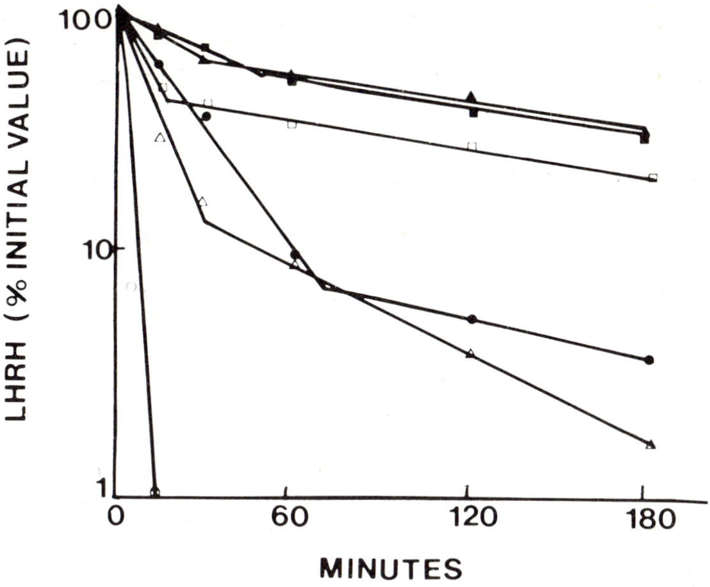

Figure 32.1 Time course of LHRH and [D-Trp^6]LHRH degradation by hypothalamic homogenates, expressed as a percentage of the initial concentration. LHRH: supernatant (○——○), particulate (●——●); LHRH in presence of [D-Trp^6]LHRH: supernatant (△——△), particulate (▲——▲). [D-Trp^6]LHRH: supernatant (□——□), particulate (■——■).

RECEPTOR BINDING

The relative contributions of resistance to degradation and enhanced receptor binding of LHRH agonists are difficult to separate since degrading enzymes are present in the receptor plasma membrane (Clayton *et al.*, 1979; Elkabes *et al.*, 1981) and may form an intrinsic component of the receptor complex. Enhanced receptor binding may be due partially to resistance to degradation and not solely increased intrinsic affinity.

We tested the effect of bacitracin (10^{-4} mol/l) and *p*-amino-mercuribenzoate (10^{-5} mol/l) on the IC_{50} of LHRH and analogs (J. Barron and R. Millar, unpublished data). At 4 °C the peptidase inhibitors reduced the specific maximal binding of ^{125}I-[D-Leu^6,Pro^9-NHEt]LHRH but the K_Ds of superactive analogs were identical in the presence and absence of the inhibitors. Unexpectedly, LHRH was less effective in displacing the labeled agonist in the presence of the peptidase inhibitors. At 37 °C binding of ^{125}I-LHRH-analogs was further decreased but was unaffected by the peptidase inhibitors. Displacement by LHRH was identical in the presence or absence of the inhibitors.

In the receptor assay we found that both [D-Trp^6]LHRH and [D-Trp^6, Pro^9-NHEt]LHRH had lower IC_{50}s than did LHRH, with the ethylamide analog showing a greater affinity for the receptor (Table 32.1). The biological

Table 32.2 Receptor binding and biological potency of LHRH and analogs

	Receptor activity[a]		*Biological potency*	
	ED_{50} (nmol/l)	*Relative potency*	b	c
LHRH	60	1	1	1
[D-Trp^6]LHRH	1.5	40	36	100
[D-Trp^6,Pro^9-NHEt]LHRH	0.79	76	144	15

[a] Determined using rat anterior pituitary membranes
[b] Data from Vale *et al.*, 1977
[c] Data from Coy *et al.*, 1976.

potency of these analogs in releasing LH from pituitary cells in culture (Vale *et al.*, 1977), corresponds with receptor binding data (Table 32.2). However, the biological potency of [D-Trp^6,Pro^9-NHEt]LHRH reported by Coy *et al.*, (1976) does not accord with these data.

METABOLIC CLEARANCE RATE IN NORMAL MEN

The major contributing factors to the potency of LHRH agonists *in vivo* are the survival time in the circulation, receptor binding activity, and the ability to stimulate cellular events leading to gonadotropin hormone release. Although *in vitro* degradation studies give an indication of the resistance of the LHRH agonists to enzymes, this may not reflect their fate or potency *in vivo*. Therefore studies on survival *in vivo* are desirable for an assessment of the biological activity of LHRH agonists and the design of future analogs.

After bolus intravenous administration of LHRH, the initial half-life ($T_{\frac{1}{2}}$) in plasma is short (3–6 min), followed by a second slower component (20–30 min) (Keye *et al.*, 1973; Arimura *et al.*, 1974; Jeffcoate *et al.*, 1974). There is no difference in the plasma $T_{\frac{1}{2}}$ (3–4 min) of LHRH and superactive analogs after bolus intravenous injection in sheep (Swift and Crighton, 1979). The major contribution to the plasma clearance after bolus administration is likely due to the movement of peptide into the extracellular fluid. This method of study does not, therefore, reflect the true metabolic fate of the peptide. The plasma $T_{\frac{1}{2}}$, after continuous i.v. infusion of LHRH in man was longer than the $T_{\frac{1}{2}}$ after bolus administration (Pimstone *et al.*, 1977; Chikamori *et al.*, 1981). For this reason [D-Trp^6]LHRH (100 μg) and LHRH (100 μg) were infused intravenously using a constant infusion pump over a period of 60 min into normal healthy men and the plasma elimination was followed after attaining constant plasma levels (Barron *et al.*, 1982). Three of the subjects received [D-Trp^6]LHRH infusions alone and five received a simultaneous infusion of both [D-Trp^6]LHRH and LHRH.

The metabolic clearance rate (MCR), steady state level (SSL) and $T_{\frac{1}{2}}$ of [D-Trp^6]LHRH was significantly different ($p<0.01$) from that of LHRH (Table 32.3). There was no difference between the MCR of [D-Trp^6]LHRH

Table 32.3 Metabolic clearance rate and half-life of LHRH and [D-Trp^6]LHRH following constant infusion in men

	n	*SSL* (ng/ml)	*MCR* (ml/min)	$T_{\frac{1}{2}}$ (min) *Rapid component*	*Slow component*	*Stripped rapid*
LHRH	5	1.09 ± 0.21[a]	1766.0 ± 404.3[a]	7.8 ± 1.2[a]	13 ± 1.4[a]	3.8[a]
[D-Trp^6]LHRH	8	3.69 ± 0.45	503.4 ± 196.4	19.0 ± 1.8	50 ± 2.1	5.3

The results are expressed as the mean ± SEM. The stripped $T_{\frac{1}{2}}$ is derived by stripping off the mean slow component of the degradation curve from the mean rapid component. Data from Barron *et al.* 1982.
[a] $p < 0.01$ for LHRH vs [D-Trp^6]LHRH

infused with or without LHRH. The MCR of LHRH when infused with [D-Trp^6]LHRH was similar to that found when LHRH was infused alone (Pimstone *et al.*, 1977; Chikamori *et al.*, 1981). The fact that [D-Trp^6]LHRH did not inhibit LHRH clearance implies that the degradation clearance systems are not saturated at the dose of the peptide infused. This constrasts with *in vitro* studies where [D-Trp^6]LHRH decreased the degradation of LHRH. The findings demonstrate that LHRH is cleared about three times more rapidly from the plasma than [D-Trp^6]LHRH.

The mean plasma disappearance curve for [D-Trp^6]LHRH and LHRH after cessation of the infusion was biphasic (Figure 32.2). This was not due to a slower elimination from the circulation of immunologically active fragments, because on reassay with antiserum 744, which requires residues Arg^8–Gly^{10} of LHRH and therefore also recognizes carboxy-terminal fragments of [D-Trp^6]LHRH, the same values were obtained. Furthermore, HPLC of the plasma showed only the intact molecule to be present. Although the absence of plasma degradation could in part account for this (Swift and Crighton, 1979; Koch *et al.*, 1974; Bennett and McMartin, 1978) these findings also suggest that any C-terminal fragments produced by tissue degradation are either completely degraded within the tissues or are rapidly further degraded in the plasma or cleared by the kidney. To examine loss through the kidney, we assayed urine collected at the end of the study from the three persons infused with [D-Trp^6]LHRH alone. At this stage, 3–14% of the peptide infused was present in the urine. The circulating levels of [D-Trp^6]LHRH 40 min after cessation of infusion indicate that approximately 30% of the total peptide infused was present in the extracellular fluid. Therefore, 60% was not accounted for and presumably was degraded or present within tissues.

After bolus administration in humans, the effects of [D-Trp^6]LHRH and [D-Trp^6,Pro^9-NHEt]LHRH in stimulating LH and FSH release were similar and the plasma LH and FSH levels achieved were from three to five times greater than for LHRH (Wass *et al.*, 1979). The same dose of [D-Trp^6]LHRH administered i.v. by constant infusion over 60 min gave a peak plasma LH response (95.3 ± 46 i.u./l) four times greater than the response to a bolus dose (J. Barron and R. Millar, unpublished results). The relative potency of LHRH and [D-Trp^6]LHRH cannot be assessed from the increases in plasma LH as dose-response studies are required. The differences in clearance between

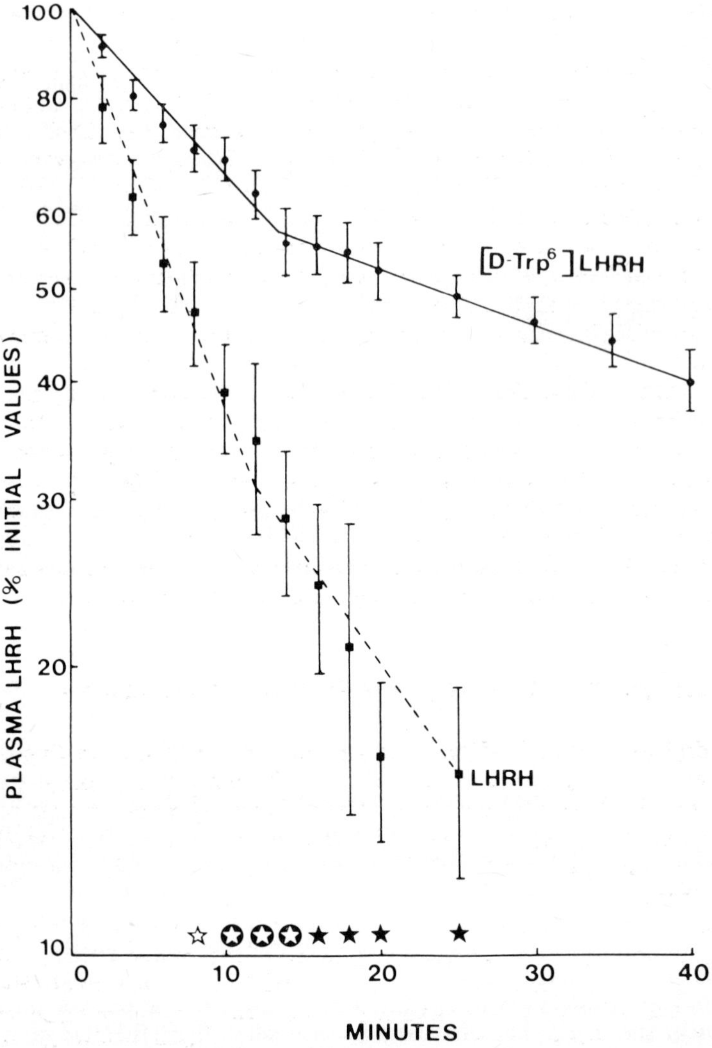

Figure 32.2 Plasma disappearance of [D-Trp6]LHRH (●——●) and LHRH (■——■) levels, expressed as a percentage of the plasma concentration at the time of cessation of the infusion. Vertical bars represent the SEM. ★, $p < 0.001$; ✪, $p < 0.01$; ☆, $p < 0.05$ (comparing LHRH and [D-Trp6]LHRH at the time intervals indicated). (From Barron *et al.*, 1982)

LHRH and [D-Trp6]LHRH shown here undoubtedly contribute to the enhanced potency of [D-Trp6]LHRH.

METABOLIC CLEARANCE RATE DURING PREGNANCY

LHRH or analogs administered to pregnant rabbits are known to prevent implantation and induce fetal resorption (Sandow *et al.*, 1982), and may find application in contraception. We therefore examined the MCR of LHRH analogs in pregnant women. Four women presenting for therapeutic abortion in the first trimester of pregnancy (6–11 weeks) gave consent for infusion of either 500 μg [D-Trp^6]LHRH or [D-Trp^6,Pro^9-NHEt]LHRH over a period of 60 min, using the protocol described previously (Barron *et al.*, 1982). The mean MCRs for [D-Trp^6]LHRH and [D-Trp^6,Pro^9-NHEt]LHRH were 300 and 269 ml/min respectively. These were lower than the MCR obtained during the infusion of 100 μg of [D-Trp^6]LHRH in men. The MCR of LHRH has been found to decrease progressively with increasing dosage (Kelch *et al.*, 1975; Huseman and Kelch, 1978) which may be due to saturation of the degradation/clearance systems. The half-lives for [D-Trp^6]LHRH and [D-Trp^6,Pro^9-NHEt]LHRH were identical to that in men. The metabolic changes associated with pregnancy do not apparently influence the clearance of LHRH analogs containing D-Trp^6. The presence of the ethylamide residue, which protects the peptide from postproline-cleaving-enzyme activity (Horsthemke *et al.*, 1981), does not lead to a prolonged survival time in pregnant women. This indicates that degradation by the postproline-cleaving-enzyme in human tissues contributes minimally to LHRH clearance. This is supported by reports that both D-Trp analogs are equipotent *in vivo* (Schally *et al.*, 1980; Wass *et al.*, 1979). However, it should be noted that antiserum 69 used in our studies would interact with the analog lacking the glycinamide.

EFFECTS ON PLASMA HORMONES IN PREGNANCY

Daily administration of LHRH or agonist in rats has resulted in an increase in progesterone and decrease in estradiol. Although bolus administration of LHRH was ineffective in changing plasma hormone levels in first trimester pregnant women (Sandow *et al.*, 1982; Rubinstein *et al.*, 1978; Sowers *et al.*, 1978), constant infusion of LHRH increased FSH levels significantly (Yoshida *et al.*, 1981).

We therefore studied the effects of two D-Trp^6 analogs in the pregnant woman. Progesterone increased 82% above basal levels 40 min following cessation of the 60 min infusion in both patients treated with 500 μg of [D-Trp^6,Pro^9-NHEt]LHRH, whereas in the two patients infused with [D-Trp^6]LHRH, progesterone increased by 37% above basal levels. FSH increased 85% above basal levels 6 h following the infusion with [D-Trp^6,Pro^9-NHEt]LHRH, whereas with the same dose of [D-Trp^6]LHRH, FSH increased by 22% above basal levels. PRL, β-hCG, HPL and estradiol were unaffected by either analog.

CONCLUDING REMARKS

The stability of peptide hormones in body fluids and tissues is an important factor in biological half-life and duration of action. The *in vivo* half-lives of [D-Trp^6]LHRH and [D-Trp^6,Pro^9-NHEt]LHRH, after constant infusion, are three times longer than that of LHRH. These analogs therefore reach higher circulating levels when infused at the same dose as LHRH and will have greater biological effects. Furthermore, these analogs have higher affinities for pituitary receptors and will therefore bind and activate these receptors at lower circulating levels than will LHRH. Thus resistance to degradation and enhanced receptor binding both contribute to the greater biological activity of these analogs.

Acknowledgements

We thank Professor M. C. Berman for his encouragement and support and C. Tobler and J. Maxwell for excellent technical assistance. Antiserum 744 was a gift from A. Arimura. The work was supported by the South African MRC, the University of Cape Town Staff Research Fund, the Harry Crossley Foundation, the Merrin Bequest and the Atomic Energy Board.

References

Arimura, A., Kastin, A. J., Gonzales-Barcena, D., Siller, J., Weaver, R. E. and Schally, A. V. (1974). Disappearance of LHRH in man as determined by radioimmunoassay. *Clin. Endocrinol.,* **3,** 421

Barron, J. L., Millar, R. P. and Searle, D. (1982). Metabolic clearance and plasma half-disappearance time of D-Trp^6 and exogenous LHRH. *J. Clin. Endocrinol. Metab.,* **54,** 1169

Bauer, K., Beier, S., Horsthemke, B., Knisatschek, H. and Sievers, J. (1980). Estrogen effects of LHRH degrading brain and pituitary enzymes. In Wuttke, W. and Horowski, R. (eds.) *Gonadal Steroids and Brain Function,* pp. 93–107. (Berlin: Springer)

Bennett, H. P. J. and McMartin, C. (1978). Peptide hormones and their analogues. *Pharmacol. Rev.,* **30,** 247

Carone, F. A., Petersen, D. R. and Flouret, G. (1982). Renal tubular processing of small peptide hormones. *J. Lab. Clin. Med.,* **100,** 1

Chikamori, K., Suchiro, F., Ogawa, T., Sato, K., Mori, H., Oshima, I. and Saito, S. (1981). Distribution volume, metabolic clearance and plasma half disappearance time of exogenous luteinizing hormone releasing hormone in normal women and women with obesity and anorexia nervosa. *Acta Endocrinol.,* **96,** 1

Clayton, R. N. and Catt, K. J. (1980). Receptor-binding affinity of GnRH analogs. *Endocrinology,* **106,** 1154

Clayton, R. N., Shakespear, R. A., Duncan, J. A. and Marshall, J. C. (1979). LHRH inactivation by purified pituitary plasma membranes: effects on receptor-binding studies. *Endocrinology,* **104,** 1484

Coy, D. H., Labrie, F., Savary, M., Coy, E. J. and Schally, A. V. (1976). LH-releasing activity of potent LHRH analogs in vitro. *Biochem. Biophys. Res. Commun.,* **67,** 576

Elkabes, S., Fridkin, M. and Koch, Y. (1981). Studies on the enzymic degradation of LHRH by rat pituitary plasma membranes. *Biochem. Biophys. Res. Commun.,* **103,** 240

Griffiths, E. C., Hooper, K. C., Jeffcoate, S. A. and Holland, D. T. (1975). The effects of gonadectomy and gonadal steroids on the activity of hypothalamic peptidases. *Brain Res.,* **88,** 384

Griffiths, E. C., Kelly, J. A., Klootivijk, W. and Visser, T. J. (1979). Enzymic inactivation of thyrotrophin releasing hormone by the hypothalamus and other areas of rat brain. *J. Physiol.,* **290,** 39P

Horsthemke, B. and Bauer, K. (1980). Characterization of a nonchymotrypsin-like endopeptidase from anterior pituitary that hydrolyzes LH-RH at the Tyrosyl-Glycine and Histidyl-Tryptophan bonds. *Biochemistry,* **19,** 2867

Horsthemke, B. and Bauer, K. (1981). Chymotryptic-like hydrolysis of LHRH by an adenohypophyseal enzyme of high molecular weight. *Biochem. Biophys. Res. Commun.,* **103,** 1322

Horsthemke, B., Knisatschek, H., Rivier, J., Sandow, J. and Bauer, K. (1981). Degradation of LHRH and analogs by adenohypophyseal peptidases. *Biochem. Biophys. Res. Commun.*, **100,** 753

Huseman, C. A. and Kelch, R. P. (1978). Gonadotrophin responses and metabolism of synthetic GnRH during constant infusion of GnRH in men and boys with delayed adolescence. *J. Clin. Endocrinol. Metab.*, **47,** 1325

Jeffcoate, S. L., Greenwood, R. H. and Holland, D. T. (1974). Blood and urine clearance of LHRH in man measured by radioimmunoassay. *J. Endocrinol.*, **60,** 305

Kelch, R. P., Clemans, L. E., Markovs, M., Westhoff, M. H. and Hawkins, D. W. (1975). Metabolism and effects of synthetic GnRH in children and adults. *J. Clin. Endocrinol. Metab.*, **40,** 53

Keye, W. R., Kelch, R. P., Niswender, G. D. and Jaffe, R. B. (1973). Quantitation of endogenous and exogenous gonadotrophin releasing hormone by radioimmunoassay. *J. Clin. Endocrinol. Metab.*, **36,** 1263

Koch, Y., Baram, T., Chobsieng, P. and Fridkin, M. (1974). Enzymic degradation of LHRH by hypothalamic tissue. *Biochem. Biophys. Res. Commun.*, **61,** 95

Millar, R. P., Denniss, P., Tobler, C., King, J., Schally, A. V. and Arimura, A. (1978). Presumptive prohormonal forms of hypothalamic peptide hormones. In Vincent, J. D. and Kordan, C. (eds.) *Cell Biology of Hypothalamic Neurosecretion,* pp. 487–510. (Paris: CNRS)

Pimstone, B., Epstein, S., Hamilton, S. M., Le Roith, D. and Hendericks, S. (1977). Metabolic clearance and plasma half disappearance time of exogenous gonadotrophin releasing hormone in normal subjects and in patients with liver disease and chronic renal failure. *J. Clin. Endocrinol. Metab.*, **44,** 356

Rubinstein, L. M., Parlow, A. F., Derzko, C. and Hershman, J. (1978). Pituitary gonadotrophin response to LHRH in human pregnancy. *Obstet. Gynecol.*, **52,** 172

Sandow, J. and Konig, W. (1978). Chemistry of the hypothalamus hormones. In Jeffcoate, S. and Hutchinson, J. (eds.) *The Endocrine Hypothalamus,* pp. 149–211. (London: Academic Press)

Sandow, J., Konig, W., Geiger, R. and Uhmann, R. (1978). Structure – activity relationship in the LHRH molecule. In Crighton, D. B., Haynes, N. B., Foxcroft, G. R. and Lamming, G. E. (eds.) *Control of Ovulation,* pp. 49–70. (London: Butterworth)

Sandow, J., Kuhl, H. and Krauss, B. (1979). Studies on enzyme stability of LHRH analogues. *J. Endocrinol.*, **81,** 157

Sandow, J., Kuhl, H., Jerzabek, G., Kille, S. and von Rechenberg, W. (1982). The reproductive pharmacology and contraceptive application of LHRH and its analogues. In Flamigni, C. and Givens, J. R. (eds.) *The Gonadotropins: Basic Science and Clinical Aspects in Females,* pp. 77–105. (London: Academic Press)

Schally, A. V., Arimura, A. and Coy, D. H. (1980). Recent approaches to fertility control based on derivatives of LHRH. *Vitam. Horm.*, **38,** 257

Sowers, J. R., Colantino, M., Fayez, J. and Jonas, H. (1978). Pituitary response to LHRH in midtrimester pregnancy. *Obstet. Gynecol.*, **52,** 685

Swift, A. D. and Crighton, D. B. (1979). Relative activity, plasma elimination and tissue degradation of synthetic LHRH and certain of its analogues. *J. Endocrinol.*, **81,** 141

Vale, W., Rivier, C. and Brown, M. (1977). Regulatory peptides of the hypothalamus. *Ann. Rev. Physiol.*, **39,** 473

Wass, J. A., Besser, G. M., Gomez-Pan, A., Scanlon, M. F., Hall, R., Kastin, A. J., Coy, D. H. and Schally, A. V. (1979). Comparison of long-acting analogues of LHRH in man. *Clin. Endocrinol.*, **10,** 419

Yoshida, T., Hattori, Y., Suzuki, H. and Noda, K. (1981). Response of FSH, prolactin and HCG to continuous LHRH infusion in pregnant women. *Tohoku J. Exp. Med.*, **135,** 255

33
Delivery systems for LHRH and analogs

S. T. ANIK, L. M. SANDERS, M. D. CHAPLIN, S. KUSHINSKY and C. NERENBERG

The delivery of polypeptide and protein drugs by a convenient and effective method is a major challenge in the development of these compounds as therapeutic agents. Due to degradation and/or lack of absorption in the gastrointestinal tract, large, uneconomical doses are required for activity following oral administration. Rectal, nasal and depot injectable preparations have been investigated for the delivery of insulin but success has been limited. The injectable route, which assures availability of drug to the patient, is still the most frequently used. Efficient absorption and low variability of absorption are among the criteria to be emphasized when developing alternative delivery systems.

Delivery of LHRH analogs across nasal, rectal and vaginal membranes is possible due to the high potency, low toxicity and relatively low molecular weight of these analogs. The very high therapeutic ratio of these compounds also makes substantial variability of absorption tolerable for some of these routes. These features were recognized at an early stage during the clinical development of these analogs. As a result, several studies exploring the metabolic profile (Fink *et al.*, 1974; Barron *et al.*, 1982), and biological responses after administration by injection (Mortimer *et al.*, 1974), or by intranasal (Fink *et al.*, 1974; Gonzalez-Barcena *et al.*, 1976), intravaginal and rectal (Saito *et al.*, 1977) routes have been reported. The relative bioavailability by vaginal, rectal, nasal and oral routes has been measured, and the utility of various absorption enhancers demonstrated (Okada *et al.*, 1982).

INJECTABLE ROUTES

The earliest studies were designed to compare the different injectable routes by monitoring LH and FSH levels. The injectable routes are generally equivalent in the magnitude and duration of the LH/FSH response (Mortimer *et al.*, 1974), although the need for a larger dose of LHRH by subcutaneous (s.c.) injection (four times intravenous) has been reported (Happ *et al.*, 1978). LH peaks are observed within 20–30 min and elevated LH levels are maintained for 3–6 h after LHRH administration. A typical LH profile after intravenous

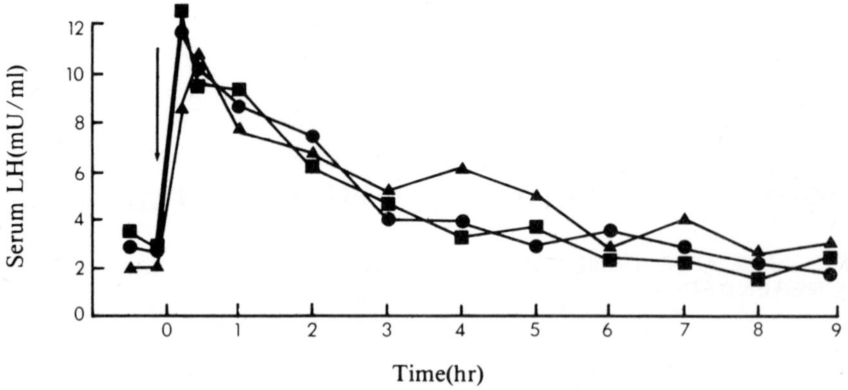

Figure 33.1 The serum LH responses in one subject following i.v. (●), i.m. (■) and s.c. (▲) injection of LHRH 100 μg. (From Mortimer *et al.*, 1974, by kind permission of Blackwell Scientific Publications Limited).

(i.v.), intramuscular (i.m.) and s.c. injection of LHRH in men is shown in Figure 33.1. The FSH response requires larger doses, is more variable and is slower, with peak levels occurring 45 min–1 h after administration and lasting 6–9 h.

Dose-response studies of the LH response after i.v. administration of LHRH indicate a linear log dose-response up to a maximal response for doses of LHRH of 50–100 μg (Haug and Torjesen, 1973). Similar results were also observed after i.m. administration of [D-Leu^6,Pro^9-NHEt]LHRH (Turner *et al.*, 1976).

A second type of study monitored the levels of LHRH in blood after i.v. administration. This profile has been characterized as a multiexponential curve to two or three phases (Figure 33.2). The half-life ($T_{\frac{1}{2}}$) of the first phase (distributive phase) is short (2–8 min), whereas the $T_{\frac{1}{2}}$ of the second phase is 20–30 min (Fink *et al.*, 1974; Seyler, 1975). Longer $T_{\frac{1}{2}}$s (50–60 min) for the second phase also have been reported but these findings are based on measurements of blood levels of labeled compound by total radioactivity which will also detect metabolic fragments (Miyachi *et al.*, 1973). A third phase with a $T_{\frac{1}{2}}$ of 130 min was reported (Fink *et al.*, 1974), with blood levels in the range of 50–100 pg/ml after a 100 μg i.v. dose.

One possible explanation for the enhanced potency of certain LHRH analogs relative to LHRH is their longer $T_{\frac{1}{2}}$. The first (α) and second (β) phases of the blood level profile for [D-Trp^6]LHRH in men had $T_{\frac{1}{2}}$s of 18.7 and 50 min respectively (Barron *et al.*, 1982). The corresponding $T_{\frac{1}{2}}$s of LHRH were 7.8 and 13 min. The metabolic clearance rate of LHRH was calculated to be three times faster than that for [D-Trp^6]LHRH. Longer half-lives have also been observed for [D-Nal(2)^6]LHRH in women and monkeys. The higher potency and longer half-lives of these analogs provide a more prolonged gonadotropic response (Happ *et al.*, 1978), and have advantages in decreased frequency of administration, and delivery system design.

Although the clearance of LHRH from the plasma is quite rapid, the

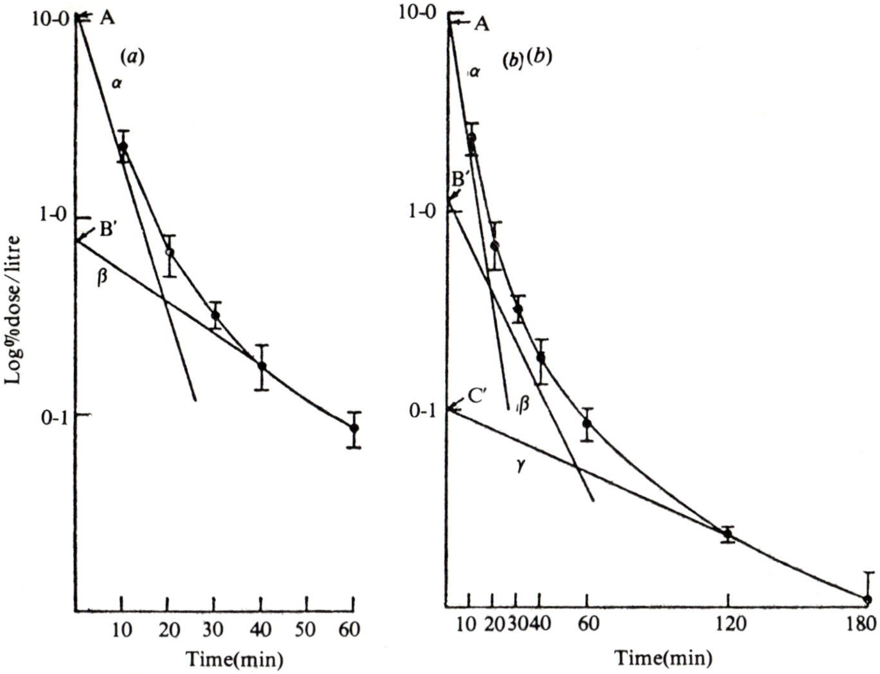

Figure 33.2 The mean ± SEM disappearance curves (log % dose/litre vs time in min) of LHRH after i.v. injection of 100 μg into four men. The curve from 10 to 60 min (*a*) could be characterized by two exponentials, but three exponentials were required to characterize the curve when values at all the times were used (*b*). (From Fink *et al.*, 1974, by kind permission of the Biochemical Society.)

LH/FSH response lasts much longer. This may be due to the longer half-lives of the gonadotropins (Marshall *et al.*, 1973). The development of delivery systems which will provide for slow release and maintenance of blood levels is strongly indicated.

TRANSMUCOSAL ROUTES

When investigating alternate delivery routes, such as nasal, vaginal and rectal, it is important to define clearly the desired blood level profile. Due to the complexity of the mechanism of action of LHRH and analogs, it is unclear whether levels of analog or the gonadotropic response should be used for studying delivery systems. Most studies have measured LH and FSH levels, although some have also included LHRH levels. Although gonadotropins are important because they are the effectors of subsequent physiological responses, there are several reasons why they should not be the exclusive indicators when comparing delivery systems. Release of LH and FSH is refractory at higher doses of analog (Fink *et al.*, 1974, Happ *et al.*, 1978) and hence the extent of absorption of the analog may not be reflected by gonadotropin levels. Desirable profiles of LH/FSH levels are still to be determined and these may vary depending on the therapeutic indication. The response can vary considerably between subjects and between men and women, and there may be interference from endogenously produced LHRH (Rebar *et al.*, 1972). Hence monitoring blood levels of the analog itself will provide a better indication of the efficiency of the delivery routes used.

Nasal administration

The nasal route has been shown to be a viable method of administering peptides, and other drugs such as propranolol (Hussain *et al.*, 1980). Nasal absorption of LHRH is quite rapid, with peak levels achieved within 15–30 min (Fink *et al.*, 1974). Blood level and LH/FSH release profiles are similar to those obtained by injection. Dose-response studies in humans indicate a linear LH peak response for doses of LHRH ranging from 0.1 to 2 mg of LHRH (Dahlen *et al.*, 1974), whereas doses above 2.5 mg did not further increase the LH response (London *et al.*, 1973). A linear relationship was also reported between dose administered and peak blood levels of LHRH (Fink *et al.*, 1974). The increases in peak blood levels, however, are not proportional to the increase in dose (i.e. a ten-times increase in dose gives a less than ten-times increase in peak height). These results cannot necessarily be extrapolated to other LHRH analogs, however, since absorption as a function of dose can vary with the analog studied.

An 80–100-fold larger dose is needed for nasal administration of LHRH, relative to the injectable route (Fink *et al.*, 1974). This dosage multiple appears to be the same whether it is based on the LH/FSH response or blood levels of LHRH. Although only about 1% of LHRH administered nasally is absorbed, the relatively low effective doses for the superactive analogs (5–25 μg by injection), make this route feasible. Furthermore, the greater lipophilicity of the more potent analogs may provide for better nasal absorption. A dosage multiple of about 20 has been reported for [D-Leu^6,Pro^9-NHEt]LHRH (Happ *et al.*, 1978) and a similar ratio has also been observed for [D-Nal(2)^6]LHRH in humans (see below).

Vaginal and rectal administration

The early success with nasal administration as well as the relative inconvenience of vaginal and rectal delivery has led to the majority of interest being in nasal systems. There have, however, been some studies on the other two routes (Okada *et al.*, 1982, 1983). The time course of the response to [D-Leu^6, Pro^9-NHEt]LHRH by rectal and vaginal administration in women was different from that following injection or nasal administration (Saito *et al.*, 1977). The onset of the LH response was slower for both vaginal and rectal administration with peak LH levels occurring at 4–6 h after dosing. The LH response after vaginal administration was quite prolonged, with elevated levels being maintained at 48 h. Based on the LH peak, the dose multiples relative to injection were 150 and 200, for vaginal and rectal administration, respectively. Although these dose multiples are larger than that found for nasal administration, the absolute doses are still quite small and delivery by these routes may be feasible. An alternative to the nasal route is desirable for such circumstances as disease of the nasal passage. Vaginal rings, for example, may provide continuous drug delivery over prolonged periods of time.

OTHER ROUTES

At least a thousandfold higher dose relative to injection was required to elicit an LH response after oral dosing of LHRH (Gonzalez-Barcena *et al.*, 1975), making this route uneconomical. Ovulation is stimulated in rats following cutaneous application of LHRH in dimethylsulfoxide (Reel *et al.*, 1975) but an acceptable means of transdermal delivery has not been reported. A comparison of many different routes of administration of [D-Trp^6,N-MeLeu^7, Pro^9-NHEt]LHRH in the rat ovulation induction model has been reported (Corbin and Bex, 1982). These results may not directly apply to other analogs due to differences in their potencies, metabolic profiles and permeability characteristics.

DELIVERY SYSTEMS FOR [D-Nal(2)^6]LHRH

Published data with other LHRH agonists suggested the nasal route to be a suitable method for routine administration of the highly potent agonistic LHRH analog [D-Nal(2)^6]LHRH (Nestor *et al.*, 1982). The low effective dose and the long term usage projected for [D-Nal(2)^6]LHRH also make it an ideal candidate for the development of a controlled release injectable product of extended duration.

Nasal delivery

Animal studies

Blood levels of [D-Nal(2)^6]LHRH (Figure 33.3) were measured by radioimmunoassay in six female rhesus monkeys receiving [D-Nal(2)^6]LHRH by the intranasal and subcutaneous routes (Nerenberg *et al.*, 1983). A pronounced non-linearity was noted between the intranasal dose administered and the levels of drug present in the blood (Table 33.1). An increase in dose from 125 μg to 270 μg resulted in an approximately eightfold increase in peak height and a $6\frac{1}{2}$-fold increase in area under the curve (AUC). Because the plasma elimination profiles were similar for all doses, the observed non-linearity is probably associated with changes in the absorption phase. Additional experiments indicated that the non-linearity in blood levels with the increase in dose was concentration dependent. At a level of 1.25 mg/ml, a twofold increase in dose resulted in a slightly greater than twofold increase in peak height. On

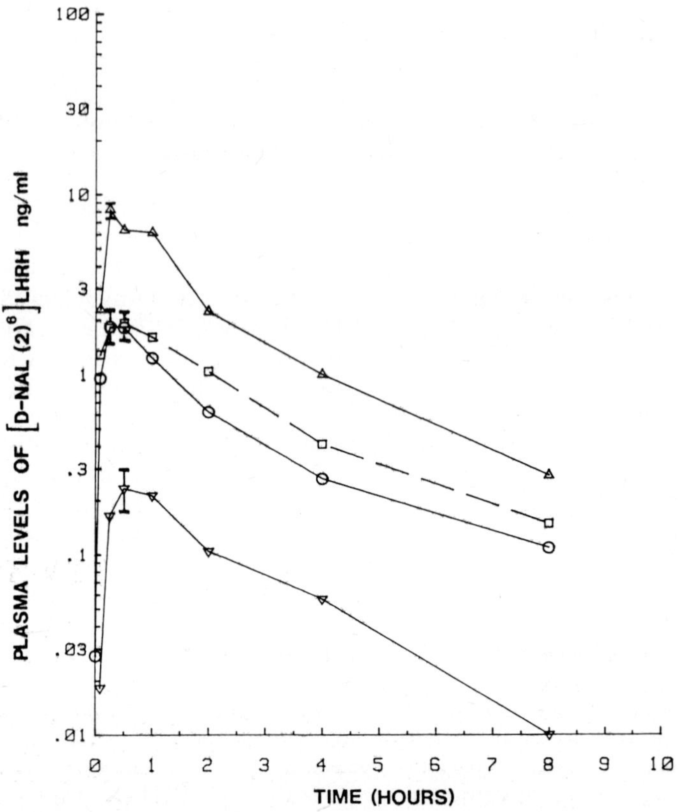

Figure 33.3 Mean concentrations (± SEM) of [D-Nal(2)^6]LHRH in plasma of monkeys after a single subcutaneous or intranasal dose. △ = 431 μg nasal; ○ = 272 μg nasal; ▽ = 133 μg nasal; □ = 5 μg subcutaneous (from Anik *et al.*, 1984, with permission).

Table 33.1 Plasma level parameters of [D-Nal(2)^6]LHRH following nasal and subcutaneous administration in rhesus monkeys.

Route	*No. of Animals*	*Conc. mg/mL*	*Dose Volume μL*	*Average Dose μg*	*Peak Height ng/mL*	*AUC ng hr/mL*
Nasal	6	0.625	213	133 (1.8)	0.23 (0.07)	0.63 (0.3)
	4	1.25	217	272 (4.1)	1.84 (0.35)	4.56 (1.1)
	4	2.5	173	431 (15.7)	8.24 (0.7)	15.9 (2.1)
	6	1.2	121	140 (10.3)	0.82 (0.28)	2.31 (0.76)
Subcutaneous	6	0.01	500	5	1.93 (0.35)	5.57 (0.97)

[1] Numbers in parentheses are standard errors.

the other hand, a twofold increase in concentration resulted in a $3\frac{1}{2}$-fold increase in peak height, for the same total doses. These observations may be due to saturation of binding sites on proleolytic enzymes which are known to be present in the nasal membrane (Hirai *et al.*, 1981).

The blood level profile obtained with the 270 μg nasal dose of [D-Nal(2)^6]LHRH was superimposable on that obtained after the 5 μg subcutaneous injection. This relative bioavailability of 2% is of the same magnitude as that documented with other analogs.

The reason for the relatively low bioavailability of these compounds by the nasal route is not known. Enzymatic degradation in the nasal membrane may be a factor, and some material may be lost via postnasal drip. The bioavailability data are in agreement with bioassay results, where the minimum effective doses for inhibition of ovulation in female rhesus monkeys were reported to be 250 μg and 5 μg daily by nasal and subcutaneous injection, respectively. Hence, the monkey serves as a useful animal for studying nasal delivery of this analog.

Human studies

Plasma levels and absorption of [D-Nal(2)^6]LHRH were determined in four women after a 500 μg single intranasal dose and a 5 μg single subcutaneous dose of the drug in an aqueous formulation. Three of the women were hysterectomized and the fourth was postmenopausal. The peak plasma levels of [D-Nal(2)^6]LHRH after the intranasal dose ranged from 1.5 to 4.3 ng/ml and were attained at 20 min after dosing (Figure 33.4). After the peak plasma level was attained, [D-Nal(2)^6]LHRH declined biexponentially with time; the rapid plasma $T_{\frac{1}{2}}$ was 54 min and the slower plasma $T_{\frac{1}{2}}$ was 3.3 h. After the single 5 μg subcutaneous dose, the peak plasma level of 0.35 ng/ml was reached 20 min after dosing and the terminal plasma $T_{\frac{1}{2}}$ was 2.4 h (Figure 33.4).

The systemic bioavailability of the intranasal dose relative to the subcutaneous dose was estimated by comparing areas under the plasma concentration-time curves (AUC values). The average relative bioavailability of the intranasal dose in these four volunteers was 5% (range 2–9%). Thus, an approximately 20-fold larger dose is required by the intranasal route to approximate the [D-Nal(2)^6]LHRH plasma AUC provided by a single 5 μg subcutaneous dose, a dose known to produce hormonal changes in women. However, additional studies are required in humans to determine the relationship between the extent of nasal absorption and the intranasal dose administered.

Controlled release injectable

A controlled release injectable preparation of an LHRH analog would afford several advantages over other means of delivering these compounds. Such a formulation would be much more convenient, would result in greater patient compliance and would probably require a lower total dose of compound compared with transmucosal modes of administration. Improved dosage accuracy would result because the variance introduced by frequent self-administration would be reduced, and variability of nasal absorption kinetics would be avoided.

Possible disadvantages of a controlled release injectable preparation are: (1) the commitment to treatment with the compound for a relatively long period

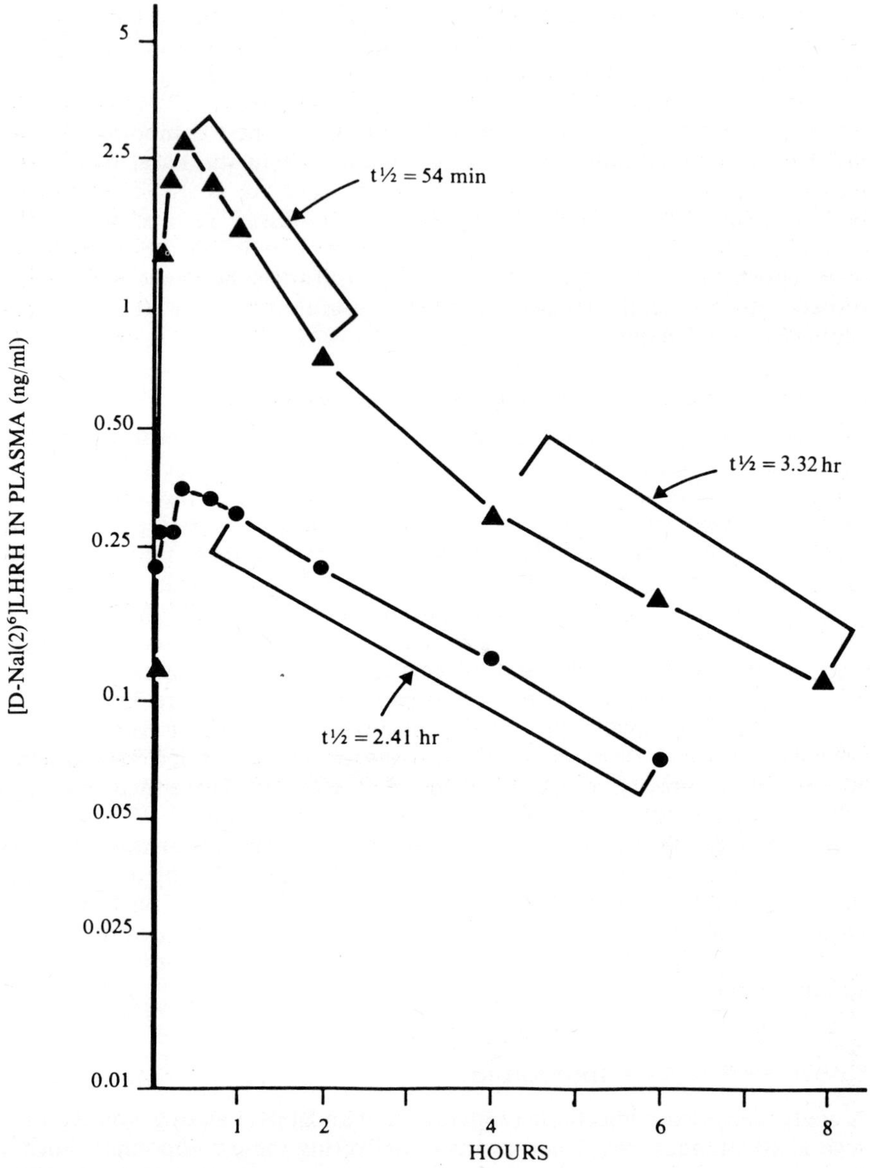

Figure 33.4 Mean concentrations (± SEM) of [D-Nal(2)^6]LHRH in plasma of female volunteers after a single subcutaneous or intranasal dose. ● = subcutaneous – 5 μg; ▲ = nasal – 486 ± 4μg, (mean + SE).

of time, since it may not be possible to terminate treatment prior to exhaustion of injected material and (2) the complexity of development of such a delivery system. Although these considerations make a controlled release injectable preparation a less than ideal choice for early studies on LHRH analogs, such a formulation may be of increasing significance in later studies, and may be critical in determining commercial viability of the compounds for some indications, such as contraception.

There are several possible approaches to developing a controlled release injectable formulation of a LHRH analog. One approach would be to microencapsulate the compound in a biocompatible polymer which will biodegrade *in vivo* at the rate required to release the compound. There are many polymers which potentially are suitable for this purpose (Heller, 1980; Thies, 1981), and some polymers such as poly (amino acids) (Anderson *et al.*, 1974; Sidman *et al.*, 1980), polyorthoesters (Heller *et al.*, 1982), polyurethanes, polyacetals, and polyketals (Pitt *et al.*, 1980), already have been examined. Polyesters are perhaps the broadest class, and include the

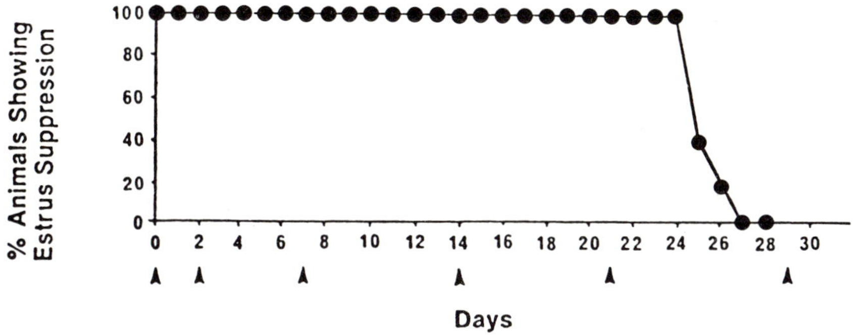

Figure 33.5 Biological profile of 50/50 PLGA microsphere containing [D-Nal(2)^6]LHRH injected subcutaneously in female rats (from Kent *et al.*, 1982, with permission).

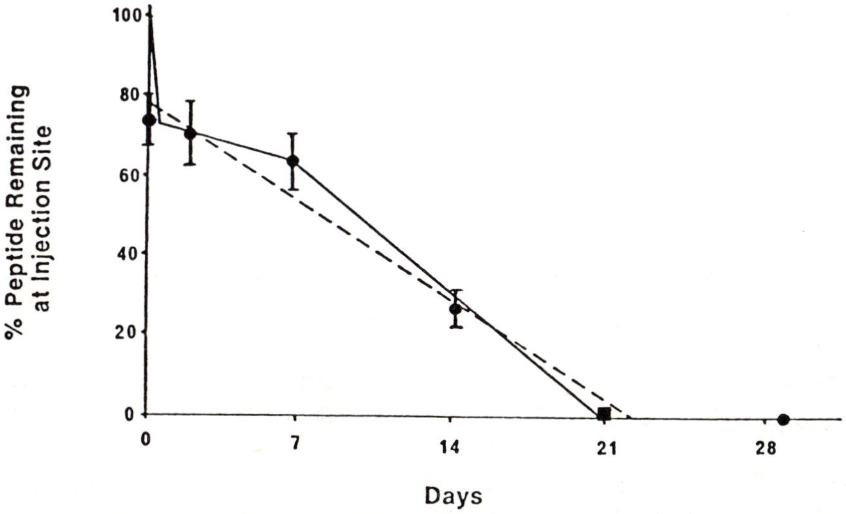

Figure 33.6 *In vivo* release profile of [D-Nal(2)^6]LHRH from 50/50 PLGA microspheres. (From Kent *et al.*, 1982, with permission).

Figure 33.7 Plasma levels of progesterone and [D-Nal(2)^6]LHRH in the rhesus monkey following a single s.c. injection of [D-Nal(2)^6]LHRH microencapsulated in 55/45 PLGA.

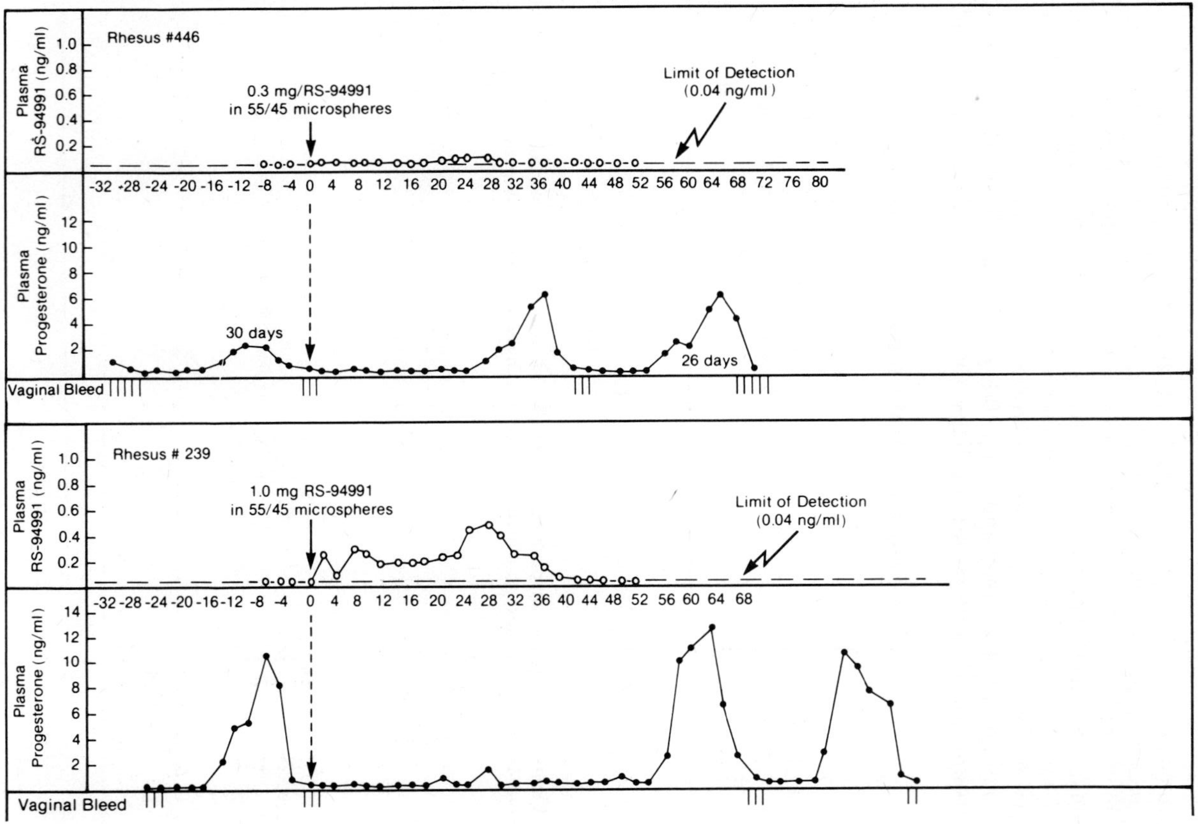

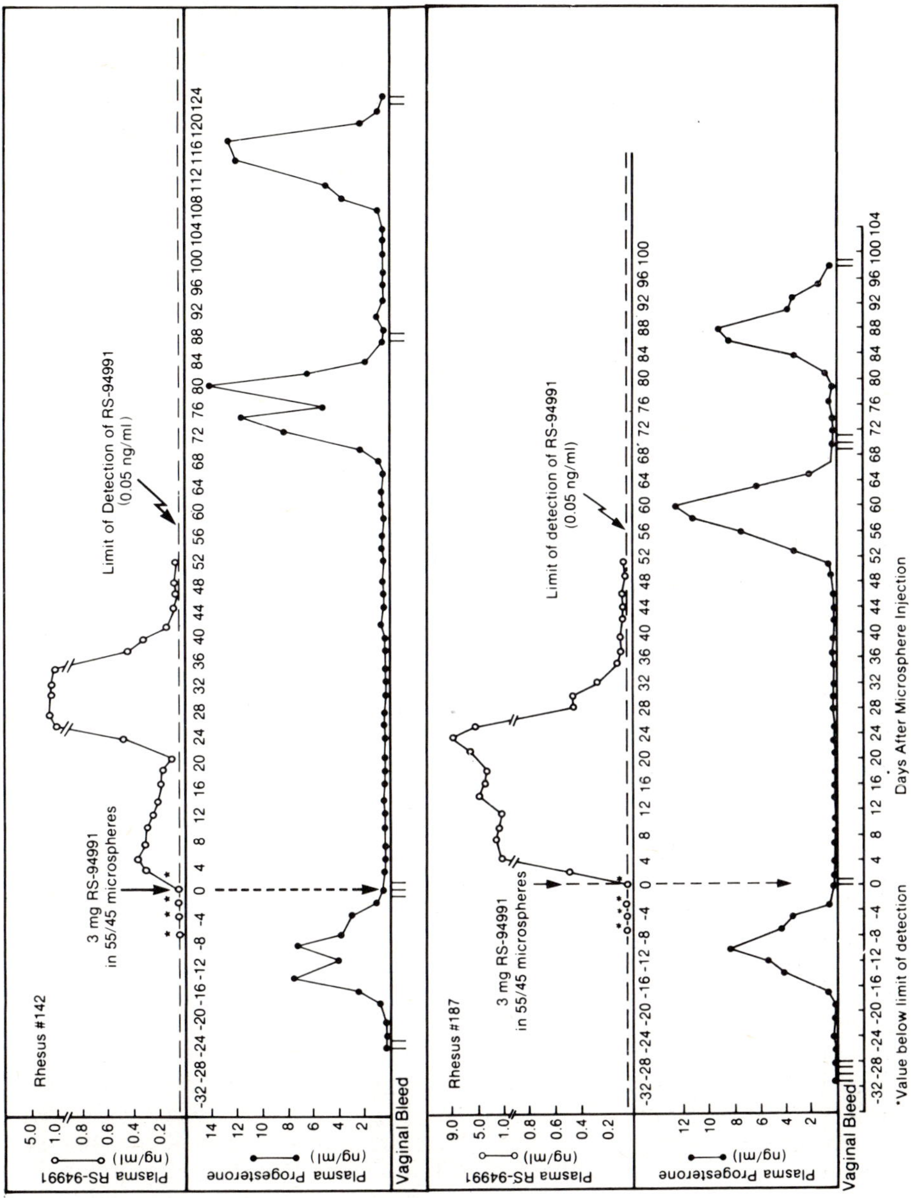
Rhesus #142
3 mg RS-94991
in 55/45 microspheres
Limit of Detection of RS-94991
(0.05 ng/ml)
Plasma RS-94991
(ng/ml)
Plasma Progesterone
(ng/ml)
Vaginal Bleed
Rhesus #187
3 mg RS-94991
in 55/45 microspheres
Limit of detection of RS-94991
(0.05 ng/ml)
Plasma RS-94991
(ng/ml)
Plasma Progesterone
(ng/ml)
Vaginal Bleed
Days After Microsphere Injection
*Value below limit of detection

extensively studied poly D,L-lactic-co-glycolic acids (PLGA) (Pitt *et al*, 1980). Most of these polymers appear to degrade homogeneously *in vivo*. Since the rate of hydration is greater than the rate of degradation, the mass of polymer hydrates, degrades and erodes at a fairly uniform rate throughout. A surface eroding polymer where the rate of hydration is slow and less than the rate of polymer hydrolysis, would be a more readily controllable system to work with since it would provide a slowly moving front of eroding polymer from the surface of the device inwards. This would allow relatively simple manipulation of the release kinetics by adjustment of the polymer's hydrophilicity, and the device's geometry. There are, however, very few examples reported in the literature of such an ideal 'surface eroding' polymer (Heller *et al.*, 1978).

There are many reasons for the wide use of poly D,L-lactic-co-glycolic acids. For example, their degradation products present a good toxicological profile. Glycolic acid and L-lactic acid are found endogenously, and D-lactic acid will be excreted without entering the metabolic pool. These polymers have a proven biocompatibility, having had years of general use as biodegradable suture material (Vicryl (Ethicon), Dexon (Davis and Geck)). The erosion kinetics and compound release profile may be readily adjusted over a broad range by manipulation of the monomer ratio and polymer molecular weight. Methods of producing the material are well known, and it has physical and chemical properties that allow its use in such procedures as micro-encapsulation.

PLGA has been successfully used in controlled release preparations of sulfadiazine (Wise *et al.*, 1978), chemotherapeutic agents (Yolles and Morton, 1978), naltrexone (Thies, 1976; Harrigan *et al.*, 1978) and norethindrone (NET) (Anderson *et al.*, 1976; Beck *et al.*, 1979). The PLGA/NET system is currently under clinical study as an injectable contraceptive with up to 6 months duration of action (Beck *et al.*, 1981).

We have prepared controlled release injectable formulations of [D-Trp^6,Pro^9-NHEt]LHRH and [D-Nal(2)^6]LHRH (Kent *et al.*, 1982) which allow compound release concurrent with polymer erosion. Microspheres containing approximately 1% of LHRH analog have been prepared in various PLGA excipients by a phase-separation process (Sanders *et al.*, 1982). They are typically 30–50 μm in diameter, and may readily be suspended to afford an injectable preparation. They have been evaluated in the female rat, in which 0.4 μg of [D-Nal(2)^6]LHRH by both continuous administration and by daily injection is sufficient to maintain suppression of the estrus cycle. The estrus suppression profiles generated following administration of 300 μg of [D-Nal(2)^6]LHRH microencapsulated at the 1% level in a 50/50 lactic/glycolic copolymer is shown in Figure 33.5. There are about 24 days of continuous release of compound, with a sharp cut-off, which is followed by resumption of normal cycling. As shown in Figure 33.6, sacrifice of groups of these animals, at the times indicated by the arrows, and subsequent analysis of the excised injection sites for remaining compound, gives a release profile that is approximately linear. There was no detectable tissue residue or 'tailing' of compound release after cessation of biological activity, which is characteristic of this particular mechanism of compound release. Similar microspheres prepared with a 55/45 lactic/glycolic copolymer were administered subcutaneously to female rhesus monkeys at doses of 0.3 mg, 1.0 mg and 3.0 mg of the analog. Plasma samples were assayed by radioimmunoassay for [D-Nal(2)^6]LHRH (Nerenberg *et al.*, 1983) and for progesterone. The data from this dose-response study are shown in Figure 33.7. With the exception of the lowest dose, progesterone levels are clearly depressed, and menstrual bleeding is eliminated while the LHRH analog is present in the plasma. There is, however, non-linearity of compound release with this particular polymer, although an abrupt termination of release is still evident.

The interactions of the contributing variables that control the behavior of this system are clearly complex, but the parameters of monomer ratio and polymer molecular weight may be manipulated to adjust the release profile of the compound. In the long term, such an approach may provide the delivery system of choice for many of the applications required for LHRH analogs.

CONCLUDING REMARKS

Considerable progress has been made in developing delivery systems for the LHRH analogs. Currently, the nasal route holds the greatest promise for routine administration of these compounds but its practicability for indications such as contraception is still under test (Bergquist *et al.*, 1982). An increase in the bioavailability by this route would be particularly desirable to minimize variability of absorption. The controlled release injectable also offers an attractive possibility as a delivery system that is particularly suited to LHRH analogs.

Delivery of peptides orally by manipulation of the formulation will always be the preferred mode of administration, and is still a challenge to the ingenuity of the pharmaceutical scientist. Additional investigations of the transport of these compounds across mucous membranes will be required before improved delivery systems for nasal, vaginal and rectal routes can be developed. The continuing development of new peptide drugs ensures that greater attention will be given to these aspects of drug delivery.

Acknowledgements

The authors are indebted to JoAnn Foreman and Nancy Chu for the metabolism work, to Karen Vitale and Jiin-Yu Hwang for the formulation work, to Brian Vickery, Georgia McRae and Ann Worden for the animal studies and to Thomas Tice and Danny Lewis of the Southern Research Institute for preparation of some of the materials.

References

Anderson, J. M., Gibbons, D. F., Martin, R. L., Hiltner, A. and Woods, R. (1974). The potential for poly-α-amino acids as biomaterials. *J. Biomed. Mater. Res. Symp.*, **5,** 197

Anderson, L. C., Wise, D. L. and Howes, J. F. (1976). An injectable sustained release fertility control system. *Contraception,* **13,** 375

Anik, S. T., McRae, G., Nerenberg, C., Worden, A., Foreman, J., Hwang, J. Y., Kuskinsky, S., Jones, R. E. and Vickery, B. (1984). Nasal absorption of nafarelin acetate or [D-Nal(2)^6]LHRH a decapeptide, in rhesus monkeys, *J. Pharm. Sci.*, (In press)

Barron, J. L., Millar, R. P. and Searle, D. (1982). Metabolic clearance and plasma half-disappearance time of D-Trp^6 and exogenous luteinizing hormone-releasing hormone. *J. Clin. Endocrinol. Metab.*, **54,** 1169

Beck, L. R., Cowsar, D. L., Lewis, D. H., Gibson, J. W. and Flowers, C. E. (1979). New long-acting injectable microcapsule contraceptive system. *Am. J. Obstet. Gynecol.*, **135,** 419

Beck, L. R., Ramos, R. A., Flowers, C. E., Lopez, G. Z., Lewis, D. H. and Cowsar, D. R. (1981). Clinical evaluation of injectable biodegradable contraceptive system. *Am. J. Obstet. Gynecol.*, **140,** 799

Bergquist, C., Nillius, S. J. and Wide, L. (1982). Long-term intranasal luteinising hormone-releasing hormone agonist treatment for contraception in women. *Fertil. Steril.*, **38,** 190

Corbin, A. and Bex, F. J. (1982). Physiology and contraceptive effects of LHRH and agonistic analogs in female animals. In Zatuchni, G. I., Shelton, J. D. and Sciarra, J. J. (eds.) *LHRH Peptides as Female and Male Contraceptives*, pp. 68–84. (Philadelphia: Harper and Row)

Dahlen, H. G., Keller, E. and Schneider, H. P. G. (1974). Linear dose dependent LH release following intranasally sprayed LRH. *Horm. Metab. Res.*, **6,** 510

Fink, G., Gennser, G., Liedholm, P., Thorell, J. and Malder, J. (1974). Comparison of plasma levels of luteinizing hormone-releasing hormone in men after intravenous or intranasal administration. *J. Endocrinol.*, **63,** 351

Gonzalez-Barcena, D., Miller M. C. III, Coy, D. H., Kastin, A. J., Schalch, D. S., Schally, A. V. and Escalante-Herrera, A. (1975). Stimulation of luteinizing hormone (LH) release after oral administration of an analogue of LH releasing hormone. *Lancet*, 6 December 1126

Gonzalez-Barcena, D., Kastin, J. A., Schalch, D. S., Coy, D. H. and Schally, A. V. (1976). Prolonged elevation of luteinizing hormone (LH) after intranasal administration of an analog of LH-releasing hormone. *Fertil. Steril.*, **27,** 1246

Happ, J., Hartmann, U., Weber, T., Cordes, U. and Beyer, J. (1978). Gonadotropin and testosterone secretion in normal human males after stimulation with gonadotropin-releasing hormone (GnRH) or potent GnRH analogs using different modes of application. *Fertil. Steril.*, **30,** 666

Harrigan, S. E., McCarthy, D. A., Reuning, R. and Thies, C. (1978). Release of naltrexone pamoate from injectable microcapsules. *Midl. Macromol. Monogr.*, **5,** 91

Haug, E., and Torjesen, P. (1973). Effect of synthetic luteinizing hormone and follicle stimulating hormone-releasing hormone (LH/FSH-RH) on serum levels of LH, FSH, thyrotropin (TSH) and growth hormone (HGH) in normal male subjects. *Acta Endocrinol.*, **73,** 465

Heller, J. (1980). Controlled release of biologically active compounds from bioerodible polymers. *Biomaterials*, **1,** 51

Heller, J., Baker, R. W., Gale, R. M. and Rodin, J. D. (1978). Controlled drug release by polymer dissolution. I. Partial esters of maleic anhydride copolymers – properties and theory. *J. Appl. Polym. Sci.*, **22,** 1991

Heller, J., Penhale, D. W. H., Helwing, R. F. and Fritzinger, B. K. (1982). Controlled release of norethindrone from poly (ortho ester). In Roseman, T. J. and Mansdorf, S. Z. (eds.) *Controlled Released Delivery Systems* (New York: Dekker)

Hirai, S., Yashiki, T. and Mima, H. (1981). Mechanisms for the enhancement of the nasal absorption of insulin by surfactants. *Int. J. Pharm.*, **9,** 173

Hussain, A., Foster, T., Hirai, S., Kashihara, T., Batenhorst, R. and Jones, M. (1980). Nasal absorption of propranolol in humans. *J. Pharm. Sci.*, **69,** 1240

Kent, J. S., Sanders, L. M., McRae, G. I., Vickery, B. H., Tice, T. R. and Lewis, D. H. (1982). In vivo controlled release of an LHRH analog from injected polymeric microcapsules. *Contracept. Deliv. Syst.*, **3,** 58

London, D. R., Butt, W. R., Lynch, S. S., Marshall, J. C., Owusu, S., Robinson, W. R. and Stephenson, J. M. (1973). Hormonal responses for intranasal luteinizing hormone-releasing hormone. *J. Clin. Endocrinol. Metab.*, **37,** 829

Marshall, J. C., Anderson, D. C., Fraser, T. R. and Hasoulis, P. (1973). Human luteinizing hormone in man: Studies of metabolism and biological action. *J. Endocrinol.*, **56,** 431

Miyachi, Y., Meckleburg, R. S., Hansen, J. W. and Lipsett, M. B. (1973). Metabolism of ^{125}I-Luteinizing Hormone-Releasing Hormone. *J. Clin. Endocrinol. Metab.*, **37,** 63

Mortimer, C. H., Besser, G. M., Hook, J. and McNeilly, A. S. (1974). Intravenous, intramuscular, subcutaneous and intranasal administration of LH/FSH-RH: The duration of effect and occurrence of asynchronous pulsatile release of LH and FSH. *Clin. Endocrinol.*, **3,** 19

Nerenberg, C., Foreman, J. and Kushinsky, S. (1983). Radioimmunoassay for (D-naphthyl alanine(2)^6)LHRH (RS-94991) in plasma or serum. *Abstr. Ann. Mtg. Endocr. Soc.*, 1983, San Antonio, Texas

Nestor, J. J. Jr., Ho, T. L., Simpson, R. A., Horner, B. L., Jones, G. H., McRae, G. I. and Vickery, B. H. (1982). The synthesis and biological activity of some very hydrophobic analogs of luteinizing hormone-releasing hormone. *J. Med. Chem.*, **25,** 795

Okada, H., Yamazaki, I., Ogawa, Y., Hirai, S., Yashiki, T. and Mima, H. (1982). Vaginal absorption of a potent luteinizing hormone-releasing hormone analog (Leuprolide) in rats I: Absorption by various routes and absorption enhancement. *J. Pharm. Sci.*, **71,** 1367

Okada, H., Yamazaki, I., Yashiki, T. and Mima, H. (1983). Vaginal absorption of a potent luteinizing hormone-releasing hormone analogue (Leuprolide) in rats II: Mechanism of absorption enhancement with organic acids. *J. Pharm. Sci.*, **72,** 75

Pitt, C. G., Marks, T. A. and Schindler, A. (1980). Biodegradable drug delivery systems based on aliphatic polyesters: application to contraceptives and narcotic antagonists. In Lewis, D. (ed.) *Controlled Release of Bioactive Materials*, pp. 19–43. (London: Academic Press)

Rebar, R., Yen, S. S. C., Vandenberg, G., Naftolin, F., Ehara, Y., Engblom, S., Ryan, K. J., Rivier, J., Amoss, M. and Guillemin, R. (1972). Gonadotropin responses to synthetic LRF: Dose response relationship in men. *J. Clin. Endocrinol. Metab.*, **36,** 10

Reel, J. R., Humphrey, R. R., Vaitkus, J. W. and Dermody, W. C. (1975). Stimulation of LH release and ovulation in the rat by cutaneous application of luteinizing hormone-releasing hormone (LH-RH) in dimethyl sulfoxide (DMSO). *Endocr. Res. Commun.*, **2,** 327

Saito, M., Kumasaki, T., Yaoi, Y., Nishi, N., Arimura, A., Coy, D. and Schally, A. V. (1977). Stimulation of luteinizing hormone (LH) and follicle-stimulating hormone by [D-Leu^6,des-Gly^{10}-NH_2] LH-releasing hormone ethylamide after subcutaneous, intravaginal, and intrarectal administration to women. *Fertil. Steril.*, **28,** 240

Sanders, L., Kent, J., McRae, G., Vickery, B., Tice, T. and Lewis, D. (1982). Controlled release of a GnRH analogue from injected polymeric microcapsules: formulation characteristics. *Arch. Androl.*, **9,** 91

Seyler, L. E. Jr., (1975). Disappearance of biologic activity of synthetic LRH in normal and hypogonadal men. *J. Clin. Endocrinol. Metab.*, **41,** 1155

Sidman, K. R., Schwope, A. D., Steber, W. D., Rudolph, S. E. and Pontin, S. B. (1980). Biodegradable, implantable sustained release systems based on glutamic acid copolymers. *J. Memb. Sci.*, **7,** 277

Thies, C. (1976). Development of injectable microcapsules for use in the treatment of narcotic addiction. In Willette, R. E., (ed.) *Research Monograph Series*, **4,** pp. 19–20

Thies, C. (1981). Biodegradable polymers for parenteral administration. *Int. J. Pharm. Tech. Prod. Mfr.*, **2,** 25

Turner, D., Turner, E. A., Aparicio, N. J., Schwarzstein, L., Coy, D. H. and Schally, A. V. (1976). Response of luteinizing hormone and follicle-stimulating hormone to different doses of D-Leucine-6-LH-RH Ethylamide in oligospermic patients. *Fertil. Steril.*, **27,** 545

Wise, D. L., McCormick, G. J., Willet, G. P., Anderson, L. C. and Howes, J. F. (1978). Sustained release of sulphadiazine. *J. Pharm. Pharmacol.*, **30,** 686

Yolles, S. and Morton, D. F. (1978). Timed-release depot for anti-cancer agents II. *Acta Pharm. Suec.*, **15,** 382

SECTION X
PERSPECTIVES

34

Prospects for LHRH analogs as contraceptives

M. J. K. HARPER

Chemical modifications to the LHRH structure have resulted in highly active agonists and several such compounds, e.g. [D-Ser(tBu)^6,Pro^9-NHEt]LHRH, [D-Trp^6,Pro^9-NHEt]LHRH and [D-Nal(2)^6]^6]LHRH have been studied clinically. Highly active antagonists were discovered more recently, e.g. [Ac-D-pCl-Phe^1,D-pCl-Phe^2,D-Trp^3,D-Arg^6,D-Ala^{10}]LHRH and [N-Ac-D-Nal(2)^1,D-pF-Phe^2,D-Trp^3,D-Arg^6]LHRH, but these are only just reaching the stage of clinical trial. There are now available sufficiently potent analogs of both types for adequate testing as contraceptive agents. There is still scope for improvement in design, e.g. increased resistance to metabolism and hence prolonged *in vivo* bioactivity may be possible. More potent compounds may be discovered, but their mode of action probably will be the same as those already described. LHRH analogs have proved non-toxic, despite their interference with endocrinological control mechanisms. It is possible to evaluate the potential of these compounds for contraception. Already certain trends are clear. Although there was hope that LHRH analogs might be contraceptive by several mechanisms (e.g. luteolytic, abortifacient and defective luteal phase), present evidence suggests that only inhibition of ovulation in the female and inhibition of spermatogenesis in the male will be effective. Even in the modalities where contraception may be achieved, it will probably be necessary to use steroids – progestins in the female and androgens in the male – as adjuncts to LHRH analog treatment.

CONTRACEPTIVE POTENTIAL IN WOMEN

Inhibition of ovulation

Clinical trials indicate that LHRH analogs can reliably inhibit ovulation in women (Nillius *et al.*, 1978; Bergquist *et al.*, 1979*a*, *b*; Schmidt-Gollwitzer *et al.*, 1981). Subcutaneous (s.c.) administration of 5 μg of buserelin to four normally menstruating women for 22–30 days inhibited ovulation (Nillius *et al.*, 1978). A dose of 400 μg per day intranasally inhibited ovulation during a

5-week trial (Bergquist *et al.*, 1979*a*). When daily treatment was continued for 3–6 months, ovulation was still suppressed, but incidence of menstrual bleeding was reduced and some women became amenorrheic (Bergquist *et al.*, 1979*b*).

Another study reported similar results; however, it was suggested that unopposed estrogenic stimulation of the endometrium during chronic daily buserelin administration might cause endometrial hyperplasia (Schmidt-Gollwitzer *et al.*, 1981). When women were given buserelin daily (400 or 600 μg, intranasally) for up to 12 months, and underwent endometrial biopsies during treatment, only atrophic or weakly proliferative endometrium was found (Bergquist *et al.*, 1981, 1982). This putative estrogenic stimulation of the endometrium therefore may not be a major problem. In a recent study, 71 regularly menstruating women used buserelin at 200, 400 or 600 μg per day intranasally for up to 21 months (Nillius and Bergquist, 1984). Of the 564 treatment months, only 3 were ovulatory, as judged by hormone levels. Even in the ten subjects receiving only 200 μg/day, ovulation was consistently suppressed. In 28 women receiving 200 μg/day of buserelin in another study, contraception was achieved, but when one woman, on her own initiative, decreased the daily dose to 100 μg, pregnancy ensued. However, 100 μg twice a day was as effective as 200 μg once daily (Schmidt-Gollwitzer *et al.*, 1984).

In all these studies a percentage of the women experienced amenorrhea; it has been suggested that this is more likely in women who had irregular cycles prior to treatment. The incidence of amenorrhea is dose-related (Schmidt-Gollwitzer *et al.*, 1984). Irregular menstrual bleeding and amenorrhea adversely affect the acceptability of any contraceptive method, and this has been noted with many of the contraceptive formulations depending on hormonal steroids, e.g. pills, implants, injections and vaginal rings (Harper, 1983).

One method to regularize the cycle is to give, in addition to the LHRH analogs, a progestational steroid, such as a progestin mini-pill. This approach prevents endometrial hyperplasia due to continuous estrogenic stimulation (Hardt *et al.*, 1984). Women were given 400 μg of buserelin daily intranasally for 22 days from the onset of menstruation, and also received 10 mg of norethisterone acetate orally on each of days 20–22. After a 6-day break this treatment was repeated. This regimen inhibited ovulation and regular menstrual-like bleeding occurred in 97% of the 101 treatment cycles (Hardt *et al.*, 1984). These preliminary results look encouraging and such a regimen may prove to be a successful compromise between the all-steroid or all-peptide treatments. However, the mere fact that steroids must be given at all, even if for only a few days, negates one of the most attractive features of the LHRH analogs.

The foregoing studies depended on continuous or daily treatment for at least 3 weeks per cycle to inhibit ovulation effectively. Obviously, treatment for only a few days per cycle would be more attractive, if ovulation could be reliably inhibited. Several attempts have been made in this direction. When buserelin is given (10 μg/day i.m.) from days 1–14 of the cycle, ovulation at the normal time is not permanently inhibited, but is delayed for approximately 2 weeks (Baumann *et al.*, 1980). Administration of buserelin (5 or 25 μg per day) for 1–5 days in the early follicular phase to 12 regularly menstruating women similarly prolonged the follicular phase (Skarin *et al.*, 1982). Thus this type of short treatment during the follicular phase with an LHRH agonist does not seem promising for providing contraception through inhibition of ovulation.

In contrast, treatment with an LHRH antagonist might be more promising, since the mode of action involves a one-time inhibition of the LH surge responsible for ovulation. With an agonist, the supramaximal stimulation seems to down regulate LH receptors, whose sensitivity to stimulation then gradually returns. Thus an agonist may need to be given chronically for a longer period than an antagonist to exert the same effect on ovulation. LHRH analogs work at both the hypothalamo-hypophyseal axis and at extra-pituitary, e.g. gonadal, sites in rats (Bex and Corbin, 1981). The mechanism of action of such peptides on human reproductive systems is not certain.

A 2 mg dose of [N-Ac-D-pCl-Phe^{1},D-pCl-Phe^{2},D-Trp^{3},D-Phe^{6},D-Ala^{10}] LHRH given to ten normally ovulating women on day 12 of the cycle inhibited ovulation in six and produced inadequate luteal function in two others (Zárate *et al.*, 1981). However, in rhesus monkeys, 1 mg of the same antagonist given i.m. on days 10–14 of the cycle only delayed ovulation in five of seven monkeys (Balmaceda *et al.*, 1981). The ability of an antagonist to consistently inhibit ovulation, and the precise timing of administration, are still not certain. The precise timing of treatment which is required to block the onset of the LH surge will cause major difficulties in human use. For contraceptive purposes, such administration will require development of satisfactory methods of predicting ovulation.

Postcoital treatment

The problem of specific timing for short or intermittent treatment with LHRH analogs would be obviated if the drug could be given by reference to a well-defined event such as coitus. The disadvantage of this approach, with the varied coital frequencies seen in different cultures, is the danger of under- or overdosage. The lack of toxicity of LHRH analogs makes overdosage a less critical question. Thus, if LHRH analogs, when given postcoitally could be shown to exert a contraceptive effect in humans as they do in rodents (Corbin *et al.*, 1979), these analogs could provide a useful and acceptable contraceptive method despite the dosage problems. Unfortunately, it has proved difficult, even in rodents, to inhibit pregnancy reliably during the preimplantation period with LHRH analogs without administration of large doses for several days (Corbin *et al.*, 1979). Short periods of treatment in primates, whether given before or after ovulation, have been similarly ineffective in preventing pregnancy.

Treatment of women with the antagonist, [N-Ac-D-pCl-Phe^{1},D-pCl-Phe^{2},D-Trp^{3},D-Phe^{6},D-Ala^{10}]LHRH, on day 12 of the cycle, when it did not inhibit ovulation, produced an inadequate luteal phase (Zárate *et al.*, 1981). In another study, injection of 50 μg per day of the agonist [D-Trp^{6},Pro^{9}-NHEt]LHRH, for 3 days from the onset of menstruation, also produced luteal phase defects and a prolonged follicular phase. Such interference with the cycle has been suggested as a possible means of achieving contraception (Sheehan *et al.*, 1982). Confirmation of this biological action was less successful. Twelve regularly cycling women were given 5 or 25 μg of buserelin s.c. for 1, 3 or 5 days starting early in the follicular phase: the luteal phase of the cycle was not altered, but the follicular phase was disrupted and ovulation postponed (Skarin *et al.*, 1982). Follicular phase administration of these analogs will not prove useful contraceptively, unless ovulation is reliably inhibited, not just postponed. This means that treatment will have to be continuous for at least 20 days. Instead of daily administration, controlled release systems, e.g. injectable preparations that would last the required period of time, might be used. Such systems are now under development as polymeric microspheres (Kent *et al.*, 1982) or cholesterol implants (Vickery *et al.*, 1983).

In summary, evidence for a luteolytic action of LHRH agonists or antagonists in a pregnant woman has yet to be provided. This may be a question of dose or length of treatment, but it suggests that postcoital treatment, whether in the follicular or luteal phase, is unlikely to provide effective or acceptable contraception.

Monthly treatment

Monthly contraceptive treatment has the advantage that it can be timed in relation to the non-appearance of an expected event – menstruation. If menstruation fails to occur when expected, whether the woman is pregnant or not, appropriate treatment to ensure menstruation can be initiated. If LHRH analogs are effective by either a luteolytic or uterotonic action, there would be tremendous interest in their use as contraceptive agents.

Animal experiments show that LHRH analogs are more effective in terminating pregnancy when given after implantation rather than before (Corbin *et al.*, 1979; Rivier *et al.*, 1979). In non-pregnant primates, a luteolytic effect can be demonstrated, with reduction in progesterone levels and early onset of menstrual bleeding (Koyama *et al.*, 1978; Lemay *et al.*, 1979*a*, *b*, 1980; Casper and Yen, 1979; Vickery and McRae, 1980*c*; Bergquist *et al.*, 1980*a*). The optimal time for production of this effect was thought to be restricted to days 1–5 after the LH surge (Lemay *et al.*, 1979*a*), but this period has been extended in more recent studies to days 7 or 8 after the LH surge (Lemay *et al.*, 1984). Unfortunately, this luteolytic action is overcome by concomitant administration of hCG (Casper *et al.*, 1980; Bergquist *et al.*, 1980*b*; Lemay *et al.*, 1984). Thus LHRH agonists are unlikely to induce a luteolytic effect in a pregnant woman, even if given during the early part of the luteal phase. From an acceptable contraceptive regimen, it would in any event be more difficult to time drug administration correctly for this application than to wait for the non-appearance of menstruation. LHRH antagonists may be no more successful than agonists as luteolytic agents.

Pregnancy interception (after a missed menses) would be an acceptable birth control method in many cultures where abortion is not interdicted.

However, experiments to date are not promising. Pregnancy was not interrupted in four women less than 54 days pregnant given 500 μg of [D-Trp^6,Pro^9-NHEt]LHRH s.c. on 2 consecutive days (Casper *et al.*, 1980) or in four women 46–69 days pregnant given 100 μg of [D-Trp^6]LHRH twice per day for 5–10 days (Tolis *et al.*, 1981*a*). The failure to induce abortion may not be due to inadequate dosage, since baboon experiments in which pellets containing 125 μg/kg of [D-Trp^6,Pro^9-NHEt]LHRH or [D-Nal(2)^6]LHRH were administered s.c. between days 14 and 21 of gestation and left *in vivo* for 18–33 days resulted in abortion in only one out of six animals within 3 weeks or less of treatment. Despite continuation of treatment, only one additional baboon aborted (Vickery *et al.*, 1981). The baboons were exposed to continuous stimulation by the agonist for weeks, yet abortion could not be consistently induced. By contrast, s.c. administration of 50 μg of the agonist [D-Ser(tBu)^6,Pro^9-NHEt]LHRH at 8 or 12 h intervals over 4–6 days to pregnant baboons at the time CG was detected (days 26–31 of the cycle) apparently resulted in abortion (Das and Talwar, 1983). These results seem at variance with those reported by others, but the timing of treatment appears important, since even these latter authors could not prevent pregnancy when the agonist was given only in the luteal phase. This is further exemplified by studies showing that an LHRH antagonist, [N-Ac-Pro^1,D-pF-Phe^2,D-Nal(2)^{3,6}]LHRH can inhibit hormonal secretion from 13-week human placental explants, but this inhibition was not apparent at 6 weeks of gestation (Siler-Khodr *et al.*, 1983). In conclusion, it is not yet certain whether LHRH analogs will be effective to induce abortion, but if they are, the timing for success may be very critical. Such a limited window for efficacy would present problems for widespread use as a birth control agent. As might be predicted by the experiments in non-pregnant women where luteolysis could not be induced in the face of exogenous hCG, it seems difficult to induce abortion in the face of endogenous CG.

CONTRACEPTIVE POTENTIAL IN MEN

Inhibition of spermatogenesis

Fewer clinical trials have been done in the male than in the female. More studies have been done with the agonists. Early animal studies showed that chronic administration of LHRH agonists reduced testicular, seminal vesicle and ventral prostate weights, reduced mating frequency and disrupted spermatogenesis (Auclair *et al.*, 1977; Corbin *et al.*, 1979; Vickery and McRae, 1979, 1980*a*). In baboons it was shown that testosterone levels reached a nadir by 26–30 days after implantation of pellets containing [D-Trp^6,Pro^9-NHEt]LHRH (Vickery and McRae, 1980*b*). Similarly, chronic daily administration of [D-Nal(2)^6]LHRH to male beagle dogs resulted in azoospermia by day 38, but testosterone and libido were also depressed: after 5 weeks of treatment no ejaculates could be obtained (Vickery *et al.*, 1984).

Rhesus monkeys have been proposed as a good model system for study of human testicular function (Nieschlag and Wickings, 1980), but they are relatively insensitive to high daily doses of LHRH agonists (Wickings *et al.*,

1981; Bint Akhtar *et al.*, 1982; Resko *et al.*, 1982; Sundaram *et al.*, 1982). Constant infusion of agonist via a minipump to rhesus monkeys, however, led to greatly depressed testosterone and LH levels and reduced testicular volume, but azoospermia was not reliably reduced (Bint Akhtar *et al.*, 1984). In most of the studies where testicular sperm production was investigated, it was found that only when androgen levels were reduced to very low levels was seminiferous tubular function also reduced. Thus the rhesus monkey may not be a suitable model for the human, due to its resistance to LHRH treatment (Bint Akhtar *et al.*, 1984).

Studies in men have found that daily treatment with LHRH agonists can suppress testosterone and LH levels (Bergquist *et al.*, 1979*c*; Linde *et al.*, 1981; Tolis *et al.*, 1981*b*; Faure *et al.*, 1982; Heber *et al.*, 1984), but that again spermatogenesis is not reliably suppressed (Bergquist *et al.*, 1979*c*; Linde *et al.*, 1981). Concomitant testosterone administration, while maintaining libido, does not potentiate the sperm-suppressing activity of the LHRH analog, and intermittent administration of the analogs is ineffective (Doelle *et al.*, 1984). The available evidence in men suggests that LHRH agonists, either alone or in combination with androgen replacement, are not effective as male contraceptives. Treatment with continuous LHRH analog administration (pellet implant, capsules or microspheres) remains to be tested. One study done in four male volunteers with a weak antagonist showed that pituitary responses to LHRH could be diminished (Gonzalez-Barcena *et al.*, 1977). More potent antagonists are now available and animal experiments look promising. With as little as 10 days treatment with [N-Ac-Δ^3-Pro^1,D-pCl-Phe^2,D-Trp^{3,6},N-MeLeu^7]LHRH, testicular weight decreased 60% and tubule diameter 47%. Spermatogenesis was completely suppressed. Unfortunately, accessory organ weights, testosterone and FSH levels were also reduced. The accessary organ weights, but not spermatogenesis, were restored with testosterone enanthate treatment (Rivier *et al.*, 1980). Clearly, such therapy with an LHRH analog will necessitate concomitant treatment with an androgen for a useful male contraceptive method. To date, no clinical studies have been done in men with such potent antagonistic analogs, and a major question to be resolved will be whether complete cessation of spermatogenesis can be achieved.

Chronic treatment with LHRH analogs will be required and suitable testosterone replacement therapy will be mandatory. Consequently, the acceptability of such a method of male contraception will be questionable. For less developed countries, the necessity for monthly injections of a testosterone ester may cause service delivery problems. A longer term injectable preparation or biodegradable implant might be more acceptable, and such development should be within the scope of available technology.

FUTURE PROSPECTS

LHRH analogs can reliably inhibit ovulation and a scheme similar to that used for oral contraceptive pills, e.g. 21 days treatment per month, may prove satisfactory without causing the cycle disruption and amenorrhea observed with chronic treatment. Whether it will prove necessary to supplement the LHRH analogs with daily progestin treatment remains to be determined, but if this is the case, then the acceptability and freedom from side-effects of the method may be severely compromised. The attraction of the LHRH analogs is that they can produce their action on ovulation without the side-effects of hormonal steroid therapy.

The prospects for developing LHRH analogs that would be contraceptive due to luteolytic activity seems remote. It may be possible to develop an analog as an abortifacient, but the timing for successful administration may be very restricted. Treatment early in the follicular phase of the cycle may also not be useful, since ovulation is only delayed, not inhibited, and luteal phase inadequacy only induced very inconsistently. Thus, present evidence suggests that LHRH analogs (either agonists or antagonists), whether given postcoitally, after ovulation or after a missed menses, may not prove effective contraceptively.

In men, the available data suggest that the agonistic analogs will not produce azoospermia reliably. The antagonists may prove more effective in this regard, but clinical data are needed. The usefulness of LHRH analogs for male contraception may well hinge on suitable delivery systems and mandatory testosterone replacement. Such combination therapy adds to the complexity of the research and development process, and increases the toxicological problems. Development of such a male method, if feasible, is not likely to reach completion in the near future.

The great promise felt for the LHRH analogs as contraceptive agents 2 years ago has yet to be realized and present evidence suggests that their impact for contraception may be less than originally thought.

References

Auclair, C., Kelly, P. A., Labrie, F., Coy, D. H. and Schally, A. V. (1977). Inhibition of testicular luteinizing hormone receptor level by treatment with a potent luteinizing hormone-releasing hormone agonist or human chorionic gonadotropin. *Biochem. Biophys. Res. Commun.*, **76,** 855

Balmaceda, J. P., Schally, A. V., Coy, D. and Asch, R. H. (1981). The effects of an LH-RH antagonist ([N-Ac-D-Trp^{1,3},D-p-Cl-Phe^{2},D-Phe^{6},D-Ala^{10}]-LHRH) during the preovulatory period of the rhesus monkey. *Contraception,* **24,** 275

Baumann, R., Kuhl, H., Taubert, H. D. and Sandow, J. (1980). Ovulation inhibition by daily i.m. administration of a highly active LH-RH analog (D-Ser[TBU]^{6}-LHRH-[1-9] nonapeptide-ethylamide). *Contraception,* **21,** 191

Bergquist, C., Nillius, S. J. and Wide, L. (1979*a*). Inhibition of ovulation in women by intranasal treatment with a luteinizing hormone-releasing hormone agonist. *Contraception,* **19,** 497

Bergquist, C., Nillius, S. J. and Wide, L. (1979*b*). Intranasal gonadotropin-releasing hormone agonist as a contraceptive agent. *Lancet,* **2,** 215

Bergquist, C., Nillius, S. J., Bergh, T., Skarin, G. and Wide, L. (1979*c*). Inhibitory effects on gonadotrophin secretion and gonadal function in men during chronic treatment with a potent stimulatory luteinizing hormone-releasing hormone analogue. *Acta Endocrinol.,* **91,** 601

Bergquist, C., Nillius, S. J. and Wide, L. (1980*a*). Effects of a luteinizing hormone-releasing hormone agonist on luteal function in women. *Contraception,* **22,** 287

Bergquist, C., Nillius, S. J. and Wide, L. (1980*b*). Luteolysis induced by a luteinizing hormone-releasing hormone agonist is prevented by human chorionic gonadotropin. *Contraception,* **22,** 341

Bergquist, C., Nillius, S. J., Wide, L. and Lindgren, A. (1981). Endometrial patterns in women on chronic luteinizing hormone-releasing agonist treatment for contraception. *Fertil. Steril.*, **36,** 339

Bergquist, C., Nillius, S. J. and Wide, L. (1982). Long-term intranasal luteinizing hormone-releasing hormone agonist treatment for contraception in women. *Fertil. Steril.*, **38,** 190

Bex, F. J. and Corbin, A. (1981). Luteinizing hormone-releasing hormone (LHRH) and LHRH agonist termination of pregnancy in hypophysectomized rats: Extrapituitary site of action. *Endocrinology,* **108,** 273

Bint Akhtar, F., Wickings, E. J., Zaidi, P. and Nieschlag, E. (1982). Pituitary and testicular functions in sexually mature rhesus monkeys under high dose LRH-agonist treatment. *Acta Endocrinol.,* **101,** 113

Bint Akhtar, F., Wickings, E. J. and Nieschlag, E. (1984). Male fertility control with LHRH agonists: primate studies. This volume, chapter 7

Casper, R. F. and Yen, S. S. C. (1979). Induction of luteolysis in the human with a long-acting analog of luteinizing hormone-releasing factor. *Science,* **205,** 408

Casper, R. F., Sheehan, K. L. and Yen, S. S. C. (1980). Chorionic gonadotropin prevents LRF-agonist-induced luteolysis in the human. *Contraception,* **21,** 471

Corbin, A., Beattie, C. W., Jones, R. and Bex, F. (1979). Peptide contraception: Antifertility properties of LH-RH analogues. *Int. J. Gynaecol. Obstet.*, **16,** 359

Das, C. and Talwar, G. P. (1983). Pregnancy-terminating action of a luteinizing hormone-releasing hormone agonist D-Ser(Bu^t)^{6}desGly^{10}ProEA in baboons. *Fertil. Steril.,* **39,** 218

Doelle, G. C., Evans, R. M., Alexander, A. N. and Rabin, D. (1984). Antifertility effects of an LHRH agonist in men. This volume, Chapter 21

Faure, N., Labrie, F., Lemay, A., Bélanger, A., Gordeau, Y., Laroche, B. and Robert, G. (1982). Inhibition of serum androgen levels by chronic intranasal and subcutaneous administration of a potent luteinizing hormone-releasing hormone (LH-RH) agonist in adult men. *Fertil. Steril.,* **37,** 416

Gonzalez-Barcena, D., Coy, D. H., Kastin, A. J., Nikolics, K. and Schally, A. V. (1977). Suppression of gonadotrophin release in man by an inhibitory analogue of LH-releasing hormone. *Lancet,* **2,** 997

Hardt, W., Genz, T. and Schmidt-Gollwitzer, M. (1984). Antifertility by discontinuous treatment with buserelin in women. This volume, Chapter 18

Harper, M. J. K. (1983). *Birth Control Technologies Prospects by the Year 2000.* (Austin: University of Texas Press and London: W. Heinemann Medical Books)

Heber, D., Swerdloff, R. S. and Henzl, M. (1984). Effects of nafarelin acetate in men. This volume, Chapter 20

Kent, J. S., Sanders, L. M., McRae, G. I., Vickery, B. H., Tice, T. R. and Lewis, D. H. (1982). In vivo controlled release of an LH-RH analog from injected polymeric microcapsules. *Contracept. Deliv. Syst.,* **3,** 58

Koyama, T., Ohkura, T., Kumasaka, T. and Saito, M. (1978). Effect of postovulatory treatment with a luteinizing hormone-releasing hormone analog on the plasma level of progesterone in women. *Fertil. Steril.,* **30,** 549

Lemay, A., Labrie, F., Bélanger, A. and Raynaud, J. P. (1979*a*). Luteolytic effect of intranasal administration of [D-Ser(TBU)^6,des-Gly-NH^{10}]-luteinizing hormone releasing hormone ethylamide in normal women. *Fertil. Steril.,* **32, 646**

Lemay, A., Labrie, F., Ferland, L. and Raynaud, J. P. (1979*b*). Possible luteolytic effects of luteinizing hormone-releasing hormone in normal women. *Fertil. Steril.,* **31,** 29

Lemay, A., Labrie, F. and Raynaud, J. P. (1980). Luteolytic activity of LHRH and [D-SER(TBU)^6,DES-GLY-NH^{10}]LHRH ethylamide: A new and physiological approach to contraception in women. *Int. J. Fertil.,* **25,** 203

Lemay, A., Faure, N., Labrie, F. and Fazekas, A. T. A. (1984). Postcoital contraception with intranasal buserelin. This volume, Chapter 17

Linde, R., Doelle, G. C., Alexander, N., Kirchner, F., Vale, W., Rivier, J. and Rabin, D. (1981). Reversible inhibition of testicular steroidogenesis and spermatogenesis by a potent gonadotropin-releasing hormone agonist in normal men. *N. Engl. J. Med.,* **305,** 663

Nieschlag, E. and Wickings, E. J. (1980). Does the rhesus monkey provide a suitable model for human testicular functions? In Serio, M. and Martini, L. (eds.) *Animal Models in Human Reproduction,* pp. 103–119. (New York: Raven Press)

Nillius, S. J., Bergquist, C. and Wide, L. (1978). Inhibition of ovulation in women by chronic treatment with a stimulatory LRH analogue – A new approach to birth control? *Contraception*, **17**, 537

Nillius, S. J. and Bergquist, C. (1984). LHRH agonists for female contraception. This volume, Chapter 16

Resko, J. A., Bélanger, A. and Labrie, F. (1982). Effects of chronic treatment with a potent luteinizing hormone releasing hormone agonist on serum luteinizing hormone and steroid levels in male rhesus monkeys. *Biol. Reprod.*, **26**, 378

Rivier, C., Rivier, J. and Vale, W. (1979). Effect of the LRF-antagonist [D-pGlu^{1},D-Phe^{2},D-Trp^{3,6}]-LRF on pregnancy in the rat. *Contraception*, **19**, 185

Rivier, C., Rivier, J. and Vale, W. (1980). Antireproductive effects of a potent gonadotropin-releasing hormone antagonist in the male rat. *Science*, **210**, 93

Schmidt-Gollwitzer, M., Hardt, W., Schmidt-Gollwitzer, K., von der Ohe, M. and Nevinny-Stickel, J. (1981). Influence of the LH-RH analogue buserelin on cyclic ovarian function and on endometrium: A new approach to fertility control. *Contraception*, **23**, 187

Schmidt-Gollwitzer, M., Hardt, W. and Schmidt-Gollwitzer, K. (1984). Risks and benefits of LHRH agonists as antifertility agents. This volume, Chapter 19

Sheehan, K. L., Casper, R. F. and Yen, S. S. C. (1982). Luteal phase defects induced by an agonist of luteinizing hormone-releasing factor: A model for fertility control. *Science*, **215**, 170

Siler-Khodr, T. M., Khodr, G. S., Valenzuela, G., Harper, M. J. K., Vickery, B. H. and Nestor, J. J. (1983). Differential inhibition of αhCG, hCG, progesterone, estrogens and prostaglandins from early and midgestational human placental cultures by a GnRH antagonist. *Proceedings of 30th Annual Meeting, Society for Gynecologic Investigation*, Washington, D.C. (Abstr. No. 154, p. 83).

Skarin, G., Nillius, S. J. and Wide, L. (1982). Early follicular phase luteinizing hormone-releasing hormone agonist administration – Effects on follicular maturation and corpus luteum function in women. *Contraception*, **25**, 31

Sundaram, K., Connell, K. G., Bardin, W., Samojlik, E. and Schally, A. V. (1982). Inhibition of pituitary-testicular function with [D-Trp^{6}] luteinizing hormone-releasing hormone in rhesus monkeys. *Endocrinology*, **110**, 1308

Tolis, G., Comaru-Schally, A. M., Mehta, A. E. and Schally, A. V. (1981*a*). Failure to interrupt established pregnancy in humans by D-Tryptophan-6-luteinizing hormone-releasing hormone. *Fertil. Steril.*, **36**, 241

Tolis, G., Mehta, A., Comaru-Schally, A. M. and Schally, A. V. (1981*b*). Suppression of androgen production by D-tryptophan-6-luteinizing hormone-releasing hormone in men. *J. Clin. Invest.*, **68**, 819

Vickery, B. H. and McRae, G. I. (1979). Effects on male rats of continuous treatment with DesGly^{10}D-Ala^{6}ProNHEt^{9}LHRH (LHRH-A). *Program and Abstracts, Proceedings of the 61st Annual Meeting of the Endocrine Society*, Bethesda, MD, The Endocrine Society, Abstr. No. 441

Vickery, B. H. and McRae, G. I. (1980*a*). Responses of the males of different laboratory species to continuous administration of an LHRH agonist. *J. Androl.*, **1**, 62 (Abstr.)

Vickery, B. H. and McRae, G. I. (1980*b*). Effects of continuous treatment of male baboons with superagonists of LHRH. *Int. J. Fertil.*, **25**, 179

Vickery, B. H. and McRae, G. I. (1980*c*). Effects of continuous treatment with superagonists of LHRH when initiated at different times of the menstrual cycle in female baboons. *Int. J. Fertil.*, **25**, 171

Vickery, B. H., McRae, G. I. and Stevens, V. C. (1981). Suppression of luteal and placental function in pregnant baboons with agonist analogs of luteinizing hormone-releasing hormones. *Fertil. Steril.*, **36**, 664

Vickery, B. H., McRae, G. I., Briones, W., Worden, A., Seidenberg, R., Schanbacher, B. D. and Falvo, R. (1984). Effects of an LHRH agonist upon sexual function in male dogs: Suppression, reversibility and effect of testosterone replacement. *J. Androl.* (In press)

Vickery, B. H., McRae, G. I. and Tallentire, D. (1983). Disparate effects of daily versus continuous administration of a potent LHRH agonist on plasma LH levels in female rhesus monkeys. *Fertil. Steril.*, **39**, 417 (Abstr.)

Wickings, E. J., Zaidi, P. and Nieschlag, E. (1981). Effect of chronic, high-dose LHRH-agonist treatment on pituitary and testicular function in rhesus monkeys. *J. Androl.*, **2**, 72

Zárate, A., Canales, E. S., Sthory, I., Coy, D. H., Comaru-Schally, A. M. and Schally, A. V. (1981). Anovulatory effect of a LHRH antagonist in women. *Contraception*, **24**, 315

35
The therapeutic potential of LHRH and LHRH analogs

R. A. EDGREN and D. R. SHEVLIN

The physiological action of luteinizing hormone releasing hormone (LHRH) depends on pulsatile patterns of secretion. Continuous stimulation of the pituitary by LHRH, which may be achieved either by high doses or by constant infusion, results in (1) desensitization of the pituitary gland, (2) failure of gonadotropin secretion, (3) involution of the gonads and (4) regression of organs, structures and functions that depend on gonadal steroids for maintenance. This paradoxical antifertility effect of LHRH can be mimicked by the administration of antagonistic analogs of LHRH, which block the effect of the parent hormone at the level of the pituitary receptors. Peripheral effects of LHRH acting directly on the gonads were described, but their physiological significance remains to be elucidated.

In addition to these antagonistic analogs, there are a number of agonistic analogs that are significantly more potent than their parent when assayed for their ability to release LH. The increased potency of at least some of these appears to result from amino acid substitutions that resist metabolic degradation and permit longer exposure of the LHRH receptors to the analog.

LHRH and its analogs have a broad range of therapeutic applications. These segregate into the effects of LHRH and agonistic analogs, which have both stimulatory and paradoxical inhibitory actions, and the effects of antagonistic analogs.

GONADOTROPIN-RELEASING EFFECTS

Induction of ovulation

One of the originally projected applications of LHRH was the induction of ovulation in infertile women. As with gonadotropin treatment, this goal has been achieved, but the pregnancy rate has been disappointing. This may be a result of inadequacies in postovulatory physiology. This approach should not, however, be abandoned until pulsatile administration with LHRH and perhaps certain short-acting analogs has been further studied.

Hypogonadotropic hypogonadism

Exciting developments in the treatment of idiopathic hypogonadotropic hypogonadism (IHH) have been reported by Hoffman and Crowley (1984), who achieved completely normal endocrine status in at least some adult male patients by administering natural LHRH in pulses paralleling the pulsatile release of LH that occurs every 90–120 min in normal men. Doses of 25 ng/kg delivered subcutaneously every 2 h by infusion pump to six adult men resulted in normal to supranormal adult levels of LH and FSH that were sustained for at least 3 months. Two subjects attained midpubertal testosterone levels, and four rapidly attained normal adult levels and a marked increase in testicular volume. Three of these achieved mature spermatogenesis, and one successfully impregnated his wife. Within 6–8 weeks, all six underwent pubertal changes: nocturnal emissions, spontaneous erections, transient breast tenderness and acne.

Attempts to slow the virilization process by reducing the doses from 25 to 10 ng/kg in six other patients resulted in increased testicular volume – simulating the early stages of puberty – but no other pubertal changes; however, reduction of the dose in one of the original patients after 9 months did not reverse the testosterone level and was followed by development of spermatogenesis. In some patients unresponsive to this therapy, increasing the doses to 100–200 ng/kg has proved successful. However, some subjects do not respond.

One patient, initially responsive, relapsed after developing antibodies to LHRH. It remains to be seen whether development of antibodies will prove to be an obstacle to the chronic replacement therapy necessary for IHH. The inconvenience of wearing a portable infusion pump day and night would appear to be unavoidable, for Hoffman and Crowley's success makes clear that the failure of earlier attempts to treat IHH with less frequent injections of longer-acting LHRH analogs (Mortimer *et al.*, 1974; Krabbe and Skakkebaek, 1977; Van Loon and Brown, 1975; Brook and Dombey, 1979; Happ *et al.*, 1975; Hashimoto *et al.*, 1975; Crowley *et al.*, 1980) was due to their failure to simulate normal intermittent release of gonadal hormones.

Efforts to capitalize upon the gonadotropin-releasing effects of LHRH and its analogs in treating various androgen deficiency states involve long term replacement therapy – that is, they attempt to mimic or restore normal conditions. In this respect, the work of Hoffman and Crowley indicates that the probable pulsatile release of LHRH from the hypothalamus must be simulated very closely indeed in order for success to be achieved with natural LHRH: the effects they achieved with pulses at an approximately 2 h frequency were reversed when dosage frequency was increased to every hour or decreased to every 3–4 h. It is also clear that determination of the proper dose levels – particularly of the long-acting LHRH analogs – will be critical in long term therapy if desensitization, leading to failure of therapy, is to be avoided. The success in the treatment of IHH, however, demonstrates the viability of LHRH replacement therapy and holds great promise for its success in other hypogonadal disorders.

Delayed puberty

The success with IHH in adults suggests that juveniles with delayed puberty might likewise respond to LHRH treatment. Preliminary work using bolus administration and high-potency LHRH analogs has achieved adult levels of testosterone in slightly better than one third of patients (Brook and Dombey, 1979; Laron *et al.*, 1981; Mies *et al.*, 1982; Happ *et al.*, 1979, 1980, 1981; Happ, 1981). However, as Happ has pointed out, therapeutic efficacy would be indistinguishable from spontaneous onset of puberty in cases where testosterone levels remain high after cessation of therapy; and since the vast majority of the reported successes fit this pattern rather than one of treatment-dependent effects, it is not certain that the therapy was responsible for triggering or accelerating pubertal development. While it is too soon to abandon these approaches, the mimicking of normal hormonal patterns with pulsatile administration would seem to offer the most promise.

Cryptorchidism

In cryptorchidism, LHRH therapy has been attempted over the past decade and has shown results comparable to those attained with human chorionic gonadotropin in stimulating the descent of testes in boys (Happ, 1984). While the success rates have varied widely among investigators, Happ concludes that, provided the doses are adequate, the treatment can be assumed to be successful in most if not all of those patients whose cryptorchidism is due to hypothalamic disturbances rather than to pituitary dysfunction or mechanical blockage; he attributes the wide variability of success rates to differences in the composition of their respective patient populations. The advantage of LHRH therapy for cryptorchidism is that it may be employed to stimulate Leydig cell function at doses that do not produce virilizing effects, which are undesirable at the age of most of the patients. The failure of LHRH or its analogs to stimulate pubertal developments in these cases is probably attributable to the fact that, as Happ points out, the doses used are clearly supraphysiologic; but since the therapeutic effect is achieved with short term administration – after only 7 days in one case – the effects of desensitization that apparently thwarted the attempts to treat IHH with longer acting LHRH analogs before the advent of pulsatile administration were fortuitously avoided.

Normogonadotropic oligospermia

A number of investigators have attempted to treat idiopathic normogonadotropic oligospermia with LHRH or its analogs. Several have reported promising improvements in various parameters of sperm quality (Zárate *et al.*, 1973; Schwarzstein *et al.*, 1975; Aparicio *et al.*, 1976; Besser *et al.*, 1978), including at least transiently improved – though still subnormal – sperm counts (Zárate *et al.*, 1973; Schwarzstein *et al.*, 1975; Levalle *et al.*, 1981). It is too early to evaluate this approach critically. Large t.i.d. doses of natural LHRH (Mandelbaum *et al.*, 1976) or b.i.d. doses of [D-Leu^6,Pro^9-NHEt]

LHRH (leuprolide) (Happ *et al.*, 1978) have resulted in desensitization. Pulsatile therapy warrants a trial in this indication also.

Hypogonadal impotence

Since LHRH increases testosterone levels, its potential in the treatment of impotence in hypogonadal males is obvious; and some receiving LHRH therapy have reported increased potency (Bergada *et al.*, 1972; Mortimer *et al.*, 1974; Davies *et al.*, 1977). However, one study found that testosterone levels did not drop despite pituitary desensitization, suggesting that the effects of LHRH on potency may in fact not be mediated exclusively by changes in serum testosterone (Davies *et al.*, 1977). Double blind trials of 100 or 500 μg by bolus injection or infused over 2 h in healthy males increased self-reported sexual arousal and well-being, but the differences between LHRH and placebo were modest (McAdoo *et al.*, 1978); another blind trial in normal males found a significant, but transient, difference 6 weeks afterward (Davies *et al.*, 1977). Again, pituitary desensitization has proved to be an obstacle to long term effectiveness, and pulsatile administration deserves a trial.

GONADOTROPIN-INHIBITORY EFFECTS

Since the paradoxical action of LHRH and its agonistic analogs will have the same ultimate result as the blocking effects of LHRH antagonists – viz. inhibiting secretion of gonadotropins and preventing effects subsequent to gonadotropins in normal sexual function – these two inhibitory approaches can be discussed together.

Precocious puberty

Several groups of investigators have demonstrated the efficacy of LHRH or its longer acting analogs in treating true precocious puberty by paradoxical inhibition of hypothalamic release of gonadotropins when continuously elevated levels of the decapeptide are maintained (Belchetz *et al.*, 1978; Crowley *et al.*, 1979; Bergquist *et al.*, 1979; Tharandt *et al.*, 1977; Linde *et al.*, 1981; Comite *et al.*, 1984). Comite and associates (1984) have studied the effect of [D-Trp^6,Pro^9-NHEt]LHRH 4 μg/kg per day administered subcutaneously for 4–16 months to 15 children (11 girls and four boys ranging in age from 2 to 8 years) with true precocious puberty, either idiopathic or secondary to hypothalamic hamartoma. In all cases, gonadotropins were suppressed within 4 months, and the patients showed complete suppression of response to stimulation with exogenous LHRH. Estradiol levels and vaginal maturation scores in the girls and testosterone levels in the boys dropped to normal prepubertal levels; and preliminary observations suggest that linear and ulnar growth were likewise lowered to normal prepubescent levels. Clinical manifestations of precocious puberty also tended to regress: among the 11 girls, breast size decreased in nine, pubic hair disappeared in five, and irregular vaginal bleeding ceased during therapy in all six in whom it had been present before treatment; among the four boys, facial and pubic hair decreased in all three in whom it had been present, and testicular size decreased in all. Suspension of therapy reversed all effects, with recovery of hypophyseal responsiveness in 10–12 weeks and reversion of clinical improvements to pretreatment (i.e. pubertal) levels. The response of gonadotropins and sex steroids to this therapy is quite uniform and may provide a diagnostic test for true precocious puberty, since steroidogenesis from an ovarian cyst in another child was found to be unresponsive to LHRH analog therapy. Thus, the use of LHRH analogs to treat precocious puberty shows great promise and should certainly be pursued.

Breast cancer

Since the progression of mammary cancers, particularly those that develop during premenopausal years, is often dependent upon estrogens of ovarian origin and responds to surgical castration, the medical castration produced by agonistic analogs of LHRH may provide an additional therapeutic modality for some patients. The animal and preliminary clinical studies published to date are reviewed by Harvey *et al.* (1984). At present, the numbers of reported patients who have received LHRH analog therapy are too small to allow assessment of success rates. Preliminary studies using [D-Ser (tBu)^6,Pro^9-NHEt]LHRH (buserelin) or leuprolide reduced estrone and estradiol to castrate levels in all cases (though some patients continued to show periodic elevations) and produced regression or stabilization of disease in four of seven patients (Klijn and De Jong, 1982; Harvey *et al.*, 1984). The absence of adverse effects, despite the use of high doses, suggests that LHRH analogs may prove to be useful adjuncts to current therapies for mammary cancer in premenopausal women.

Prostatic cancer

Prostatic cancer has received more attention than mammary cancer as a potential therapeutic application of LHRH hormonal suppression. Since prostatic cancer is usually androgen-dependent, the inhibition of testosterone secretion would be expected to produce remission of the disease. And, indeed, several trials in patients with prostatic cancer have demonstrated that LHRH agonists can achieve long term inhibition of testosterone tantamount to chemical castration. Most studies have employed leuprolide or buserelin administered subcutaneously or intranasally. A 95% reduction in testosterone was reported by Warner *et al.* (1982), who used injected leuprolide; and a 75% reduction was reported by Tolis *et al.* (1982), who used intranasal buserelin or subcutaneous leuprolide. Faure *et al.* (1982) found great individual variation in response to intranasal buserelin 500 μg b.i.d.

Borgmann *et al.* (1982) demonstrated the efficacy of beginning the treatment with mega-doses of subcutaneously injected buserelin 1 mg b.i.d. for 3 days, followed by chronic treatment with the more convenient intranasal spray of buserelin 0.6–1.2 mg t.i.d. (of which $\simeq 5\%$ is absorbed); the testosterone levels of the nine patients dropped to within the castrate range within 3 weeks and remained there for the 6 month duration of the study. In a subsequent study employing 23 patients treated initially with subcutaneous injections of buserelin (1 mg b.i.d. or 500 μg t.i.d. for 6 days), Borgmann and co-workers found that during the subsequent long term intranasal administration, a daily dose of 1200 μg (400 μg t.i.d.) was necessary to maintain testosterone levels consistently at values equivalent to those of surgically castrated controls (< 1 ng/ml) (V. Borgmann, R. Hagel, W. Hardt and M. Schmidt-Gollwitzer, unpublished results, 1983).

These results are confirmed by Faure *et al.* (1984), who found that initial subcutaneous administration of mega-dose buserelin (500 μg t.i.d.) for 3–7 days followed by chronic intranasal application (400 μg t.i.d.) thereafter for up to 5 months increased the rapidity and profundity of testosterone suppression – with levels of <1 ng/ml after 4 weeks in 13 out of 18 patients. Santen *et al.* (1984) have reported the administration of megadoses of leuprolide (1 or 10 mg/day) to a large group of intact patients, whose testosterone levels fell to those of castrated men.

While these megadoses of the LHRH agonist suppressed LH, testosterone, dihydrotestosterone, and, to a lesser extent, FSH, they did not significantly alter prolactin or cortisol levels during chronic administration; and, indeed, the hormonal suppression attained by LHRH agonists would appear to be notably free of side-effects other than those of castration.

Complete suppression of testosterone is not, of course, a guarantee of clinical success, for a certain percentage of prostatic tumors are refractory to surgical castration. However, the clinical success of LHRH agonist therapy appears to be equivalent to that of surgical castration. Tolis *et al.* (1982) reported a rapid improvement in clinical symptoms in all of 10 patients with advanced disease who were treated with buserelin. Borgmann and co-workers reported marked or adequate tumor regression in 14 of 17 patients treated with buserelin for 6–15 months, and stable disease in the other three (V. Borgmann, R. Hagel, W. Hardt and M. Schmidt-Gollwitzer, unpublished results, 1983). Faure *et al.* (1984) reported a decrease of subjective and objective symptoms in 16 (73%) of 22 patients treated with intranasal buserelin for 2–28 months, while ten (56%) of 18 with bone pain noted improvement. Most encouraging are the results of the large Phase I trial with megadose therapy reported by Santen *et al.* (1984): in males with inoperable prostatic cancer who had had no prior treatment, 53% experienced objective remission after 4 months of treatment; 34% were stabilized, and 13% progressed. In patients who had previously been treated with diethylstilbestrol or Tace, 19% achieved remission, 33% stabilized, and 48% progressed at 10 weeks, with 64% progressing by 4 months. Predictably, patients who had been surgically castrated failed to respond, with 94% progressing and only 6% stabilized.

There seems to be no doubt that agonistic analogs of LHRH are extremely useful agents in the treatment of prostatic carcinoma. The functional castration that is achieved is more acceptable to many patients than surgical castration, and the putative atherosclerotic and cardiac side-effects of estrogen treatment will presumably be avoided. Further studies will, of course, be needed to determine such matters as the optimal dosages for the various analogs, their comparative efficacy, and the possible role of adjunctive therapy.

CONCLUSION

The ability of LHRH and its agonistic analogs to release LH and FSH provides a range of new therapeutic possibilities in certain cases of infertility, delayed puberty, sexual infantilism and other conditions associated with hypothalamic–pituitary failure. The preliminary results reported in therapy for anovulation, hypogonadism, cryptorchidism, impotence and normogonadotropic oligospermia are encouraging. Extensive future studies will be required to provide a full understanding of the potentials and limitations of this modality.

The antagonistic analogs of LHRH and the paradoxical effects of LHRH agonists provide the physician with a pharmacological mechanism for reversibly shutting down the pituitary–gonadal axis. The early reports of the use of these agents in such gonad-dependent conditions as precocious puberty and mammary and prostatic carcinoma indicate success, though therapeutic details, problems and limitations await the completion of more extensive studies.

Therapy with LHRH agonistic analogs is normally accompanied by increases in pituitary gonadotropins and gonadal steroids before desensitization occurs and results in suppressed levels. The clinical impact of this initial stimulation remains to be evaluated; however, LHRH antagonists are expected not to have this effect and may, as a result, have greater value in suppressive therapy.

The therapeutic potential of LHRH agonists and antagonists should be evident. It remains only for us to refine our approaches in order to utilize these drugs to their fullest potential.

References

Aparicio, N. J., Schwarzstein, L. and Turner, E. A. (1976). Treatment of idiopathic normogonadotropic oligoasthenospermia with synthetic luteinizing hormone-releasing hormone. *Fertil. Steril.*, **27**, 549

Belchetz, P. E., Plant, T. M., Nakai, Y., Keogh, E. J. and Knobil, E. (1978). Hypophysial responses to continuous and intermittent delivery of hypothalamic gonadotropin-releasing hormone. *Science*, **202**, 631

Bergada, C., Mancini, R. E., Vilar, O., Rivarola, M. A., Calamera, J. C., Bianculli, C., Schally, A. V. and Kastin, A. J. (1972). Effect of chronic administration of synthetic LH-RH-FSH-RH on prepubertal boys and in hypogonadotropic hypogonadism. In *Serono Research Foundation, Proceedings of a Conference*, p. 299. June 29–July 1, Acapulco, Mexico

Bergquist, C., Nillius, S. J. and Wide, L. (1979). Reduced gonadotropin secretion in postmenopausal women during treatment with a stimulatory LRH analogue. *J. Clin. Endocrinol. Metab.*, **49**, 472

Besser, G. M. and Mortimer, C. H. (1978). Gonadotropin-releasing hormone therapy in hypothalamic-pituitary dysfunction. In *Hypothalamic Hormones – Chemistry, Physiology and Clinical Applications*, p. 589. Proceedings of the 2nd European Colloquium on Hypothalamic Hormones, July 1976, Tübingen. (Weinheim: Verlag Chemie)

Borgmann, V., Hardt, W., Schmidt-Gollwitzer, M., Adenauer, H. and Hagel, R. (1982). Sustained suppression of testosterone production by the luteinizing-hormone releasing-hormone agonist buserelin in patients with advanced prostate carcinoma. *Lancet*, **1**, 1097

Brook, C. G. and Dombey, S. (1979). Induction of puberty: Long-term treatment with high-dose LHRH. *Clin. Endocrinol.*, **11**, 81

Comite, F., Cutler, G. B. and Loriaux, D. L. (1984). LHRH analog therapy of precocious puberty. This volume, Chapter 24

Crowley, W. F., Vale, W., Beitins, I. Z., Rivier, J., Rivier, C. and McArthur, J. (1979). Chronic administration of a long-acting LRF agonist (D-Trp^6-Pro^9-NEt-LRF), in hypogonadotropic hypogonadism: The critical nature of dosage and frequency in enhancement, extinction and restoration of gonadotropin responsiveness. *Endocrine Soc. Abstr.*, **16**, 76

Crowley, W. F., Jr., Beitins, I. Z., Vale, W., Kliman, B., Rivier, J., Rivier, C. and McArthur, J. W. (1980). The biologic activity of a potent analogue of gonadotropin-releasing hormone in normal and hypogonadotropic men. *N. Engl. J. Med.*, **302**, 1052

Davies, T. F., Gomez-Pan, A., Watson, M. J., Mountjoy, C. Q., Hanker, J. P., Besser, G. M. and Hall, R. (1977). Reduced 'gonadotropin response to releasing hormone' after chronic administration to impotent men. *Clin. Endocrinol.*, **6**, 213

Faure, N., Labrie, F., Lemay, A., Bélanger, A., Gourdeau, Y., LaRoche, B. and Robert, G. (1982). Inhibition of serum androgen levels by chronic intranasal and subcutaneous administration of a potent luteinizing hormone-releasing hormone (LH-RH) agonist in adult men. *Fertil. Steril.*, **37**, 416

Faure, N., Lemay, A., Tolis, G., Labrie, F., Bélanger, A. and Fazekas, A. T. A. (1984). Buserelin therapy for prostatic carcinoma. This volume, Chapter 26

Happ, J. (1981). *Therapie mit Gonadotropin-Releasing-Hormon-Untersuchungen zur Anwendung bei Hypogonadismus, Pubertas tarda und Kryptorchismus.* (Munich: Urban & Schwartzenberg)

Happ, J. (1984). Correction of infertility with LHRH agonists in the male. This volume, Chapter 23

Happ, J., Neubauer, M., Egri, A., Demisch, K., Schoffling, K. and Beyer, J. (1975). GnRH therapy in males with hypogonadotrophic hypogonadism. *Horm. Metab. Res.*, **7**, 526

Happ, J., Hartmann, U., Weber, T., Cordes, U. and Beyer, J. (1978). Gonadotropin and testosterone secretion in normal human males after stimulation with gonadotropin-releasing hormone (GnRH) or potent GnRH analogs using different modes of application. *Fertil. Steril.*, **30**, 666

Happ, J., Schmitz, V., Cordes, U., Krause, U., von der Ohe, M. and Beyer, J. (1979). Intervalltherapie mit Gonadoliberin und einem potenten Gonadoliberin-Analogen bei männlichen Patienten mit idiopathischer Pubertas tarda und mit Kallmann-Syndrom. *Hoppe-Seyler's Z. Physiol. Chemie*, **360** (9), 1154

Happ, J., Deigentasch, V., Schmitz, V., Krause, U., Beyer, J. and von der Ohe, M. (1980). Intermittent pernasal gonadotropin-releasing hormone therapy in male patients with delayed puberty. In Voelter, W. and Weitzel, G. (eds.), *Structure and Activity of Natural Peptides*, p. 483. (Berlin: de Gruyter)

Happ, J., Benner, A., Krause, U. and Beyer, J. II (1981). Treatment of delayed puberty with a potent Gn-RH analog: Effectiveness of low-dose regimen. *Acta Endocrinol.*, **96** (Suppl. 240), 112

Harvey, H. A., Lipton, A. and Max, D. T. (1984). LHRH analogs for human mammary carcinoma. This volume, Chapter 25

Hashimoto, T., Miyai, K., Onishi, T., Matsumoto, K. and Kumahara, Y. (1975). Comparison of short and long-term treatment with synthetic LH-releasing hormone and clomiphene citrate in male hypothalamic hypogonadism. *J. Clin. Endocrinol. Metab.*, **41**, 905

Hoffman, A. and Crowley, W. F., Jr. (1984). LHRH therapy for hypogonadotropic hypogonadal men. This volume, Chapter 22

Klijn, J. G. and De Jong, F. H. (1982). Treatment with a luteinizing-hormone-releasing-hormone analog (buserelin) in premenopausal patients with metastatic breast cancer. *Lancet*, **1**, 1213

Krabbe, S. and Skakkebaek, N. E. (1977). Gonadotropin-releasing hormone (LH-RH) and human chorionic gonadotropin in the treatment of two boys with hypogonadotrophic hypogonadism. *Acta Paediatr. Scand.*, **66**, 361

Laron, Z., Dickerman, Z., Ben Zeev, Z., Prager-Lewin, R., Comaru-Schally, A. M. and Schally, A. V. (1981). Long-term effect of D-Trp^6-luteinizing hormone-releasing hormone on testicular size and luteinizing hormone, follicle-stimulating hormone and testosterone levels in hypothalamic hypogonadotropic males. *Fertil. Steril.,* **35,** 328

Levalle, O., Tropea, L., Aparicio, N., Guitelman, A., Mancini, R., Comaru-Schally, A. M. and Schally, A. V. (1981). D-tryptophan-6-LH-RH at low doses in the treatment of male subfertility. *Andrologia,* **13,** 207

Linde, R., Doelle, G. C., Alexander, N., Kirchner, F., Vale, W., Rivier, J. and Rabin, D. (1981). Reversible inhibition of testicular steroidogenesis and spermatogenesis by a potent gonadotropin-releasing hormone agonist in normal men: An approach toward the development of a male contraceptive. *N. Engl. J. Med.,* **305,** 663

McAdoo, B. C., Doering, C. H., Kraemer, H. C., Dessert, N., Brodie, H. K. and Hamburg, D. A. (1978). A study of the effects of gonadotropin-releasing hormone on human mood and behaviour. *Psychosom. Med.,* **40,** 199

Mandelbaum, J., Gayral, M. N. and Piette, F. (1976). Immunisation contre le LHRH de synthèse utilisée à titre thérapeutique en administration prolongée. *Nouv. Presse Med.,* **5** (34), 2256

Mies, R., Fischer, H. and von der Ohe, M. (1982). The efficacy of an LHRH analog in the treatment of delayed puberty. *Acta Endocrinol.,* **99** (Suppl. 246), 90

Mortimer, C. H., McNeilly, A. S., Fisher, R. A., Murray, M. A. F. and Besser, G. M. (1974). Gonadotrophin-releasing hormone therapy in hypogonadal males with hypothalamic or pituitary dysfunction. *Br. Med. J.,* **4,** 617

Santen, R. J., Warner, B., Demers, L. M., Dufau, M. and Smith, J. A. Jr. (1984). Leuprolide therapy for prostatic carcinoma. This volume, Chapter 27

Schwarzstein, L., Aparicio, N. J., Turner, D., Calamera, J. C., Mancini, R. and Schally, A. V. (1975). Use of synthetic luteinizing hormone-releasing hormone in treatment of oligospermic men: A preliminary report. *Fertil. Steril.,* **26,** 331

Tharandt, L., Schulte, H., Benker, G., Hackenberg, K. and Reinwein, D. (1977). Treatment of isolated gonadotropin deficiency in men with synthetic LH-RH and a more potent analogue of LH-RH. *Neuroendocrinology,* **24,** 195

Tolis, G., Ackman, D., Stellos, A., Mehta, A., Labrie, F., Fazekas, A. T. A., Comaru-Schally, A. M. and Schally, A. V. (1982). Tumor growth inhibition in patients with prostatic carcinoma treated with luteinizing hormone-releasing hormone agonists. *Proc. Natl. Acad. Sci. USA,* **79,** 1658

Van Loon, G. R. and Brown, G. M. (1975). Secondary drug failure occurring during chronic treatment with LHRH: Appearance of an antibody. *J. Clin. Endocrinol. Metab.,* **41,** 640

Warner, B., Santen, R. and Demers, L. (1982). Effects of [D-Leu^6-Des-Gly NH_2^{10} Pro-Ethylamide^9]-GnRH (leuprolide) on steroidogenesis when used to treat prostatic carcinoma. *J. Androl.,* **3,** 14

Zárate, A., Valdés-Vallina, F., Gonzáles, A., Pérez-Ubierna, C., Canales, E. S. and Schally, A. V. (1973). Therapeutic effect of synthetic luteinizing hormone-releasing hormone (LH-RH) in male infertility due to idiopathic azoospermia and oligospermia. *Fertil. Steril.,* **24,** 485

36
Epilog

E. S. E. HAFEZ

Naturally occurring LHRH has a very short biological $t_{1/2}$ due to enzymatic cleavage and normal clearance processes. Analogs of LHRH with very high *in vivo* agonistic (Nestor, 1984; Nestor *et al.*, 1984) or antagonistic potencies (Rivier *et al.*, 1984; Nestor *et al.*, 1984; Nekola and Coy, 1984) are available. The most potent agonists contain D-hydrophobic amino acid substitutions at position 6 to reduce enzymatic degradation and increase receptor affinity (Schally *et al.*, 1981; Yen, 1984). Deletion (Monahan *et al.*, 1972) or, more importantly, replacement of the His residue in position 2 of LHRH by D-*p*-halo-Phe (Beattie *et al.*, 1975; Nekola and Coy, 1984) gives LHRH antagonists. Similar 6-position substitutions to those enhancing agonistic potency are incorporated into the antagonists, but more recently D-Arg (Coy *et al.*, 1982; Nekola and Coy, 1984; Rivier *et al.*, 1984) and D-hArg(Et_2) substitutions (Nestor *et al.*, 1984) are giving highly potent and long-acting antagonists. Further substitution by D-hydrophobic amino acids at positions 1 and 3 gives increased antagonistic potency (Nekola and Coy, 1984).

BIOASSAYS

Several *in vitro* and *in vivo* bioassays were used to evaluate the potency of LHRH analogs (Hahn *et al.*, 1984). *In vitro* testing has usually involved the stimulation of LH release from monolayers of dispersed pituitary cells in culture for agonists or inhibition of LH release in this system for antagonists. Receptor binding assays were developed (Clayton, 1984) using pituitary membrane preparations or whole cells (Loumaye *et al.*, 1982). These binding assays use enzymatically stable, radiolabeled superagonist analogs as ligands and offer a reproducible approximation of potency. These assays do not reflect the metabolic and dispositional aspects of *in vivo* activity, however. The radioligand may also be used in a radioreceptor assay to determine the population of receptors on cells. This makes possible the study of the regulation of receptor numbers in response to hormonal treatments and provides evidence for the autoregulation of LHRH receptors (Clayton, 1984). Thus the number of LHRH receptors reflects the prior exposure of the pituitary to LHRH.

Currently, the most used *in vivo* assays for the agonists (Hahn *et al.*, 1984) are ovulation induction, uterine weight gain, and LH release in immature male rats (Arimura *et al.*, 1974), and disruption of estrous cyclicity (Nestor *et al.*, 1982). The last assay reflects the paradoxical antifertility activities of the potent agonists caused by pituitary and/or ovarian desensitization/down-regulation, while the other assays measure the more acute profertility effects of LHRH or its analogs. The effects of the vehicle used can be quite important in the *in vivo* assays (Hahn *et al.*, 1984).

APPLICATIONS OF LHRH ANALOGS

Some aspects of the use of LHRH analogs for contraceptive (Harper, 1984) and therapeutic applications (Edgren and Shevlin, 1984) were reviewed in detail. Table 36.1 condenses some of the clinical parameters for these and other applications in a tabular form for convenience.
Table 36.2 presents a listing of observations in response to LHRH or LHRH agonist treatment which illustrate the present and possible future applications of LHRH analogs.

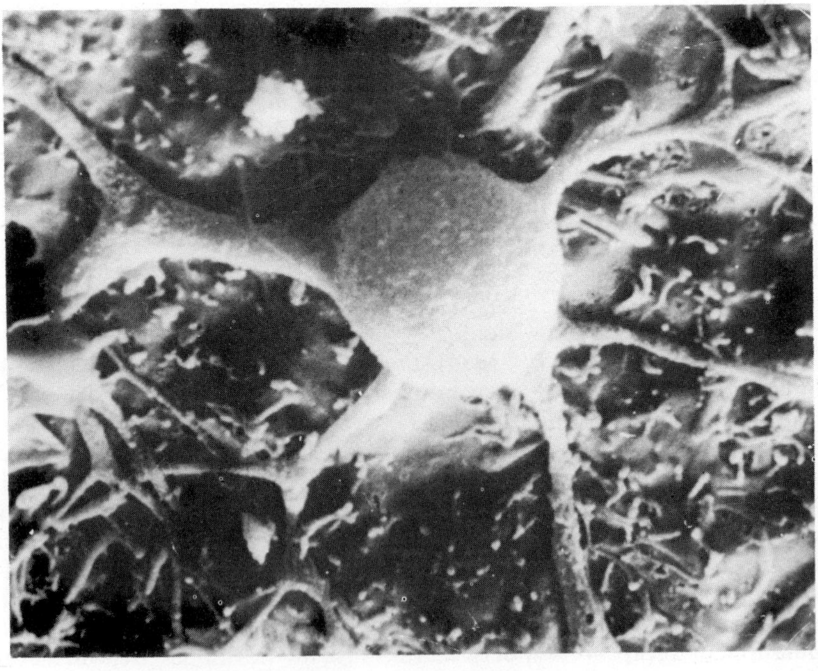

Figure 36.1 Scanning electron micrograph of the hypothalamic cell in the third ventricle. Note dendrites which release neurosecretory material to the portal system of the anterior pituitary gland.

Table 36.1 Summary of clinical experience with LHRH agonistic analogs

Syndrome	*Clinical observations in response to LHRH agonists*
Cryptorchidism	FSH levels rise initially, then decline. LH levels increase progressively. Complete or partial descent of testes occurs within 4 weeks of treatment in most patients without mechanical obstruction.
Precocious puberty	Daily subcutaneous injections of 4 $\mu g\, kg^{-1}\, day^{-1}$ of [D-Trp^6]LHRH ethylamide caused marked reduction of pituitary-ovarian activity, reversed pubertal stages up to Tanner IV. Slowed bone growth and postponed epiphyseal closure resulted.
Delayed puberty	Pulsatile infusion of LHRH or alternate day injection of agonists stimulates pituitary/gonadal function.
Idiopathic hypogonadotropic hypogonadism/secondary amenorrhea	LHRH agonists give short lived stimulation followed by refractoriness. Pulsatile administration of LHRH over long term very successful for both testicular and ovarian function and fertility.
Endometriosis	Daily injection or insufflation of LHRH agonists rapidly (3–6 months) regress lesions and symptoms including dysmenorrhea and dyspareunia and will probably lead to enhanced fertility.
Polycystic ovarian disease	Androstenedione, testosterone and estrogens declined to castrate levels in response to LHRH agonist; adrenal function unaffected. Menstrual cyclicity restored in a percentage of patients after one month of daily therapy.
Prostatic carcinoma	Transitory rise in gonadotropin and androgen levels; steroids falling to castrate levels within 4 weeks of agonist treatment. Metastatic primary tumour regression appears similar to orchidectomy. Will probably be superior to DES therapy.
Mammary carcinoma	Limited studies in premenopausal metastatic carcinoma consistent with effects of ovariectomy. May be useful against tumors with steroid receptors.

DIAGNOSTIC TESTS

The functional capacity of the anterior pituitary gonadotropic cells can be assessed by measurement of LH and FSH levels in the peripheral blood after a bolus of subcutaneous or intravenous LHRH. The LH response is dose-dependent up to a specific level. A specific dose is used to stimulate the pituitary with clearly readable but less than maximal LH response in normal patients. Subtle changes in pituitary function, particularly in hypogonadotropic patients, can be detected.

The range of normal baseline LH levels varies with the patient and in different laboratories and clinical centers. Proper interpretation of this diagnostic test requires an understanding of the hypothalamic–pituitary–gonadal physiology, the clinical status of the patient, and fam-

Table 36.2 Summary of the effects and uses of LHRH analogs

Clinical uses	*Sex*	*Effect*
Antifertility	Males	Inhibition of spermatogenesis Inhibition of sperm motility Disruption of semen characteristics
	Females	Direct effect on granulosa cells Inhibition of ovulation Premature luteinization of follicles Induction of luteal insufficiency Postcoital contraception Termination of pregnancy
Profertility	Males	Stimulation of spermatogenesis Control of Leydig cell function Treatment of idiopathic hypogonadotropic hypogonadism and idiopathic normogonadotropic oligozoospermia Stimulation of potentia/libido Correction of cryptorchidism
	Females	Induction of follicular maturation Induction of ovulation Synchronization of ovulation in follicular cohorts for *in vitro* fertilization and transfer Synchronization of estrus (farm animals) Maintenance of corpus luteum functions Delayed puberty Therapy for polycystic ovarian disease
Other therapeutic uses	Males	Suppression of prostatic carcinoma Protection against gonadotropic effects of cancer chemotherapy
	Females	Correction of dysfunctional menstrual bleeding Control of dysmenorrhea/premenstrual tension Inhibition of mammary and other gonadal endocrine dependent syndromes
Diagnostic uses	post-hypophysectomy	complete partial radiation therapy with or without hypophysectomy
	idiopathic syndromes	prepubertal panhypopituitarism postpubertal panhypopituitarism hypogonadotropic hypogonadism
	other syndromes	anorexia nervosa craniopharyngioma pituitary trauma Kallman syndrome Sheehan syndrome Prader–Willi syndrome

iliarity with the normal ranges and the standards used in the laboratory performing the LH assays. For example exogenous *factors* (androgens, estrogens, and progestins) affect both the basal level of serum LH and the serum LH response to LHRH. This response is altered by doses of sex steroid administration, the temporal relationship between the drug administration and the LHRH testing, and the *in vivo* endocrine environment at the time of administration and testing. Tests with a normal response indicate the presence of functional pituitary gonadotropes. This diagnostic response is useful for patients with suspected gonadotropin deficiency, whether isolated or in combination with deficiencies of other pituitary hormones. The test is also employed to evaluate residual gonadotropic function following surgical or radiation therapy of the pituitary. LHRH tests, performed concomitantly with other post-treatment evaluations, complement the clinical examination and other laboratory tests used to conform or substantiate hypogonadotropic hypogonadism.

The single dose injection test does not measure pituitary gonadotropic reserve which requires prolonged or repeated administration. The single injection test is not used to differentiate pituitary from hypothalamic anomalies. Although allergic and hypersensitivity reactions have been reported with other polypeptide hormones, these reactions are not encountered after a single dose of LHRH. Chronic administration of large doses of LHRH, however, may cause some antibody formation. These tests are not indicated in pregnancy and in patients receiving preparations containing androgens, estrogens, progestins or glucocorticoids, which affect pituitary secretion of gonadotropins.

CONCLUDING REMARKS

The extensive clinical trials already under way with LHRH agonists, especially in the therapeutic areas, indicate that this class of drug has a place in medicine. The LHRH antagonists are only now approaching extensive clinical trials, but appear promising for indications where rapid and complete suppression of sexual function is required. The list of potential therapeutic applications for LHRH analogs (Table 36.2) has not been fully explored, and an even brighter future for these agents may be anticipated.

References

Arimura, A., Vilchez-Martinez, J. A. and Schally, A. V. (1974). *In vivo* comparison of LH-RH and FSH-RH activities of [DES-GLY^{10}] [PRO^{9}-ethylamide]-LH-RH, [DES-GLY^{10}] [PRO^{9}-propylamide]-LH-RH, and LH-RH using immature male rats. *Endocrinology*, **95**, 1174

Beattie, C. W., Corbin, A., Foell, T. J., Garsky, V., McKinley, W. A., Rees, R. W. A., Sarantakis, D. and Yardley, J. P. (1975). Luteinizing hormone-releasing hormone. Antiovulatory activity of analogs substituted in positions 2 and 6. *J. Med. Chem.*, **18**, 1247

Clayton, R. N. (1984). Pharmacological regulation of pituitary LHRH receptors. This volume, Chapter 4

Comite, F., Cutler, G. B., Jr. and Loriaux, D. L. (1984). LHRH analog therapy of precocious puberty. This volume, Chapter 24

Coy, D. H., Horvath, A., Nekola, M. V., Coy, E. J., Erchegyi, J. and Schally, A. V. (1982). Peptide antagonists of LH-RH: Large increases in antiovulatory activities produced by basic D-amino acids in the six position. *Endocrinology*, **110**, 1445

Edgren, R. A. and Shevlin, D. R. (1984). Prospects for LHRH analogs as therapeutical agents. This volume, Chapter 35

Faure, N., Lemay, A., Tolis, G., Labrie, F., Belanger, A. and Fazekas, A. T. A. (1984). Buserelin therapy for prostatic carcinoma. This volume, Chapter 26

Hahn, D. W., McGuire, J. L., Vale, W. W. and Rivier, J. (1984). Biological assays utilized to characterize LHRH and its analogs. This volume, Chapter 5

Happ, J. (1984). Correction of infertility with LHRH agonists in the male. This volume, Chapter 23

Harper, M. J. K. (1984). Prospects for LHRH analogs as contraceptives. This volume, Chapter 34

Loumaye, E., Naor, Z. and Catt, K. J. (1982). Binding affinity and biological activity of gonadotropin-releasing hormone agonists in isolated pituitary cells. *Endocrinology,* **111,** 730

Laron, Z., Prager-Lewin, R. and Dickerman, Z. (1984). Diagnostic uses of LHRH. This volume, Chapter 28

Meldrum, D. R., Chang, R. J., Lu, J., Vale, W., Rivier, J. and Judd, H. L. (1982). 'Medical oophorectomy' using a long-acting GnRH agonist—a possible new approach to the treatment of endometriosis. *J. Clin. Endocrinol. Metab.,* **54,** 1081

Monahan, M. W., Rivier, J., Vale, W. and Guillemin, R. (1972). [Gly^2]LRF and des-His^2-LRF. The synthesis, purification, and characterization of two LRF analogues antagonistic to LRF. *Biochem. Biophys. Res. Commun.,* **47,** 551

Nekola, M. and Coy, D. H. (1984). LHRH antagonists in females. This volume, Chapter 10.

Nestor, J. J., Jr. (1984). Development of LHRH analogs. This volume, Chapter 1

Nestor, J. J., Jr., Ho, T. L., Simpson, R. A., Horner, B. L., Jones, G. H., McRae, G. I. and Vickery, B. H. (1982). Synthesis and biological activity of some very hydrophobic superagonist analogues of luteinizing hormone-releasing hormone. *J. Med. Chem.,* **25,** 795

Nestor, J. J., Jr., Ho, T. L., Tahilramani, R., Horner, B. L., Simpson, R. A., Jones, G. H., McRae, G. I. and Vickery, B. H. (1984). LHRH agonists and antagonists containing very hydrophobic amino acids. This volume, Chapter 3

Rivier, J., Rivier, C., Perrin, M., Porter, J. and Vale, W. W. (1984). LHRH analogs as antiovulatory agents. This volume, Chapter 2

Schally, A. V., Arimura, A. and Coy, D. H. (1981). Recent approaches to fertility control based on derivatives of LHRH. *Vitam. Horm.,* **38,** 257

Yen, S. S. (1984). Clinical applications of gonadotropin-releasing hormone and gonadotropin-releasing hormone analogs. *Fertil. Steril.,* **39,** 257

Subject Index

J. J. NESTOR Jr